Guidebook to Dermatologic Diagnosis

Guidebook to Dermatologic Diagnosis

Susan Burgin, MD
Associate Professor of Dermatology
Harvard Medical School
Attending Dermatologist
Brigham and Women's Hospital
Boston, Massachusetts

New York   Chicago   San Francisco   Athens   London   Madrid   Mexico City
Milan   New Delhi   Singapore   Sydney   Toronto

1 2 3 4 5 6 7 8 9   DSS   25 24 23 22 21 20

ISBN 978-0-07-173875-0
MHID 0-07-173875-4

This book was set in Minion Pro by Cenveo® Publisher Services
The editors were Karen Edmonson and Christie Naglieri.
The production supervisor was Richard Ruzycka.
Project management was provided by Garima Poddar, Cenveo Publisher Services.
The cover designer was W2 Design.

Library of Congress Cataloging-in-Publication Data

Names: Burgin, Susan, editor.
Title: Guidebook to dermatologic diagnosis / editor, Susan Burgin.
Description: New York : McGraw-Hill Education, [2020] | Includes index.
Identifiers: LCCN 2019001035 | ISBN 9780071738750 (adhesive–soft : alk.
  paper)
Subjects: | MESH: Skin Diseases—diagnosis | Diagnosis, Differential
Classification: LCC RL105 | NLM WR 141 | DDC 616.5/075—dc23 LC record available at
https://na01.safelinks.protection.outlook.com/?url=https%3A%2F%2Flccn.loc.gov%
2F2019001035&data=01%7C01%7Cleah.carton%40mheducation.com%7C7b1b-
f67a34d14612130408d677109dea%7Cf919b1efc0c347358fca0928ec39d8d5%7C0&s
data=nan2Sot2mTzd%2BuBAcXqqgwVG8h5sUvNFUwqfr78mRpQ%3D&reserved=0

McGraw Hill books are available at special quantity discounts to use as premiums and sales promotions, or for use in corporate training programs. To contact a representative, please visit the Contact Us pages at www.mhprofessional.com.

For my family and for my extended family
of teachers, colleagues, and friends

Contents

Preface

I am a diagnostician at heart. Through my years of study and practice in dermatology, I have worked to develop a system that elucidates a fundamental approach to dermatologic diagnosis.

I trained in South Africa where the multitude of diseases we came across guaranteed a vigorous clinical training. Each week, our chief, Dr. Joy Schultz, would quiz us on clinical cases, determined to teach us how to appreciate even the most subtle clues that the skin can proffer. On a dermatology elective in Cape Town, I encountered a methodological approach to diagnosis for the first time. Dr. Paul Strauss, in between seeing his atopic dermatitis patients in a pediatric clinic one day, began to show me how the morphology of primary lesions, their grouping and distribution, as well as the history of the patient could guide one step by step to a differential diagnosis. I thank him for introducing me to this interactive way of thinking that was the genesis for what I have called the wheel of diagnosis.

I repeated a dermatology residency after moving to the United States. There, I was fortunate to be mentored by Dr. Michael Fisher, a master of differential diagnosis. Dr. Fisher introduced me to the concept of the reaction patterns that I have expanded upon in this book. At the Albert Einstein College of Medicine in the Bronx, we practiced differential diagnosis at Grand Rounds each week. We were not permitted to ask a history from the patients, except for three questions: "Does it itch?" "Does it burn?" and "Does it hurt?" Our eyes would have to do the rest diagnostically, and the residents built impressive lists of differential diagnoses in the discussions that followed.

In my subsequent years as an attending physician at New York University Medical Center, Beth Israel Deaconess Medical Center, and now at Brigham and Women's Hospital, honing my own diagnostic skills and teaching these skills to residents and students has remained my passion. I have learned so much from the incisive questions the residents have asked in our myriad interactive sessions; first at NYU and now here at Harvard. I have also worked to expand the original ideas of the wheel of diagnosis and the reaction patterns to encompass other useful algorithms and pathways to teach a comprehensive approach to differential diagnosis. *A Guidebook to Dermatologic Diagnosis* is an embodiment of this work.

Introduction

"Listen to the patient, he is telling you the diagnosis." This quotation, attributed to Sir William Osler, emphasizes what every medical student learns in medical school: history is more than 80 percent of diagnosis. To this, I would like to add, "Look at the skin, it reveals the diagnosis."

At its core, the Guidebook addresses how to diagnose in dermatology. Cognitive psychologists have shown that diagnostic reasoning takes place through activation of "scripts." Scripts describe the memory structure of clinical medical knowledge. They are networks of relevant knowledge and experience that direct selection and interpretation of new information. Expert dermatologists have, through experience, amassed a repository of scripts and have encountered a myriad of patterns on the skin. Imagine a patient presenting with an itchy linear rash after gardening. Instantly, knowledge of acute contact dermatitis pops into the clinician's mind. Accompanying this knowledge is a script of physical examination findings that confirm diagnosis and a script of treatment options, both based on the clinician's prior experience. Next, a patient presents with a longstanding rash over the elbows and knees, and joint pain. The prior script leaves active memory and is replaced by knowledge of psoriasis. Pattern recognition is another powerful processing strategy employed in dermatology. Seasoned clinicians have a repository of visual scripts that, in the absence of history, can direct diagnoses.

In the examples above, seeing linear erythematous plaques with vesicles, or well-demarcated plaques with silvery scale on the elbows and knees, with no history at all, will instantaneously call out acute contact dermatitis and psoriasis to the experienced clinician. For the novice, no such internal pathways exist. The novice needs to acquire knowledge of presentations and disease, as well as a set of rules to determine actions based on this knowledge. Even experts have not encountered the entirety of clinical presentations and can be stumped. When they encounter a novel or unusual eruption, they too need a way to stimulate further thought, a way to activate pre-existing scripts. The algorithms and pathways in this book are the tools or "rules" that can be used to guide one to a differential diagnosis, until such time as experience is accrued, and scripts and pattern recognition can take over.

There are two ways to create differential diagnostic lists. The first is to use an etiologic classification. Here, diseases are grouped according to whether they are inherited or acquired. If acquired, we subdivide them according to whether they are infectious, inflammatory, neoplastic, or drug-induced by nature. Other categories here include metabolic/depositional, vascular, or traumatic.

Another way to classify dermatoses, and the one heavily used in this book, is on morphologic grounds: we group diseases that look the same together. For example, all vesicobullous diseases, whether they may be caused by infection or an inflammatory process, such as autoimmunity, can be grouped together. We would then distinguish these diseases by clinical features, such as the depth of the bulla (informed by how many intact bullae versus erosions are seen, and whether the bullae are tense or flaccid) and the associated secondary lesions present (bullae and urticarial plaques, for example, connote bullous pemphigoid, whereas bullae, erosions, and vegetating plaques connote pemphigus vegetans). We would then look at the grouping of lesions (annular vesicles connote linear IgA disease, whereas herpetiform vesicles suggest herpes simplex, herpes zoster, dermatitis herpetiformis, or pemphigus herpetiformis); their distribution (dermatitis herpetiformis likes extensor aspects of extremities, a variant of bullous pemphigoid resides on the palms and soles, and pemphigus foliaceus can be found in the seborrheic areas); and how the scalp, hair, nails, mucous membranes, and lymph nodes are affected (oral involvement is always seen in pemphigus vulgaris, but it is less frequent in bullous pemphigoid; mucous membrane pemphigoid may cause scarring alopecia on the scalp; and there may be enlarged lymph nodes palpable in paraneoplastic conditions, such as paraneoplastic pemphigus). This morphologic classification requires an intimate knowledge of dermatologic diseases and the way they present. It also requires a framework. The elements of wheel of diagnosis (outlined above), the reaction patterns, and the differential diagnostic lists outlined in this Guidebook provide this framework.

To start off, in Chapter 1, the concept of the wheel of diagnosis is introduced. We then delve into ways to think about the primary lesions in Chapter 2 and discuss the diagnostic clues that secondary lesions can offer in Chapter 3. Color is a powerful diagnostic determinant, explored in depth in Chapter 4. In Chapter 5, reaction patterns are outlined and summarized. A reaction pattern refers to the lesions the skin produces in disease and comprises those dermatoses that have the same characteristic morphologic findings. For example, the papulosquamous reaction pattern connotes those dermatoses that manifest with scaly papules and plaques. In Chapters 6 through 10, each of the reaction patterns is reviewed at length, bringing in elements of the diagnostic wheel. The wheel of diagnosis, the reaction patterns, and color differentials may be used in sum or in part to create a differential diagnosis. By Chapters 11 and 12, we have moved on to discussing the grouping and configuration, and the distribution of lesions, respectively. The scalp, hair, mucous membranes, and nails yield important diagnostic clues, and examination of these areas is vital. Chapter 13 is devoted to discussing these clues. Bedside diagnostic maneuvers are another tool in the diagnostician's toolbox. The scrape of a Q-tip or a wipe of mineral oil can bring out features of diagnostic significance, for example, and we explore these in the last chapter, Chapter 14.

Whether you are a medical student or a dermatology resident encountering the field of dermatologic diagnosis for the first time, an internist or family practitioner looking to develop your approach to dermatology, or a seasoned clinician-dermatologist looking to augment your methodology of teaching differential diagnosis, this book is intended to be your guide, your authority, and your companion.

Acknowledgments

I would like to thank my mentors. Professor Joy Schulz, your lessons are indelible. Dr. Michael Fisher, this book is an extension of all that you taught me and my gift back to you. To all my other teachers and colleagues and also to the residents and students I have taught over the years, thank you. You all have taught and inspired me. You've challenged me to think through new knowledge and concept areas. I feel privileged and proud to have been a part of many great institutions over the years—the University of the Witwatersrand in Johannesburg, South Africa; New York University (NYU) and the Albert Einstein College of Medicine in New York; and Beth Israel Deaconess Medical Center and Brigham and Women's Hospital in Boston. To my dermatology teachers at the University of Witwatersrand in South Africa—Professor Deepak Modi and Drs. Richard Nevin, David Klevansky, Hansa Ratanjee, Vivian Berro, Vivian Jacques, and Rob Weiss—your love of dermatology and your knowledge are with me still. Professor Modi, thank you too for your image contributions to the Guidebook. To my co-registrar group in South Africa—Drs. Steven Glassman, Eric Bue, Jacques Malan, Barbara Fine, and Pholile Mpofu—you were phenomenal teachers. Warm South African gratitude also goes to my esteemed colleague, Professor Ncoza Dlova. Thank you for your image contributions to this book, and for your inspiration, dear friendship, and our ongoing work together. In 1996, Dr. Irwin Freedberg, the chair of dermatology at the Ronald O Perelman Department of Dermatology of NYU, changed my life's course when I was asked to become a senior resident there. I subsequently completed a full second dermatology residency in the Division of Dermatology at Einstein, where Dr. Fisher was the chair. Dr. Freedberg, Dr. Fisher, and the faculty, residents, and students of NYU and of Einstein embraced me as a colleague and teacher. Dr. Miguel Sanchez, thank you for allowing the inclusion of images from the patients we saw at the time. Dr. Ken Katz, I will always remember when you were a first-year resident and you told me that you had just diagnosed a new case of in-transit melanoma metastases based on what you learned in my class only a few days prior. Thanks also go to my co-residents at Einstein for some wonderful shared years. You helped to make New York City my home. To Dr. Andrea Cambio, thank you for your unwavering friendship. To Dr. Barry Smith, thank you for your image contribution. To Dr. Todd Minars, thank you being one of the first to want to read this book. I hope your patience will now finally be rewarded.

Since 2005, I have been part of the medical community at Harvard and its affiliated hospitals, initially at Beth Israel Deaconess Medical Center where Dr. Robert Stern was chair, and subsequently at Brigham and Women's Hospital under Dr. Tom Kupper's leadership. The vibrancy of this academic community continues to inspire my work, and I have forged many strong working relationships and friendships here—Drs. Marissa Heller, Anthony Cukras, Ruth Ann Vleugels, Erin Wei, and Charlie Taylor, and Lori Newman, to name but a few. To Drs. Adam Lipworth and Molly Plovanich, first residents and now colleagues, thank you for your image contributions. I have also had the opportunity to work with a wonderful team at VisualDx. To Dr. Elena Hawryluk, also resident and now valued colleague, thank you for your brilliant naming of the GIFTs box on the wheel of diagnosis. To Professor Lowell Goldsmith, thank you for your invaluable advice when this book was in its nascence. To Dr. Art Papier and the entire VisualDx team, my gratitude knows no bounds. To all my wonderful dermatology colleagues and friends in the United States, you have enriched my life in myriads of ways. I am grateful to be your colleague.

This book is dedicated as well to my own family. Mom, you were a force. My book will join your chemistry textbook on our bookshelf at home. I miss you. Dad, you are a true giant among people. You are an amazing doctor, a mensch, and an inspiration to everyone around you, every day. We love you forever. Ruth, Danni, Yoni, and Davidi Aharon, you guys are the best! To Walt Friedman, my one true love—what a gift to be able to spend my life with you! To our daughter, Orli, with all my love and blessings—you are our greatest joy. And to all my friends—I am so grateful to you.

To Anne Sydor who saw this book in my initial work, profound thanks. And to Karen Edmonson and your amazing team, equally profound thanks for your ongoing patience and support. We made it!

Thank you to New York University School of Medicine, Department of Dermatology for contributing the following figures:

Figure 1.6A and D

Figure 1.7F

Figure 1.9 (some of the images)

Figure 1.10

Figure 2.22

Figure 3.5, 8, 12, 20, 24

Figure 4.3C, 4.4A, 4.17C

Figure 6.8B, 6.33C and D, 6.34C

Figure 7.22, 23, 25

Figure 8.8

Figure 9.14, 15, 25, 26, 37, 41, 43, 51, 52

Figure 10.14 and 20

Figure 11.9, 16, 17, 23, 29, 30, 33, 36, 38, 41

Figure 12.21, 25, 30, 32, 38, 65

Figure 13.32

The Wheel of Diagnosis

The "wheel of diagnosis," as depicted in Figure 1.1, encompasses the salient clinical features of skin lesions that can be used to make a diagnosis. The "spokes" or diagnostic boxes on this virtual wheel are the fundamental clinical features that render diagnostic information:

- Identifying primary (and associated secondary) lesions
- Grouping and configuration of these lesions
- Studying the distribution of these lesions
- Examining the lesions and gleaning information from the scalp, hair, nails, mucous membranes, and lymph nodes
- Contextualizing these findings to the patient's history

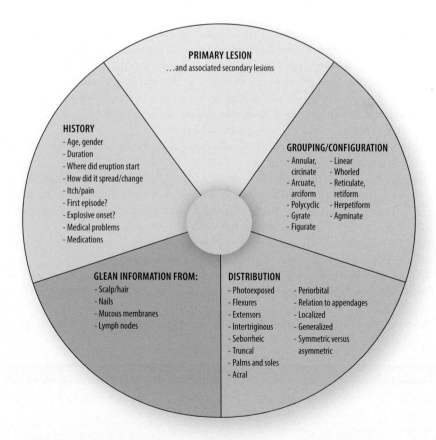

FIGURE 1.1 · The Wheel of Diagnosis.

You may need to go through each diagnostic box on the wheel to make a diagnosis. Sometimes, however, one particular characteristic of a rash is so striking that this, by itself, may generate a differential diagnosis, such as grouping of primary lesions or their distribution. In this context, any of the other diagnostic boxes may be used to either confirm or narrow down a diagnosis. This chapter delves into each of the diagnostic boxes of the wheel in depth.

PRIMARY LESIONS

Primary lesions are those lesions that the body produces in any given eruption. They are the main determinants of diagnosis. In any widespread eruption, a vital first step is to seek out the primary lesions as this will determine the next diagnostic pathway that you choose. The primary lesions and their definitions are summarized as follows:

- **Macule** (Figure 1.2A): A *macule* is a circumscribed, flat lesion. It is a flat area that differs from the surrounding skin only with respect to its color. Red, brown, purple, and white are the usual colors of macules, but exogenous pigments of almost any color may be found in tattoos, for example.
- **Plaque** (Figure 1.2B): A *plaque* is a solid raised or depressed lesion that measures at least 1 cm in diameter. Raised plaques, as opposed to nodules, are broader than they are tall; that is, their surface area is greater than their height. Plaques may be scaly or smooth.
- **Patch**: The term *patch* is used to connote any portion of skin that is different in appearance or character from its surroundings. In practice, dermatologists have used this term variably. Some restrict its use to mean large macules (those greater than 1 cm), and others use it to refer to relatively thin but large plaques. In general, accurate description can almost always be better served by employing the more precise terminology, such as a "large macule" or a "thin plaque." You will see that this term is therefore not included in the wheel.
- **Papule** (Figure 1.2C): A *papule* is a solid, circumscribed elevated or depressed lesion that measures less than 1 cm.
- **Nodule** (Figure 1.2D): A *nodule* is similar in configuration to a papule, but it measures 1–5 cm. It may be elevated about the skin surface, or it may be deep and palpable. Nodules may involve the epidermis and dermis, the dermis and subcutaneous fat, or subcutaneous fat alone.
- **Tumor**: A *tumor* is a solid mass that measures more than 5 cm. The term *tumor*, used in this context, does not imply benignity or malignancy.
- **Vesicle and bulla** (Figure 1.2E): A *vesicle* is a small, circumscribed, raised lesion that contains fluid. It measures less than 1 cm. A *bulla* measures 1 cm or greater.
- **Pustule** (Figure 1.2F): A *pustule* is a small, circumscribed raised lesion that contains pus.

The Primary Lesions

• Macule	• Nodule	• Bulla
• Plaque	• Tumor	• Pustule
• Papule	• Vesicle	

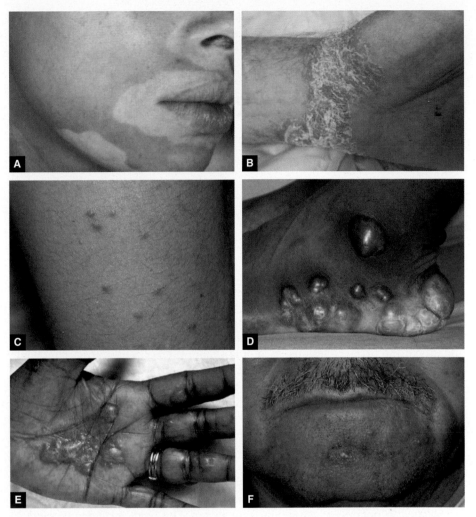

FIGURE 1.2 • Primary lesions. (A) White macules of vitiligo; (B) scaly plaque of psoriasis; (C) erythematous non-follicular papules on a limb: an arthropod assault; (D) skin-colored nodules of late stage erythema elevatum diutinum (Used with permission from Dr. Miguel Sanchez, New York University, New York, NY.); (E) vesicles and bullae of severe dyshidrotic eczema; (F) pustules (and papules) of folliculitis.

The dermatology lexicon also includes combination terms. The term *papulovesicle* refers to the presence of a vesicle that is superimposed on a papule. A papulovesicular eruption comprises both papules and vesicles. *Papulonodule* refers to a lesion that is around 1 cm and could be classified as either a papule or a nodule, and a papulonodular eruption comprises both. Finally, the term *maculopapular* connotes the presence of both macules and papules in an eruption. This term was used in the past to denote the findings in an exanthematous drug eruption or a viral exanthem, for example. This term is currently out of vogue, given that it was frequently used imprecisely. As a result, maculopapular drug eruption has become an exanthematous drug eruption, and for eruptions that consist of macules and papules, it is preferred that these be described as such.

Primary lesions hold key diagnostic information that can be appreciated visually, such as their size, color, shape, surface characteristics (contour and scales), and border. Consistency, tenderness, and depth are further important diagnostic features that are best appreciated through palpation.

Diagnostic Determinants of Primary Lesions	
Visual	**Tactile**
• Size	• Depth
• Color	• Consistency
• Shape	• Tenderness
• Surface characteristics: contour and scales	
• Border	

Size as a diagnostic determinant can often be inferred from the type of primary lesion present; for example, a papule is less than 1 cm and a nodule is 1 cm or greater. Color is another salient diagnostic determinant that can help to formulate differential diagnoses. Red, pink, and white are the most commonly encountered colors in the skin, but the skin can appear purple, maroon, gray, yellow, orange, black, and even green and blue. Further visual diagnostic determinants of the primary lesions, including shape, surface, and border characteristics, as well as the tactile determinants, are summarized in Tables 1.1 and 1.2, respectively.

Regarding shape, very few macules and plaques are completely round. The terms *nummular* and *discoid* are synonymous with round. Fixed drug eruption, pityriasis rotunda, and nummular eczema are classically round. While the macules and thin plaques of erythema migrans are usually oval or annular, they may be round. Externally applied devices can create a round indentation on the skin, such as is seen in the circles of petechiae that are caused by the practice of cupping. Single primary lesions, like configurations of lesions, may also be annular, arcuate (arc-shaped; a portion of an annulus), or linear. The term *serpiginous* refers to the presence of a wavy, snake-like line, such as may be seen in larva currens or urticarial vasculitis. Other shape descriptors include polygonal (papules of lichen planus), oval or ovoid (a classic shape for plaques of pityriasis rosea), and digitate (resembling fingers, such as digitate dermatosis). *Target lesions* may be macules or plaques. They are classically composed of a central dusky macule or bulla surrounded by a lighter pink rim and a third red ring. Targetoid macules and plaques comprise two color zones rather than three. The central zone is usually dusky or darker than the surrounding zone. It is this dusky center that allows for the specific targetoid designation, rather than the more generic term, *annular*, of which *targetoid* is a subset.

> **Clinical Tip** *Annular* and *targetoid* both connote lesions with two zones of color. *Targetoid* lesions are that subset of all *annular* or ring-shaped lesions that have dusky centers.

TABLE 1.1. Visual Properties of Primary Lesions

SHAPE
- Round: nummular, discoid
  - Fixed drug eruption
  - Pityriasis rotunda
  - Nummular eczema
  - Erythema migrans of Lyme disease
  - Circles of petechiae caused by cupping
- Annular
  - Granuloma annulare
  - Leprosy
  - Lichen planus
- Arcuate
  - Erythema annulare centrifugum
  - Necrolytic migratory erythema
- Linear
  - Hypomelanosis of Ito
  - Linear and whorled hypermelanosis
  - Larva currens
- Serpiginous
  - Larva currens
- Polygonal
  - Lichen planus
- Oval or ovoid
  - Pityriasis rosea
- Digitate: like fingers
  - Digitate dermatosis
- Target or iris lesion
  - Erythema multiforme
- Targetoid lesions
  - See Table 10.1 for a complete list
- Stellate
  - Plaques of Vohwinkel syndrome
  - Depressed plaques of livedoid vasculopathy
- Geometric
  - Poison ivy
  - Phytophotodermatitis
- Phylloid
  - Ash-leaf macule of tuberous sclerosis
  - Phylloid hypomelanosis

SURFACE CHARACTERISTICS
- Contour
  - Verrucous
    - Warts
    - Warty plaques other than viral warts; see Table 6.2 for a complete list
  - Acuminate
    - Condyloma acuminata
  - Filiform
    - Warts

(Continued)

TABLE 1.1. Visual Properties of Primary Lesions (continued)

- Vegetating
  - See Table 6.2 for a complete list
- Bosselated
  - Dermatofibrosarcoma protuberans (DFSP)
- Mammillated
  - Sweet syndrome
- Papillated
  - Linear verrucous epidermal nevus
- Dome-shaped
  - Molluscum contagiosum
- Umbilicated
  - Molluscum contagiosum
  - Herpetic infections
- Peau d'orange appearance
  - Lymphedema
- Scales
  - See Chapter 6 for a complete discussion of scales

BORDER CHARACTERISTICS
- "Coast of Maine"
  - McCune–Albright syndrome
- "Coast of California"
  - Neurofibromatosis
- Geographic
  - Erythrokeratoderma variabilis
- Well-demarcated
  - Psoriasis
- Ill-defined or "smudged"
  - Patch stage of mycosis fungoides
- "Islands of sparing"
  - Mycosis fungoides
  - Pityriasis rubra pilaris
- "Cliff-drop" sign
  - Atrophoderma of Pasini and Pierini
- Scalloped
  - Herpes simplex infection

Stellate means star-shaped. Confluent retiform purpura, the depressed plaques of livedoid vasculopathy, and the keratotic plaques of Vohwinkel syndrome are typically stellate. The term *geometric* implies a shape with right angles or straight or curved borders. Geometric shapes are usually formed from externally applied allergens (acute contact dermatitis) or chemicals (chemical burn, phytophotodermatitis). A *phylloid* shape resembles a leaf. The ash leaf macules of tuberous sclerosis are phylloid. Phylloid hypomelanosis is a form of cutaneous mosaicism that is seen in trisomy 13. Broad leaf-shaped hypopigmented macules cover the skin surface.

Examples of Shapes

- Round: nummular, discoid
- Annular: ring-shaped
- Arcuate: part of a ring, arc-shaped
- Linear: forms a line
- Serpiginous: wavy, snake-like
- Polygonal: has five sides
- Oval: ovoid
- Digitate: like fingers

- Target or iris lesion: resembles a target or bull's eye; has three color zones
- Targetoid: resembles a target, has two color zones
- Stellate: resembles a star
- Geometric shape: with right angles or straight or curved borders
- Phylloid: resembling a leaf

TABLE 1.2. Tactile Properties of Primary Lesions

DEPTH
- Dermatofibrosarcoma protuberans

CONSISTENCY
- Hard
  - Calcium
  - Bone
  - Foreign bodies
- Very firm to hard
  - Dermatofibroma
- Firm
  - Most papules and nodules
- Soft
  - Acrochordon
  - Neurotized nevus
  - Neurofibroma
  - Nevus lipomatosus
  - Lipoma
- Fluctuant
  - Abscess
  - Infected or inflamed cyst
- Boggy
  - Lipedema of the scalp
  - Sweet syndrome

TENDERNESS
- Infections
  - Bacterial (eg, furunculosis, carbuncles, infected cysts)
- Inflammatory conditions
  - Sweet syndrome
- Necrosis
  - Epidermal necrosis (eg, Stevens Johnson syndrome /toxic epidermal necrolysis–SJS/TEN)
  - Dermal necrosis (eg, calciphylaxis, coumadin necrosis, and other thrombotic disorders, or venomous bites)

Surface characteristics include contour (or topography) and scales. Both papules and plaques may have distinctive contours. Papules may be *dome-shaped*; this implies a rounded, convex surface, like a dome. *Umbilicated* refers to the presence of a central dell. An example of a dome-shaped, umbilicated papule is molluscum contagiosum. Vesicles, too, may be umbilicated, such as those of herpes simplex, varicella, or zoster. The papules of lichen planus are classically described as being flat-topped. Warts may have an *acuminate* (pointed) or *filiform* (thread-like) contour. The term *verrucous* is used to connote a wart-like papule or plaque that is covered in wart-like projections (a more general term that may encompass acuminate and/or filiform presentations). A verrucous contour is seen in warts and other warty plaques, such as chromomycosis and other deep fungal infections, tuberculosis verrucosa cutis (a warty tuberculide), and the verrucous stage of incontinentia pigmenti. Further regarding plaques, the term *vegetating* or *vegetation-like* implies an exophytic growth with an undulating surface. *Undulating* implies a continuous up-and-down shape. Vegetating plaques may be moist and eroded or dry. They may also be verrucous. Examples of vegetating plaques include those of pemphigus vegetans or verrucous carcinomas. *Papillated* is used to describe a contour with small, nipple-like projections, such as the surface of a linear verrucous epidermal nevus. *Mammillated* also implies the presence of small rounded nipple-like projections. These projections are blunter or flatter than those seen in papillated surfaces. The plaques of Sweet syndrome (acute febrile neutrophilic dermatosis) are typically described as mammillated. *Bosselated* refers to the presence of larger protuberances on the surface of a primary lesion. *Bosses* are typically convex. Examples of bosselated plaques include those seen in cutaneous Rosai–Dorfman disease and dermatofibrosarcoma protuberans. The term *rippled* implies small undulations that resemble waves. Lichen amyloid typically has a rippled surface. A *peau d'orange* appearance describes plaques that resemble the skin of an orange, such as those seen in breast lymphedema caused by carcinomatous lymphatic invasion. The term implies a dimpled or pitted appearance.

Examples of Contour

Papules
- Dome-shaped: round, convex like a dome
- Umbilicated: having a central dell
- Flat-topped
- Acuminate: pointed
- Filiform: thread-like
- Verrucous: wart-like

Plaques
- Verrucous: wart-like
- Vegetating: vegetation-like

- Papillated: surface having many small nipple-like projections that resemble papillae of the tongue
- Mammillated: surface having many blunt round nipple-like projections
- Bosselated: surface having many round protuberances
- Rippled: small undulations
- Peau d'orange: resembles an orange peel

The lesion border may also hold diagnostic information. For example, borders of macules include the *coast of Maine* outline of those café-au-lait macules seen in McCune–Albright syndrome (these manifest jagged or serrated borders) and the *coast of California* outline of those seen in neurofibromatosis (these have smooth borders). For purpuric macules, angulated borders connote the presence of retiform purpura. For plaques, the term *geographic* is used to describe a complex edge that comprises convex and concave borders. The fixed scaly erythematous plaques of erythrokeratoderma variabilis may have geographic borders, as may the plaques of urticarial vasculitis. Typically, the plaques of psoriasis are well defined with sharp borders and the borders of patch stage mycosis fungoides are ill-defined, indistinct, or *smudged.* They fade off into normal skin. *Islands of sparing* is a phrase that refers to areas of normal skin (the *islands*) that are surrounded by a widespread rash. Typically, pityriasis rubra pilaris and mycosis fungoides are described as having plaques that surround *islands* of normal skin. Atrophoderma of Pasini and Pierini is a variant of morphea with depressed plaques that typically present on the backs of young women. The plaques in this condition are separated from normal skin by a border that drops vertically downward like the side of a cliff—the so-called *cliff-drop* sign. As the grouped vesicles of herpes simplex become erosions, the confluent convex outline so formed gives rise to a *scalloped* border, which is characteristic of the condition.

Examples of Diagnostically Suggestive Borders

- Café au lait macules:
  - "Coast of Maine": McCune-Albright syndrome
  - "Coast of California": neurofibromatosis
- Angulated borders: retiform purpura
- Geographic borders: erythrokeratoderma variabilis
- Well-demarcated: psoriasis
- Ill-defined: patch-stage mycosis fungoides
- "Islands of sparing": pityriasis rubra pilaris, mycosis fungoides
- "Cliff drop" sign: atrophoderma of Pasini and Pierini
- Scalloped: herpes simplex virus

While most morphologic features are appreciated visually, important diagnostic information can also be gathered through touch.

Clinical Tip Palpation allows appreciation of the following:
- Depth
- Consistency
- The presence of tenderness

Nodules and tumors may be deep-seated, and their full extent may be appreciated only through palpation. Dermatofibrosarcoma protuberans is a low-grade sarcoma that is sometimes likened to an iceberg; just a small part of the tumor is visible on the skin surface, but palpation will reveal the larger, deeper part of the tumor. Consistency of lesions proffers further diagnostic clues. Examples here include the hard consistency of calcinosis cutis or osteoma cutis or the firm to hard consistency of a dermatofibroma. A firm consistency implies a dense dermal process; this is the most common consistency of papules and nodules. Acrochordons, neurofibromas, nevus lipomatosus, neurotized nevi, and lipomas are usually soft. The term *fluctuant* implies the presence of fluid such as pus, as in an abscess or an infected or inflamed cyst. The term *boggy* implies that lesions, usually plaques, feel compressible but are not fluctuant. Synonyms include *spongy* or *doughy.* A rare dermatosis that presents with boggy plaques is lipedema of the scalp. It is a condition affecting older females where there is thickening of the scalp secondary to an increase in the subcutaneous fat layer along

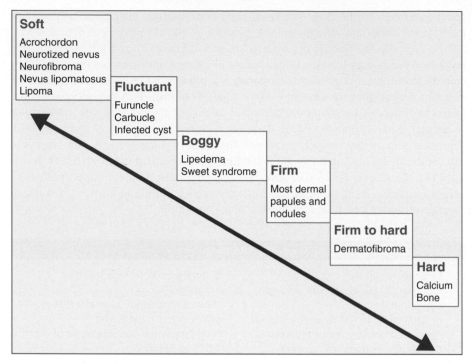

Soft
Acrochordon
Neurotized nevus
Neurofibroma
Nevus lipomatosus
Lipoma

Fluctuant
Furuncle
Carbucle
Infected cyst

Boggy
Lipedema
Sweet syndrome

Firm
Most dermal
papules and
nodules

Firm to hard
Dermatofibroma

Hard
Calcium
Bone

FIGURE 1.3 • The consistency spectrum.

with diffuse alopecia. Conditions with neutrophils and edema in the dermis also feel boggy—such as Sweet syndrome. Figure 1.3 is a conceptual representation of consistency as a continuum, with examples of each included.

Tenderness implies infection (as in furuncles or carbuncles) or necrosis (epidermal, in Stevens–Johnson syndrome/toxic epidermal necrolysis (SJS/TEN); or dermal as in ischemia from vasculitis or a thrombotic vasculopathy). Sweet syndrome presents with one or more tender, juicy plaques. It is postulated that cytokines released from neutrophils are responsible for this clinical sign. Similarly, rheumatoid neutrophilic dermatosis and neutrophilic eccrine hidradenitis are tender to the touch.

> **Clinical Tip** Tenderness implies the following conditions:
> • Infection (eg, furuncles or carbuncles)
> • Necrosis
>   • Epidermal, in Stevens-Johnson syndrome/toxic epidermal necrolysis
>   • Dermal, in ischemia from intraluminal occlusion of blood vessels, such as in calciphy-
>   laxis or a thrombotic vasculopathy
> • Neutrophilic inflammation (eg, Sweet syndrome)

In the box on primary lesions in the wheel, I have included an allusion to secondary lesions. Secondary lesions result when primary lesions resolve or when primary lesions are modified by the patient, through scratching, for example. Secondary lesions are incorporated into the wheel because of the diagnostic clues that they may proffer. An example is the presence of round erosions as a footprint of preceding vesicles, such as is seen in some of the more superficial autoimmune blistering diseases, such as the pemphigus group. Chapter 3 is dedicated to secondary lesions and their inherent diagnostic clues.

> **Clinical Tip** Secondary lesions may also hold diagnostic clues.

REACTION PATTERN

The term *reaction pattern* is used to describe a specific cluster of morphologic findings that groups of dermatoses have in common. The papulosquamous reaction pattern is defined by the presence of papules, plaques, or nodules with scale. The vesicobullous reaction comprises those dermatoses that present with vesicles and bullae. The eczematous reaction pattern houses the lesions of acute, subacute, and chronic eczema. Diseases in the dermal reaction pattern present with smooth papules, nodules, or plaques. Their surfaces are devoid of other characteristics. The vascular reaction pattern (also known as the "red reaction pattern") includes macules and thin and more substantive plaques whose defining characteristic is the color red. They may be blanchable or nonblanching. If they do not blanch, the term *purpura* is used.

As such, by definition, reaction pattern is not a diagnostic determinant of a primary lesion, but rather a diagnostic determinant of more than one primary lesion or a mixture of primary and secondary lesions. It can be layered onto the wheel of diagnosis as is shown in Figure 1.4. Reaction patterns in general are covered in Chapter 5.

Reaction Patterns

- Papulosquamous: see Chapter 6
- Vesicobullous: see Chapter 7
- Eczematous: see Chapter 8
- Dermal: see Chapter 9
- Vascular: see Chapter 10

GROUPING AND CONFIGURATION OF LESIONS

The manner in which lesions are grouped may be characteristic of a given eruption. The term *grouping* may be used synonymously with *arrangement*. The term *configuration* refers to the shape formed by confluent grouped lesions. For example, papules may be grouped together to form an annular configuration, as is seen in granuloma annulare.

Configuration can be contrasted with the term *shape*: *configuration* refers to the shape or outline of more than one primary lesion, as opposed to *shape*, which refers to the outline of a single lesion.

> **Clinical Tip** Configuration is the outline formed by more than one shape. Shape is the outline of a single lesion.

An illustrative example here is lichen planus; individual papules of lichen planus may have a polygonal shape, but they may be arranged in a linear configuration, as is seen with the Koebner phenomenon, or in a ring or annulus. A primary lesion may have a linear shape, too, such as the hypopigmented macules of hypomelanosis of Ito. Similarly, an annulus may occur not as the result of grouped lesions, but rather as the result of different parts of a primary lesion being at different stages of morphologic development,

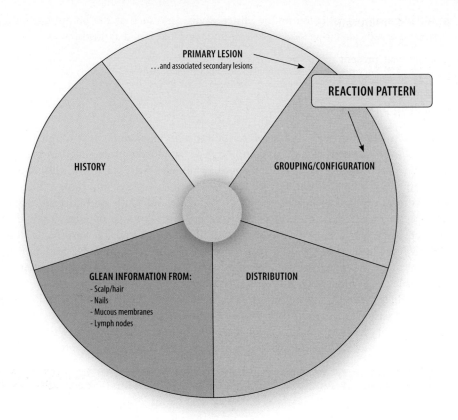

FIGURE 1.4 • The Wheel of Diagnosis, with reaction pattern added.

such as is seen in fixed drug eruption. In the early stages, a red ring may surround the round purplish macules of a more well-developed part of this eruption. The annuli of granuloma annulare may be composed of either a grouping of papules, in which case this would be defined as a configuration, or a single, usually atrophic, annular plaque.

> **Clinical Tip** Primary lesions may have an annular or linear shape. Similarly, primary lesions may be arranged in an annular or linear configuration.

Further configurations include arcuate, polycyclic, gyrate, figurate, whorled, and reticulate. Herpetiform and agminate are groupings or arrangements of primary lesions. Grouping and configuration of lesions is discussed here and again in more depth in Chapter 11.

Grouping and Configuration of Lesions

• Annular, circinate	• Gyrate	• Reticulate, retiform
• Arcuate, arciform	• Figurate	• Herpetiform
• Concentric	• Linear	• Agminate
• Polycyclic	• Whorled	

Annular Configuration

The term *circinate* is used synonymously with *annular*. Commonly encountered dermatoses that present with annuli include tinea corporis, cruris and faciei, pityriasis rosea, psoriasis, granuloma annulare, erythema annulare centrifugum, and lichen planus (Figure 1.5). A clinical hallmark of tinea corporis, cruris and faciei is that scales sit on

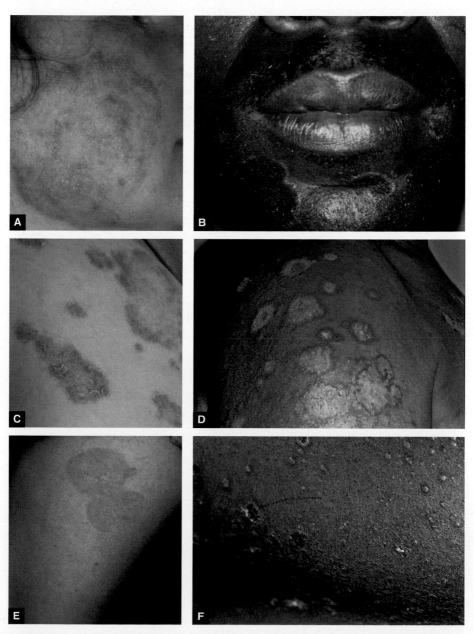

FIGURE 1.5 • The annular grouping. (A) An annular scaly plaque on the face: Tinea faciei; (B) "nickles and dimes" of secondary syphilis; (C) annular plaques of psoriasis; (D) subacute cutaneous lupus erythematosus; (E) erythema annulare centrifugum; (F) annular plaques of lichen planus.

top of the annulus, whereas in erythema annulare centrifugum, scales trail behind the leading annular edge of the plaque ("trailing scale"). Pityriasis rosea has ovoid "medallions", also with trailing fine scale. Lichen planus may have plaques that are annular only or annular and atrophic. A rare variant of pustular psoriasis is known as recurrent circinate erythema. It is a subacute form of pustular psoriasis that presents, usually in children, with erythematous annuli and annular arrays of pustules. Tumid lupus and the annular polycyclic variant of subacute cutaneous lupus are more rarely encountered diseases that present with annuli. The incidence of syphilis is on the rise again in many parts of the world and should be considered as a "do not miss" diagnosis in any atypical annular eruption. The "nickels and dimes" presentation of syphilis refers to annular plaques on the face that are nickel- and dime-sized.

Dermatoses may be classified according to the more traditional etiologic classification, or by a morphologic approach. With the morphologic classification, diseases are classified according to the physical examination findings, as opposed to the textbook chapter. Table 1.3 provides an encapsulated list of dermatoses that commonly present with annuli, based on an etiologic classification. Table 1.4 displays an annular list that has been transformed into a morphologic classification. We can intuit that other diagnostic determinants may be important in refining this list further; the color of lesions would be important (eg, the purple of lichen planus vs the salmon pink of psoriasis), as would the distinction between scaly papules or plaques and nonscaly papules or plaques. (For example, most of the conditions listed in the plaque category of Table 1.4 are scaly, but tumid lupus, borderline leprosy, and the annular/polycyclic variant of subacute cutaneous lupus are not.) Scales define the papulosquamous reaction pattern. Scales may

---

TABLE 1.3. Annular Differential Diagnosis by Etiology

INFECTIOUS
- Tinea corporis, cruris and faciei
- Secondary syphilis
- Tertiary syphilis: "nodular syphilide"
- Leprosy: polar tuberculoid (TT), borderline tuberculoid (BT) and borderline (BB) types

INFLAMMATORY
- Psoriasis: including recurrent circinate erythema
- Pityriasis rosea
- Lichen planus
- Tumid lupus
- Subacute cutaneous lupus erythematosus (SCLE), annular polycyclic variant
- Erythema annulare centrifugum
- Granuloma annulare
- Benign pigmented purpura, Majocci type
- Linear IgA disease and chronic bullous disease of childhood
- Eosinophilic folliculitis of Ofuji

NEOPLASTIC/PARANEOPLASTIC
- Mycosis fungoides
- Necrolytic migratory erythema

DRUG-RELATED
- Drug-induced SCLE

TABLE 1.4. The Annular List That Has Been Transformed into a Morphologic Classification

MACULES
- Benign pigmented purpura, Majocci type

PLAQUES
- Tine corporis (Figure 1.5A), tinea cruris and faciei
- Secondary syphilis (Figure 1.5B) and tertiary syphilis
- Leprosy
- Psoriasis (Figure 1.5C)
- Pityriasis rosea
- Tumid lupus, SCLE (including drug-induced SCLE; Figure 1.5D)
- Erythema annulare centrifugum (Figure 1.5E)
- Mycosis fungoides
- Necrolytic migratory erythema
- Lichen planus (Figure 1.5F)

PAPULES
- Granuloma annulare

VESICLES AND BULLAE
- Linear IgA disease/chronic bullous disease of childhood

PUSTULES
- Eosinophilic folliculitis of Ofuji

---

also be seen in the eczematous reaction pattern. Extensive differential diagnostic lists for each grouping based on morphologic grounds, including reaction patterns and color, as well as the wheel of diagnosis can be built, as will be seen later in the book.

As we learn to hone our eyes to look for diagnostic clues, we will also accustom our minds to create differential diagnostic lists based on morphology. So, from here on, lists based on morphologic features will be included. Lists based on etiopathogenesis are also very useful, as many of us think in these categories reflexively. So, etiologic classifications will be included as well, whenever they can add value.

> **Clinical Tip** Diagnostic lists can be created via an etiologic or a morphologic approach.

Arcuate or Arciform Configurations

Many diseases that form annuli present with curvilinear plaques or arcs that are parts of a ring or annulus. Papules may be configured to form these plaques as well. Erythema annulare centrifugum classically presents with arcuate or annular plaques. Necrolytic migratory erythema, the distinctive eruption of glucagonoma, is a more rarely encountered dermatosis that presents with arcuate and annular plaques. Urticaria and urticarial vasculitis may display arcuate plaques as well as papules that coalesce to form an arcuate configuration.

Concentric Configuration

The term *concentric* in the present context refers to the presence of one ring inside another. Erythema gyratum repens is an extremely rare paraneoplastic eruption occurring secondary to solid-organ malignancies. Concentric smooth or scaly plaques appear to spiral around each other. A similar appearance, usually scaly, is seen in tinea imbricata (also known as *Tokelau*). This is a superficial fungal infection caused by *Trichophyton concentricum* that is endemic to islands of the Southern Pacific Ocean, including Tokelau. Concentric scaly plaques resembling woodgrain are seen. A gyrate appearance may also be seen. Rarely, tinea corporis exhibits concentric rings (more commonly, arcuate plaques may be seen in the middle of the annular plaque). This finding is also rare in erythema annulare centrifugum.

Polycyclic Configuration

The term *polycyclic* refers to a shape that is formed from more than one ring. Urticaria, especially urticaria multiforme, and urticarial vasculitis may have polycyclic plaques. The annular, polycyclic form of subacute cutaneous lupus erythematosus (SCLE) presents with fixed annular and polycyclic plaques.

Gyrate Configuration

The term *gyrate* refers to a rarely encountered configuration. It refers to plaques that seem to spiral or whirl around each other. Erythema gyratum repens and tinea imbricata classically exhibit this phenomenon.

Figurate Configuration

Figurate is a more general term, meaning "figure-forming." The term *figurate erythemas* refers to a group of erythemas that form annuli and arcuate, gyrate, polycyclic, or serpiginous configurations. Sometimes reticulate, geographic, and bizarre shapes and configurations are seen. These include early erythema annulare centrifugum, deep gyrate erythema, erythema migrans, erythema gyratum repens, erythema marginatum of rheumatic fever, and annular erythema of infancy. *Figurate* also describes any other eruption that manifests more than one configuration simultaneously, including mycosis fungoides, necrolytic migratory erythema, urticarial vasculitis, serum sickness and serum sickness–like reactions, and eosinophilic annular erythema.

Linear Configuration

The differential diagnosis of linear lesions can be broadly divided into those caused by external factors (colloquially known as an "outside job") and those caused by irregularities in anatomic structure (an "inside job").

- **Outside job**: Examples here include allergic contact dermatitis to poison ivy, phytophotodermatitis (Figure 1.6A), scabetic burrows (Figure 1.6B), and excoriations secondary to scratching.
- **Inside job**: Here, dermatoses may follow blood vessels, such as in thrombophlebitis; cutaneous sensory nerves, as in zoster (Figure 1.6C); embryonic developmental lines, such as Blaschko lines, as in incontinentia pigmenti; and Futcher lines (lines of pigmentary demarcation; Figure 1.6D).

> **Clinical Tip** The linear configuration may be caused by external factors ("outside job") or they may follow internal anatomic lines ("inside job").

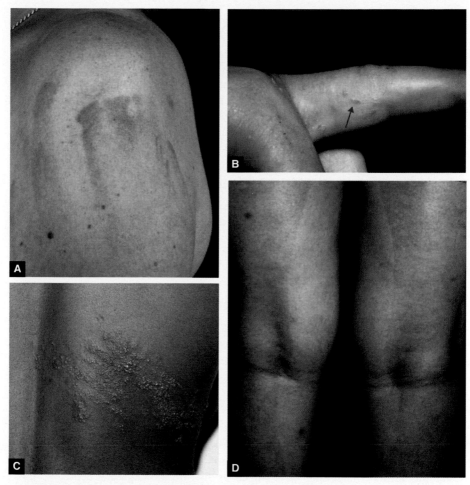

FIGURE 1.6 • The linear grouping. (A) Phytophotodermatitis from limes; (B) a linear burrow in scabies; (C) zoster in a thoracic dermatome; (D) Futcher lines of pigmentary demarcation.

Whorled Configuration

Whorled is another term meaning spiraled or swirled. Whorls of color are seen in blaschkoid disorders such as linear and whorled hypermelanosis and hypomelanosis of Ito. The whorls of hyper- or hypopigmentation respectively interleave between macules of normal skin color.

Reticulate or Retiform Configuration

The terms *reticulate* and *retiform* refer to a net-like or lacy configuration of macules, papules, or plaques. Many reticulate dermatoses follow the pattern of the superficial vascular network that supplies the cutaneous surface, including livedo reticularis, livedo racemosa, livedoid vasculopathy, and retiform purpura. Other net-like arrays arise independently of this vasculature, such as the lacy eruption seen in erythema infectiosum (also known as fifth disease).

> **Clinical Tip** Reticulate, retiform = net-like, lacy.

Herpetiform Configuration

The adjective *herpetiform* is used to describe grouped lesions on an erythematous base. These lesions may be papules, vesicles, erosions or crusts. Herpes simplex and herpes zoster are commonly seen and are the classic examples of this. More rarely encountered dermatoses that manifest herpetiform grouping include impetigo herpetiformis (pustular psoriasis in pregnancy), which presents with herpetiform pustules; pemphigus herpetiformis, which displays grouped vesicles and erosions; and dermatitis herpetiformis, which manifests grouped urticarial papules, vesicles, and erosions.

> **Clinical Tip** The word *herpetiform* can be defined as grouped lesions on an erythematous base.

Agminate or Agminated Configuration

The terms *agminate* and *agminated* refer to the fact that lesions are clustered in a particular site. Spitz nevi, pyogenic granulomas, melanoma metastases, and leiomyomas can manifest in this way.

> **Clinical Tip** Agminate = clustered.

DISTRIBUTION

The distribution of an eruption may be so characteristic as to suggest a diagnosis. Let us begin to explore some of the more common distribution areas and the eruptions that tend to reside there. Chapter 12 will cover distribution in greater depth.

Distribution of Primary Lesions	
• Photoexposed	• Acral
• Flexures	• Periorbital
• Extensors	• Relation to appendages: follicular or eccrine
• Intertriginous	
• Seborrheic	• Localized
• Truncal	• Generalized
• Palms and soles	• Symmetric or asymmetric

Photoexposed Areas

Sites that are most commonly affected include the face, neck, the "V" of the chest, the upper back, and the dorsal arms and hands. Sun-covered areas are spared, including eyelid creases, the area of the upper neck that is in shadow from the chin, and Wilkinson's triangle (a triangular area behind the earlobe). In contrast, these areas are not spared in eruptions induced by airborne allergens, such as an airborne allergic contact dermatitis. The etiologic and morphologic classifications of the photoexposed areas appear

TABLE 1.5. Etiologic Classification of Photo-exposed Eruptions

INHERITED CONDITIONS

- Xeroderma pigmentosum
- Rothmund–Thompson syndrome (poikiloderma congenitale)
- Cockayne syndrome
- Bloom syndrome
- Trichothiodystrophy

ACQUIRED CONDITIONS

INFLAMMATORY CONDITIONS

- Subacute cutaneous lupus (SCLE), systemic lupus (SLE)
- Chronic actinic dermatitis, actinic reticuloid
- Actinic prurigo
- Porphyria cutanea tarda, erythropoietic protoporphyria, variegate porphyria, hereditary coproporphyria
- Polymorphous light eruption (PMLE)
- Hydroa vacciniforme
- Solar urticaria

NUTRITIONAL CONDITIONS

- Pellagra

DRUG-INDUCED CONDITIONS

- Phototoxic eruptions
- Photoallergic eruptions
- Photolichenoid drug: hydrochlorothiazide, tetracyclines, furosemide
- Photoaccentuated pigmentation from drugs
  - Slate-gray: amiodarone, tricyclic antidepressants
  - Blue-gray: phenothiazines, minocycline
  - Brown-gray: antimalarials
  - Magenta: gold

in Tables 1.5 and 1.6, respectively. Many dermatoses that occur in photoexposed areas are rarely encountered. Some are rare genetically inherited syndromes. Phototoxic and photoallergic eruptions are more common, and medications as a cause, or underlying lupus or some of the porphyrias should always be borne in mind.

> **Clinical Tip** Sun-covered areas are not involved in photoexposed eruptions, including the upper eyelid creases, the upper neck that is in shadow from the chin, and the triangular area behind the earlobe (Wilkinson's triangle).

Flexures

This classification includes the antecubital and popliteal fossae. Common dermatoses with a predilection for these areas include atopic dermatitis and allergic contact dermatitis to formaldehyde. Erythrasma, a *Corynebacterium* infection, presents as scaly brown macules that favor intertriginous and flexural regions of the body. More rarely encountered dermatoses with flexural involvement include pseudoxanthoma elasticum and fibroelastolytic papulosis (these present as yellow or white papules that involve

TABLE 1.6. Morphologic Classification of Photoexposed Eruptions

ERYTHEMATOUS MACULES
- Cockayne syndrome
- Trichothiodystrophy
- Phototoxic eruption
- SLE

RETICULATE ERYTHEMA
- Bloom syndrome

WHEALS
- Solar urticaria
- Erythropoietic protoporphyria

OTHER URTICARIAL PLAQUES
- Tumid LE
- Annular polycyclic variant of SCLE
- Reticulate erythematous mucinosis (REM)
- Polymorphic light eruption (PMLE)

PSORIASIFORM PLAQUES
- SCLE
- Photo exacerbated psoriasis

PAPULES, PAPULOVESICLES
- PMLE
- Hydroa vacciniforme

ECZEMATOUS
- PMLE, eczematous type
- Actinic prurigo
- Photoallergic dermatitis
- Chronic actinic dermatitis
- Actinic reticuloid

BULLAE WITH SCARRING
- Porphyria cutanea tarda
- Variegate porphyria
- Hereditary coproporphyria
- Hydroa vacciniforme

FLAKY, DESQUAMATING
- Pellagra

LICHENOID PAPULES AND PLAQUES
- Photolichenoid eruption from tetracyclines, hydrochlorothiazide, furosemide

PIGMENTARY CHANGES
- Slate-gray: amiodarone, tricyclic antidepressants
- Blue-gray: phenothiazines, minocycline
- Brown-gray: antimalarials
- Magenta: gold

POIKILODERMA
- Rothmund–Thompson syndrome (poikiloderma congenitale)

DYSCHROMIA
- Xeroderma pigmentosum

the neck, axillae, and antecubital fossae among other areas) and reticulate pigmented anomaly of the flexures (Dowling–Degos disease), an autosomal dominant dermatosis that presents with pigmented macules of flexural areas and the neck.

> **Clinical Tip** Flexures include the antecubital and popliteal fossae.

Extensors

The *extensor aspects* include the elbows and knees as well as adjacent skin. Dermatoses with a propensity for these areas include those listed in Table 1.7. Common eruptions that involve the elbows and knees include psoriasis and granuloma annulare. Frictional lichenoid dermatitis, erythema multiforme, dermatomyositis, tuberous xanthomas, rheumatoid nodules, palisaded and neutrophilic granulomatous dermatitis, erythema elevatum diutinum, and dermatitis herpetiformis are more rarely seen. Frictional lichenoid dermatitis typically presents as slightly violaceous plaques over the elbows in a child. Erythema multiforme presents with typical targets lesions or raised atypical targets (central bulla with surrounding zone of erythema) in the case of herpes simplex virus–induced disease. Extensor aspects of the extremities including dorsal hands and feet are classic sites of involvement. One of the cutaneous findings in dermatomyositis is violaceous linear macules that extend down the forearms from the elbows and up the thighs from the knees. Tuberous xanthomas are yellow papules and nodules that favor elbows and knees. Rheumatoid nodules are skin-colored or reddish deep nodules. Palisaded neutrophilic and granulomatous dermatitis is similar to granuloma annulare, but papules are discrete and are rarely annular. This entity is seen in the setting of connective tissue disease. Erythema elevatum diutinum comprises red-brown papules, plaques, and nodules that favor extensor aspects. In dermatitis

---

TABLE 1.7. Dermatoses That Favor the Extensor Aspects by Primary Lesion

MACULES
- Dermatomyositis

PLAQUES
- Psoriasis
- Frictional lichenoid dermatitis
- Erythema multiforme

PAPULES AND NODULES
- Tuberous xanthomas
- Rheumatoid nodules

PAPULES AND PLAQUES
- Granuloma annulare
- Palisaded and neutrophilic granulomatous dermatitis

PAPULES, PLAQUES, AND NODULES
- Erythema elevatum diutinum

PAPULES, VESICLES, AND EROSIONS
- Dermatitis herpetiformis

herpetiformis, urticarial plaques with grouped vesicles or erosions are seen on elbows, knees, scalp, and buttocks.

> **Clinical Tip** Extensors include elbows, knees, and adjacent skin.

Intertriginous Areas

The *intertriginous areas* are those locations where two skin areas contact each other, such as the inguinal or axillary folds, the intergluteal area, and the inframammary areas (Figure 1.7). Many diseases have a predilection for these areas. Tables 1.8 and 1.9 display succinct lists of diseases by etiologic and morphologic classification, respectively. Intertrigo refers to the irritant reaction that results from friction between the two closely opposed skin surfaces. Heat, moisture, ill-fitting undergarments, and obesity are predisposing factors. Shiny, thin, ill-defined pink plaques are seen. Intertrigo may be a manifestation of seborrheic dermatitis. Irritant dermatitis in the axillae from deodorant use is similar in appearance to intertrigo. Inverse psoriasis presents as well-demarcated, salmon pink plaques that may be shiny or macerated. Beefy red plaques with outlying satellite papules or pustules are diagnostic of a candida intertrigo. Other rarer causes of thin plaques in the intertriginous areas include Hailey–Hailey disease (benign familial pemphigus), erythrasma, acrodermatitis enteropathica, and systemic drug-related intertriginous and flexural exanthema (SDRIFE). Hailey–Hailey disease manifests as macerated intertriginous plaques with linear erosions (linear "rents") that may develop a verrucous surface. Erythrasma presents as asymptomatic brown, scaly macules in intertriginous zones, the antecubital fossae or the lower abdomen. In acrodermatitis enteropathica, a "do not miss" diagnosis, which is associated with zinc deficiency, vesicles, bullae, crusted and psoriasiform plaques, occurs periodically and in the inguinal creases. In SDRIFE, there is well-demarcated erythema of the buttocks, thighs, and intertriginous areas, following exposure to systemic drugs, such as β-lactams and mercury. Mycosis fungoides favors in the sun-covered area between the posterior axillary fold and the axilla. Vegetating plaques in the folds connote either pemphigus vegetans or extramammary Paget disease. Pemphigus vegetans is the intertriginous variant of pemphigus vulgaris. It presents as vegetating plaques with superficial erosions. Extramammary Paget disease, another "do not miss" entity, typically presents as a solitary vegetating plaque on the suprapubic skin or the skin in and around the inguinal folds. Velvety plaques in the axillae signify acanthosis nigricans. The differential diagnosis of papules in the intertriginous areas includes three rare diseases: pseudoxanthoma elasticum, fibroelastolytic papulosis, and Fox–Fordyce disease. The former two disorders of elastic tissue present as asymptomatic 2–3 mm yellowish papules whereas Fox–Fordyce disease presents with perifollicular/periapocrine papules in the axillae. Hidradenitis suppurativa presents as tender erythematous nodules that may drain, along with sinus tract formation and cribriform scarring, and this is more commonly seen.

Finally in this category is another rare disease, Dowling–Degos disease, which presents with reticulate pigmentation in the intertriginous zones as well as the flexures.

Seborrheic Areas

The *seborrheic distribution* comprises the following areas: scalp, eyebrows, glabella, nasolabial folds, presternal region, in the ears, and behind the ears. The intertriginous areas may also be involved. Seborrheic dermatitis is the most common eruption that

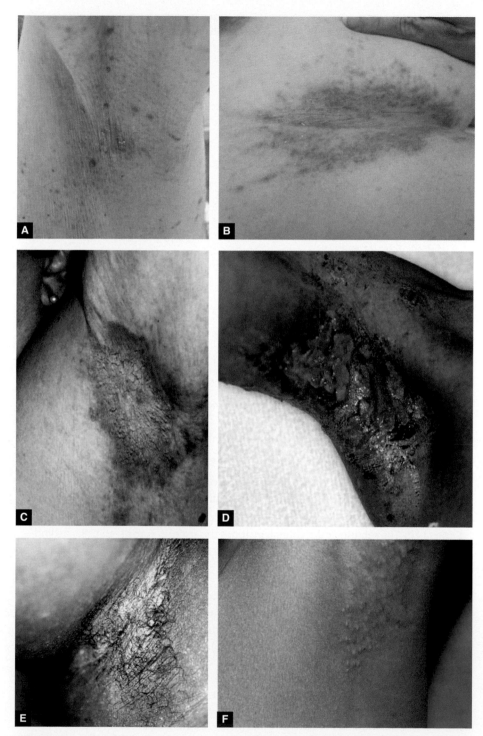

FIGURE 1.7 • The intertriginous distribution. (A) Intertrigo in seborrheic dermatitis; (B) candidal intertrigo with outlying satellite papules; (C) Hailey-Hailey disease with linear erosions; (D) pemphigus vegetans, early; (E) acanthosis nigricans in the axilla; (F) regularly spaced papules of Fox-Fordyce disease.

TABLE 1.8. Etiologic Classification of Intertriginous Eruptions

INHERITED
- Pseudoxanthoma elasticum
- Hailey–Hailey disease
- Dowling–Degos disease

ACQUIRED
- Infectious
  - Candidal intertrigo
  - Erythrasma
- Inflammatory
  - Intertrigo
  - Irritant dermatitis
  - Inverse psoriasis
  - Pemphigus vegetans
  - Hidradenitis suppurativa
- Degenerative
  - Fibroelastolytic papulosis
- Nutritional
  - Acrodermatitis enteropathica
- Neoplastic/paraneoplastic
  - Acanthosis nigricans
  - Fox–Fordyce disease
  - Mycosis fungoides
  - Extramammary Paget disease
- Drug-induced
  - Systemic drug-related intertriginous and flexural exanthema (SDRIFE)
  - Toxic erythema of chemotherapy

---

occurs in this distribution. Darier disease (keratosis follicularis), pemphigus foliaceus, and the rash of vitamin B_6 deficiency also typically occur in this distribution.

> **Clinical Tip** The seborrheic distribution includes the scalp, eyebrows, glabella, behind the ears, in the ears, the presternal region, and the intertriginous areas.

Truncal Areas

Whereas many dermatoses favor the extremities, others preferentially occur on the trunk. Viral exanthems, exanthematous drug eruptions, drug reactions with eosinophilia and systemic symptoms (DRESS), and SJS/TEN begin on the trunk. SJS/TEN presents with tender macules on the chest that then spread centrifugally. The central chest is a site of predilection for seborrheic dermatitis, and the lower back is a site of predilection for psoriasis. Dermatitis herpetiformis preferentially involves buttocks along with elbows, knees, and scalp. Grover disease (transient acantholytic dermatosis) occurs in older individuals with lighter skin phototypes. The convex aspects of the back and upper abdomen are sites of predilection. Scaly papules and sometimes vesicles are seen. It is generally an extremely pruritic condition, but not all cases are pruritic. Seabather's eruption is a hypersensitivity

TABLE 1.9. Morphologic Classification of Intertriginous Eruptions

RETICULATE MACULES
- Dowling–Degos disease

SCALY MACULES
- Erythrasma

THIN PLAQUES
- Intertrigo, including seborrheic dermatitis (Figure 1.7A)
- Irritant dermatitis
- Inverse psoriasis
- Candidal intertrigo (Figure 1.7B)
- Systemic drug-related intertriginous and flexural exanthema (SDRIFE)
- Toxic erythema of chemotherapy
- Hailey–Hailey disease (Figure 1.7C)
- Acrodermatitis enteropathica
- Mycosis fungoides

VEGETATING PLAQUES
- Pemphigus vegetans (Figure 1.7D)
- Extramammary Paget disease

VELVETY PLAQUES
- Acanthosis nigricans (Figure 1.7E)

PAPULES
- Fox–Fordyce disease (Figure 1.7F)
- Pseudoxanthoma elasticum
- Fibroelastolytic papulosis

NODULES, SINUSES
- Hidradenitis suppurativa

reaction to nematocysts of the sea anemone or jellyfish. These organisms become trapped in the fabric of bathing suits and cause a self-limited erythematous papular eruption on the trunk.

Palms and Soles

A myriad of dermatoses, both common and rare, favor the palms and soles (Figure 1.8). Table 1.10 contains a short list, by etiology, and Table 1.11, by morphology. Dyshidrotic hand eczema, other eczemas, viral warts, psoriasis, tinea pedis, and erythema multiforme are among the most commonly encountered dermatoses in this location. Dyshidrotic hand eczema presents with "tapioca-like" vesicles in the lateral aspects of fingers, fingertips, and on the palms and soles, and hyperkeratotic plaques present in more longstanding cases. Keratolysis exfoliativa is the name given to mild dyshidrotic eczema that has more scaling and fewer vesicles than its congener. Allergic contact dermatitis initially involves the dorsal aspects of the hands but palms may also be involved in severe cases. Tinea pedis is common, and tinea manuum is rarer. In early tinea pedis, only one foot is involved. In later-stage disease, both feet may be involved, and the presence of a "one hand, two foot" scaly dermatosis is a classic presentation of tinea pedis

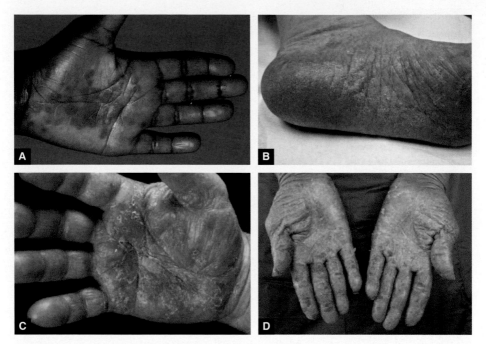

FIGURE 1.8 · Palms and soles. (A) Violaceous scaly papules of secondary syphilis; (B) powdery scales and a background of erythema of moccasin-type tinea pedis; (C) hyperkeratotic plaques and "tapioca-like" vesicles (fingertips) of longstanding dyshidrotic eczema; (D) hyperkeratotic plaques of mycosis fungoides.

and manuum. Look for powdery scale with small collarettes, and possible nail dystrophy as well. Erythema multiforme presents with typical target lesions or raised atypical targets (central bulla with surrounding zone of erythema) in the case of herpes simplex virus–induced disease. Extensors, including dorsal hands, are one pattern of presentation, and a palmoplantar presentation may also be seen. Psoriasis may present as a typical plaque form with hyperkeratosis in this anatomic location. Lichen planus, discoid lupus, lupus erythematosus/lichen planus (LE/LP) overlap, and pityriasis rubra pilaris are also causes of an inflammatory palmar or plantar keratoderma. Palmoplantar pustular psoriasis is a not infrequently encountered presentation; here, look for pustules, flat brown incipient crusts, and collarettes of scale. More rarely encountered conditions on palms and soles include keratodermas, porokeratosis, and the pigmented macules of vitamin B$_{12}$ deficiency. Inherited keratodermas may be diffuse, focal, or punctate. Keratodermas may be associated with ichthyosis, such as the hyperlinear palms that are seen in ichthyosis vulgaris. The palmoplantar ectodermal dysplasias include a group of diseases where palmoplantar keratoderma is just one of many findings. An example is pachyonychia congenita. Here, a focal palmoplantar keratoderma is accompanied by wedge-shaped nails, follicular hyperkeratosis (especially over the knees), and natal teeth and steatocystoma multiplex in some forms. The palmoplantar subtype of porokeratosis presents as multiple flat hyperkeratotic papules with thread-like raised rims. Brown macules may be a normal finding, especially in people with darker phototypes, but new onset pigmented macules should prompt a search for a vitamin B$_{12}$ deficiency.

Classic drug eruptions in this anatomic location include acral erythema and the hyperkeratotic hand–foot reaction that is seen with the newer multikinase inhibitors

TABLE 1.10. Etiologic Classification of Diseases That Favor the Palms and Soles

INFECTIOUS
- Viral warts
- Secondary syphilis
- Rocky Mountain spotted fever
- Tinea pedis and tinea manuum
- Tinea nigra
- Septic vasculitis
- Scabies
- Crusted scabies

INFLAMMATORY
- Erythema multiforme
- Focal palmoplantar peeling
- Dyshidrotic hand eczema
- Keratolysis exfoliativa
- Reactive arthritis
- Inflammatory keratodermas
  - Psoriasis
  - Lichen planus
  - Discoid lupus
  - Lupus erythematosus/lichen planus overlap
  - Pityriasis rubra pilaris
- Pustular psoriasis

NONINFLAMMATORY
- Primary keratodermas
- Keratodermas associated with ichthyoses
- Palmoplantar ectodermal dysplasias

NUTRITIONAL
- Vitamin B_{12} deficiency

NEOPLASTIC/PARANEOPLASTIC
- Porokeratosis of the palms and soles
- Acral lentiginous melanoma
- Amelanotic melanoma
- Mycosis fungoides
- Bazex syndrome (acrokeratosis paraneoplastica)
- Tripe palms
- Diffuse or punctate keratoderma

DRUG-INDUCED
- Acral erythema
- Hand–foot syndrome from multikinase and BRAF inhibitors

(sunitinib, sorafenib) and the BRAF inhibitors (vemurafenib, dabrafenib). Acral erythema (also known as the hand–foot syndrome) is seen from traditional chemotherapeutic agents such as doxorubicin or 5-fluorouracil. There are tender lichenoid papules and plaques on palms and soles that extend to the lateral aspects of fingers and toes, and sometimes to the dorsal hands and feet. Acral erythema may be part of a more

TABLE 1.11. Morphologic Classification of Eruptions on Palms and Soles

PURPURIC MACULES
- Septic vasculitis
- Rocky Mountain spotted fever

PIGMENTED MACULES
- Tinea nigra: usually single
- Vitamin B_{12} deficiency: usually multiple

SMOOTH ERYTHEMATOUS PLAQUES
- Acral erythema
- Secondary syphilis, early (Figure 1.8A)

SCALY ERYTHEMATOUS PLAQUES
- Inflammatory keratodermas
  - Psoriasis
  - Lichen planus
  - Discoid lupus
  - Lupus erythematosus/lichen planus overlap
  - Pityriasis rubra pilaris
- Tinea pedis (Figure 1.8B) and tinea manuum
- Bazex syndrome

SCALY PLAQUES
- Longstanding dyshidrotic eczema (Figure 1.8C)
- Diffuse keratodermas
- Reactive arthritis
- Mycosis fungoides (Figure 1.8D)
- Keratolysis exfoliativa
- Tinea pedis and tinea manuum

NONSCALY PLAQUES
- Tripe palms

PAPULES
- Porokeratosis of palms and soles
- Punctuate keratodermas

NODULES
- Hand–foot syndrome from multikinase inhibitors
- Pachyonychia congenita

VESICLES
- Dyshidrotic eczema

PUSTULES
- Pustular psoriasis

generalized eruption known as toxic erythema of chemotherapy, where intertriginous areas are also involved with erythema or violaceous erythema. The hand–foot reaction that occurs with newer targeted anticancer agents presents as painful hyperkeratotic plaques and nodules with an erythematous rim on weight-bearing areas or in areas of friction.

There are many "do not miss" diseases that should be borne in mind when looking at palms and soles. These are also rare. "Do not miss" infections include secondary syphilis and Rocky Mountain spotted fever. In secondary syphilis, tender violaceous papules and plaques present on palms and soles. *Ollendorff sign* refers to the tenderness that patients feel when pressure is applied to secondary syphilis lesions in this location. In Rocky Mountain spotted fever, palms and soles are involved early on; petechiae and purpura are seen. Tinea nigra is a rarely encountered fungal infection that presents as a dark brown to black macule on the sole or palm that simulates melanoma. Scabies burrows are classically seen in webspaces and along wrists, and in crusted scabies, crusts or fine sheets of powdery scale are seen in these locations or more generally. In septic vasculitis, macular or palpable purpura is seen, especially on the fingertips, and occasionally on the palms. In mycosis fungoides there may be thick scaly plaques or thinner erythematous scaly plaques in the Sezary syndrome. Another rare "do not miss" infection is reactive arthritis (Reiter syndrome): keratoderma blennorhagicum refers to hyperkeratotic plaques with an ostracious (oyster-like) scale that is seen on the soles. Paraneoplastic "do not miss" items are the extremely rare "tripe palms" presentation of acanthosis nigricans on the palms and acrokeratosis paraneoplastica (Bazex syndrome). In tripe palms, the palms are thickened and velvety with accentuation of skin markings. In acrokeratosis paraneoplastica, there are acral psoriasiform papules and plaques that may also be violaceous. Occasionally an acquired diffuse or punctate keratoderma is a paraneoplastic phenomenon. The most deadly neoplasm in this anatomic location is acral lentiginous melanoma. Be aware that many melanomas on palms and soles may be amelanotic, and consider this diagnosis for any new skin-colored or pink papule or nodule arising in this location.

Acral Areas

The term *acral* refers to the distal parts of the body. This distribution encompasses not only the digits, palms, and soles but also the nose, ears, and penis. Examples of eruptions that are found in an acral distribution include cryoglobulinemia and the even rarer cryofibrinogenemia. Cocaine levamisole toxicity also favors these sites. The term *acral* has been used more loosely in our literature to refer to conditions that are located on palms and soles only—a partial acral distribution.

Periorbital Areas

A number of dermatoses can be found in a periorbital location, as can be seen in Tables 1.12 and 1.13. Common diseases in this location include allergic contact dermatitis and atopic dermatitis. Syringomas are frequently found on the lower eyelid. Periorificial dermatitis is more frequently found around the lips, but periorbital involvement may occur. Look for 1–2 mm pink and reddish papules in this location. A granulomatous variant is rarer; here, the papules will be more substantive. For substantive brownish papules, the diagnosis of micropapular or papular sarcoidosis should be considered. The periorbital skin is a site of predilection for vitiligo. Rare and important "do not miss" entities that occur in this location include dermatomyositis, primary amyloidosis, and lipoid proteinosis. A common and pathognomonic finding in dermatomyositis is the presence of a heliotrope rash. Typically, violaceous erythema is seen. The heliotrope rash is most commonly bilateral, and asymmetric forms may occur. While the heliotrope is usually smooth, scales or erosions may be seen. Edema may also be present. In primary amyloidosis, the skin is infiltrated diffusely with amyloid. Waxy papules may be seen on the eyelid margins along with purpuric

TABLE 1.12. Etiologic Classification of Periorbital Dermatoses

INFECTIOUS
- Hordeolum

INFLAMMATORY
- Eyelid dermatitis: atopic, allergic, or irritant
- Blepharitis, including seborrheic dermatitis and rosacea
- Periorbital dermatitis
- Vitiligo
- Heliotrope rash of dermatomyositis
- Chalazion

DEPOSITIONAL
- Amyloid (waxy, eyelid margin)
- Lipoid proteinosis (waxy, eyelid margin)
- Colloid milium
- Sarcoidosis
- Xanthomas, plane xanthomas
- Necrobiotic xanthogranuloma

NEOPLASTIC
- Acrochordons
- Seborrheic keratoses
- Syringomas
- Eccrine and apocrine hidrocystomas
- Trichoepitheliomas, trichilemmomas
- Melanocytic nevus
- Sebaceous carcinoma

macules ("pinch purpura"). In lipoid proteinosis, beaded waxy papules are seen on the eyelid margins and periorally, along with warty papules on the lateral aspects of fingers and over the knees. For single papules along the lid margin, consider hordeolum or chalazion, melanocytic nevus, and sebaceous carcinoma. Hordeola may be internal or external. An external hordeolum or external stye is usually a bacterial infection of a follicle on the lid margin. An internal hordeolum is an infection of meibomian glands on the inner aspect of the eyelid. These are both tender. A chalazion represents chronic inflammation of an eyelid gland, such as if an internal hordeolum does not resolve. This is seen as a red or skin-colored eyelid margin papule that is nontender.

Sebaceous carcinoma has a predilection for the eyelid margin, especially the upper lid. It presents as a reddish brown or yellowish painless papule that is slow-growing. It may resemble a chalazion, and therefore diagnosis may be delayed.

Relation to Appendages: Follicular or Eccrine

These dermatoses comprise papules, pustules, and occasionally nodules or very superficial vesicles. The hallmark of these lesions is that they are evenly spaced with respect to each other:

- **Follicular differential diagnosis**: This is extremely broad and will be covered in greater detail when follicular papules are discussed in Chapter 2.

TABLE 1.13. Morphologic Classification of Periorbital Dermatoses

PAPULES
- Single: eyelid margin
  - Hordeolum
  - Chalazion
  - Nevus
  - Sebaceous carcinoma
  - Apocrine hidrocystoma
- Single or multiple
  - Acrochordons
  - Seborrheic keratoses
- Multiple
  - Periorbital dermatitis
  - Syringomas
  - Eccrine hidrocystomas
  - Trichoepitheliomas, trichilemmomas

PAPULES AND PLAQUES
- Amyloid (waxy, eyelid margin)
- Lipoid proteinosis (waxy, eyelid margin)
- Colloid milium
- Sarcoidosis
- Xanthomas, plane xanthomas
- Necrobiotic xanthogranuloma

PLAQUES
- Eyelid dermatitis: atopic, allergic, or irritant
- Heliotrope rash of dermatomyositis

MACULES
- Blepharitis
- Vitiligo
- Heliotrope rash of dermatomyositis

- **Eccrine differential diagnosis**: This includes the miliaria group (miliaria crystallina, rubra, pustulosa, and profunda), and can be invoked when multiple tumors arise from eccrine ducts and coils (such as in eccrine hidrocystomas and syringomas).

Localized Areas

A localized distribution may be a random phenomenon, such as a cluster of insect bites on an extremity; however, it may also represent preferential involvement of a body site by an eruption. The truncal and periorbital distributions are examples of localized distribution areas. Chapter 12 is dedicated to a comprehensive discussion of dermatoses by distribution, including categorization by preferential body part involved.

Generalized Areas

Certain eruptions occur on all or most body parts. These may start in one location and progress to involve all locations. Examples include viral exanthems, such as measles or rubella; and drug eruptions, such as the exanthematous drug eruption. Global involvement of all or almost all the skin is termed *erythroderma*. Causes of erythroderma will be discussed in Chapters 6 and 10.

Symmetric or Asymmetric Distribution

Symmetry implies an exact mirror-image distribution on the left and right sides of the body. Symmetric eruptions usually imply the existence of an internal cause, such as erythema multiforme or leukocytoclastic vasculitis. Some inherent dermatoses may be symmetric or asymmetric, such as psoriasis and granuloma annulare. Tinea pedis is usually asymmetric at the beginning with preferential involvement of one foot. Both feet may be similarly involved in a more longstanding case. Unilateral laterothoracic exanthema (also known as asymmetric periflexural exanthem of childhood) comprises erythematous papules and plaques that begin near intertriginous folds on one side of the body. After 2 weeks, the eruption may become more generalized. Cellulitis on the lower extremity is unilateral and asymmetric. Bilateral lower-extremity cellulitis is exceedingly rare, and other diagnoses should always be considered in the presence of bilateral erythema of the legs.

> **Clinical Tip** Bilateral lower-extremity cellulitis is exceedingly rare, and other diagnoses should always be considered in the presence of bilateral erythema of the legs.

More on Distribution

Other distributions that are characteristic of specific dermatoses may be seen "One hand, two foot" is another typical distribution of tinea pedis and tinea manuum. Pityriasis rosea typically has a "T-shirt and shorts" distribution, where distal extremities, palms and soles, and neck and face are spared. Exuberant cases do not always respect this distribution. Interestingly, sometimes configurations have been termed *distributions*, such as zoster being described as grouped vesicles on an erythematous base in a dermatomal distribution. Strictly speaking, dermatoses in dermatomes are *configured* that way. *Distribution*, as we will see, refers to body location, so zoster of a thoracic dermatome can be described as "grouped vesicles on an erythematous base in a dermatomal configuration on the trunk." This terminology also holds for dermatoses following Blaschko lines.

EXAMINING AND GLEANING INFORMATION FROM SCALP, HAIR, NAILS, MUCOUS MEMBRANES, AND LYMPH NODES

These so-called "hidden areas" may hold a wealth of diagnostic information and should be examined routinely when creating a differential diagnosis, or when narrowing it down, as is outlined here and discussed in more depth in Chapter 13.

- **Scalp**: A classic finding on the scalp may help clinch a diagnosis, such as perifollicular scale and scarring alopecia in lichen planus, or orange-brown plaques and scarring alopecia in sarcoidosis. In general, the approach is to differentiate scarring from nonscarring alopecia, and to look for the accompanying clinical features.
- **Hair**: Many hair shaft disorders are inherited. However, hair shaft abnormalities are also seen in acquired dermatoses and may hold clues to the diagnosis of scalp disorders specifically. Examples include the broken-off hairs and "black dots" of *Trichophyton tonsurans* tinea capitis and the exclamation point hairs of alopecia areata.
- **Nails**: Knowledge of the way inflammatory dermatoses present in the nail, and spending time examining the nails, are two important tools in the diagnostician's

armamentarium. Examples include the fine pits of alopecia areata, the alternating red and white lines (so-called "sandwich sign") of Darier disease, and the "oil spots" of psoriasis.

- **Mucous membranes**: A wealth of diagnostic information is housed in the mouth. Other mucous membranes include the conjunctivae, the vulva and vagina, and the urethra. Later in the book, we explore the differential diagnosis or oral ulcers, orogenital ulcers, and marginal gingivitis, among other disorders.
- **Lymph nodes**: These may be enlarged and reactive in erythroderma from any cause or in the drug hypersensitivity syndrome (DRESS) or enlarged and neoplastic in mycosis fungoides and the Sezary syndrome or in lymphomas.

> **Clinical Tip** The scalp, hair, nails, mucous membranes, and lymph nodes may hold a wealth of diagnostic information and should be examined routinely when creating a differential diagnosis, or when narrowing it down.

CONTEXTUALIZING THESE FINDINGS TO THE PATIENT'S HISTORY

As discussed in the introduction, the importance of taking a thorough history cannot be understated. The top box on the wheel of diagnosis is the beginning of the clinical examination, namely, the primary lesion. By the time the patient is being examined, we do already have a history to guide us. After completing a comprehensive examination, we loop back to reconsider the patient's history in the context of their clinical findings. So, history comes before and after the examination. Specifically, the patient's demographics, environmental exposures, past medical history, and current medications will inform or give context to the clinical findings and help narrow down a differential diagnosis.

> **Clinical Tip** History taking comes before, during, and after the clinical examination. The patient's demographics, environmental exposures, past medical history, and current medications will inform or give context to the clinical findings and help narrow down a differential diagnosis.

Pruritus as a symptom can provide extremely useful diagnostic information and should also be sought on history. While this is a subjective symptom, the majority of dermatoses are accompanied by itch. Some dermatoses are typically accompanied by severe pruritus. Scabies is one of these. Itch occurs throughout the day and is worst at night just after the patient gets into bed. The itch of scabies is defined as being so severe that patients cannot avoid scratching in front of you during the office visit. Dermatitis herpetiformis is similarly so pruritic that the associated vesicles that arise deep in the epidermis may be completely excoriated at the time of presentation. Grover disease is usually itchy and sometimes severely so. Other typically itchy conditions include the eczema family. While urticaria is itchy, urticarial vasculitis burns or is painful, and the urticarial eruption of Schnitzler syndrome (urticaria, M protein, and bone pain) is neither itchy nor painful. Psoriasis is seldom itchy but occasionally may be. Generalized pruritus without a rash should prompt a search for underlying systemic disease, including renal, thyroid, and liver disease, as well as lymphoma or HIV disease. Localized pruritus without rash may be caused by neuropathic itch, such as when itch is localized to the upper-limb girdles, in which case cervical spine pathology should be suspected.

A PRIMER ON USING THE WHEEL

As previously discussed, sometimes a single attribute of an eruption is so characteristic as to suggest a diagnosis. In these situations, only a part of the diagnostic wheel will need to be used. As the practitioner accrues experience, this will become the case more frequently. On the other hand, when an eruption is not immediately recognizable, the entire wheel may need to be flexed.

Figure 1.9 shows an example of lichen planus. Sometimes the primary lesion is overtly flat-topped and violaceous enough to suggest the diagnosis. If these features are

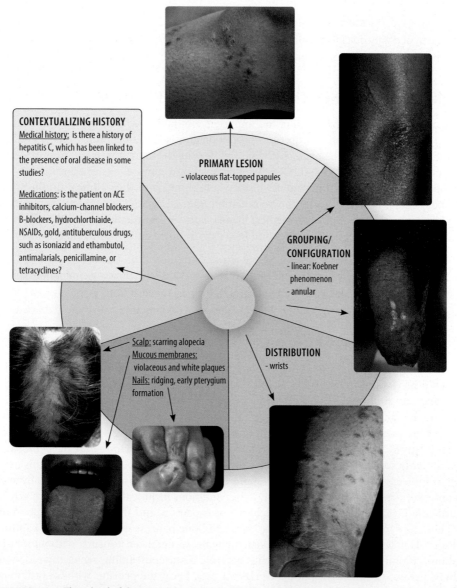

CONTEXTUALIZING HISTORY
Medical history: is there a history of hepatitis C, which has been linked to the presence of oral disease in some studies?

Medications: is the patient on ACE inhibitors, calcium-channel blockers, B-blockers, hydrochlorthiaide, NSAIDs, gold, antituberculous drugs, such as isoniazid and ethambutol, antimalarials, penicillamine, or tetracyclines?

PRIMARY LESION
- violaceous flat-topped papules

GROUPING/ CONFIGURATION
- linear: Koebner phenomenon
- annular

Scalp: scarring alopecia
Mucous membranes: violaceous and white plaques
Nails: ridging, early pterygium formation

DISTRIBUTION
- wrists

FIGURE 1.9 • The wheel of diagnosis: the example of lichen planus.

not immediately recognizable, the presence of the Koebner phenomenon and annular plaques (groupings) may alert one to the diagnosis. The typical distribution on the wrists, flexor forearms, and ankles may provide additional information. Examination of the scalp may yield perifollicular scaly papules with scarring alopecia; nails may show longitudinal ridging or pterygium formation; and mucous membranes may manifest whitish plaques on the lips, a reticulate buccal network, or an erosive pattern on the tongue. If so, the practitioner can narrow the differential diagnosis down quite dramatically. At this point, after successfully diagnosing lichen planus, reexamining the patient's medical history and medications is vital to ensure that this is not a lichenoid drug eruption, and, in cases of oral involvement (in some parts of the world), that there is no associated underlying hepatitis C.

Figure 1.10 shows an eruption of nonscaly papules. As will be seen in later chapters, lack of surface change on a lesion connotes the dermal differential diagnosis, which conjures up a very broad differential diagnosis, including sarcoidosis, granuloma annulare, and palisaded and neutrophilic granulomatous dermatitis, among other eruptions. On closer inspection, these papules are seen to be configured into annuli. Our differential diagnosis is subsequently narrowed to the annular differential. We then pay attention to the distribution of the papules (the extensor aspects of the arm), and the differential diagnostic list is narrowed once more. On the basis of typical grouping and the distribution of the primary lesions, the diagnosis of granuloma annulare can be made.

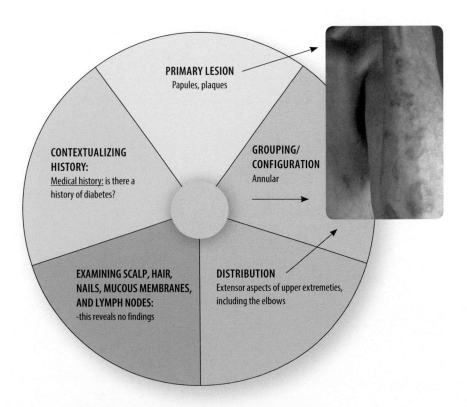

FIGURE 1.10 · The wheel of diagnosis: the example of granuloma annulare.

In this case, the scalp, hair, nails, and mucous membranes, as well as the lymph nodes, do not hold further clues. There may be an association with diabetes in a minority of cases that needs to be investigated.

In the remaining chapters, further concepts will be introduced that will allow us to granulate physical findings further and enable us to create differential diagnoses and then narrow them down as much as possible.

SUMMARY

- The diagnostic boxes of the wheel of diagnosis define the attributes of a dermatosis that can guide diagnosis or the creation of a differential diagnosis.
- Reaction patterns are properties of groups of primary lesions, or a cluster of primary and secondary lesions.
- This chapter explores each diagnostic box in detail and discusses examples of dermatoses that present with each finding.

An Approach to Primary Lesions   2

In this chapter, a customized approach to each primary lesion, using the diagnostic boxes of the wheel of diagnosis and additional algorithmic decision points, will be introduced. The approach is based on the study of the diagnostic determinants of the primary lesions, the number of lesions present, their grouping or configuration, and the distribution they tend to follow, harnessing additional diagnostic pointers from the scalp, hair, nails, and mucous membranes, and from the history. As mentioned in chapter 1, diagnostic determinants include both visual and tactile features. These are revisited in the textbox below and discussed for each primary lesion, where relevant.

Diagnostic Determinants of Primary Lesions

Visual
- Size
- Color
- Shape
- Surface characteristics: contour and scales
- Border

Tactile
- Depth
- Consistency
- Tenderness

The approach to macules, papules, and pustules is presented in its entirety here. For white macules, a supplemental in-depth discussion of various approaches can be found in Chapter 4. For some of the primary lesions, a fuller discussion will be found in Chapters 6–10. Examples include a comprehensive discussion of the approach to vesicles and bullae in Chapter 7 and a discussion of nodules based on their reaction pattern, either dermal (Chapter 9) or papulosquamous (Chapter 6). For plaques, which can be categorized into many of the reaction patterns, the global overview presented here is supplemented by reaction pattern–specific information in each respective chapter.

MACULES

Macules may be categorized primarily according to their color. Other diagnostic determinants, such as size or shape of the macule, may also provide useful information (Table 2.1).

The initial decision point in approaching white macules is whether they are depigmented or hypopigmented. An example of this distinction is shown in Figure 2.1,

---

Color as the Major Diagnostic Determinant of Macules

- White
- Purple
- Pink, red
- Maroon
- Brown
- Black
- Blue
- Blue-gray
- Gray

TABLE 2.1. Diagnostic Determinants of Macules

COLOR
- White, purple, pink, red, maroon, brown, black, blue, blue-gray, gray

SIZE
- *White*: Differential diagnosis of guttate white macules
  - Confetti-like macules of tuberous sclerosis
  - Idiopathic guttate hypomelanosis
  - Leukodermic macules of Darier disease
  - Associated with keratosis punctata
  - Pinta
  - Seborrheic keratoses in a dark skin
  - Flat warts and epidermodysplasia verruciformis in a dark skin
  - Arsenic exposure
  - Pityriasis alba
  - Multiple tumors of the follicular infundibulum
- *Brown*: The café-au-lait macules of McCune–Albright syndrome are large; those of neurofibromatosis are small
- *Red*: Petechiae (<1 mm) and purpura (>1 mm) may have different diagnostic connotations; see Chapter 10.

SHAPE
- Round
  - Red, purple, gray
    - Fixed drug eruption
  - Red, maroon
    - Petechiae left behind after cupping
  - Pink, red
    - Erythema migrans
- Linear
  - White
    - Nevus depigmentosus/hypomelanosis of Ito
    - Fourth stage of incontinentia pigmenti
    - Koebner phenomenon in vitiligo
    - Segmental vitiligo
  - Brown
    - Linear and whorled hypomelanosis
    - Postinflammatory: flagellate erythema, phytophotodermatitis
  - Red
    - Flagellate erythema
  - Maroon
    - Vibices (traumatic purpura)
    - Koebner phenomenon seen in leukocytoclastic vasculitis
  - Purple
    - Linear macules extending from joints in dermatomyositis
- Segmental
  - White
    - Segmental vitiligo
  - Brown
    - McCune–Albright syndrome
    - Becker nevus

(Continued)

TABLE 2.1. Diagnostic Determinants of Macules (continued)
SHAPE (CONT.)

- Geometric
  - Phytophotodermatitis or postinflammatory hyperpigmentation from dermatitis artefacta
- Whorled
  - White
    - Hypomelanosis of Ito
    - Fourth stage of incontinentia pigmenti
  - Brown
    - Linear and whorled hypomelanosis
- Annular
  - White
    - Lepromatous leprosy
  - Brown
    - Postinflammatory hyperpigmentation after tinea corporis

which depicts the depigmented macules of vitiligo and the hypopigmented macules of tinea versicolor. This differential may or may not be clinically obvious, and a Wood's lamp can be employed in cases of doubt. A *Wood's lamp* is an ultraviolet lamp that emits light at 365 nm. In a dark room, under Wood's lamp, depigmented macules will appear bright white or "milk-white," whereas hypopigmented macules will have a muted yellowish-white color. Subclassifications of white macules can be made according to whether there is one or more than one macule present, by macule shape (linear or phylloid, ie, leaf-like) or size (guttate, ie, raindrop-like or larger) and by groupings. More information about the approach to white macules can be found in the chapter dedicated to color (Chapter 4).

> **Clincal Tip** A Wood's lamp can assist in deciding if a macule is de- or hypopigmented.

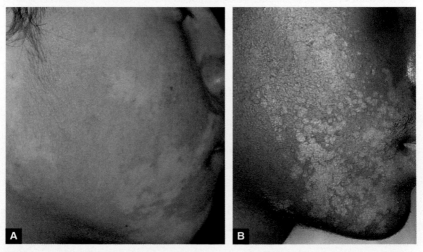

FIGURE 2.1 • **(A) Depigmented macules of vitiligo** (Used with permission from Dr. Miguel Sanchez, New York University, New York, NY.); **(B) hypopigmented macules of tinea versicolor.**

The differential diagnosis of purple macules is a shorter list that comprises the duskiness of early epidermal necrosis, lichenoid and interface dermatitides (including dermatomyositis and resolving lichen planus), fading erythema, and the patch stage of Kaposi sarcoma.

Differential Diagnosis of Purple Macules

- Fading erythema that appears violaceous
- Interface dermatitis: dermatomyositis
- Lichenoid processes: resolving lichen planus
- Early epidermal necrosis that appears dusky or violaceous
- Patch-stage Kaposi sarcoma

Pink and red macules are discussed in detail in the vascular reaction pattern chapter (Chapter 10). To summarize, they can be categorized as those that blanch and those that do not (in which case they are termed *purpura*). Purpura may be maroon-colored, as may other macules, such as a port-wine stain. In general, maroon represents a vascular proliferation, vasculitis, or vasculopathy.

Brown macules are usually a postinflammatory phenomenon. Their shape and size can provide clues as to the preceding dermatosis. For example, truncal ovoid brown macules following lines of cleavage signify postinflammatory change from pityriasis rosea. Flagellate erythema of chemotherapy leaves behind persistent linear macules in its wake. Linear and geometrically shaped brown macules may be seen in the persistent pigmentation after a phytophotodermatitis resolves. Brown macules may also connote primary lesions, such as café-au-lait macules, lentigines, junctional nevi, melanoma in-situ or early invasive melanoma (one color or variegated brown with or without other colors) urticaria pigmentosa (brown-red), or the benign pigmented purpuras (cayenne-pepper- or rust-colored) (Figure 2.2). Drug-induced pigmentation may be brown, brown-gray, blue-gray, slate-gray, violet-brown, or reddish-brown.

Differential Diagnosis of Brown Macules

Primary lesions or dermatoses
- Café-au-lait macules, lentigines, junctional nevi
- Melanoma in-situ or early invasive melanoma (brown, variegated brown, with or without black, pink, red, white)
- Urticaria pigmentosa (brown-red)
- Benign pigmented purpura (cayenne-pepper- or rust-colored)
- Drug-induced pigmentation

Secondary lesions: postinflammatory hyperpigmentation
- After pityriasis rosea: truncal ovoid brown macules following lines of cleavage
- Phytophotodermatitis: linear, geometric
- Flagellate erythema of bleomycin toxicity: linear

A black macule may be an ink-spot lentigo, a deeply pigmented junctional nevus, a pigmented spindle cell tumor of Reed, a melanoma in-situ or rarely an invasive melanoma.

Discrete blue-gray macules are seen on the lower back and sacral area in congenital dermal melanocytosis (formerly known as *Mongolian spots*). Nevus of Ota is a deeper

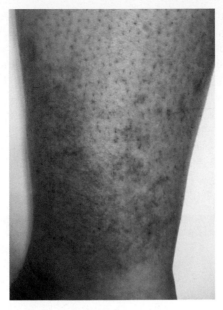

FIGURE 2.2 • Benign pigmented purpura, Schamberg-type, showing cayenne-pepper/rust-colored macules.

color than congenital dermal melanocytosis and is classically seen in the V1 and V2 distribution of the trigeminal nerve. Nevus of Ito occurs on the upper back near the shoulder. Blue nevi may appear blue or blue-gray, and these may be macular. Acquired dermal melanocytosis presents in adulthood as similarly colored blue-gray macules on the bilateral aspects of the forehead. Drug-induced pigmentation may be gray, blue-gray, or purple-gray. Gray as a postinflammatory phenomenon connotes the prior presence of an interface dermatitis. For example, the postinflammatory macules that lichen planus leaves in its wake are gray. This color is also seen when fixed drug eruption resolves. Medical tattoos, such as for radiation therapy fields, may appear black, blue or dark gray. Decorative tattoos may be any color.

Differential Diagnosis of Blue-Gray and Gray Macules

- Congenital dermal melanocytosis
- Nevus of Ota
- Nevus of Ito
- Blue nevi
- Acquired dermal melanocytosis
- Drug pigmentation
- Old interface dermatitis

Other diagnostic determinants of macules include their border, size, and shape and whether they are tender or not. The border of café-au-lait macules may render diagnostic information. If there are café-au-lait macules with jagged or serrated borders that are reminiscent of the coast of Maine, consider the diagnosis of McCune–Albright syndrome. If these have smooth borders that resemble the coast of California, consider the diagnosis of neurofibromatosis in the presence of other diagnostic criteria. Similarly, size of macules may be diagnostic. In McCune–Albright syndrome, the café-au-lait macules are large, whereas those in neurofibromatosis are smaller. The shapes of macules, as alluded to above, may be significant. Perfectly round macules are a rare finding. They may be seen in fixed drug eruption or may result from external causes, such as from cupping. Erythema migrans may also manifest perfectly round macules or thin plaques. Linear and whorled macules connote a dermatosis that follows Blaschko lines. Examples include linear and whorled hypermelanosis or if hypopigmented, nevoid hypomelanosis or the fourth stage of incontinentia pigmenti. An additional diagnostic clue is the number of macules present. A single macule is usually seen in nevus anemicus and segmental vitiligo. In fixed drug eruption, one or more macules can be present. Multiple macules are typically seen in postinflammatory hyperpigmentation from pityriasis rosea, secondary syphilis, or other rashes. Finally, if macules are tender, the specter of epidermal necrosis should be raised, as in early toxic epidermal necrolysis or Stevens–Johnson syndrome, or in fixed drug eruption.

Diagnostic Determinants of Macules		
Visual:	• Size	**Tactile:**
• Color	• Shape	• Tender or nontender
• Border	• Quantity	

As can be seen in Table 2.1, the shape of macules may be annular or linear. The grouping of macules may also be linear, as is summarized in Table 2.2. Small grouped brown macules in a dermatomal distribution signify postinflammatory hyperpigmentation from zoster.

The distribution of macules can add diagnostic information, which is summarized in Table 2.3. Sunburn and phototoxicity from medications manifest red tender photodistributed macules. Photosensitivity in systemic lupus erythematosus or dermatomyositis is seen as erythema in photoexposed areas. The photosensitive erythema in dermatomyositis may have a violaceous hue. Many rare inherited syndromes display photosensitivity, including Bloom syndrome, Cockayne syndrome, and Rothmund–Thomson syndrome. In the early stages of xeroderma pigmentosum,

TABLE 2.2. Grouping of Macules

BROWN
- Herpetiform
  - Postinflammatory hyperpigmentation after zoster
- Linear
  - Postinflammatory hyperpigmentation after zoster
- Reticulate
  - Erythema ab igne
  - Bloom syndrome

PINK/RED
- Herpetiform
  - Early macular HSV or zoster
- Reticulate
  - Livedo reticularis
  - Livedo racemosa
  - Erythema infectiosum (fifth disease)

TABLE 2.3. Distribution of Macules

PHOTOEXPOSED
- Brown
  - Postinflammatory hyperpigmentation after phytophotodermatitis
  - Xeroderma pigmentosum
- Pink/red
  - Sunburn
  - Phototoxic reactions due to drugs
  - Phototoxicity that accompanies connective tissue disease, including SCLE, SLE, and dermatomyositis
  - Cockayne syndrome
  - Trichothiodystrophy
  - Bloom syndrome: photodistributed reticulate erythema
  - Rothmund–Thomson syndrome
- Purple
  - Photosensitivity in dermatomyositis may have a violaceous hue

FLEXURES
- Brown
  - Postinflammatory hyperpigmentation from atopic eczema
  - Erythrasma
  - Tinea versicolor
  - Dowling–Degos disease

EXTENSORS
- White
  - Vitiligo
- Red/pink
  - Toxic erythema of chemotherapy

INTERTRIGINOUS
- Brown
  - Axillary freckling of neurofibromatosis
  - Dowling–Degos disease
- Pink/red
  - Toxic erythema of chemotherapy
  - SDRIFE

SEBORRHEIC
- White
  - Postinflammatory hypopigmentation from seborrheic dermatitis
  - Tinea versicolor
- Brown
  - Tinea versicolor
- Red/pink
  - Tinea versicolor

PALMS AND SOLES
- White
  - Raynaud disease
- Brown

(Continued)

TABLE 2.3. Distribution of Macules (continued)

PALMS AND SOLES (CONT.)
- Single
  - Talon noire
  - Tinea nigra
  - Melanocytic nevi: one or few
  - Acral melanoma
- Multiple
  - Normal variant in darker skin type
  - Postinflammatory hyperpigmentation from a preceding eruption, such as secondary syphilis
  - Vitamin B$_{12}$ deficiency
- Pink/red
  - Palmar erythema
  - Raynaud disease
  - Raynaud phenomenon
  - Acral erythema from chemotherapy
  - Kawasaki disease
  - Erythromelalgia
  - Complex regional pain syndromes
  - Acrodynia
  - Erythema multiforme
- Red/maroon
  - Leukocytoclastic vasculitis: palmar involvement not common
  - Septic vasculitis
    - Distal asymmetric purpura
    - Janeway lesions
  - Lymphocytic vasculitis
- Blue/purple
  - Acrocyanosis
  - Raynaud disease
  - Blue toe syndrome: blue toes occur from microvascular occlusion caused by thromboembolic disease, or abnormal circulating blood constituents
  - Acral erythema of toxic erythema of chemotherapy—can appear violaceous
- Black
  - Talon noire
  - Tinea nigra
  - Acral melanoma

ACRAL
- Maroon/purple
  - Type 1 cryoglobulinemia
  - Cryofibrinogenemia

PERIORBITAL
- White
  - Vitiligo
- Purple
  - Heliotrope of dermatomyositis

FOLLICULAR
- Repigmentation of vitiligo
- Perifollicular retention of pigment in the vitiligo-like macules of scleroderma

another rare inherited disorder of DNA repair, freckling and larger lentigines are seen in photo exposed areas.

Flexural pigmentation may be seen as a postinflammatory phenomenon from atopic dermatitis. Erythrasma and tinea versicolor may appear macular, and the antecubital fossae is a frequent site of involvement for these. Dowling–Degos disease is a rare inherited pigmentary disorder that presents with reticulate brown macules in the flexures and intertriginous areas.

With respect to extensor-distributed macules, vitiligo typically occurs over bony prominences of extensor aspects of the extremities, as well as distal digits and periorbitally. Red macules over the elbows and knees may be seen in toxic erythema of chemotherapy, as this is a less frequent site of involvement than the typical acral and intertriginous involvement. Symmetric drug-related intertriginous and flexural exanthema (SDRIFE) is a similar eruption that occurs secondary to other drugs, such as antibiotics. In the baboon syndrome, erythema involves the buttocks as well. Brown intertriginous macules are seen in axillary freckling, which is one of the diagnostic criteria for neurofibromatosis.

Macules in the seborrheic distribution connote tinea versicolor or postinflammatory change from seborrheic dermatitis. Other truncal macules include Becker nevus and progressive macular hypomelanosis. Becker nevus is seen in young men as a brown macule on the upper trunk. It may sometimes be raised and have hair egressing from it. It represents a smooth-muscle hamartoma. Progressive macular hypomelanosis is rare. Hypopigmented macules with no preceding dermatosis occur on the lower trunk most frequently. *Propionibacterium acnes* is thought to play a role in the pathogenesis.

Color changes on palms and soles signify Raynaud disease or Raynaud phenomenon if white gives way to blue and then to red. In Raynaud disease, symmetric episodic, vasospasm occurs secondary to cold exposure. Fingers and sometimes palms turn white, then blue, then red. In Raynaud phenomenon, similar changes to Raynaud disease occur in the setting of connective tissue disease, usually in scleroderma. Vasospasm is typically asymmetric, nail fold capillary changes may be seen, and digital necrosis may occur. In terms of brown or black coloration on palms or soles, the differential diagnosis of a single brown or black macule in this location includes a melanocytic nevus and talon noire. Talon noire is a single dark brown, red, or black macule that represents hemorrhage within the stratum corneum. Tinea nigra is less frequently seen. It is a superficial dermatophyte infection that presents as a brown or black macule of any size on the palm or sole. It is more frequently encountered in the tropics or subtropics. A "do not miss" diagnosis is acral melanoma. Acral melanoma may appear a flesh-colored, pink, brown, black, or variegated macule, plaque, or nodule. Multiple brown macules on palms or soles may represent a normal finding in a darker-skin phototype, postinflammatory change from a prior dermatosis such as secondary syphilis, or they may represent a cutaneous finding of vitamin B_{12} deficiency. The differential diagnosis of diffusely red palms is broad. The most common cause is palmar erythema, which may be seen in liver disease, pregnancy, or autoimmune disease. Raynaud disease and phenomenon manifest red palms as their final color manifestation after vasospasm passes. Acral erythema that occurs as part of toxic erythema of chemotherapy may present with pink or violaceous smooth or scaly plaques with or without paresthesiae. One of the diagnostic criteria for Kawasaki disease is erythema and edema of palms and soles. Fever, lymphadenopathy, a polymorphic rash, and conjunctival and oropharyngeal involvement are further criteria. Erythromelalgia is a rare cause of palmar erythema; here, there is episodic occurrence of erythema and burning of bilateral feet, more frequently than hands, which is worse at night. Complex regional pain syndromes cause pain in an affected limb that may be accompanied by red or purplish discoloration, textural changes in skin, and abnormally profuse sweating. Acrodynia is now very rarely seen. There is painful erythema of palms and soles that occurs in children in the setting of mercury poisoning. Palms and soles may be edematous, and fingertips may also be involved. Other causes of pink or red macules on the palms or soles include erythema multiforme (target lesions), septic vasculitis, lymphocytic vasculitis of Rocky Mountain spotted fever, thrombotic vasculopathy, or leukocytoclastic vasculitis (a rare site of involvement). In septic vasculitis, there are distal asymmetric stellate purpura that involve tips and pulps of digits. Janeway lesions, a sign of acute bacterial endocarditis, are painless macules that are usually found on the thenar and hypothenar eminences. In Rocky Mountain spotted fever, although palms and soles are a classic site of involvement, not all patients develop lesions there. Initially there are blanching macules; later in the disease course, these become petechial or purpuric.

Blue or purple retiform macules on palms and/or soles signify impending ischemia from thrombotic vasculopathies, septic vasculitis, or vascular thrombosis. In acrocyanosis, the distal extremities appear bluish or purplish secondary to a cold-sensitive, vasospastic circulation.

The acral distribution includes distal extremities, nasal tip, ears, and the tip of the penis. Cryoglobulinemia can give rise to purple macules in these locations.

Periorbital macules include vitiligo and the heliotrope rash of dermatomyositis. Regarding the follicular distribution, there is perifollicular retention of pigment in the vitiligo-like depigmentation of scleroderma. Perifollicular repigmentation occurs in treated vitiligo; this occurs randomly as opposed to the grid-like regular pattern of perifollicular retention of pigment in scleroderma.

The clinical signs that may be seen on the scalp, hair, nails, and mucous membranes in macular dermatoses are listed in Table 2.4. Please also refer to the vascular reaction pattern chapter (Chapter 10) for supplemental information in this regard for red macules. In broad terms, in this category, history should encompass age of onset of any photosensitive disorder, an appraisal of any systemic connective tissue disease symptoms, a history of HIV disease (in the case of patch stage Kaposi sarcoma), and a thorough drug history.

In summary, the important decision points in appraising macules are seen in the textbox below. These points can also be applied to the wheel of diagnosis, as is seen in Figure 2.3.

Approach to Macules: Summary

- What color are they?
- Are there any diagnostic border characteristics?
- What is their size?
- What is their shape?
- Are there one, few, or many of them?
- Are they tender?
- What is their grouping?
- What is their distribution?
- Are there any further diagnostic clues from scalp, hair nails, mucous membranes, or lymph nodes?
- Augment physical findings with a thorough history.

TABLE 2.4. Additional Diagnostic Clues That Can Be Found in Macular Dermatoses

HAIR
- Nonscarring alopecia
  - Anagen effluvium may be seen in patients receiving chemotherapy
  - Telogen effluvium may be seen in connective tissue disease appearance
  - Rothmund–Thomson: sparse hair, premature graying
- Hair shaft abnormalities
  - Trichothiodystrophy: brittle hair, trichorrhexis nodosa, trichoschisis, alternating light and dark bands, known as "tiger-tail banding," under light microscopy

NAILS
- Rothmund–Thomson: atrophic nails
- Trichothiodystrophy: brittle, thin nails, onychorrhexis, yellow nails, onychoschisis, and onychogryphosis
- Subungual melanoma: Hutchinson sign is extension of pigment from the nail matrix onto the proximal or lateral nail fold; this sign is seen in advanced subungual melanomas
- Connective tissue disease: periungual erythema, nail fold capillary changes (especially dermatomyositis), ragged cuticles, nail fold infarcts

MUCOUS MEMBRANES
- Systemic lupus erythematosus: oral ulcers
- Dermatomyositis: ovoid palatal patch
- Kaposi sarcoma: intraoral involvement should prompt a search for gastrointestinal involvement

LYMPH NODES
- Examine lymph nodes basins in xeroderma pigmentosum patients with a history of melanoma or squamous cell cancer
- Generalized lymphadenopathy may be seen in HIV

PLAQUES

The shape of plaques can hold important diagnostic information. For example, the plaques of pityriasis rosea are typically oval. Round plaques include nummular eczema, pityriasis rotunda, and the plaques of fixed drug eruption. Erythema migrans may also present with perfectly round macules or smooth thin plaques. Plaques may be linear as in dermatoses that follow Blaschko lines (such as epidermal nevi and inflammatory linear verrucous epidermal nevus) or annular (such as in lichen planus or leprosy). Color may render diagnostic information as in the purple of lichen planus, the yellow of plane xanthomas, and the orange of pityriasis rubra pilaris.

Regarding surface characteristics, plaques may be scaly (Figure 2.4) or smooth (Figure 2.5). The presence or absence of scales can assist with categorizing a rash into a reaction pattern. An approach to scaly plaques is discussed in the papulosquamous reaction pattern chapter (Chapter 6) and supplemented by a discussion of subacute and chronic eczema in Chapter 8. Nonscaly plaques fall into either the dermal reaction pattern or the vascular reaction pattern, and these will be discussed in Chapters 9 and 10, respectively.

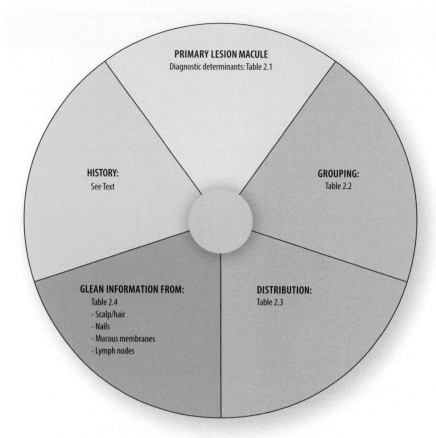

FIGURE 2.3 • The wheel of diagnosis, customized to macules.

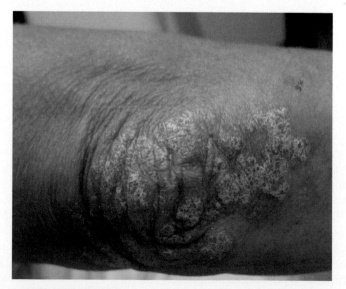

FIGURE 2.4 • A scaly plaque of psoriasis.

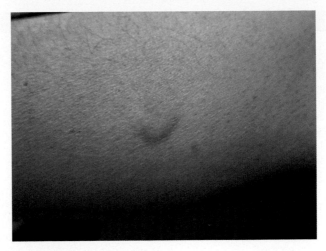

FIGURE 2.5 • A smooth plaque (wheal) of urticaria.

> **Clinical Tip**
> • Scaly plaques = papulosquamous or eczematous reaction pattern
> • Smooth plaques = dermal or vascular reaction pattern

Contour is also a useful feature in diagnosis. Plaques are usually raised, but they may be depressed, such as in scars, morphea, or other sclerotic conditions. The plaques of Sweet syndrome (acute febrile neutrophilic dermatosis) are mammillated. Examples of bosselated plaques include those seen in cutaneous Rosai–Dorfman disease and dermatofibrosarcoma protuberans (DFSP). A verrucous contour is seen in warts and other warty plaques, such as chromomycosis and other deep fungal infections, tuberculosis verrucosa cutis (a warty tuberculide), and the verrucous stage of incontinentia pigmenti. Vegetating plaques may be moist and eroded or dry. They may also be verrucous. Examples of vegetating plaques include those of pemphigus vegetans or verrucous carcinomas.

The border of plaques may be a characteristic diagnostic feature of an eruption. Psoriatic plaques are well demarcated. The patches (thin plaques) of mycosis fungoides typically have ill-defined or "smudged" borders. The "cliff-drop sign" refers to the borders of depressed plaques that extend perpendicularly down from the skin surface, like a cliff. The sign is characteristic of atrophoderma of Pasini and Pierini, a variant of morphea that typically presents on the backs of young women. The expression "islands are sparing" refers to areas of normal skin (the "islands") that are surrounded by a widespread rash. Pityriasis rubra pilaris and mycosis fungoides are classic eruptions that display "islands" of normal skin.

Palpation of plaques is an important diagnostic maneuver. Tender plaques are seen with epidermal necrosis in Stevens–Johnson syndrome and toxic epidermal necrolysis. Tenderness may imply dermal necrosis as well such as in brown recluse spider bites and ischemia from vasculitis or vasculopathies. Tender substantive plaques are characteristic of Sweet syndrome and rheumatoid neutrophilic dermatosis.

The grouping and configuration of plaques are summarized in Table 2.5. Annular plaques comprising papules are seen in granuloma annulare, subacute cutaneous lupus erythematosus (SCLE), and reticulate erythematous mucinosis. Urticaria, urticarial

TABLE 2.5. Grouping and Configuration of Plaques

ANNULAR
- Granuloma annulare
- Urticaria multiforme
- Urticarial vasculitis
- Necrolytic migratory erythema
- Subacute cutaneous lupus erythematosus
- Reticulate erythematous mucinosis
- Erythema marginatum
- Erythema gyratum repens
- Deep gyrate erythema

ARCUATE
- Urticaria multiforme
- Urticarial vasculitis
- Necrolytic migratory erythema
- Erythema marginatum

POLYCYCLIC
- Urticaria multiforme
- Urticarial vasculitis

RETICULATE
- Retiform purpura
- Erythema marginatum

GYRATE
- Erythema gyratum repens
- *Trichophyton concentricum*

LINEAR
- Linear verrucous epidermal nevus
- ILVEN
- Linear psoriasis
- Linear lichen planus
- Lichen striatus
- Blaschkitis

vasculitis, necrolytic migratory erythema, and the figurate erythemas display many configurations, including annular, arcuate, and polycyclic. Erythema gyratum repens and tinea imbricata display concentric or gyrate plaques. Linear plaques are seen in many dermatoses that follow Blaschko lines, and these are mentioned in Table 2.5.

The distribution of plaques is summarized in Table 2.6. Photodistributed plaques include the wheals of solar urticaria, the scaly or smooth plaques of discoid and subacute lupus erythematosus, and the lichenified plaques of chronic actinic dermatitis, a photosensitive eczematous reaction that develops predominantly in men. Flexural plaques include those seen in atopic and formaldehyde contact dermatitis. The differential diagnosis of intertriginous plaques is broad, as seen in Table 2.6. Additional diagnostic clues seen in scalp, hair, nails, mucous membranes, and lymph nodes, and the important aspects of history in diseases presenting with plaques will be summarized in the relevant reaction pattern chapters later in the book.

In summary, the diagnostic questions to be answered with respect to plaques is seen in the textbox given on the next page and depicted in the wheel of diagnosis in Figure 2.6.

TABLE 2.6. Distribution of Plaques

PHOTOEXPOSED
- Solar urticaria
- Erythropoietic protoporphyria
- Discoid lupus erythematosus
- Tumid lupus erythematosus
- Subacute cutaneous lupus erythematosus
- Reticulate erythematous mucinosis
- Polymorphic light eruption
- Photoallergic dermatitis
- Chronic actinic dermatitis
- Actinic reticuloid

FLEXURES
- Atopic dermatitis
- Formaldehyde contact dermatitis

EXTENSORS
- Psoriasis
- Frictional lichenoid dermatitis
- Erythema multiforme
- Granuloma annulare
- Palisaded and neutrophilic granulomatous dermatitis
- Erythema elevatum diutinum

INTERTRIGINOUS
- Intertrigo, including seborrheic dermatitis
- Irritant dermatitis
- Inverse psoriasis
- Candida intertrigo
- Systemic drug-related intertriginous and flexural exanthema (SDRIFE)
- Toxic erythema of chemotherapy
- Hailey–Hailey disease
- Acrodermatitis enteropathica
- Mycosis fungoides
- Pemphigus vegetans
- Extramammary Paget disease
- Acanthosis nigricans

SEBORRHEIC
- Seborrheic dermatitis
- Pemphigus foliaceus
- Rash of vitamin B_6 deficiency, seborrheic dermatitis–like

PALMS AND SOLES
- Inherited and acquired keratodermas
- Inflammatory keratodermas
  - Psoriasis
  - Lichen planus
  - Discoid lupus
  - Lupus erythematosus/lichen planus overlap
  - Pityriasis rubra pilaris

(Continued)

TABLE 2.6. Distribution of Plaques (continued)

PALMS AND SOLES (CONT.)
- Tinea pedis
- Acral erythema of chemotherapy
- Secondary syphilis
- Bazex syndrome
- Mycosis fungoides
- Longstanding dyshidrotic eczema
- Contact dermatitis
- Tripe palms

ACRAL
- Cocaine levamisole toxicity

PERIORBITAL
- Allergic contact dermatitis
- Atopic dermatitis
- Heliotrope rash of dermatomyositis

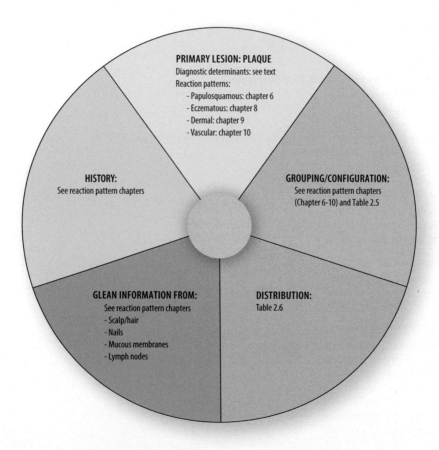

FIGURE 2.6 • The wheel of diagnosis, customized to plaques.

> **Approach to Plaques: Summary**
> - What shape are they?
> - What color are they?
> - Are they scaly?
> - What reaction pattern are they?
> - Can any diagnostic information be gleaned from their contour?
> - Are there any diagnostic border characteristics?
> - Are they tender?
> - What is their distribution?
> - Are there any further diagnostic clues from scalp, hair, nails, mucous membranes, or lymph nodes?
> - Augment physical findings with a thorough history.

PAPULES

The initial decision point in appraising a papule is whether it is follicularly-based. Figure 2.7 illustrates this approach. Follicular papules center around a hair and are usually regularly spaced. However, it may be difficult to see fine vellus hairs (a dermatoscope can help), and regular spacing of papules is neither a specific (miliaria may also be regularly spaced) nor a sensitive finding.

> **Clinical Tip** Look for a hair in the center of a papule to help differentiate follicular from nonfollicular papules. A dermatoscope can help.

Furthermore, some dermatoses are not primarily follicular, but they display follicular prominence. Examples include discoid lupus erythematosus and lichen sclerosus. Therefore, sometimes, clinically, there may be doubt that requires the creation of a differential diagnosis with both nonfollicular and follicular papules. Discussions of each will follow.

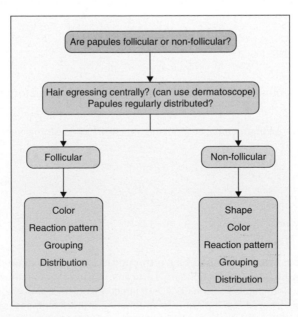

FIGURE 2.7 · An approach to papules.

For nonfollicular papules, color is a useful feature. Table 2.7 summarizes the differential diagnosis of papules of each color. The shape of a papule can hold important diagnostic information, such as the polygonal papules of lichen planus. The contour of a papule may also be characteristic of a diagnosis; for example, dome-shaped, umbilicated papules are characteristic of molluscum or molluscum-like papules. This physical

Differential Diagnosis of Umbilicated Papules

Molluscum contagiosum
Disseminated molluscum-like eruptions:
• Cryptococcosis

• Histoplasmosis
• Coccidioidomycosis
• *Penicillium marneffei* infection

TABLE 2.7. The Color of Papules

WHITE
• Milia, small cysts, calcinosis, gouty tophus, white fibrous papulosis of neck

YELLOW
• Eruptive xanthomas, xanthelasma, necrobiotic xanthogranuloma, xanthoma disseminatum, Fordyce spots, sebaceous hyperplasia, juxtaclavicular beaded lines (follicle-based papules), pseudoxanthoma elasticum, fibroelastolytic papulosis

ORANGE
• Xanthogranuloma, benign progressive histiocytosis, pityriasis rubra pilaris (follicle-based papules)

PURPLE
• Lichen planus, any inflamed dermatosis in a dark skin, pyogenic granuloma, bacillary angiomatosis, hemangiomas, Kaposi sarcoma, cutaneous metastases, angiosarcoma, lymphoma or leukemia cutis

GRAY
• Granuloma faciale

BROWN
• Urticaria pigmentosa, sarcoidosis, nevi, melanoma, seborrheic keratosis

BLUE
• Epidermal cyst, pilomatricoma, eccrine and apocrine hidrocystoma, venous lake, blue nevus

GREEN
• Chloroma

BLACK
• Foreign body, nevi, melanoma

RED
• Exanthematous drug eruption, scabies, arthropod reaction (papular urticaria), dermal hypersensitivity reaction, cholinergic urticaria, miliaria rubra, chilblains, lupus chilblains, pseudo-chilblains from COVID-19 infection, polymorphous light eruption, pruritic urticarial papules and plaques of pregnancy, prurigo pigmentosa, cercarial dermatitis, seabather's eruption, palpable purpura of leukocytoclastic vasculitis

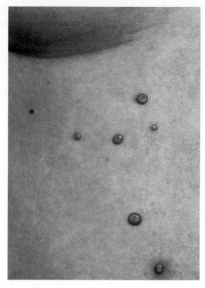

FIGURE 2.8 • Dome-shaped umbilicated papules of molluscum contagiosum. (Reproduced with permission from Kang S, Amagai M, Bruckner AL, et al: *Fitzpatrick's Dermatology*, 9th ed. New York, NY: McGraw Hill; 2019.)

feature is depicted in Figure 2.8 (molluscum contagiosum) and Figure 2.9 (molluscum-like papules in histoplasmosis). Shape and surface characteristics of papules and the diseases for which they are characteristic are listed in Table 2.8.

Another diagnostic determinant of nonfollicular papules, and some follicular papules, is reaction pattern. This may be difficult to discern, depending on the size of the papules. However, reaction pattern should always be considered as it can guide differential diagnosis. Table 2.9 gives a comprehensive list of papules by reaction pattern. Each of these dermatoses will be discussed in more detail in their respective reaction pattern chapters. Palpating a papule provides information about consistency as seen in Table 2.10.

The differential diagnosis of follicular papules is very broad. Follicular papules can be classified according to the etiologic classification, and subclassified by morphology. For example, papules that are primarily inflammatory in nature may be subclassified

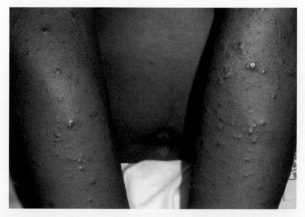

FIGURE 2.9 • Molluscum-like papules in a case of disseminated histoplasmosis in an HIV-positive patient. (Used with permission from Dr. Adam Lipworth, Lahey Hospital & Medical Center, Burlington, MA.)

TABLE 2.8. Shape and Surface Characteristics of Papules

SHAPE
- Polygonal
  - Lichen planus
- Oval
  - Pityriasis rosea

CONTOUR
- Flat-topped
  - Flat warts and lichen planus
- Dome-shaped
  - Molluscum contagiosum and molluscum-like eruptions
- Umbilicated
  - Molluscum contagiosum and molluscum-like eruptions
- Acuminate (pointed)
  - Warts
- Filiform (thread-like)
  - Warts
- Verrucous
  - Warts

TABLE 2.9. Differential Diagnosis of Papules by Reaction Pattern

PAPULOSQUAMOUS
- Follicular
  - Spiny papules
    - Lichen spinulosus
    - Keratosis pilaris group
    - Pityriasis rubra pilaris
    - Reactive perforating folliculitis
    - Phrynoderma
- Nonfollicular
  - Papular pityriasis rosea
  - Guttate psoriasis
  - Secondary syphilis
  - Lichen planus
  - Lichen striatus
  - Viral warts
  - Epidermodysplasia verruciformis
  - Confluent and reticulated papillomatosis of Gougerot–Carteaud
  - Acrokeratosis verruciformis of Hopf
  - Darier disease (Figures 2.39 and 2.40)
  - Pityriasis lichenoides chronica and pityriasis lichenoides et varioliformis acuta
  - Acrokeratosis paraneoplastica
  - Cutaneous horn
  - Actinic keratoses

ECZEMATOUS
- Follicular
  - Follicular eczema
  - Recurrent and disseminate infundibulofolliculitis

(Continued)

TABLE 2.9. Differential Diagnosis of Papules by Reaction Pattern (continued)

ECZEMATOUS (CONT.)
- Nonfollicular
  - Subacute eczema (eg, allergic contact dermatitis)
  - Papular seborrheic dermatitis
  - Frictional lichenoid dermatitis

VESICOBULLOUS
- Grover disease (transient acantholytic dermatosis; also classifiable as papulosquamous reaction pattern) (Figure 2.42)
- Hailey–Hailey disease (benign familial pemphigus)
- Early pemphigus herpetiformis
- Early dermatitis herpetiformis
- Gianotti–Crosti disease

DERMAL
- Sarcoid: micropapular, popular, and lichenoid variants
- Granuloma annulare: papules make up annuli and are diffusely distributed in the generalized variant
- Erythema elevatum diutinum
- Generalized eruptive histiocytosis
- Papulonecrotic tuberculide
- Lichen myxedematosus and scleromyxedema
- Acral persistent papular mucinosis

- Self-healing papular mucinosis
- Lipoid proteinosis
- Colloid milium
- Gout
- Mucopolysaccharidosis
- Osteoma cutis
- Calcinosis cutis
- Xanthoma disseminatum
- Anetoderma

VASCULAR
- Exanthematous drug eruption
- Scabies
- Arthropod reaction (papular urticaria)
- Dermal hypersensitivity reaction
- Cholinergic urticaria
- Miliaria rubra
- Chilblains
- Lupus chilblains
- Pseudo-chilblains from COVID-19 infection
- Polymorphous light eruption
- Pruritic urticarial papules and plaques of pregnancy
- Prurigo pigmentosa
- Cercarial dermatitis
- Seabather's eruption
- Palpable purpura of leukocytoclastic vasculitis

TABLE 2.10. Consistency of Papules

- Soft
  - Acrochordon, neurofibroma, myxoma, neurotized nevus
- Firm
  - Most papules are firm
- Firm to hard
  - Dermatofibroma, keloidal papules
- Hard
  - Calcinosis cutis, osteoma cutis, foreign body, pilomatricoma

according to whether pustules are present and are spiny. Table 2.11 displays this classification.

Infectious causes of follicular papules (folliculitis) usually give rise to pustules in association. *Staphylococcus aureus* is a frequent cause of folliculitis. Staphylococcal folliculitis is also known as impetigo of Bockhart (Figure 2.10). Sycosis barbae is the term given to a staphylococcal infection of the beard area. Gram-negative folliculitis may present as a centrofacial eruption in acne patients on chronic tetracyclines or isotretinoin therapy. *Klebsiella* or *Proteus* spp. are responsible. Hot-tub folliculitis is another type of Gram-negative folliculitis; it is usually caused by *Pseudomonas* and occurs within a day or two of hot-tub exposure, usually on the trunk. Pustules may be large with a prominent erythematous base (Figure 2.11). Herpetic folliculitis from

TABLE 2.11. Follicular Differential Diagnosis

INFECTIOUS (WITH PUSTULES)
- Folliculitis
  - Bacterial
    - *Staphylococcus aureus*: also known as impetigo of Bockhart
    - Gram-negative folliculitis
      - In acne patients on tetracyclines or isotretinoin
      - Hot-tub folliculitis
  - Viral
    - Herpes simplex folliculitis
    - Chickenpox or zoster folliculitis
  - Fungal
    - *Pityrosporum* folliculitis
    - Majocchi granuloma
    - Disseminated histoplasmosis
    - Cryptococcosis
  - Parasitic
    - *Demodex* folliculitis

INFLAMMATORY
- With pustules; with or without comedones
  - Occlusive folliculitis
  - Acne
  - Rosacea
  - Pyoderma faciale

(Continued)

TABLE 2.11. Follicular Differential Diagnosis (continued)

INFLAMMATORY (CONT.)
- Pseudofolliculitis barbae
- Acne keloidalis nuchae
- Behcet disease
- Neonatal cephalic pustulosis
- Eosinophilic pustular folliculitis of infancy
- Eosinophilic pustular folliculitis of Ofuji
- Eosinophilic pustular folliculitis of HIV disease
- With spines
  - Keratosis pilaris group:
    - Keratosis pilaris
    - Ulerythema ophryogenes (KP atrophicans facei)
    - Keratosis follicularis spinulosa decalvans
    - Folliculitis spinulosa decalvans
  - Pityriasis rubra pilaris
  - Lichen spinulosus
  - Reactive perforating folliculitis
  - Phrynoderma
  - Erythromelanosis follicularis faciei
- Papules only
  - Follicular eczema
  - Recurrent and disseminate infundibulofolliculitis
  - Lichen planopilaris
  - Graham–Little–Piccardi–Lassueur syndrome
  - Follicular mucinosis
  - Lichen scrofulosorum
  - Fox–Fordyce disease

POSTINFLAMMATORY
- Papular acne scars

NEOPLASTIC
- Benign tumors of the hair follicle:
  - Trichilemmomas
  - Trichoblastomas
  - Trichoepitheliomas
  - Trichofolliculomas
  - Fibrofolliculomas
  - Trichodiscomas
  - Basaloid follicular hamartomas
  - Pilomatricomas
- Cysts
  - Milia
  - Epidermal inclusion cyst
  - Pilar cyst
  - Eruptive vellus hair cyst
  - Steatocystoma multiplex
- Follicular mucinosis

DRUG
- Drug-induced/exacerbated acne
- Drug-induced papulopustular eruption

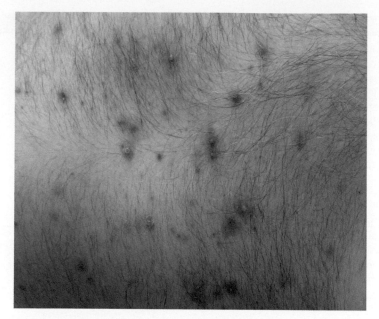

FIGURE 2.10 • Follicular papules and pustules in bacterial folliculitis.

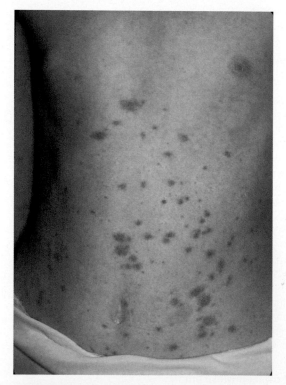

FIGURE 2.11 • Hot-tub folliculitis from *Pseudomonas*.

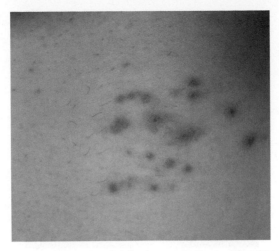

FIGURE 2.12 · Herpes zoster presenting with follicular papules (zoster folliculitis).

HSV is seen in the beard area but may also occur in other hair-bearing sites. Varicella zoster virus manifests more frequently than herpes simplex as a folliculitis in both chickenpox and zoster (Figure 2.12). A broad range of fungal dermatoses may manifest with folliculitis. *Pityrosporum* folliculitis is a very itchy eruption of the face, chest, back, shoulders, and neck. Pinpoint papules and pustules are seen. It may be seen in acne patients on long-term oral antibiotic therapy (Figures 2.13 and 2.14). Majocchi granuloma is a fungal folliculitis, usually caused by *Trichophyton rubrum*. In histoplasmosis, follicular and acneiform presentations of disseminated disease have been described. In cryptococcosis, acneiform presentations have been described. *Demodex* folliculitis presents with facial papules and pustules without other signs of rosacea, usually in immunosuppressed patients, such as those with HIV disease.

Inflammatory causes of papules can be categorized as those that occur with pustules, those that are spiny, or those that occur without pustules or spines. Pustules frequently accompany many conditions in the inflammatory group:

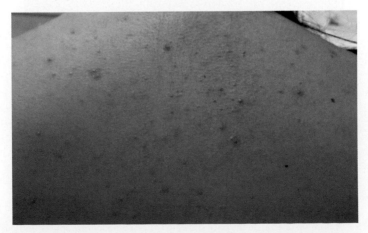

FIGURE 2.13 · Pityrosporum folliculitis in a patient on long-term doxycycline for acne.

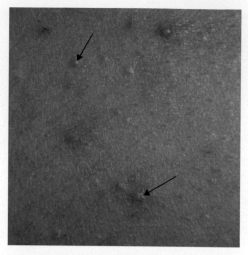

FIGURE 2.14 • Pityrosporum folliculitis: close-up of pinpoint pustules atop papules.

In occlusive folliculitis, small papules and pustules are seen in areas of tight-fitting clothing. No comedones are present. In acne, comedones, papules, pustules, cysts, and nodules may be seen in the seborrheic areas (Figure 2.15). The scalp may be involved. In rosacea, papules and pustules are seen in concert with erythema, flushing, and te-langiectasia, but without comedones. The face is commonly involved, but scalp and chest involvement may be seen. Pyoderma faciale, also known as rosacea fulminans, is a severe variant of rosacea, in which large inflammatory papules, pustules, and nodules erupt centrofacially (Figure 2.16). In pseudofolliculitis barbae, perifollicular papules and pustules occur in the beard area and other areas where hair has been shaved or waxed, due to an inflammatory reaction caused by an ingrowing hair (Figure 2.17). In acne keloidalis nuchae, papules and pustules from a pseudofolliculitis eventuate into

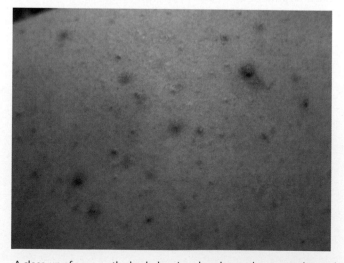

FIGURE 2.15 • A close-up of acne on the back showing closed comedones, papules, and pustules.

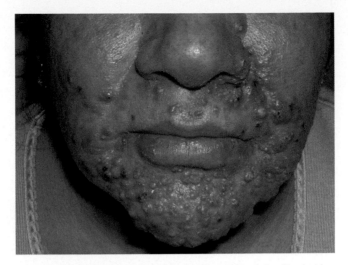

FIGURE 2.16 • Pyoderma faciale showing papules, pustules, and nodules. (Used with permission from Dr. Miguel Sanchez, New York University, New York, NY.)

keloidal papules, plaques, and nodules, on the occipital scalp. Behcet disease is a rare cause of pustules, which are reported to be both follicular and nonfollicular (Figure 2.18). Recurrent oral aphthae is a required criterion for this diagnosis, along with genital aphthae, eye findings, or a positive pathergy test.

In neonates, follicular eruptions also occur. Neonatal cephalic pustulosis is commonly seen. It represents neonatal acne, but no comedones are present. *Malassezia* spp. have been implicated in the pathogenesis. Eosinophilic pustular folliculitis of infancy is rare. It presents as itchy papules and pustules on the scalp and face and less commonly in a more widespread distribution. Onset is within the first few weeks of life. Two other forms of eosinophilic pustular folliculitis occur. Eosinophilic pustular folliculitis of Ofuji presents with follicular pustules on the upper trunk and proximal extremities in young females from Japan. Circinate plaques with central clearing are a feature, and

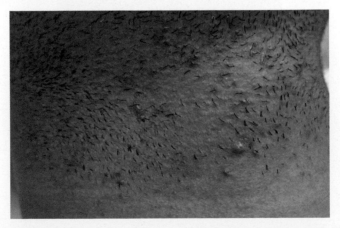

FIGURE 2.17 • Pseudofolliculitis barbae showing ingrown hairs with surrounding inflammatory papules.

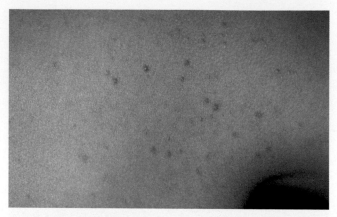

FIGURE 2.18 • Behcet disease showing follicular and nonfollicular pustules. (Used with permission from Dr. Miguel Sanchez, New York University, New York, NY.)

the palms and soles may be involved. Eosinophilic pustular folliculitis may also be associated with HIV disease. This presents typically when the CD4 count is less than 200 cells per microliter (µL). Itchy urticarial papules and pustules occur on the face (Figure 2.19), upper trunk, and upper extremities.

Spiny papules occur in commonly encountered and rarer dermatoses. Keratosis pilaris is most frequently encountered in this group. Here, follicular keratotic plugs occur on upper arms, thighs, and more widely. In the inflammatory variant, there is a rim of erythema at the base of each plug (Figure 2.20). Other variants of keratosis pilaris are less frequently encountered. In ulerythema ophryogenes [also known

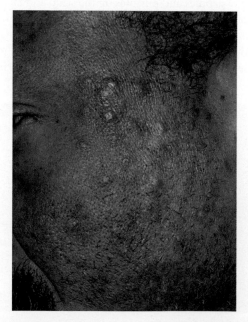

FIGURE 2.19 • Eosinophilic pustular folliculitis of HIV. Excoriated follicular papules on the face. (Used with permission from Dr. Miguel Sanchez, New York University, New York, NY.)

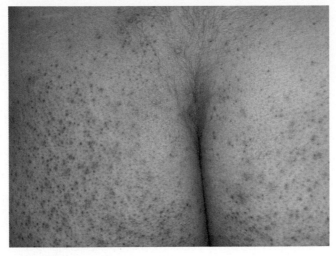

FIGURE 2.20 • Inflammatory keratosis pilaris. (Used with permission from Dr. Miguel Sanchez, New York University, New York, NY.)

as *keratosis pilaris atrophicans faciei* (KPAF)], follicular plugs are seen facially, including lateral eyebrows, where scarring alopecia may eventuate. In keratosis follicularis spinulosa decalvans (KFSD), follicular plugs with erythematous rims lead to scarring alopecia, including scalp, eyelashes, and eyebrows. Palmoplantar keratoderma and keratitis are associated. It is inherited in an X-linked recessive manner. In folliculitis spinulosa decalvans, the manifestations of KFSD are accompanied by follicular pustules. An autosomal dominant inheritance pattern is seen. In the classic adult type of pityriasis rubra pilaris, follicular papules coalesce to form plaques (Figure 2.21). These start on the upper trunk and progress downward. In the classic, limited childhood form, follicular papules are limited to elbows and knees. Lichen spinulosus manifests as

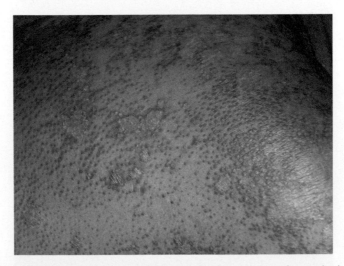

FIGURE 2.21 • Pityriasis rubra pilaris with follicular papules that coalesce to form scaly plaques. (Used with permission from Dr. Miguel Sanchez, New York University, New York, NY.)

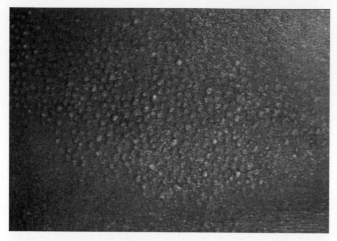

FIGURE 2.22 · Lichen spinulosus showing groupings of follicular papules with spines.

grouped follicular papules with central keratotic spines on the trunk and extremities. It is usually nonpruritic (Figure 2.22). Other dermatoses that manifest papules with spines are more rarely encountered. Reactive perforating folliculitis is a rare type of transepidermal elimination that occurs in relation to hair follicles. It is seen in young adults. Phrynoderma is seen in vitamin A deficiency and leads to large follicular keratotic plugs on the extensor aspects of the extremities. Plugs are cone-shaped and leave pits when removed. Erythromelanosis follicularis faciei is a very rare disorder with follicular spiny papules of the lateral cheeks and sometimes the neck. These overlie erythematous and brown macules. This disorder is usually seen in individuals from Japan.

Follicle-based papules without pustules or spines are encountered most frequently in follicular eczema. Here, itchy erythematous papules are seen, often in patients with an atopic diathesis (Figure 2.23). Recurrent and disseminate infundibulofolliculitis is a pruritic eruption of substantive perifollicular papules that is usually seen on the trunk

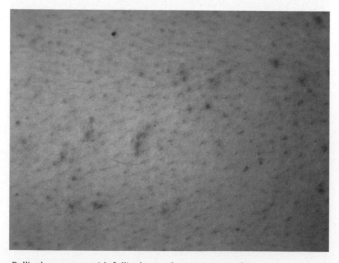

FIGURE 2.23 · Follicular eczema with follicular erythematous papules.

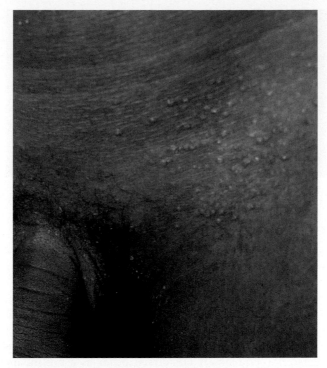

FIGURE 2.24 • Recurrent and disseminate infundibulofolliculitis on the trunk of a young man.

of in young males (Figure 2.24). In lichen planopilaris, perifollicular violaceous papules with perifollicular scale eventuate in a scarring alopecia. Scalp and other body sites may be affected (Figure 2.25). Graham–Little–Piccardi–Lassueur syndrome comprises follicular lichen planus on and off the scalp with scarring alopecia of the scalp, which is often accompanied by other mucocutaneous findings of lichen planus. Follicular

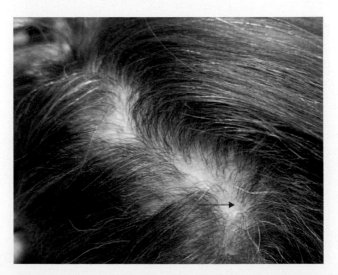

FIGURE 2.25 • Lichen planopilaris showing the classic perifollicular scale and a scarring alopecia.

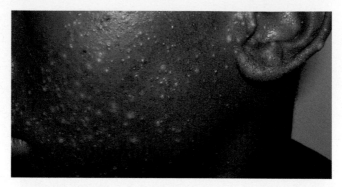

FIGURE 2.26 • Lichen scrofulosorum. (Used with permission from Professor Ncoza Dlova, University of KwaZulu-Natal, Durban, South Africa.)

mucinosis is a more rarely encountered dermatosis. It is also known as *alopecia mucinosa*. Primary forms occur in children and young adults where there are grouped follicular papules and/or plaques on the head and neck with alopecia. The cutaneous T-cell lymphoma-associated form is seen in older adults and manifests more widespread follicular papules and plaques. Lichen scrofulosorum is a tuberculide that manifests as widespread, small, lichenoid, perifollicular papules on the trunk, and proximal extremities (Figure 2.26). These may be grouped to form annular plaques.

Papular acne scars (perifollicular elastolysis) occur as a postinflammatory phenomenon and represent perifollicular anetoderma. These are white to yellow-white papules that occur at sites of old acne papules. They are usually seen on the upper trunk (Figure 2.27)

In the neoplastic category, benign tumors of the hair follicle include trichilemmomas, trichoblastomas, trichoepitheliomas, trichofolliculomas, fibrofolliculomas (Figure 2.28), trichodiscomas, basaloid follicular hamartomas, and pilomatricomas. Milia are small epidermal inclusion cysts that arise around vellus hairs. Epidermal inclusion

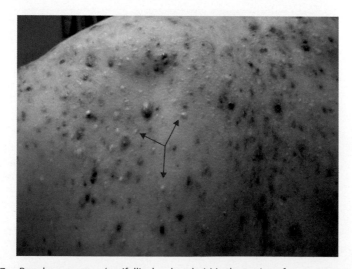

FIGURE 2.27 • Papular acne scars (perifollicular elastolysis) in the setting of severe acne.

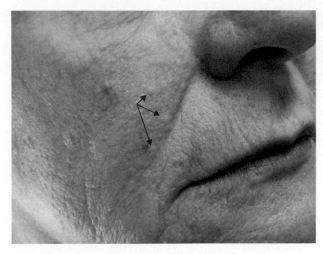

FIGURE 2.28 · Fibrofolliculomas in a patient with Birt–Hogg–Dube syndrome.

cysts arise from the infundibulum of the hair follicle, or, they may be nonfollicular, through implantation of the epidermis. Pilar cysts, also known as trichilemmal cysts, arise from the isthmus of the hair follicle and show trichilemmal keratinization. Eruptive vellus hair cysts are 1–4-mm flesh-colored cystic papules that contain numerous vellus hairs (Figure 2.29). Steatocystoma multiplex are slightly larger papules. They are usually multiple and occur truncally. They are lined by epithelium with sebaceous differentiation and may be associated with pachyonychia congenita.

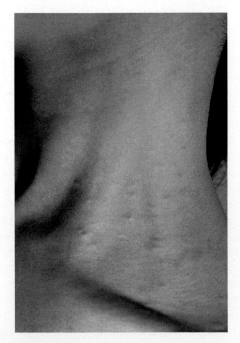

FIGURE 2.29 · Eruptive vellus hair cysts.

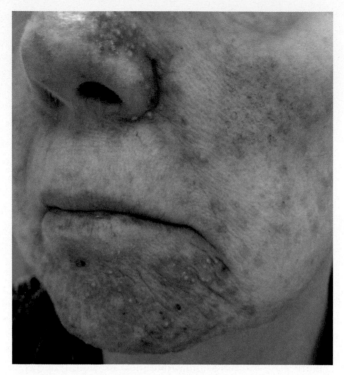

FIGURE 2.30 · Papulopustular eruption caused by cetuximab.

Drug-induced follicular papules and pustules are seen in drug-induced/exacerbated acne from corticosteroids, anabolic steroids, isoniazid, lithium, and anticonvulsants and in the drug-induced papulopustular eruption from epidermal growth factor receptor (EFGR) inhibitors and MEK inhibitors (Figure 2.30).

For follicular papules, their color and reaction pattern might hold further diagnostic clues, such as the orange color and papulosquamous reaction pattern of pityriasis rubra pilaris (PRP). Spiny follicular papules, such as those seen in lichen spinulosus, may also be classified as papulosquamous reaction pattern.

After examining the clinical features of papules closely, we can take a step back and look at their configuration or grouping, which can add value (Table 2.12). The annular list is categorized by reaction pattern, which is a convenient subdivision. The linear differential diagnosis can be conceptualized in many ways. Linear papules are subcategorized by whether they are induced from the outside (so-called "outside job"), or from the inside (so-called "inside job"). This is one of the clinically more applicable decision points. Herpetiform papules are seen prior to vesiculation in herpetiform eruptions. In herpes simplex and varicella zoster infections, lesions classically progress from macules, through papules, vesicles (and sometimes pustules), and ulcers to crusts. Most dermatoses that display agminated (clustered) lesions comprise papules (Table 2.12).

The distribution of papules holds further diagnostic clues. Table 2.13 provides extensive differential diagnostic lists of various classic distributions, including generalized, periorbital, facial, dorsal hand, lateral aspects fingers, and palmoplantar distributions. All these sites may be affected by numerous papular dermatoses. In the periorbital and

TABLE 2.12. Grouping and Configuration of Papules

ANNULAR
- Papulosquamous reaction pattern: lichen planus, psoriasis, secondary syphilis
- Eczematous reaction pattern: seborrheic dermatitis
- Dermal reaction pattern: granuloma annulare, sarcoidosis
- Follicular papules: lichen scrofulosorum, Majocchi granuloma

LINEAR
- "Outside job"
  - Allergic contact dermatitis for example, to poison ivy
  - Koebner phenomenon: psoriasis, lichen planus, leukocytoclastic vasculitis, Kaposi sarcoma
  - Autoinoculation: mollusca, flat warts
  - Dermatitis artefacta
  - Bug bites ("breakfast-lunch-dinner")
- "Inside job"
  - Lymphocutaneous (sporotrichoid) spread: *Mycobacterium marinum, Sporothrix schenckii, Francisella tularensis,* melanoma in-transit metastases
  - Dermatomal: zoster
  - Pseudodermatomal: zosteriform metastases
  - Following Blaschko lines: incontinentia pigmenti, chondrodysplasia punctata, ichthyosis hystrix and epidermal nevus syndrome, Darier disease, benign familial pemphigus, linear verrucous epidermal nevus, ILVEN, nevus sebaceous, lichen striatus, linear lichen planus, nevus comedonicus (follicular papules)

HERPETIFORM
- Herpes simplex
- Herpes zoster
- Early dermatitis herpetiformis
- Early pemphigus herpetiformis

AGMINATE
- Leiomyomas
- Spitz nevi
- Pyogenic granulomas
- Melanoma metastases
- Cutaneous metastases from internal malignancies
- Lymphangioma circumscriptum
- Angiokeratoma circumscriptum

facial differential lists, most of the conditions fall into the dermal reaction pattern. As these lists are fairly lengthy, they are subdivided by etiology in Table 2.13.

Palmoplantar papules may be conceptualized as pits, keratoses, scaly papules, purpuric papules, and target lesions.

Palmoplantar Papules Can Be:

- Pits
- Keratoses
- Scaly
- Purpuric
- Target lesions

TABLE 2.13. Distribution of Papules

PHOTOEXPOSED
- Polymorphous light eruption
- Solar urticaria
- Photoallergic dermatitis

INTERTRIGINOUS, ESPECIALLY GROIN
- Condyloma lata (Figure 2.48)
- Condyloma accuminata
- Papular acantholytic dyskeratosis
- Darier disease
- Hailey–Hailey disease

PERIORBITAL
- Infectious
  - External hordeolum
  - Internal hordeolum
- Inflammatory
  - Granulomatous rosacea (follicle-based)
  - Granulomatous perioral and periorbital dermatitis (follicle-based)
  - Sarcoidosis
  - Chalazion
- Depositional
  - Primary amyloidosis (waxy papules on eyelid margin)
  - Lipoid proteinosis (waxy papules on eyelid margin)
  - Xanthelasma, plane xanthoma, necrobiotic xanthogranuloma, orbital xanthogranu-loma, Erdheim–Chester disease
- Adnexal tumors
  - Syringomas (infraorbital)
  - Apocrine hidrocystomas (single, eyelid margin)
  - Eccrine hidrocystomas (multiple, periorbital, and can be more widespread)
- Other benign neoplasms
  - Acrochordons
  - Seborrheic keratoses
  - Melanocytic nevi
- Malignant neoplasms
  - Sebaceous carcinoma (eyelid margin)
  - Basal cell cancer

FACIAL PAPULES: MULTIPLE
- Inflammatory
  - Papular eczema
  - Granulomatous rosacea
  - Granulomatous perioral and periorbital dermatitis
  - Lupus miliaris disseminata faciei
  - Sarcoidosis
- Depositional
  - Amyloid
  - Lipoid proteinosis
  - Xanthelasma, plane xanthoma, necrobiotic xanthogranuloma
  - Osteoma cutis

(Continued)

TABLE 2.13. Distribution of Papules (continued)

FACIAL PAPULES: MULTIPLE (CONT.)
- Benign neoplasms
  - Intradermal nevi
  - Syringomas
  - Fibrous papules (centrofacial)
  - Apocrine and eccrine hidrocystomas
  - Trichilemmomas (scattered over face, lip margin): suggestive of Cowden syndrome
  - Trichoepitheliomas (centrofacial)
  - Adenoma sebaceum (centrofacial): suggestive of tuberous sclerosis
  - Brooke–Spiegler syndrome
  - Trichodiscomas, fibrofolliculomas: suggestive of Birt–Hogg–Dube syndrome

EXTENSORS
- Frictional lichenoid dermatitis
- Pityriasis rubra pilaris
- Recurrent and disseminate infundibulofolliculitis
- Granuloma annulare
- Erythema elevatum diutinum
- Palisaded and neutrophilic granulomatous dermatitis
- Papulonecrotic tuberculide
- Psoriasis
- Eruptive xanthomas
- Rothmund–Thompson syndrome

PALMS AND SOLES
- Keratoses
  - Spiny keratoderma
  - Arsenical keratoses
  - Porokeratosis of palms and soles
  - Verrucae
  - Cowden syndrome
- Pits
  - Punctate keratoderma
  - Keratosis punctata of creases
  - Pitted keratolysis
  - Darier disease
  - Hailey–Hailey disease
  - Basal cell nevus syndrome
  - Naegeli–Franceschetti–Jadassohn syndrome
  - Dermatopathia pigmentosa reticularis
- Scaly papules
  - Warts
  - Secondary syphilis
  - Reactive arthritis
- Purpuric papules
  - Leukocytoclastic vasculitis
  - Septic vasculitis
  - Rocky Mountain spotted fever
- Target lesions
  - Erythema multiforme

(Continued)

TABLE 2.13. Distribution of Papules (continued)

IN RELATION TO APPENDAGES
- Eccrine
  - Miliaria rubra
- Apocrine
  - Fox-Fordyce disease
- Follicular (see Table 2.10)

FLEXURES
- Atopic dermatitis
- Formaldehyde contact dermatitis

DORSAL HANDS
- Flat warts
- Flat seborrheic keratoses
- Granuloma annulare
- Atrophic dermal papules of dermatomyositis (formerly Gottron papules)
- Acrokeratosis verruciformis of Hopf
- Darier disease
- Acral persistent papular mucinosis
- Cowden syndrome
- Poikiloderma congenitale (Rothmund–Thompson syndrome)
- Multicentric reticulohistiocytosis
- Actinic keratoses
- Multinucleate cell angiohistiocytoma

LATERAL ASPECTS, FINGERS
- Dyshidrotic eczema
- Warts
- Lipoid proteinosis
- Rothmund–Thompson syndrome
- Cowden syndrome
- Acrokeratoelastoidosis of Costa
- Focal acral hyperkeratosis

Among the punctate keratodermas, there are two subtypes with *pits*. Punctuate keratoderma of the palmar creases is inherited in an autosomal dominant fashion. There are 1–2-mm pits, translucent papules, and keratotic papules that are confined to palmar creases. In diffuse punctuate keratoderma, which is also autosomal dominantly inherited, pits and translucent and keratotic papules are seen diffusely on the palms and soles. These may coalesce to form hyperkeratotic or verrucous plaques in wear-and-tear areas. Further with respect to palmar pits, Darier disease displays keratin-filled pits and keratotic papules on palms and soles. In Gorlin–Goltz syndrome (also known as basal cell nevus syndrome), palmoplantar pits occur in association with multiple basal cell cancers (which may resemble nevi), facial milia, and epidermal inclusion cysts. In pitted keratolysis, a corynebacterial infection, tiny keratotic pits that may coalesce to form larger pitted plaques occur in a background of hyperhidrotic soles. In Naegeli–Franceschetti–Jadassohn syndrome, punctuate keratotic papules on the palms and soles occur in concert with reticulate hyperpigmentation, hypohidrosis, and nail dystrophy.

In terms of *keratoses*, verrucae are perhaps the most commonly encountered. In spiny keratoderma, there are thread-like keratotic spines that arise from palmoplantar keratotic papules. It is either an autosomal dominant condition or sporadic. In porokeratosis of palms and soles (a subset of porokeratoses that are limited to palms and soles), translucent and keratotic 1–2-mm papules are seen. A thready rim may be evident clinically. Rarer conditions include arsenical keratoses from arsenic exposure (these are similar papules that arise in association with dappled pigmentary changes, and an increased risk for squamous cell carcinoma in situ) and the keratotic papules of Cowden syndrome. These occur frequently on palms and soles and are also seen on dorsal hands and over the hands and feet more generally. Trichilemmomas and sclerotic fibromas are also classically associated.

In the *scaly* papule group, warts are the most frequently encountered. Secondary syphilis displays erythematous or violaceous papules and plaques on palms and soles. Lesions may be tender to palpation (a positive *Ollendorff sign*) and scaly (including collarettes of scale). In reactive arthritis (formerly known as Reiter disease), keratoderma blennorrhagica (also known as *keratoderma blennorrhagicum*) is the finding of brownish hyperkeratotic papules and plaques on the soles. Brownish incipient scale crust and frank pus may also be seen.

In the *purpuric* papule differential, septic vasculitis displays purpuric macules and papules on the fingertips, palms, and soles. In leukocytoclastic vasculitis, palpable purpura may infrequently be seen on the palms and soles. In Rocky Mountain spotted fever, macules, papules, and petechiae are seen on the palms and soles, and may be widespread around the wrists and ankles.

Finally, *target lesions* may be papular. In erythema multiforme, palms are frequently involved.

Regarding papules that are related to appendageal structures, miliaria rubra is caused by obstruction of eccrine ducts. It presents as tiny erythematous papules on areas of increased sweating from overheating, occlusive clothing, or fever. It is usually seen on the trunk and neck.

Intertriginous involvement is also seen. Fox–Fordyce disease, also known as apocrine miliaria, occurs in apocrine-rich areas, including axillae, groin, and circumareolar skin. It manifests as flesh-colored follicular papules. Women predominantly are affected. Flexural papules occur in atopic dermatitis and formaldehyde contact dermatitis, two conditions with predilection for the antecubital and popliteal fossae.

The differential diagnosis of papules on the dorsal aspects of the hands includes common and rarer conditions. Flat warts and papular seborrheic keratosis are frequently seen. The dorsal hands are a site of predilection for actinic keratoses, which present as gritty thin papules. Granuloma annulare is not too infrequently encountered. Here, annular dermal plaques occur on the dorsal hands and over the metacarpophalangeal joints (MCPs). Atrophic dermal papules of dermatomyositis (formerly known as *Gottron papules*) present as violaceous papules and plaques occur over the MCPs and interphalangeal joints. Other papular dermatoses are more rarely seen in this location; in acrokeratosis verruciformis of Hopf, flat wart-like papules are seen on the dorsal aspects of the hands in young individuals. Hyperkeratosis of the elbows may ensue later. Mutations in the ATP2A2 gene are reported, as in Darier disease. The two diseases are thought to be allelic. Darier disease also manifests acrokeratosis verruciformis–like papules. In acral persistent papular mucinosis, flesh-colored to whitish papules are seen on dorsal hands and extensor forearms. In Cowden syndrome, acral verrucous keratoses are found on dorsal hands and feet. Poikiloderma congenitale (Rothmund–Thompson syndrome) also displays acral verrucous keratosis on the elbows, knees, hands, and feet, along with photo exposed poikiloderma.

In multicentric reticulohistiocytosis, multiple papules that are red- or yellow-brown occur acrally, including dorsal hands and dorsal fingers. Periungual clusters of papules are described as "coral beading." A very rare diagnosis in this location is multinucleate cell angiohistiocytoma; this occurs most commonly on the face and dorsal hands of older women. Clinically there are multiple dull-red papules, which display fibrohistiocytic proliferation of factor XIIIa–positive cells, with abundant bizarre multinucleate cells and vascular hyperplasia.

Papules on the lateral aspects of the fingers occur in dyshidrotic eczema and warts, and less frequently in acral verrucous keratoses (such as in Cowden syndrome, Rothmund–Thomson syndrome, and lipoid proteinosis) and keratotic papules of a keratoderma are seen. In acrokeratoelastoidosis (AKE) of Costa, inherited in an autosomal fashion, or sporadic, there are keratotic papules with pits at the junction of palm with dorsal hand, and sole with dorsal foot. Histopathologically there is loss and degeneration of elastic fibers in the dermis. Focal acral hyperkeratosis is a similar disorder to AKE but without elastic fiber changes.

Diagnostic Determinants of:	
Nonfollicular papules can be classified according to: • Shape • Contour • Consistency • Color • Reaction pattern • Grouping • Distribution	Follicular papules can be classified according to: • Color • Reaction pattern • Grouping • Distribution

The clinical signs that should be looked for on the scalp, hair, nails, and mucous membranes are listed in Table 2.14.

Finally, for all papules, we loop back around to history. Elicit prior and current medical history, and scrutinize any drugs being taken. Do not overlook a history of systemic sarcoidosis, HIV disease (eosinophilic pustular folliculitis, warts, epidermodysplasia verruciformis, mollusca, molluscum-like disseminated cryptococcosis, histoplasmosis, coccidioidomycosis, or *Penicillium marneffei*), and renal failure (perforating dermatoses). Psoriasis exacerbations may be provoked by β-blockers, lithium, antimalarial agents, and the tumor necrosis factor-α antagonists. The most common culprits of a lichenoid drug eruption include nonsteroidal anti-inflammatory drugs (NSAIDs), angiotensin-converting enzyme inhibitors, antimalarials, β-blockers, gold, lithium, methyldopa, penicillamine, ethambutol, and sulfonylurea agents. Imatinib mesylate, the statins, the tumor necrosis factor-α antagonists, sildenafil, the proton pump inhibitors, and interferon are newer offenders. Search for environmental exposures. For example, a history of drinking well water in certain parts of the world may give insight into possible arsenic exposure and the finding of arsenical keratoses; and a history of recent hospitalization and being bedridden may explain an exacerbation of Grover disease.

TABLE 2.14. Additional Diagnostic Clues That Can Be Found in Papular Dermatoses

SCALP/HAIR
- Scarring alopecia
  - Lichen planopilaris or frontal fibrosing alopecia with lichen planus
  - sarcoidosis
- Nonscarring alopecia
  - Alopecia mucinosa, follicular mucinosis
  - Secondary syphilis (which has a characteristic "moth-eaten" appearance)

NAILS
- Psoriasis
  - "Oil-drop sign": an orange-brown semicircular or circular discoloration of the nail bed that connotes incipient onycholysis
  - Coarse irregular pits
  - Onycholysis
  - Subungual hyperkeratosis
  - Splinter hemorrhages
  - In acrodermatitis continua of Hallopeau, there is peri- and subungual pustulation, loss of nails, and scarring of nail beds
- LP: longitudinal ridging, pterygium
- PRP: subungual hyperkeratosis
- Darier disease: brittle nails, longitudinal ridging, the "sandwich sign" (alternating white and red bands), single red band, multiple white lines, distal V-shaped nicking
- Hailey–Hailey disease: longitudinal white bands.

MUCOUS MEMBRANES
- LP: reticulate pattern on the buccal mucosa, white plaques tongue and lips, erosive variant displays oral ulcers, especially on the tongue
- Secondary syphilis: mucous patches, "snail-track ulcers"
- Darier disease: "cobblestoning" is the finding of white corrugated plaques on the palate

LYMPH NODES
- May be enlarged in mycosis fungoides and tuberculosis

In summary, the important decision points in the approach to papules are seen in the textbox below. These points can also be applied to the wheel of diagnosis, as is seen in Figure 2.31.

Approach to Papules: Summary

- Are they follicular or nonfollicular?
- If follicular, are pustules present as well?
- Are there spines?
- What is their shape?
- What is their color?
- What are their surface characteristics?
- What is their consistency?
- What reaction pattern is present?
- What is their grouping?
- What is their distribution?
- Are there any further diagnostic clues from scalp, hair, nails, mucous membranes, or lymph nodes?
- Augment physical findings with a thorough history.

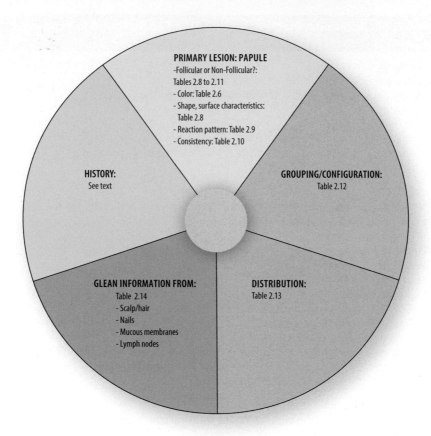

FIGURE 2.31 • The wheel of diagnosis, customized to papules.

NODULES AND TUMORS

Nodules and tumors may be categorized by reaction pattern (Figure 2.32). Most are smooth and fall into the dermal reaction pattern (Chapter 9). Scaly nodules such as squamous cell cancers, including keratoacanthomas, will be discussed in the papulosquamous reaction pattern chapter (Chapter 6). Prurigo nodularis are scaly eczematous nodules that will be discussed in the eczematous reaction pattern chapter (Chapter 8).

> **Clinical Tip**
> • Smooth nodules = dermal reaction pattern
> • Scaly nodules = papulosquamous or eczematous reaction pattern

Scaly nodules may have a verrucous or vegetating surface as well. If a smooth nodule has a central punctum, the diagnosis of epidermal inclusion cyst can be made.

Another visual diagnostic determinant of nodules and tumors is their color. While many solitary nodules in particular (such as cysts and adnexal neoplasms) are

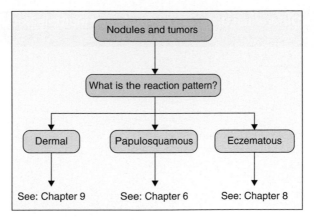

FIGURE 2.32 • Approach to nodules and tumors.

flesh-colored, vascular nodules may be red, maroon, or purple. Other "purple plums" (purple nodules) include Kaposi sarcoma, amelanotic melanoma, and lymphoma or leukemia cutis. A complete differential diagnosis of purple plums is seen in Table 9.3. Red nodules imply bacterial infection if tender. Nodular melanoma can be amelanotic, pink, purple, brown, or black. The number of nodules present can assist with diagnosis. Table 2.15 lists a broad differential diagnosis of conditions that present with nodules, subdivided by etiology and by whether there is a solitary nodule or more than one nodule.

Palpation of dermal nodules for their depth, consistency, or tenderness adds further diagnostic information that can guide diagnosis. Regarding depth, DFSP may be palpable for the most part, with a protuberant nodule on top of a deeper plaque. Bone and calcium are hard, and lipomas are soft. Cysts may be firm or rubbery (especially pilar cysts). Tenderness implies infection or possibly necrosis within a malignancy. The borders of nodules are also usually palpable rather than visible. Benign neoplasms are typically mobile, and their borders are well demarcated. Malignant nodules may be fixed to underlying structures, and borders may be difficult to palpate. Lipomas are described as having a "rolling" edge; the edges roll under the fingertips. DFSPs may have irregular or "craggy" borders. These attributes are also discussed in Chapter 9.

Diagnostic Determinants of Nodules

Visual	Tactile
• Color	• Depth
• How many?	• Consistency
	• Tender or not tender
	• Border

With respect to grouping or configuration of nodules, confluent nodules may have a bosselated surface. Nodules that are configured in lines signify lymphocutaneous, or sporotrichoid spread. After a nodule develops at the inoculation site,

TABLE 2.15. Differential Diagnosis of Single and Multiple Nodules, by Etiology

SINGLE
- Infectious
  - Furuncle
  - Carbuncle
  - Abscess
  - Atypical mycobacterial infections
  - Sporotrichosis
  - Blastomycosis
  - Histoplasmosis
  - Lobomycosis
- Inflammatory
  - Prurigo nodularis
  - Pseudolymphoma
  - Bursitis
- Depositional
  - Nodular amyloid
  - Calcinosis cutis
- Hyperproliferative
  - Keloid
- Neoplastic
  - Benign
    - Epidermal inclusion cyst
    - Pilar cyst
    - Lipoma
    - Mixed tumor
    - Osteoma
    - Pilomatricoma
    - Cylindroma
    - Ganglion cyst
    - Dermatofibroma
    - Dermatomyofibroma
    - Plexiform neurofibroma
    - Vascular malformations
    - Eccrine angiomatous nevus
  - Malignant potential uncertain
    - Proliferating trichilemmal tumor
  - Malignant
    - Basal cell cancer
    - Keratoacanthoma
    - Squamous cell cancer
    - Nodular melanoma
    - Merkel cell cancer
    - Cutaneous metastasis
    - Cutaneous lymphoma

(Continued)

TABLE 2.15. Differential Diagnosis of Single and Multiple Nodules, by Etiology (continued)

SINGLE (CONT.)
- Primary cutaneous anaplastic large cell lymphoma: usually solitary
  - Dermatofibrosarcoma protuberans
  - Leiomyosarcoma
  - Angiosarcoma
  - Other soft tissue sarcomas
  - Cutaneous metastasis

MULTIPLE
- Infectious
  - Multiple furuncles, carbuncles
  - Atypical mycobacterial infections
  - Sporotrichosis
  - Lobomycosis
- Inflammatory
  - Prurigo nodularis
  - Panniculitides
  - Medium vessel vasculitides
  - Erythema elevatum diutinum
  - Subcutaneous sarcoidosis
  - Rheumatoid nodules
  - Cutaneous Rosai–Dorfman disease
- Depositional
  - Tuberous xanthomas
  - Gouty tophi
  - Cutaneous Rosai–Dorfman disease
- Neoplastic
  - Benign
    - Blue rubber bleb nevus syndrome
    - Neurofibromatosis
    - Brooke–Spiegler syndrome
    - Gardner syndrome: lipomas, epidermal inclusion cysts, desmoid tumors, pilomatricomas
    - Other syndromes with lipomas: eg, Proteus syndrome
    - Maffucci syndrome: enchondromas and vascular malformations
    - Myotonic dystrophy: multiple pilomatricomas
  - Malignant
    - Kaposi sarcoma
    - Tumor stage mycosis fungoides
    - Cutaneous B-cell lymphoma
    - Other lymphomas
    - Leukemia cutis
    - Cutaneous metastases

usually on an extremity, *Mycobacterium marinum* and *Sporothrix schenckii* travel up lymphatics in this manner. In-transit metastases from melanoma may also appear sporotrichoid. A complete list of dermatoses with sporotrichoid spread is seen in Table 9.10. Table 2.16 presents the differential diagnosis of nodules by distribution.

Additional diagnostic signs seen in scalp, hair, nails, mucous membranes, and lymph nodes, and the important items on history in diseases presenting with nodules

TABLE 2.16. Distribution of Nodules

PHOTOEXPOSED
- Actinic prurigo
- Basal cell cancer
- Squamous cell cancer
- Keratoacanthoma
- Nodular melanoma

EXTENSORS
- Tuberous xanthomas
- Erythem elevatum diutinum
- Gouty tophi
- Rheumatoid nodules
- Olecranon bursa

PALMS AND SOLES
- Eccrine poroma
- Kaposi sarcoma

DIGITS
- Maffucci syndrome
- Giant cell tumor of tendon sheath

will be summarized in the relevant reaction pattern chapters later in the book. To summarize, the diagnostic questions to be answered for nodules are listed in the textbox below and depicted in the wheel of diagnosis in Figure 2.33.

Approach to Nodules: Summary

- What is their color? What reaction pattern is present?
- What are their surface characteristics?
- How many of them are there?
- Are they deep?
- What is their consistency?
- Are they tender?
- Do they have a border?
- What is their grouping?
- What is their distribution?
- Are there any further diagnostic clues from the scalp, hair, nails, mucous membranes, or lymph nodes?
- Augment physical findings with a thorough history.

VESICLES AND BULLAE

A comprehensive approach based on the diagnostic determinants of these primary lesions and their associated secondary lesions may be found in Chapter 7 (vesicobullous reaction pattern).

PUSTULES

As with papules, a key diagnostic determinant of pustules is the presence or absence of an associated hair follicle. This is the initial decision point diagnostically (Figure 2.34), and, as with papules, it may not always be so easy to discern. The follicular differential diagnostic list for pustules recapitulates the follicular infectious and inflammatory lists found

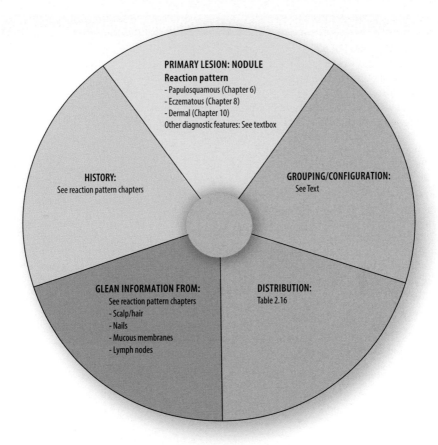

FIGURE 2.33 • The wheel of diagnosis, customized to nodules.

in Table 2.11. Additional causes of follicular pustules include the inflammatory presentations of tinea capitis, including kerion; Majocchi granuloma, a fungal folliculitis caused by a dermatophyte; and pyoderma gangrenosum, which may begin as a tense or flaccid large perifollicular pustule that arises on a bright red or violaceous base. Pseudomonal folliculitis may display greenish pus (from production of pyoverdins and pyocyanins).

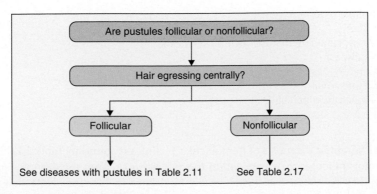

FIGURE 2.34 • Approach to pustules.

TABLE 2.17. Differential Diagnosis of Nonfollicular Pustules

SUBCORNEAL PUSTULES
- Impetigo
- Subcorneal pustular dermatosis
- Pustular psoriasis variants
  - Generalized pustular psoriasis of von Zumbusch
  - Pustular flare within chronic plaque psoriasis
  - Annular pustular psoriasis
  - Impetigo herpetiformis
  - Palmoplantar pustulosis
  - Acrodermatitis continua of Hallopeau
- Acute generalized exanthematous pustulosis (AGEP)
- IgA pemphigus, subcorneal variant
- Tinea corporis
- Cutaneous candidiasis
- Infantile acropustulosis (later lesions)
- Transient neonatal pustular melanosis
- Erythema toxicum neonatorum
- Miliaria pustulosa

INTRAEPIDERMAL PUSTULES
- Spongiform pustules
  - Pustular psoriasis variants
  - AGEP
  - Amicrobial pustulosis of the folds
- Herpes simplex
- Varicella and zoster infections
- Smallpox
- Monkeypox
- Erythema toxicum neonatorum
- Infantile acropustulosis (early lesions)
- IgA pemphigus, intraepidermal neutrophilic type
- Fire ant bites
- Miliaria pustulosa
- Halogenodermas (including bromoderma, iododerma, fluoroderma)

DERMAL PUSTULES
- Leukocytoclastic vasculitis
- Septic vasculitis
- Disseminated gonococcemia
- Candidemia
- Bowel-associated dermatosis–arthritis syndrome
- Behcet disease
- Halogenodermas
- Malignant syphilis
- Papulonecrotic tuberculide

The differential diagnosis of nonfollicular pustules is found in Table 2.17. Pustules that are not follicular may arise within the epidermis or from the dermis. Epidermal pustules may be subcorneal histologically or deeper in location. Note that subcorneal pustules are flaccid. The most common example of a dermatosis with subcorneal

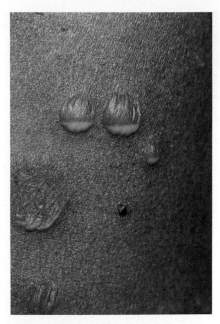

FIGURE 2.35 • Subcorneal pustular dermatosis showing pus-fluid levels. (Image appears with permission from VisualDx. Copyright VisualDx.)

pustulation is impetigo, where pustules rapidly rupture to form honey-colored crusts. In cutaneous candidiasis, beefy-red plaques occur in intertriginous sites with outlying flaccid satellite papules and pustules. In dermatophytosis, tiny subcorneal pustules are infrequently seen. Inflammatory causes of subcorneal pustules are more rarely encountered. In subcorneal pustular dermatosis, annular arrays of superficial pustules are seen in the axillae and groin. A pus-fluid level may be seen (Figure 2.35), which is a specific diagnostic sign. Lesions resolve with collarettes of scale, and then new crops occur. The subcorneal variant of IgA pemphigus is indistinguishable clinically from subcorneal pustular dermatosis.

> **Clinical Tip** A pus-fluid level connotes the diagnosis of subcorneal pustular dermatosis.

There are six distinct pustular psoriasis variants:

1. In generalized pustular psoriasis of von Zumbusch, there are widespread pustules and "lakes" of pus on a background of erythema. Patients have a high fever and feel unwell. Young males are frequently affected.
2. Pustules may be seen in a pustular flare of chronic plaque psoriasis. This may occur in disease flares or in association with strong topical steroid, oral steroid, or topical tar use.
3. Annular pustular psoriasis is a third variety. Thin annular plaques show tiny flaccid pustules at their borders and central desquamation.
4. Impetigo herpetiformis is pustular psoriasis in pregnancy, which may be associated with hypocalcemia. Annular configuration of pustules may be seen (Figure 2.36).
5. In palmoplantar pustulosis, large pustules resolve with brown incipient crusts on palms and soles (Figure 2.37).

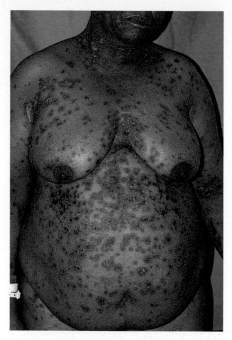

FIGURE 2.36 • Impetigo herpetiformis (pustular psoriasis in pregnancy), showing subcorneal pustules in annular arrays.

6. Finally, in acrodermatitis continua of Hallopeau, one or more distal fingers are involved with chronic pustulation. There may be subungual pustulation, which leads to nail dystrophy and loss of the nail plate.

Acute generalized exanthematous pustulosis (AGEP) displays tiny pustules that erupt rapidly atop widespread erythematous plaques (Figure 2.38). "Lakes" of pus

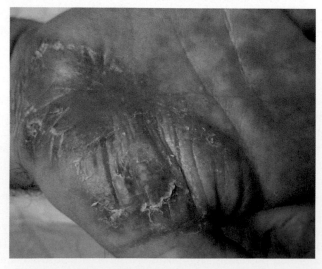

FIGURE 2.37 • Palmoplantar pustular psoriasis with pustules and brown incipient crusts.

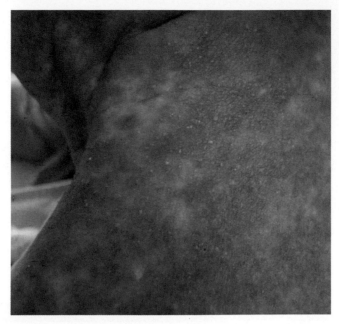

FIGURE 2.38 • Acute generalized exanthematous pustulosis, showing erythematous plaques studded with superficial pustules.

may be seen, and AGEP may resemble pustular psoriasis, especially the von Zumbusch variety. Common drug culprits include a wide array of antibiotics, including antifungals. In erosive pustular dermatosis of the scalp, superficial flaccid pustules and lakes of pus give way to eroded plaques with thick overlying crust. Pustules are sterile. Affected areas are usually chronically sun-exposed, and the contributing etiology of liquid nitrogen and other treatments for actinic keratosis has also been suggested.

> **Clinical Tip** Lakes of pus are seen in generalized pustular psoriasis of von Zumbusch, acute generalized erythematous pustulosis, and erosive pustular dermatosis of the scalp.

Subcorneal pustules may be seen in tinea corporis. In infancy, subcorneal pustules may be seen in the later lesions of infantile acropustulosis, where crops of acral pustules and vesicles occur at around 3–6 months of age and recur with waning frequency up to age 3. In transient neonatal pustular melanosis, superficial pustules are present at birth and rapidly resolve with collarettes of scale and hyperpigmentation. The face and trunk and less commonly the palms and soles may be involved. In erythema toxicum neonatorum, erythematous macules, papules, pustules, and vesicles are seen within a day or two of birth, and last up to 14 days. They start on the head and generalize to involve the trunk and limbs (Figure 2.39). Miliaria pustulosa can occur at all ages; tiny pustules occur in this more chronic variant of miliaria rubra.

Erythema toxicum neonatorum, transient neonatal pustular melanosis, acropustulosis of infancy, and miliaria pustulosa may all display both subcorneal and

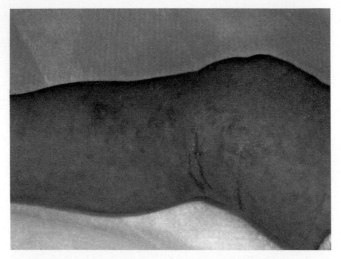

FIGURE 2.39 • Erythema toxicum neonatorum, showing tiny pustules on the leg.

Differential Diagnosis of Pustules in Infancy

At Birth or within First Few Days of Life:
- Congenital infections: listeriosis, candidiasis, herpes simplex or neonatal varicella
- Erythema toxicum neonatorum
- Transient neonatal pustular melanosis

At Birth or within First Few Weeks of Life:
- Eosinophilic pustular folliculitis

A Few Weeks after Birth, Peaking at 3 Months:
- Neonatal cephalic pustulosis

At 3-6 Months:
- Acropustulosis of infancy

intraepidermal pustules under the microscope. Another subset of diseases within the intraepidermal group includes those that form spongiform pustules. A *spongiform pustule* is defined as a collection of neutrophils in the granular and spinous layers that are separated by degenerated, necrotic keratinocytes. The pustular variants of psoriasis (see Table 2.17), amicrobial pustulosis of the folds and acute generalized exanthematous pustulosis (AGEP), may all manifest spongiform pustules histologically. Amicrobial pustulosis of the folds is a rare disorder. Recurrent sterile pustules occur in the folds periodically and on the scalp in patients with SLE and other autoimmune diatheses. Another rare cause of intraepidermal pustules is monkeypox. After a prodromal phase, a widespread popular eruption becomes vesicular, then pustular, and then crusts over. Smallpox has been eradicated globally; it presented with flaccid, widespread, nonfollicular pustules that eventuated from papules and healed with depressed, punched-out, "varioliform" scars. In IgA pemphigus, intraepidermal neutrophilic type, clinical manifestations resemble those of the subcorneal type of IgA pemphigus. A classic finding is the annular arrangement of flaccid vesicles and pustules known as the "sunflower configuration." Fire ant bites, common in the southeastern United States, are painful and itchy papules and pustules that are seen on exposed sites. Halogenodermas (including bromoderma, iododerma, fluoroderma) present with pustules or vegetating plaques. Pustules may or may not be follicular. Follicular pustules are acneiform. Early nonfollicular pustules have intraepidermal pustules.

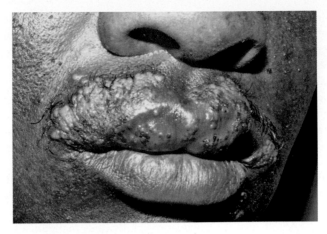

FIGURE 2.40 • Herpes simplex showing secondary pustules.

Finally, in the intraepidermal group, pustules may be a secondary rather than a primary lesion, when there is a secondary migration of neutrophils into a primary vesicle. Examples of this include dyshidrotic eczema, herpes simplex (Figure 2.40), and varicella zoster infections (Figure 2.41).

> **Clinical Tip** A pustule may be a secondary lesion, when it occurs secondary to longstanding vesicles in herpetic infections and dyshidrotic eczema.

Dermal pustules may arise on a purpuric base, such as in pustular leukocytoclastic vasculitis, septic vasculitis, disseminated gonococcemia, candidemia, bowel-associated dermatosis-arthritis syndrome, Behcet disease, and halogenodermas. In leukocytoclastic vasculitis, palpable purpura occur symmetrically on the shins. Individual lesions may progress to form pustules. Eruption may also extend up the

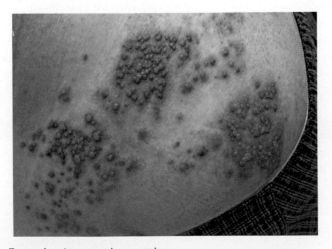

FIGURE 2.41 • Zoster showing secondary pustules.

thighs and involve the buttocks, forearms, and trunk. In septic vasculitis, bacterial or fungal organisms are seeded from an internal source to the fingertips, toes, and other acral sites. Disseminated gonococcemia is a type of septic vasculitis with few asymmetric distally located pustules. They may or may not arise on a purpuric base. In candidemia, patients are usually immunocompromised, such as after receiving chemotherapy. Pustules may be scattered in a widespread distribution. In bowel-associated dermatosis-arthritis syndrome, crops of papules and papulopustules occur on the extensor arms and trunk in patients who have undergone bowel bypass surgery or who have inflammatory bowel disease. Behcet disease displays both follicular and non-follicular pustules (as is seen in Figure 2.17) as well as pustular vasculitis (pustules on a purpuric base). Dermal pustules may be seen in halogenodermas, in both early and late lesions. Other causes of dermal pustules are rare and include secondary syphilis and papulonecrotic tuberculide. In secondary syphilis, pustules are a rare finding; these can be follicular on nonfollicular. In malignant syphilis (lues maligna, a fulminant form of secondary syphilis that usually is seen in the setting of HIV infection), ulcerated plaques and nodules are preceded by the onset of pustules. In papulonecrotic tuberculide, a hypersensitivity reaction that occurs in the setting of tuberculosis, a symmetric eruption of firm papules and papulopustules over the extensor aspects of extremities, face, and ears is seen. Papules ulcerate, crust, and leave varioliform scars.

Dermatoses That Manifest Both Follicular and Nonfollicular Pustules

- Behcet disease
- Secondary syphilis
- Halogenodermas
- Dermatophytosis
  - Nonfollicular in tinea corporis
  - Follicular in tinea capitis and Majocchi granuloma

As with papules, the diagnostic boxes on the wheel can yield important diagnostic information (Figure 2.42). Besides the follicular or nonfollicular location and the close association of flaccid pustules with a superficial epidermal location, diagnostic determinants include the contents of the pustule, size of pustules, and whether they arise on normal skin.

The grouping and distribution of pustules are shown in Tables 2.18 and 2.19. Annular pustules may signify subcorneal pustular dermatosis or IgA pemphigus, dermatophytosis (an uncommon finding), impetigo herpetiformis, or eosinophilic pustular folliculitis of Ofuji. Fire ant bites are caused by the red fire ant, *Solenopsis invicta*. Red fire ants are

---

Diagnostic Characteristics of Pustules

- Greenish pus: *Pseudomonas* infection
- Pinpoint pustules: *Pityrosporum* folliculitis
- Flaccid pustules and "lakes of pus": generalized pustular psoriasis variants, AGEP, and erosive pustular dermatosis of the scalp
- Pus-fluid level: subcorneal pustular dermatosis
- Pustules on a purpuric base: leukocytoclastic vasculitis, septic vasculitis, disseminated gonococcemia, candidemia, pyoderma gangrenosum, pustular vasculitis (Behcet disease)

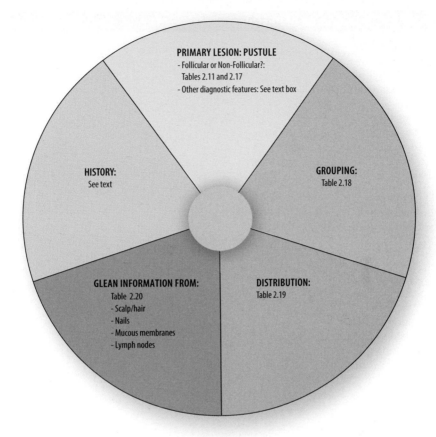

FIGURE 2.42 • The wheel of diagnosis, customized to pustules.

endemic to South America and may also be encountered in the southern and southwestern United States. Their bites are painful and are typically pustular. Lines of pustules may be seen when there are multiple bites. The herpetiform pustular differential diagnosis includes herpes simplex, zoster, and impetigo herpetiformis.

TABLE 2.18. Groupings of Pustules

- Annular
  - Subcorneal pustular dermatosis
  - IgA pemphigus
  - Dermatophytosis
  - Impetigo herpetiformis
  - Eosinophilic pustular folliculitis of Ofuji
- Linear
  - Fire ant bites
  - Herpes zoster
- Herpetiform
  - Herpes simplex
  - Herpes zoster
  - Impetigo herpetiformis

TABLE 2.19. Distribution of Pustules

SEBORRHEIC

- Infectious
  - Bacterial folliculitis
  - *Pityrosporum* folliculitis
  - Zoster
- Inflammatory
  - Acne
  - Neonatal cephalic pustulosis
  - Eosinophilic pustular folliculitis of HIV
  - Halogenodermas

EXTENSORS

- Bowel-associated dermatosis–arthritis syndrome
- Papulonecrotic tuberculide

INTERTRIGINOUS

- Infectious
  - Cutaneous candidiasis
  - Folliculitis
- Inflammatory
  - Pseudofolliculitis
  - Subcorneal pustular dermatosis
  - IgA pemphigus
  - Eosinophilic pustular folliculitis of Ofuji
  - Amicrobial pustulosis of the folds

PALMS AND SOLES

- Infectious
  - Septic vasculitis: distal, acral, purpuric
  - Disseminated gonococcemia
  - Candidemia
  - Herpetic whitlow
  - Herpes simplex, zoster
  - Scabies: secondarily infected
- Inflammatory
  - Infantile acropustulosis
  - Transient neonatal pustular melanosis—rarely seen on palms and soles
  - Eosinophilic pustular folliculitis of infancy
  - Eosinophilic pustular folliculitis of Ofuji (20% of patients)
  - Palmoplantar pustular psoriasis
  - Acrodermatitis continua of Hallopeau: can involve palmar aspects of fingers and plantar aspects of toes
  - SAPHO syndrome (synovitis, acne, pustulosis, hyperostosis, osteitis)
  - Papulonecrotic tuberculide
  - Longstanding eczema (eg, dyshidrotic and contact eczema) where vesicles become cloudy because of the influx of neutrophils

FINGERS

- Infectious
  - Blistering distal dactylitis
  - Acute paronychia

(Continued)

TABLE 2.19. Distribution of Pustules (continued)

FINGERS (CONT.)
- Cat scratch disease
- *Mycobacterium marinum* infection
- Disseminated gonococcemia
- Septic vasculitis
- Candidemia
- Herpetic whitlow
- Milker's nodule
- Inflammatory
- Dyshidrotic eczema
- Palmoplantar pustular psoriasis
- Acrodermatitis continua of Hallopeau
- Fire ant bites
- Acropustulosis of infancy
- Transient neonatal pustular melanosis

In terms of distribution, the pustules are usually infectious or inflammatory in nature. An interesting differential diagnosis is that of pustules that occur on the fingers. In adults, acute paronychia is perhaps the most frequent cause. A bacterial infection of the lateral nail fold gives rise to a deep-seated painful pustule. Initially erythema is appreciated. Pus may drain out from the free edge of the cuticle, and a pustule may also be appreciated before the pus drains. A herpetic whitlow occurs secondary to inoculation of herpes simplex on the finger. Grouped vesicles or pustules may be seen. Cat scratch disease, caused by *Bartonella henselae*, gives rise to a papule or pustule at the site of the bite within weeks of a cat scratch. *Mycobacterium marinum* is another organism that may give rise to a papule or pustule at the site of inoculation. It is an atypical mycobacterium that may contaminate swimming pools or fish tanks. A rarer cause of a similar morphological picture is a "milker's nodule," caused by the pseudocowpox virus. In a sick patient, septicemia with septic vasculitis or candidemia may be culprits. In disseminated gonococcemia, patients have associated fever and arthralgias. Blistering distal dactylitis is more common in children than adults. A flaccid cloudy bulla is seen secondary to a Gram-positive infection.

Regarding inflammatory causes of pustules on a finger, dyshidrotic eczema with its secondary pustules is perhaps most commonly encountered; palmoplantar pustular psoriasis is almost as common. Acrodermatitis continua of Hallopeau is rare. Fire ant bites are common in endemic areas.

Table 2.20 provides a summary of the clinical signs that can be seen in the scalp, hair, nails, mucous membranes, and lymph nodes.

Finally, review the patient's history in light of the clinical findings, including present and past medical history and medication lists. Think about systemic bacterial or fungal infections in adults who are systemically ill with disseminated pustules. Pustules are few in number and are scattered with tenosynovitis in gonococcemia; scattered on a purpuric base in candidemia; and occur along with crusted papules or deep-seated nodules, fever, and arthralgias in chronic meningococcemia. Follicular and acneiform variants of disseminated histoplasmosis have been reported, as has an acneiform presentation of disseminated cryptococcosis. In patients with disseminated fungal infections and in those with eosinophilic pustular folliculitis, evaluate for underlying HIV disease.

TABLE 2.20. Additional Diagnostic Clues That Can Be Found in Pustular Dermatoses

SCALP AND HAIR
- No alopecia
  - Bacterial folliculitis
  - Acne
  - Rosacea
  - Zoster
  - Eosinophilic pustular folliculitis of infancy
  - Acropustulosis of infancy: scalp is occasionally involved
  - Neonatal cephalic pustulosis: scalp may be involved
- Nonscarring alopecia
  - Pustules may be seen in tinea capitis infections
  - Amicrobial pustulosis of the folds: while scalp involvement is common, nonscarring alopecia is seen in a minority of cases
- Scarring or nonscarring alopecia
  - Kerion presents with one or more boggy plaques with pustules or sinuses; it is caused by a robust host response to a zoophilic dermatophyte, such as *Microsporum canis*, or to an anthropophilic organism, such as *Trichophyton tonsurans*, in which a hypersensitivity response develops; scarring alopecia may develop in longstanding untreated cases
- Scarring alopecia
  - Folliculitis decalvans: pustules on the scalp lead to a scarring alopecia; some authors classify folliculitis decalvans as an inflammatory form of central centrifugal cicatricial alopecia
  - Acne keloidalis nuchae: papules and pustules from pseudofolliculitis lead to keloidal papules, plaques, and nodules on the lower occiput
  - Erosive pustular dermatosis: recurrent pustules on the scalp of elderly individuals lead to scarring alopecia
  - Folliculitis spinulosa decalvans (see Table 2.10)

PUSTULES CAN HAVE ASSOCIATED NAIL FINDINGS
- Psoriasis
  - "Oil-drop" sign: an orange-brown semicircular or circular discoloration of the nail bed that connotes incipient onycholysis
  - Coarse irregular pits
  - Onycholysis
  - Subungual hyperkeratosis
  - Splinter hemorrhages
  - In acrodermatitis continua of Hallopeau, there is peri- and subungual pustulation, loss of nails, and scarring of nail beds
- Eczema
  - Coarse irregular nails pits may be seen if there is proximal nail fold involvement
- Septic vasculitis
  - Splinter hemorrhages

MUCOUS MEMBRANES
- Pustular psoriasis variants: geographic tongue
- Reiter syndrome: geographic tongue
- Behcet disease: oral and genital aphthous ulcers

(Continued)

TABLE 2.20. Additional Diagnostic Clues That Can Be Found in Pustular Dermatoses (continued)

LYMPH NODES
- Generalized lymphadenopathy may be seen in HIV disease.
- Reactive lymphadenopathy is seen in inflammatory types of tinea capitis, including kerion

Consider the diagnosis of Behcet disease in patients with oral and genital aphthae who also have arthritis, pustules, erythema nodosum, pustular vasculitis, eye findings, or neurologic involvement. AGEP is caused by a wide range of drugs, including antibiotics (macrolides, cephalosporins, β-lactams, quinolones, sulfonamides), terbinafine, diltiazem, and antimalarial drugs. Excess medicinal exposure to iodides, bromides, and fluoride can cause halogenoderma. An important category in pustules is the age of the patient. Congenital infections with pustules (listeriosis, candidiasis, herpes simplex, or neonatal varicella) appear at birth or within the first few days of life. Erythema toxicum neonatorum and transient neonatal pustular melanosis present at or shortly after birth. Eosinophilic pustular folliculitis of infancy develops at birth or in the first few weeks of life. Neonatal cephalic pustulosis develops at around 3 weeks of life and peaks at 2 months. Infantile acropustulosis typically presents at 3–6 months of age.

To summarize this section, as can be seen in the textbox below and Figure 2.42, the diagnostic approach to pustules is to decide, as with papules, whether they arise in relation to a follicle. Nonfollicular flaccid pustules imply a superficial location of pustules, and this can guide the differential diagnosis further. The grouping or distribution of pustules may be the most striking aspect of a pustular eruption, and these wheel diagnostic boxes provide further entry points for creating a differential diagnosis.

Approach to Pustules: Summary

- Are they follicular or nonfollicular?
- Are the pustules flaccid? Are there "lakes" of pus?
- What is their size?
- What is the color of the pus?
- Do they arise on a purpuric base?
- Is there a pus-fluid level?
- What is their grouping?
- What is their distribution?
- Are there any further diagnostic clues from scalp, hair, nails, mucous membranes, or lymph nodes?
- Augment physical findings with a thorough history.

SUMMARY

- Each primary lesion can be approached using the wheel of diagnosis.
- The entire wheel of diagnosis for macules, papules, and pustules is discussed in this chapter.
- Plaques and nodules will be covered in detail in the relevant reaction pattern chapters later in the book, and an overview is given here.
- Vesicles and bullae are covered in their entirety in the vesicobullous reaction pattern chapter later in the book.

Diagnostic Clues from Secondary Lesions and Postinflammatory Pigmentary Change

3

Secondary lesions are those lesions that are left behind when primary lesions resolve, or when primary lesions are altered through scratching or rubbing, for example. Secondary lesions may hold morphologic clues that can be leveraged to make a diagnosis, even in the absence of primary lesions. This chapter summarizes secondary lesions and the diagnostic information that they can offer. In this chapter, reference will also be made to the hypo- or hyperpigmented postinflammatory macules that are left behind after lesions resolve and the diagnostic clues that they provide.

SECONDARY LESIONS

Scales

Scales represent a heterogeneous group. Some may be an inherent part of the primary lesion (and not a secondary lesion, by its strict definition), such as when they lie atop papules and plaques. In this situation, scales can render a wealth of diagnostic information. Examples include the silvery scales of psoriasis, or the gritty scale of an actinic keratosis. Chapter 6 provides more details about *primary scales*, including a comprehensive morphological list as seen in Table 6.3. On the other hand, scales may be true secondary lesions, when they are seen after resolution of primary lesions. An example is the superficial *desquamative scale* that may be seen after an exanthematous drug eruption. Desquamative scale is also seen when infections resolve, such as in a treated cellulitis or erysipelas. The term *peeling* can also be applied to the desquamation that it seen when an inflammatory disorder resolves. Superficial scales can be peeled off the skin surface. *Sheets of scale* can be peeled off in staphylococcal scalded skin syndrome. This is a toxin-mediated process, where the exotoxins produced by phage group II staphylococci cleave desmoglein 1 in between keratinocytes. Sheets of superficial epidermis can be peeled away. This appearance is also known as *exfoliative scale*. Exfoliative scales are seen in pemphigus foliaceus following rapid rupture and repair of superficial bullae. Sheets of desquamative scale can also sometimes be peeled off when severe sunburn resolves.

> **Clinical Tip**
> - *Desquamative scale* may imply resolution of a prior inflammatory or infectious process.
> - Sheets of desquamative scale are termed *exfoliative scale*.

Another example of a secondary scale is the collarette. The term *collarette* refers to a circumferential margin of fine scale that is loosely adherent peripherally and centrally detached. Its presence implies a preexisting inflammatory papule or plaque, or vesicle or bulla.

> **Clinical Tip** A *collarette of scale* implies a preceding inflammatory papule or plaque, or a preceding vesicle or bulla.

Collarettes are seen when the superficial bullae of bullous impetigo resolve, or in any of the superficial autoimmune blistering diseases (see Chapter 7), such as pemphigus vulgaris.

Examples of Secondary Scales

- Desquamation/peeling: Fine superficial scales that peel off the skin surface
- Exfoliative scale: Sheets of desquamative scale
- Collarette: A circumferential margin of fine scale that is adherent peripherally and centrally detached

Atrophy

This is thinning of the skin, which may affect the epidermis, dermis, or subcutaneous fat. Normal aging leads to an atrophic epidermis. The skin surface appears wrinkled, and the underlying dermal vasculature is easily seen. A thinned epidermis is also encountered in mycosis fungoides. The characteristic appearance of the patch stage of mycosis fungoides is a thin plaque with a shiny, wrinkled, or cigarette-paper-like surface (Figure 3.1). The wrinkling can be accentuated by sidelighting: holding a penlight or dermatoscope parallel to the skin surface. Epidermal atrophy is a feature of lichen sclerosus. Figure 3.2 displays a wrinkled plaque on the trunk in a case of extragenital lichen sclerosus. Atrophic scarring of the epidermis is seen at the end stage of discoid lupus erythematosus. These plaques are shiny and usually slightly depressed with respect to the surrounding skin. There is an associated depigmentation with a rim of hyperpigmentation in many cases (Figure 3.3).

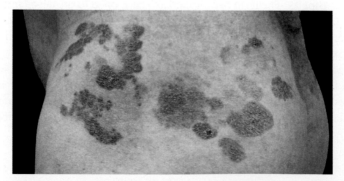

FIGURE 3.1 • Patch-stage mycosis fungoides with a classic wrinkled appearance. (Reproduced with permission from Wolff K, Johnson RA, Saavedra AP, et al: *Fitzpatrick's Color Atlas and Synopsis of Clinical Dermatology*, 8th ed. New York, NY: McGraw Hill; 2017.)

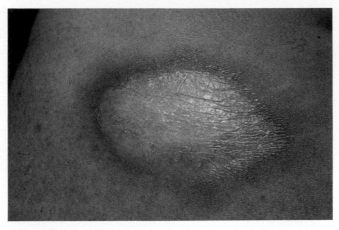

FIGURE 3.2 · Extragenital lichen sclerosus, displaying a wrinkled shiny plaque. (Image appears with permission from VisualDx. Copyright VisualDx.)

The atrophic variant of confluent and reticulated papillomatosis of Gougerot and Carteaud has an atrophic epidermis with wrinkled scaly plaques (Figure 3.4). Prolonged use of topical steroids also leads to a thinned epidermis. The epidermis appears shiny and wrinkled. Chronic topical steroid use also produces neovascularization, and so telangiectasias and superficial purpura are frequently seen.

> **Clinical Tip** The signs of epidermal atrophy include wrinkling, a shiny appearance, and prominence of dermal vasculature.

Poikiloderma comprises four features: epidermal atrophy, telangiectasia, hyperpigmentation, and hypopigmentation. Poikiloderma may be seen in the setting of a variety of congenital and acquired conditions, as is summarized in Table 3.1.

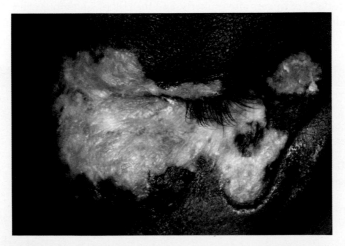

FIGURE 3.3 · Discoid lupus erythematosus, late stage, with atrophic scarring, central depigmentation, and a surrounding rim of hyperpigmentation.

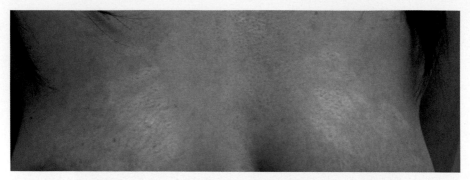

FIGURE 3.4 • Atrophic variant of confluent and reticulated papillomatosis of Gougerot and Carteaud with wrinkled shiny plaques.

Poikiloderma Consists of:

- Atrophy
- Telangiectasia
- Hyperpigmentation
- Hypopigmentation

The congenital causes of poikiloderma are rarely encountered; dyskeratosis congenita (Zinsser–Engman–Cole syndrome) is an X-linked, recessive disorder. Clinically there is poikiloderma on the neck, face, trunk, and upper thighs. Acrally, hyperkeratosis, acrocyanosis, dystrophic nails with ridging, and pterygia may be seen. Oral leukoplakia and the propensity to develop oral squamous cell carcinomas are further manifestations along with a Fanconi-type pancytopenia. Rothmund–Thompson syndrome (also known as *poikiloderma congenitale*) is an autosomal recessive disorder that presents in infancy. Individuals are photosensitive, and the initial edema and erythema on sun exposure is superseded by poikiloderma in these sun-exposed areas. Additional cutaneous signs include acral verrcuous keratoses that develop on the palms and lateral aspects of fingers after puberty, and the risk of squamous cell cancer. Other signs include short stature, absent thumbs, and hypoplastic radii. Other associated

---

TABLE 3.1. Differential Diagnosis of Poikiloderma

CONGENITAL
- Dyskeratosis congenita
- Rothmund–Thomson syndrome
- Kindler–Weary syndrome

ACQUIRED
- Poikiloderma of Civatte
- Chronic radiation dermatitis
- Connective tissue disease
  - Dermatomyositis
  - SLE
- Chronic graft-versus-host disease

malignancies include osteosarcoma and fibrosarcoma. Kindler–Weary syndrome is very rare. Vesicopustules develop on the hands and feet as early as the first months of life to late childhood. During this time there is the gradual onset of a diffuse poikiloderma with striate and reticulate atrophy that spares the face, scalp, and ears, and this persists into adulthood. Other cutaneous findings include keratotic papules on the hands, feet, elbows, and knees (onset is in early childhood) before 5 years and photosensitivity that diminishes with age. Affected individuals may exhibit finger and toe webbing and mucosal involvement leading to stenoses and ectropion.

The acquired forms of poikiloderma are more common, especially poikiloderma of Civatte, which occurs on the upper lateral neck, upper chest, and sometimes the lateral cheeks of women more than men. Ultraviolet light and photodynamic substances in cosmetics are thought to play important roles in the pathogenesis. Reddish-brown reticulate pigmentation is more prominent in this form of poikiloderma than is telangiectasia or atrophy (Figure 3.5). Chronic radiation dermatitis also may manifest poikiloderma (Figure 3.6). Connective tissue diseases are a further association, and in this category, dermatomyositis is a more common cause than SLE (Figure 3.7). In dermatomyositis, poikiloderma may eventuate from violaceous macules or from abraded skin, and in SLE, it may be seen in a longstanding malar rash or in the late stages of generalized erythema. Poikiloderma atrophicans vasculare equates to a type of patch-stage mycosis fungoides. Poikilodermatous plaques are seen (Figure 3.8). Finally, poikiloderma is a common finding in chronic graft-versus-host disease (Figure 3.9).

Dermal atrophy may also present with wrinkled plaques, such as is seen in middermal elastolysis. In this condition, there is loss of elastic fibers that is localized to the middermis (Figure 3.10). A variant presentation of mid-dermal elastolysis is plaques with a peau d'orange appearance. Alternatively, dermal atrophy may manifest as soft,

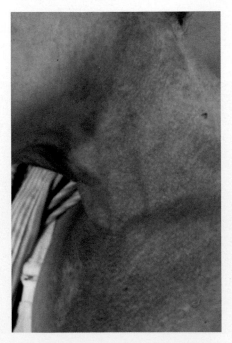

FIGURE 3.5 • Poikiloderma of Civatte, displaying a prominent telangiectatic component.

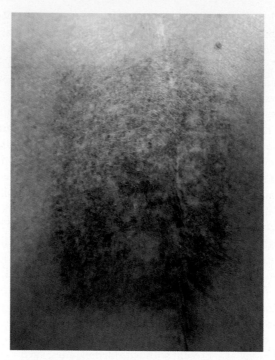

FIGURE 3.6 • Poikiloderma occurring after radiation therapy.

wrinkled sac-like papules, plaques, or nodules that feel as though you are placing your finger through a buttonhole, as is seen in anetoderma. In anetoderma, there is focal loss of elastic tissue in the papillary and midreticular dermis, which may be primary or secondary to a range of disorders, including the antiphospholipid syndrome, HIV disease, Stevens–Johnson syndrome, granuloma annulare, and leprosy. Atrophoderma of

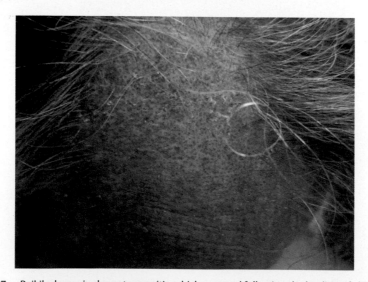

FIGURE 3.7 • Poikiloderma in dermatomyositis, which occurred following the healing of abraded skin.

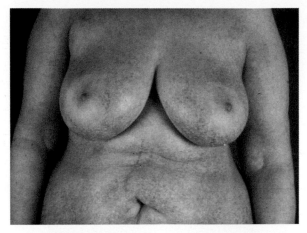

FIGURE 3.8 • Poikiloderma atrophicans vasculare with poikilodermatous plaques.

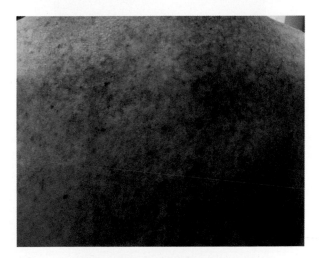

FIGURE 3.9 • Poikiloderma in chronic graft-versus-host disease.

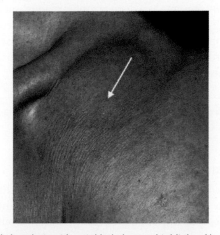

FIGURE 3.10 • Middermal elastolysis with wrinkled plaques, highlighted by the arrow.

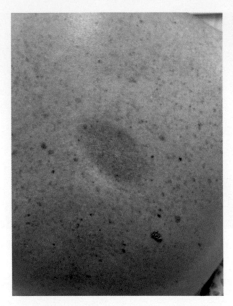

FIGURE 3.11 · Atrophoderma of Pasini and Pierini with light brown depressed plaques with "cliff-drop borders."

Pasini and Pierini is a disorder of collagen where asymptomatic, atrophic plaques occur on the back, typically in young women. The plaques appear light brown with a sharp cutoff from the surrounding normal skin: the so-called cliff-drop sign (Figure 3.11). The dermis is mildly thinned when compared to normal surrounding skin, and collagen bundles may be thickened or clumped. The etiology is unknown.

> **Clinical Tip** In dermal atrophy, wrinkled plaques, depressed plaques or soft, sac-like protrusions may be seen.

Subcutaneous atrophy presents as a deep atrophic plaque, such as is seen in localized involutional lipoatrophy at an injection site. Deeply depressed plaques may be sclerotic, rather than atrophic, which would suggest other diagnoses (such as scleroderma or sclerodermoid disorders; see differential diagnosis of sclerosis in Chapter 9). In the case of sclerosis, plaques feel firm or hard, rather than soft.

> **Clinical Tip** Depressed plaques may be atrophic or sclerotic. If plaques are firm to palpation, consider sclerotic conditions.

Erosions and Excoriations

The term *erosion* connotes the superficial loss of epidermis. Erosions are not associated with scarring. They are usually round. A round erosion holds valuable diagnostic information; its presence implies a preceding vesicle or bulla, such as those seen

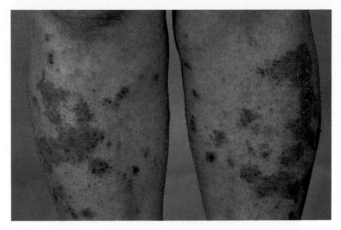

FIGURE 3.12 • Nummular eczema in the subacute stage showing diagnostic round erosions and round crusts.

in subacute eczema or autoimmune blistering diseases, for example. In the case of subacute eczema, the finding of round erosions, as seen in Figure 3.12, immediately differentiates the eruption from other scaly eruptions (all other papulosquamous diseases).

> **Clinical Tip** A round erosion signifies a preceding vesicle or bulla, such as is seen in subacute eczema or any blistering disease. It is a marker of an "inside job."

An *excoriation* is a type of erosion. It is linear or angulated and is caused by scratching. It is therefore a nonspecific indicator of an itchy eruption.

> **Clinical Tip** An excoriation is linear or angulated. It indicates that the eruption is itchy. Excoriations are made on the outside rather than the inside.

Fissure

This is a linear crack in the epidermis, such as those seen with hand eczema (Figure 3.13). Fissures may be erosions or deeper, in which case they may be classified as ulcers.

Ulcer

An *ulcer* is a deep erosion resulting from loss of epidermis as well as part of the dermis. It often heals with a scar. Diagnostic information can be gleaned from the ulcer's associated symptoms, its shape, its edge or the ulcer base, and its location, as well as the surrounding skin.

> **Clinical Tip** Diagnostic information can be gleaned from an ulcer's symptoms, shape, edge, base, location, and the surrounding skin.

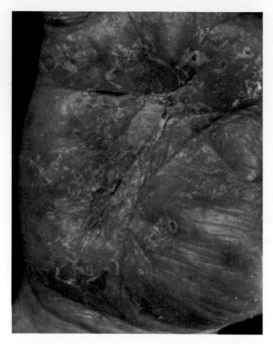

FIGURE 3.13 • Hand eczema displaying fissures and a background of hyperkeratotic scale.

Table 3.2 summarizes this diagnostic information. Painless ulcers are typical of the primary chancre of syphilis and the ulcers of granuloma inguinale. With respect to a primary chancre, it is usually solitary, but few chancres may be present at once. It has a clean base and a border that is indurated and is slightly raised above the ulcer. It feels firm. Primary chancres heal spontaneously within a couple of weeks. Granuloma inguinale also causes a painless ulcer. However, the ulcer continues to expand slowly if it is untreated. It has a beefy-red, bleeding, friable base and raised, rolled borders. Chancroid ulcers are painful and deep. It is common to see more than one ulcer. The edges are ragged and may be undermined. They are soft (so-called "soft chancre"). The base is friable, and it may be covered with a grayish exudate.

A noduloulcerative basal cell cancer has raised rolled borders. Those of an ulcerated squamous cell cancer (SCC) are described as being firm and indurated. Both these skin cancers arise in chronically sun-damaged skin. SCC may also arise in chronic wounds or other chronic skin conditions. The ulceroglandular form of tularemia begins as a small papule that breaks down to form an ulcer with a raised, rolled border and often, an over-lying eschar. The ulcers of established pyoderma gangrenosum may have raised, rolled borders (Figure 3.14). They also have undermined borders. *Undermined* means that the ulcer extends laterally under the ulcer edge. To diagnose this, place a probe, such as a Q-tip under the edge of the ulcer, and move it gently outward away from the ulcer—the probe will sink into the undermined portion. In the early stages of pyoderma gangre-nosum, the ulcer border appears violaceous; this color implies that the disease is active (Figure 3.15). The base may develop a yellow exudate, or necrosis may be present. It is typically painful and may spread rapidly, especially in the early stages. The ulcers of leish-maniasis may have similar appearance (Figure 3.16), as may those of other infections. A clinical pearl, therefore, is that in all cases where pyoderma gangrenosum is being

TABLE 3.2. Characteristic Features of Ulcers

SYMPTOMS
- Painless
  - Primary chancre of syphilis
  - Ulcers of granuloma inguinale
- Ulcer edge
- Raised, rolled
  - Basal cell cancer: noduloulcerative subtype
  - Granuloma inguinale has raised, rolled, heaped-up borders
  - Tularemia
  - Pyoderma gangrenosum
- Undermined
  - Pyoderma gangrenosum
  - Chancroid ulcers classically have both ragged and undermined borders
- Violaceous
  - Pyoderma gangrenosum
  - Leishmaniasis
- Punched-out
  - Neurotrophic ulcers
  - Arterial ulcers
  - Gummas of tertiary syphilis
  - Genital ulcers of Behcet disease
- Indurated
  - Primary chancres of syphilis are often described as having indurated borders
  - Squamous cell carcinoma

SHAPE
- Scalloped
  - Herpes simplex
  - Zoster
- Retiform
  - Retiform ulcers are caused by retiform purpura (see Chapter 10)
- Round
  - Subepidermal blistering diseases
  - An externally applied noxious substance, such as a cigarette burn
  - Calciphylaxis may present as a round painful ulcer on the penis
- Linear or geometric
  - The presence of linear or geometric ulcers implies the preceding application of an external object, such as a thermal burn from a heating pack or self-induced excoriations

BASE
- Friable, beefy-red, bleeding granulation tissue on genital skin is characteristic of granuloma inguinale
- The presence of granulation tissue in the base of an ulcer implies that it is healing

CHANGES IN SURROUNDING SKIN
- Venous stasis: hemosiderin deposition, varicose veins, champagne bottle sign of liodermatosclerosis, porcelain white small plaques of atrophie blanche
- Arterial insufficiency: hairless, dry skin, increased capillary refill time, poor peripheral pulses
- Peripheral neuropathy: symmetric diminished peripheral sensation
- Signs of dermatologic disease
  - Yellow atrophic plaques: necrobiosis lipoidica
  - Retiform purpura: causes in Chapter 10
  - Cribriform scars: seen after pyoderma gangrenosum has healed
  - Signs of lymphatic spread: sporotrichoid spread is seen in sprorotrichosis and *Mycobacterium marinum* infection, among others

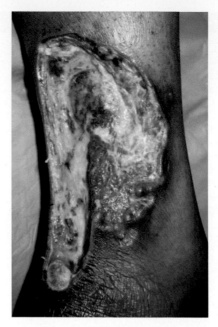

FIGURE 3.14 • Pyoderma gangrenosum with raised, rolled, undermined borders.

considered, it is important to rule out mycobacterial and fungal infections, as well as leishmaniasis, and perform tissue cultures as part of the initial workup.

Neurotrophic ulcers (also known as *mal perforans*) occur in diabetic patients secondary to peripheral neuropathy. These ulcers are seen on weight-bearing parts

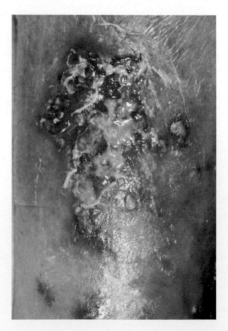

FIGURE 3.15 • Pyoderma gangrenosum at an earlier stage, showing active violaceous borders.

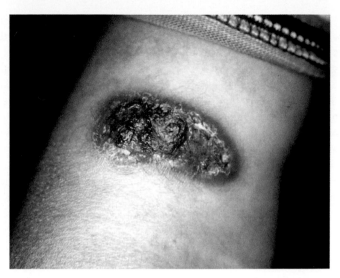

FIGURE 3.16 • Leishmaniasis with a raised, violaceous border that is reminiscent of pyoderma gangrenosum.

of the foot. They are classically punched-out (ulcers edges are well-demarcated and vertical), are painless (owing to the neuropathy), and may be seen in association with callus or callus and hemorrhage. Arterial ulcers are seen in patients with arterial insufficiency. They may be found on the feet or lateral lower extremities. As opposed to neurotrophic ulcers, they are painful. They have a punched-out appearance. Gummas of tertiary syphilis are rubbery nodules. These may ulcerate. The borders of gummatous ulcers are also classically punched-out. The genital ulcers of Behcet disease are typically described as punched-out.

The shape of ulcers can render important diagnostic information. The presence of a scalloped border implies herpetic infection, either herpes simplex or herpes zoster, as a cause. This shape is made from preceding grouped vesicles, which then give way to grouped erosions. Retiform ulcers are caused by retiform purpura. A complete differential diagnosis of retiform purpura is seen in the vascular reaction pattern chapter (Chapter 10), and in general this pattern is caused either by a thromboembolic disorder or by a vasculitis. A round ulcer implies the presence of a deeper blistering disorder, such as junctional or dystrophic epidermolysis bullosa or epidermolysis bullosa acquisita. In the absence of primary blisters, and if the ulcers are monomorphic, the possibility of something that has been externally applied, such as cigarette burns, should be considered. Calciphylaxis, while usually retiform in shape, may present as a round painful ulcer on the penis.

Some ulcers characteristically have eschars (see section titled "Oozing and Crusting," below and Table 3.4). Further diagnostic clues can be harnessed from changes in the surrounding skin. Signs of venous stasis include brown macules due to hemosiderin deposition, varicose veins, induration, the champagne bottle sign of lipodermatosclerosis, and porcelain white small plaques of atrophie blanche. Signs of arterial insufficiency include hairless, dry skin, increased capillary refill time, and poor peripheral pulses. Signs of peripheral neuropathy include diminished sensation peripherally and symmetrically. Signs of associated, causative dermatoses may also be present. For example, ulcers of necrobiosis lipoidica may have yellow, atrophic plaques either surrounding or separate from them. Retiform ulcers signify the differential diagnosis of retiform purpura, as discussed. Pyoderma gangrenosum manifests cribriform scarring, in which the scars have a perforated appearance. Signs of lymphatic spread are seen in those disorders that manifest lymphocutaneous (sporothrichoid) spread. This differential diagnosis comprises many uncommonly encountered infections as well as lymphatic spread of melanoma. The comprehensive differential diagnosis may be found in the dermal reaction pattern chapter (Chapter 9).

Inguinal lymphadenopathy is seen in primary syphilis and chancroid. In primary syphilis, there are unilateral, painless, rubbery enlarged lymph nodes. In chancroid, the lymphadenopathy is painful and unilateral. Regional lymphadenopathy is a common concomitant of primary herpes simplex infections. Lymphadenopathy is also seen in ulceroglandular tularemia. The differential diagnosis of ulceroglandular disease (an ulcer with accompanying lymphadenitis) is given in Table 3.3. Lymphadenopathy in the setting of an advanced squamous cell cancer implies metastastic spread. This lymphadenopathy is seldom tender, as opposed to the tender nodes that occur in lymphadenitis.

Oozing and Crusting

Oozing is the accumulation of moist serum over a damaged epidermis. It often overlies erosions. A *crust* is the accumulation of dried serum or pus over a damaged epidermis. Again, this often overlies erosions and is seen in the setting of vesicles,

---

TABLE 3.3. Differential Diagnosis of Ulceroglandular Disease

- **Gram-Positive Bacteria**
  - Staphylococcal lymphadenitis associated with ecthyma

- **Gram-Negative Bacteria**
  - Chancroid (*Haemophilus ducreyi*)
  - Lymphogranuloma venereum (*Chlamydia trachomatis*)
  - Tularemia (*Francisella tularensis*)
  - Cat scratch disease (*Bartonella henselae*)
  - *Pasteurella multocida* infection (from an animal bite)
  - Bubonic plague (*Yersinia pestis*)
  - Melioidosis (*Burkholderia pseudomallei*)
  - Glanders (*Burkholderia mallei*)
  - Rat bite fever from *Spirillum minus* (Sodoku)

- **Treponemal**
  - Primary syphilis

- **Mycobacterial**
  - Primary inoculation tuberculosis

- **Viral**
  - Herpes simplex virus

- **Deep Fungal**
  - Sporotrichosis (*Sporothrix schenckii*)

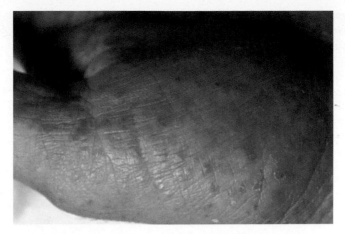

FIGURE 3.17 • Dyshidrotic eczema displaying typical vesicles and brown incipient crusts.

bullae, and pustules. In dyshidrotic eczema and palmoplantar pustular psoriasis, small light brown round macules similar in size to the associated vesicles or pustules are seen (Figure 3.17). These represent resolving vesicles or pustules in a thicker stratum corneum. In other areas of the body, small crusts would eventuate, but here full resorption of vesicle or pustule contents may occur before a crust is formed. These brown macules may be referred to as "brown incipient crusts," and they are a diagnostic hallmark of the two aforementioned dermatoses. Brown incipient crusts may be seen in any other vesicular or pustular dermatosis of palms and soles as well, such as bullous tinea pedis, for example.

> **Clinical Tip** Small brown macules on palms and soles represent incipient crusts. They may be seen in any vesicular or pustular process on the palms or soles, such as dyshidrotic eczema or palmoplantar pustular psoriasis.

An *eschar* is a black crust. It represents the end stage of necrosis and is formed when the necrotic tissue begins to slough. Table 3.4 lists the diseases that may manifest an eschar. These may be infectious, inflammatory, or ischemic in nature. The eschars of rickettsialpox, calciphylaxis, and pityriasis lichenoides et varioliformis acuta (PLEVA) are shown in Figures 3.18, 3.19, and 3.20, respectively. Figure 3.21 shows an eschar overlying a chronic ulcer caused by cytomegalovirus (CMV) in an immunosuppressed child.

The term *papulonecrotic* implies the presence of a papule with a central dark or necrotic crust. Papulonecrotic tuberculide is a type III hypersensitivity reaction to *Mycobacterium tuberculosis*. It presents as a symmetric eruption over the extensor aspects of the extremities (Figure 3.22) and on the ears. Palms may occasionally be involved, and widespread involvement has also been reported. Initially, there are papules, pustules, and occasionally nodules. These develop a central crust and resolve with varioliform scars. In pityriasis lichenoides et varioliformis acuta (PLEVA; also known as Mucha–Habermann disease), widespread papules with central necrotic or hemorrhagic crusting are seen on the proximal extremities and trunk. A third eruption that is described as papulonecrotic is that of lymphomatoid papulosis (LYP). In LYP, a

TABLE 3.4. Dermatoses That Frequently Manifest an Eschar

INFECTIOUS
- Bacterial
  - Ecthyma due to *Staphylococcus* or *Streptococcus*
  - Ecthyma gangrenosum: usually *Pseudomonas*, also other Gram-negative bacilli
  - Necrotizing fasciitis
  - Tularemia: *Francisella tularensis*
  - Glanders: *Burkholderia mallei*
  - Plague: *Yersinia pestis*
  - Tropical ulcer (phagedenic ulcer): a mixed infection with anerobes and/or Gram-negative bacilli
  - Anthrax: *Bacillus anthracis*
  - Rat bite fever: *Spirillum minus*
- Mycobacterial
  - Lucio phenomenon in leprosy: a necrotizing vasculitis that ensues when bacilli of *M. leprae* invade the endothelium in cases of lepromatous leprosy
- Viral
  - Herpes simplex
  - Orf virus
  - Milker's nodule
  - Cowpox
- Rickettsial
  - Rickettsialpox: *Rickettsia akari*
  - Boutonneuse fever: *Rickettsia conori*
  - African tick bite fever: *Rickettsia africae*
  - Scrub typhus: *Orientia tsutsugamushi*
  - Tickborne lymphadenopathy: *Rickettsia slovaca*
  - Cat flea rickettsiosis: *Rickettsia felis*
- Fungal
  - Aspergillosis
  - Fusariosis
  - Mucormycosis

INFLAMMATORY
- Brown recluse spider bite
- Pityriasis lichenoides et varioliformis acuta
- Medium vessel vasculitis
  - Polyarteritis nodosa
- Occlusive vasculopathies
  - Purpura fulminans
  - Antiphospholipid syndrome
  - Coumadin necrosis
  - Heparin necrosis
  - Calciphylaxis
  - Cryoglobulinemia
  - Cocaine levamisole toxicity
  - Cholesterol emboli

SECONDARY TO ISCHEMIA
- Mal perforans: diabetic foot ulcer
- Other bed sores

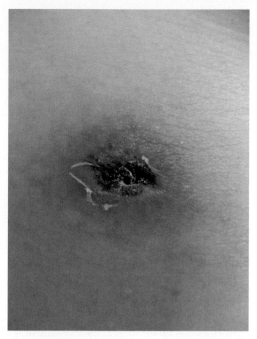

FIGURE 3.18 • **Eschar of rickettsialpox.** (Used with permission from Dr. Miguel Sanchez, Bellevue Hospital, New York University School of Medicine, New York, NY.)

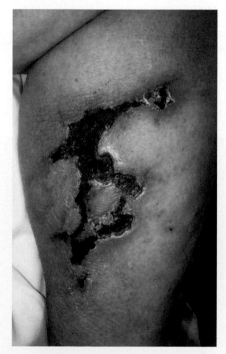

FIGURE 3.19 • **Calciphylaxis, displaying retiform eschar.** (Used with permission from Dr. Molly Plovanich, University of Rochester, Rochester, NY.)

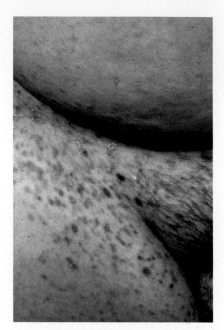

FIGURE 3.20 · Pityriasis lichenoides et varioliformis acuta (PLEVA) with small eschars and reddish papules.

lymphoproliferative disorder, crops of papules and nodules undergo central ulceration and crusting and heal with hypopigmented or atrophic scars.

Diseases with Papulonecrotic Lesions

- Papulonecrotic tuberculide
- PLEVA
- LYP

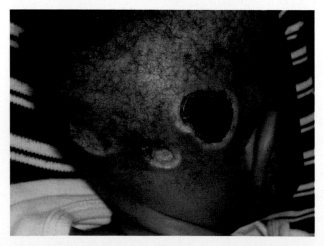

FIGURE 3.21 · Eschar overlying cytomegalovirus infection in a child with HIV. (Used with permission from Professor Ncoza Dlova, University of KwaZulu-Natal, Durban, South Africa.)

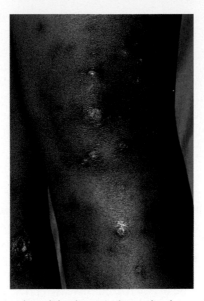

FIGURE 3.22 · Papulonecrotic tuberculide, showing ulcerated and crusted papules.

Lichenification

Lichenification is the term given to thickened skin with accentuated surface markings. This finding is caused by chronic rubbing and scratching, and its presence therefore implies itch. Atopic dermatitis presents with lichenification more frequently than other forms of eczema (Figure 3.23). Lichen simplex chronicus (LSC) presents

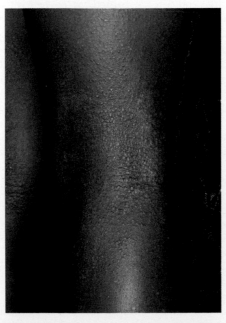

FIGURE 3.23 · Lichenification, as seen in a case of severe atopic dermatitis. (Reproduced with permission from Wolff K, Johnson RA, Saavedra AP, et al: *Fitzpatrick's Color Atlas and Synopsis of Clinical Dermatology*, 8th ed. New York, NY: McGraw Hill; 2017.)

on characteristic body sites (nape of neck, scalp, around the ankles) as a solitary lichenified plaque. LSC is initiated by cutaneous itch, which may be continuous or sporadic. Scratching or rubbing leads to enhanced symptomatology, and an itch–scratch cycle is set up, ultimately giving rise to lichenification. Noneczematous dermatoses that are itchy may also appear lichenified. Psoriasis may be pruritic and may be secondarily lichenified. Scaling, excoriations, and hypo- and hyperpigmentation may all accompany lichenification. Pigmentary changes may occur secondary to the disruption of the basement membrane zone during scratching, or from chronic topical steroid use.

Scar

A *scar* is the replacement by fibrous tissue of another tissue that has been destroyed by injury or disease. A hypertrophic scar is raised and confined to the original borders of the scar. A *keloid* is a hypertrophic scar that has spread beyond the original scar borders. Striae are atrophic scars that occur after a growth spurt (seen on the backs of teenagers in horizontal rows) or after rapid weight gain (upper thighs, arms, and elsewhere) or in pregnancy (lower abdomen). The appearance of scars may, in some cases, be characteristic of a particular disease entity. Table 3.5 categorizes diseases by their signature scar, and includes varioliform, pitted, ice pick (Figure 3.24), cribriform, and vermiculate subtypes.

TABLE 3.5. Scar Types and Their Associated Diseases

SCAR TYPE	DESCRIPTION	DISEASE
Varioliform scar	Resembles the scars of smallpox; these are small and punched out	Smallpox PLEVA (pitysiasis lichenoides et varioliformis acuta): crusted papules heal with varioliform scars Papulonecrotic tuberculide: a symmetric eruption of papules and pustules occurs on the extensor aspects of the extremities and buttocks; scars are typically small and punched out Atrophoderma maculosa varioliformis cutis: a rare, idiopathic disorder where asymptomatic varioliform and linear scarring appears on the cheeks and other areas of the face of young individuals
Pitted scars	Resemble pits; smaller than varioliform scars	Acne Follicular atrophoderma (Bazex–Dupré–Christol syndrome)
Ice-pick scar	A large pitted scar with a jagged shape, resembling an ice pick	Severe acne
Cribriform scar	Scar has a perforated appearance	Pyoderma gangranosum: classically heals with cribriform scarring
Vermiculate scar	"Worm-like": usually a series of pitted scars that coalesce in wavy lines	Atrophoderma vermiculata: a form of keratosis pilaris that occurs on the lateral cheeks, leaving depressed scars Discoid lupus erythematosus: papular forms heal with vermiculate scars

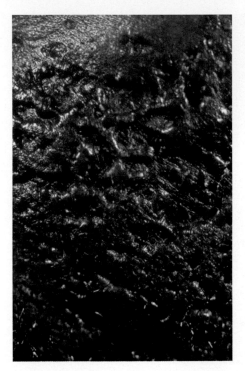

FIGURE 3.24 • A close-up of ice-pick scarring on the cheek following severe acne.

Sinus

A sinus is a tract leading from a suppurating cavity to the skin surface. Sinuses occur secondary to chronic inflammatory nodules and abscesses in hidradenitis suppurativa (Figure 3.25). Sterile sinus tracts are also seen in cutaneous Crohn disease, both in peri-anal disease and in sites distant from the gastrointestinal tract (metastatic Crohn disease). In both forms, sinuses may be seen within violaceous plaques, vegetating nodules or ulcers or arising in normal skin. One or more sinus tracts may be present. Sinuses are seen in botryomycosis, actinomycosis and mycetoma. In botryomycosis, a chronic staphylococcal infection, vegetating or ulcerated plaques or nodules with sinus tracts and sometimes fistulae to underlying muscle of bone are seen. Actinomycosis presents with suppurating nodules containing sinus tracts. In mycetoma, the affected (usually lower) limb is diffusely swollen and indurated with accompanying sinuses. Bacterial (actino-mycetoma) and fungal (eumycetoma) forms are recognized. Granules of different colors are extruded through these sinus tracts. In general, bacterial granules are white, yellow, or red. Fungal granules may be black or white. These represent colonies of organisms.

A cutaneous sinus of dental origin is formed when a periapical tooth abscess erodes into the skin. This presents as a soft, friable pyogenic granuloma-like papule or nodule on the lower face. A high index of suspicion is needed for diagnosis.

POSTINFLAMMATORY PIGMENTARY ALTERATION

Postinflammatory pigmentary changes, both hypo- and hyperpigmentation, may be left behind when eruptions resolve. Some dermatoses typically leave hypopigmenta-tion in their wake and others, hyperpigmentation.

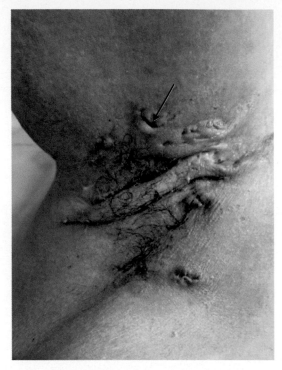

FIGURE 3.25 • Advanced case of hidradenitis suppurativa with sinuses (one highlighted by the arrow), and scarring.

Seborrheic dermatitis tends to resolve with *hypopigmentation*. This is particularly prominent in darker skin phototypes. The hypopigmented macules will occupy the same characteristic distribution of the original dermatitis and so, may be diagnostic of what went before. Pityriasis lichenoides chronica is an eruption that comprises small lichenoid scaly thin papules. These occur in crops on the extensors and trunk, and they leave behind postinflammatory hypopigmentation. Hypopigmentation may be the predominant finding of certain disease states as well, including in pityriasis alba and hypopigmented mycosis fungoides. Pityriasis alba is commonly seen in individuals with an atopic diathesis. Fine scales give way to hypopigmented macules on the face and outer arms. In hypopigmented mycosis fungoides, widespread hypopigmented macules may be accompanied by occasional scale. Note also that hypopigmentation may signify primary disease as well, including the hypopigmented forms of sarcoid and leprosy. Progressive macular hypomelanosis is seen on the trunk of younger individuals. It is hypothesized that the *Proprionibacterium acnes* that is identified on Wood's lamp examination is causative. Subacute lupus erythematosus and neonatal lupus erythematosus may leave depigmented macules in their wake (Figure 3.26).

Tinea versicolor may leave hypo- or hyperpigmentation behind when it heals. The color change may take weeks to normalize. Many other dermatoses eventuate in *hyperpigmentation*, and this is usually more prominent in darker skin phototypes. Acne typically causes hyperpigmentation, especially in darker skin types. (In lighter phototypes, purplish macules may be seen.) In infants, transient neonatal pustular melanosis will do the same. Zoster will leave behind grouped brown macules in a dermatomal distribution.

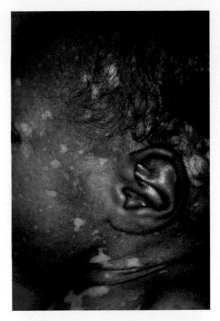

FIGURE 3.26 · Neonatal lupus erythematosus resolving with depigmented macules.

Excoriations from any itchy eruption can leave brown linear macules in their wake, typically seen in darker skin phototypes, as may eczema (Figure 3.27). Phytophotodermatitis is a phototoxic reaction caused by contact with a furocoumarin-containing plant or fruit of the Apiaceae family in the presence of sunlight. The erythema of the reaction resolves

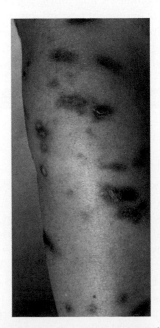

FIGURE 3.27 · Brown color of postinflammatory hyperpigmentation following eczema on an extremity. Note the active scaly plaques still present.

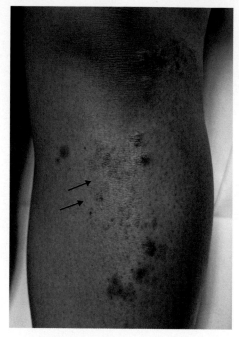

FIGURE 3.28 • Gray color of postinflammatory hyperpigmentation that eventuates after lichen planus resolves (highlighted by arrow), with active lichen planus around it.

with a prominent brown color that can be appreciated in any skin phototype. These macules are usually linear or geometric and follow the original pattern of contact (see Figure 1.6A). Another cause of prominent postinflammatory linear macules is the flagellate erythema that occurs in the setting of bleomycin toxicity. Here, this may be preceded by a pruritic erythematous eruption of linear or flagellate plaques (resembling marks caused by a whip) or this initial inflammatory phase may pass unnoticed.

Postinflammatory Linear Macules are Seen After
• Excoriations
• Zoster: grouped macules in a dermatomal distribution
• Phytophotodermatitis
• Flagellate erythema from bleomycin toxicity

Annular postinflammatory hyperpigmentation may be seen in tinea corporis, pityriasis rosea, or urticarial vasculitis. Regarding clues from distribution patterns, pityriasis rosea also may hyperpigment when it resolves. Here, the classic ovoid macules in a "Christmas tree" distribution are seen. Atopic dermatitis will leave hyperpigmentation in its wake, which again may lend diagnostic clues if flexural. The differential diagnosis of brown macules on palms and soles includes a normal finding in a darker phototype, postinflammatory hyperpigmentation, such as from a dermatosis that favors palms and soles (eg, secondary syphilis), or vitamin B_{12} deficiency.

Differential Diagnosis of Multiple Brown Macules on Palms or Soles

- Normal pigmentation in a darker skin phototype
- Postinflammatory hyperpigmentation from any rash involving palms and soles
- A sign of vitamin B_{12} deficiency

An important diagnostic distinction is to determine whether the color of the hyperpigmentation is brown or gray. A gray color signifies prior interface dermatitis, such as is seen after lichen planus (Figure 3.28), erythema dyschromicum perstans, or a fixed drug eruption.

> **Clinical Tip** Gray postinflammatory macules signify preceding interface dermatitis, such as lichen planus, erythema dyschromicum perstans, or fixed drug eruption.

SUMMARY

- Secondary lesions hold a plethora of diagnostic clues.
- Diagnostic clues can also be garnered from postinflammatory pigmentary alteration, including shape, number, and color of macules.

Color as a Diagnostic Determinant

4

As we have seen, the characteristics of primary lesions, and sometimes, secondary lesions as well, can be used to create, or narrow, differential diagnoses. This chapter focuses on color as a diagnostic determinant. Color is a powerful tool that can be harnessed to create differential diagnoses. Pink, red, brown, and white are the most common colors of primary and secondary lesions that are manifest in the skin. But the skin may house other colors as well, including yellow, orange, purple, maroon, gray, blue, green, and black. In this chapter, comprehensive differential diagnoses will be discussed for each color using the wheel of diagnosis. Additionally, the causes of generalized color changes will be outlined. While tattoo artists may introduce any of these colors into the skin, this chapter will focus only on those color changes that are endogenously produced or acquired through disease states.

It is important to note that the color of skin lesions is influenced by the color of the skin in which they arise.

> **Clinical Tip** The color of skin lesions may be influenced by the background color of the skin they arise in.

The color of normal skin is determined predominantly by the amounts of eumelanin and phaeomelanin that are present, but oxyhemoglobin, deoxyhemoglobin, and carotenoid concentrations also play a role. In darker skin, pink and red colors may be masked, or they may appear purple or brownish. In very light skin, the purple color of lichen planus and other interface dermatitides may not be appreciable, and these papules and plaques may appear pink.

> **Clinical Tip** In darker skin, pink and red colors may be masked. In lighter skin, the color purple may appear pink.

PINK AND RED

The term *erythematous* is frequently employed to describe lesions in this category. It is useful to differentiate pink from red, and the quality of the red or pink color may connote a specific disease in some instances. Examples include the deep red appearance of infections, such as furuncles and carbuncles, the (sometimes faint) pink color of urticaria (Figure 4.1A), the cherry-red color of cherry angiomas, and the shiny ruby-red color of superficial basal cell cancers. Psoriatic plaques are often described as having a salmon-pink color (Figure 4.1B); cutaneous candidiasis is described as appearing "beefy-red" (Figure 4.1C), and the bright red erythema of an exanthematous drug eruption is known as "drug-red" (Figure 4.1D).

Types of Red and Pink

- Deep red: furuncles, carbuncles
- Pink: urticaria
- Cherry-red: cherry angiomas
- Ruby-red: superficial basal cell cancers

- Salmon-pink: psoriasis
- Beefy-red: candidiasis
- Drug-red: bright red color of an exanthematous drug reaction

The differential diagnosis of pink and red lesions is almost limitless. Infections, inflammatory and neoplastic conditions, and drug eruptions may all present with primary lesions in this color spectrum. It is also useful to approach red and pink lesions using the diagnostic boxes on the wheel of diagnosis. The differential diagnosis of red

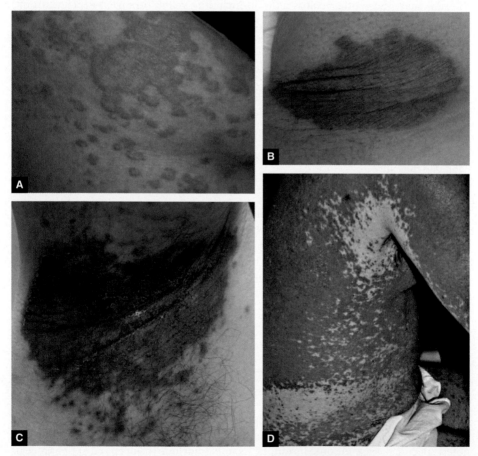

FIGURE 4.1 • Examples of pink and red dermatoses: (A) Urticaria, showing the classic pink color of wheals; (B) psoriasis, showing a well-demarcated salmon-pink plaque; (C) cutaneous candidiasis with a "beefy-red" appearance and outlying satellite papules; (D) an exanthematous drug eruption displaying a bright red or "drug-red" color.

groupings and configurations, as well as the distribution, is immense. These will be identified and described in each relevant reaction pattern chapter later in the book. A general approach to pink and red primary lesions is presented here.

Pink and red macules can be conceptualized as generalized or localized. A generalized reddish discoloration to the skin is seen in emphysema, where the work of compensatory hyperventilation causes a pinkish blush to the skin. High levels of carboxyhemoglobin impart a generalized cherry-red color in carbon monoxide poisoning.

> **Clinical Tip** Causes of generalized erythema include emphysema and carbon monoxide poisoning.

Discrete pink or red macules are categorized and differentiated in the vascular (or red) reaction pattern chapter (Chapter 10). As will be seen, these macules can be differentiated by size, shape, number, and whether they are tender. The differential diagnosis of papules is reviewed in detail in Chapter 2. Conceptually, papules may be follicular or nonfollicular, and each category comprises a different differential diagnosis. Examples of red papules that are follicle-based include folliculitis and pseudofolliculitis. Nonfollicular red papules include an arthropod reaction and chilblains. Pink or red papules, plaques, and nodules are scaly and are discussed in the papulosquamous reaction pattern chapter (Chapter 6). Examples of diseases that present with red, scaly papules include pityriasis rubra pilaris and Grover disease (transient acantholytic dermatosis). Examples of scaly plaques include psoriasis and pityriasis rosea. Keratoacanthomas and squamous cell carcinomas may appear as scaly nodules. Smooth pink and red papules, nodules, and plaques are enumerated in the dermal reaction pattern chapter (Chapter 9). Furuncles and carbuncles are included in this category, along with cutaneous metastases or amelanotic melanoma, for example. Smooth pink and red plaques may also be categorized in the vascular (or red) reaction pattern (Chapter 10). Examples here include urticaria and urticarial dermatoses (such as urticarial vasculitis and eosinophilic cellulitis).

BROWN

The wheel of diagnosis provides a useful framework for thinking through the differential diagnosis of brown in the skin as seen in Figure 4.2. Table 4.1 displays the differential diagnosis of brown by primary lesion. Brown macules may be generalized or localized. The term *hyperpigmented* is used synonymously with brown in this context. In Addison disease a diffuse hyperpigmentation may be a result of an increased production of melanocyte-stimulating hormones (MSH) by the pituitary. Pigmentation of the areolae and genital skin as well as that in palmar creases and flexures may be even more prominent. The mucous membranes may also be pigmented. In chronic renal insufficiency there is decreased clearance of β-MSH, which confers a brown color that is most accentuated in the chronically exposed areas. In hemochromatosis, the skin may have a tanned or bronze appearance, which is most marked on the convex surfaces of the face. Histopathologically, deposition of hemosiderin around eccrine glands, along with increased melanin in the basal layer, is seen. In primary biliary cirrhosis, a brown pigmentation that is most prominent in photoexposed areas may occur along with jaundice. Increased melanin is seen in the epidermis, including melanin found in layers higher than the basal layer. The mechanism of this finding is not fully elucidated.

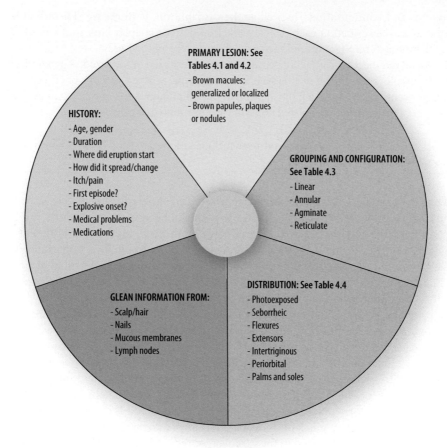

FIGURE 4.2 · The wheel of diagnosis, customized to brown.

In scleroderma, both sclerotic and nonsclerotic skin may display hyperpigmentation. This is accentuated on the face and in areas of friction. In POEMS syndrome (polyneuropathy, organomegaly, endocrinopathy, M protein, skin changes), hyperpigmentation is a frequent finding. This may be generalized or localized. In a recent study, its presence was correlated with the presence of an IgG gammopathy. While the high levels of vascular endothelial growth factor (VEGF) in POEMS have been correlated with the vascular abnormalities in this syndrome (such as the glomeruloid hemangiomas), hyperpigmentation has not, and the cause of hyperpigmentation in POEMS is not well-studied. Generalized hyperpigmentation is a rare finding in vitamin B_{12} deficiency. Prominent flexural and palmoplantar crease pigmentation may be seen. Hyperpigmented macules may also be seen over dorsal aspects of the hands and feet.

Diseases That Cause Generalized Hyperpigmentation

- Addison disease
- Hemochromatosis
- Chronic renal insufficiency
- Primary biliary cirrhosis
- Scleroderma
- POEMS syndrome
- Vitamin B_{12} deficiency

TABLE 4.1. Brown, by Primary Lesion

MACULES
- Melanocytic
  - Simple lentigo, solar lentigo
  - Café-au-lait macule
  - Junctional nevus
  - Malignant melanoma in situ
  - Nevus spilus
- Melasma
- Exogenous ochronosis
- Drug-induced pigmentation
  - Antimalarials
  - Clofazimine
  - Minocycline
- Macular amyloid
- Tinea nigra
- Urticaria pigmentosa
- Postinflammatory hyperpigmentation

PAPULES AND/OR NODULES
- Melanocytic
  - Compound nevi
  - Melanoma
- Dermatofibroma
- Pigmented basal cell cancer
- Urticaria pigmentosa
- Granulomatous conditions
  - Granuloma annulare
  - Sarcoidosis
  - Lupus vulgaris
  - Granulomatous rosacea
  - Lupus miliaris disseminatus faciei
- Secondary syphilis: "copper-colored"
- Erythema elevatum diutinum

PAPULES AND/OR PLAQUES
- Melanocytic
  - Compound nevi
  - Melanoma
- Seborrheic keratosis
- Granuloma faciale
- Confluent and reticulated papillomatosis of Gougerot and Carteaud (CARP)
- Keratodermas with transgrediens
- Epidermal nevi

PLAQUES
- Morphea
- Atrophoderma of Pasini and Pierini
- Acanthosis nigricans
- Erythrokeratodermia variabilis

Junctional nevi, lentigines, and postinflammatory hyperpigmentation are some of the more commonly seen entities that present as localized or discrete brown macules. Malignant melanoma in situ presents as a variegated brown macule. Melanoma in situ may also appear as a homogenous light, mid-, or dark brown macule. Some non-melanocytic dermatoses are also brown. Macular amyloid presents as solid or rippled brown macules on the back or shins. Tinea nigra is a superficial fungal infection that presents as a solitary brown macule on the palm or sole. It is caused by *Piedraia hortae*. Urticaria pigmentosa (Figure 4.3A) presents as multiple brown or red-brown macules or papules. This is the most common form of mastocytosis in the skin. Darier sign (wheal formation on firm stroking of involved skin) may be positive, especially in cases of more recent onset. Postinflammatory hyperpigmentation is seen with the resolution of many dermatoses, especially in individuals with darker skin. Some dermatoses that classically leave postinflammatory hyperpigmentation in their wake are transient neonatal pustular melanosis, acne, atopic dermatitis, and pityriasis rosea.

Drug pigmentation is also macular. It may appear brown, brown-gray, blue-gray, slate-gray, violet-brown, or reddish-brown. Table 4.2 lists drugs that cause gray, blue, or brown pigmentation. Antimalarial agents are associated with photoaccentuated brown, brown-gray, or blue-gray pigmentation. Clofazamine initially produces a reddish pigmentation. This is superceded by blue-gray, violet, violet-brown discoloration. This is typically localized to sites of prior and current inflammation, but it may also be

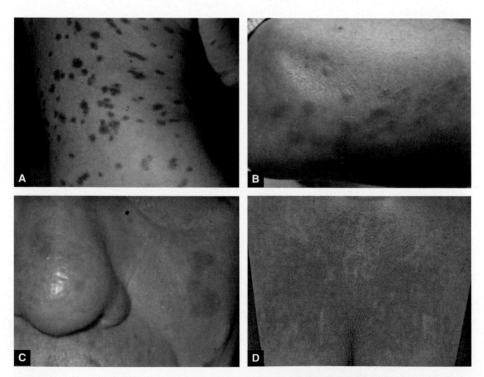

FIGURE 4.3 · Examples of brown dermatoses: (A) Urticaria pigmentosa with small brown and red-brown macules and papules; (B) granuloma annulare displaying a yellow-brown color; (C) granuloma faciale with brown-gray plaques; (D) confluent and reticulated papillomatosis of Gougerot and Carteaud showing light brown acanthotic plaques. (Image (D) used with permission from Dr. Miguel Sanchez, Bellevue Hospital, New York University School of Medicine, New York, NY.)

TABLE 4.2. Drug-Related Pigmentation

DRUG COMPOUND	CLINICAL FINDINGS	HISTOPATHOLOGIC FINDINGS
Silver (argyria)	Generalized slate-gray pigmentation is seen with accentuation in photodistributed areas (especially forehead, nose, and hands). Nails, sclera, and mucous membranes may be involved.	Silver granules are seen in the dermis (especially near the basal lamina of sweat glands), around elastic fibers, in eccrine secretory cells, and in mast cells.
Gold (chrysiasis)	Sun-exposed areas and sclerae are blue-gray to purple in color.	Gold granules are seen in dermal macrophages around blood vessels and within fibroblasts.
Bismuth	Resembles that of argyria. A blue-black line is seen at the gingival margin.	Dermal deposition of bismuth granules is seen.
Amiodarone	Sun-exposed areas are involved preferentially with a blue-gray, slate-gray, or purple pigmentation.	Brown-yellow granules are contained in dermal macrophages (degraded drug bound to lipofuscin is found in membrane-bound dense lysosomal bodies)
Antimalarials	A blue-gray or brown-gray pigmentation affects shins preferentially. Nose, cheeks, ears, hard palate, and nails may also be involved. Pigmentation is accentuated in photoexposed areas.	Drug binds to melanin and is deposited in the dermis.
Clofazamine	Blue-gray, violet, violet-brown discoloration appears in sites of cutaneous inflammation, as seen in the plaques of treated leprosy.	Foamy macrophages contain brownish granules that represent lipofuscin from drug pigment.
Tricyclic antidepressants: desipramine, imipramine	There is a slate-gray pigmentation in photoexposed areas.	Golden-brown granules are seen within histiocytes and fibroblasts and lying free in the dermis. Ultrastructurally, these are seen to be complexed to melanosomes.
Phenothiazines; chlorpromazine	There is a purple-gray pigmentation in sun-exposed skin.	Golden-brown granules representing drug are found within perivascular histiocytes and lying free in the dermis. Ultrastructurally, these are seen to be complexed to melanosomes.
Minocycline	Type I: blue-black discoloration in sites of prior inflammation. Type II is large blue-gray or blue-black discoloration on shins and forearms. Type III appears as muddy brown color in sun-exposed areas.	Type I: intra- and extracellular drug-hemosiderin complex. Type II: pigment granules that may contain melanin or iron seen in the dermis and fat. Type III: increased melanin in macrophages in the dermis and in the epidermis.

generalized. Minocycline is a lipophilic drug that is preferentially taken up by macrophages and is responsible for three types of dyspigmentation:

- Type I is the blue-black discoloration that appears in sites of prior inflammation, such as that seen in acne scars. Histopathologically, there is intra- and extracellular drug-hemosiderin complex.
- Type II is the large blue-gray and sometimes blue-black discoloration that occurs on the shins and forearms. In this type, pigment granules that may contain melanin or iron are seen in the dermis and fat.
- Type III appears as a muddy brown color in sun-exposed areas. In this subtype, there is increased melanin in macrophages in the dermis and in the epidermis.

In cases of photoexposed drug-induced pigmentation in general, it has been shown that drug metabolites react with light to produce free radicals, which then bind to melanin. Numerous chemotherapeutic agents also cause hyperpigmentation in the skin. This varies from a generalized hyperpigmentation (5-fluorouracil, cyclophosphamide) to photoaccentuated erythema (daunorubicin), to accentuation of skin creases (bleomycin), to a supravenous serpentine hyperpigmentation (5-fluorouracil and vinorelbine). Bleomycin also causes flagellate erythema that resolves with prominent hyperpigmentation, or that may present as such. Reticulate hyperpigmentation has been reported after 5-fluorouracil administration.

> **Clinical Tip** Drug pigmentation may appear as brown, brown-gray, blue-gray, slate-gray, violet-brown, or reddish-brown macules. These may or may not be photodistributed. Other patterns include linear, serpentine, and reticulate macules.

In summary, brown macules may be caused by infections (tinea nigra), inflammation (postinflammatory hyperpigmentation), benign conditions (nevi, other benign melanocytic lesions, and mastocytosis), malignancy (melanoma), or medications (drug hyperpigmentation).

Brown papules, nodules, or plaques may be melanocytic neoplasms or seborrheic keratoses. Compound nevi are light brown or midbrown papules. Melanomas may be darkly pigmented or variegated papules, plaques, or nodules that may have black, white, red, and gray areas, or melanomas may be amelanotic. Dermatofibromas may be skin-colored, brown, or pink. They are firm to hard papules or occasionally nodules that dimple on lateral pressure. Pigmented basal cell cancers may have a stippled or solid brown, black, or gray appearance. Granulomatous conditions may appear brown, red-brown, orange-brown, yellow-brown, or sometimes a maroon color (see section titled "The Purple Spectrum" below). The most frequently encountered of these is granuloma annulare (Figure 4.3B). Sarcoidosis and lupus vulgaris, variants of cutaneous tuberculosis, are rarer. Granulomatous rosacea presents with small red-brown papules on the central face. Lupus miliaris disseminatus faciei (also known as acne agminata) displays similar papules on the convex surfaces of the face and around the eyelids. It is thought that this condition is a variant of granulomatous rosacea, and it responds well to tetracyclines.

> **Clinical Tip** Granulomatous papules, plaques, and nodules appear brown, red-brown or orange-brown, yellow-brown, or maroon.

Granuloma faciale (Figure 4.3C) presents on the face as brown-gray or red-brown plaques. It is considered by some to represent a chronic form of leukocytoclastic vasculitis. No granulomas are seen histopathologically, but there is a dense infiltrate of neutrophils, eosinophils, lymphocytes, and plasma cells in the dermis. The fibrotic stage of erythema elevatum diutinum, another form of chronic leukocytoclastic vasculitis, appears as brown nodules over extensor aspects. The papules of secondary syphilis are classically described as being copper or "ham-colored." The indurated plaques of morphea may appear brown, yellow-brown, or white. In atrophoderma of Pasini and Pierini, there are softer, slightly depressed plaques with a "cliff-drop edge." The plaques appear light brown. This condition usually occurs on the back. Some authors believe that this entity represents a late stage of morphea, and others believe it to be a superficial variant of morphea. Finally, acanthotic conditions, such as acanthosis nigricans and confluent and reticulated papillomatosis of Gougerot and Carteaud (CARP) (Figure 4.3D), and conditions with a thickened stratum corneum, such as keratodermas with transgrediens, appear brown, especially in darker skin types. CARP lesions may be raised and ridged (papillated) or atrophic. It is a disorder of uncertain etiology that occurs on the upper trunk and less frequently on the neck. In erythrokeratodermia variabilis, figurate erythematous plaques are seen in childhood. As the patient ages, fixed brown hyperkeratotic plaques begin to appear especially on the trunk and limbs, sparing the folds. A generally thickened epidermis, as is seen in epidermal nevi, also renders a brown color to the constituent papules and plaques.

Brown Papules, Nodules, or Plaques may be seen in:

- Melanocytic neoplasms
- Other benign and malignant neoplasms
- Granulomatous conditions
- Granuloma faciale, erythema elevatum diuntinum
- Secondary syphilis
- Sclerotic conditions
- Mast cell proliferation as in urticaria pigmentosa
- Conditions with thickened stratum corneum

Table 4.3 summarizes brown groupings and configurations. Annular brown patterning occurs with postinflammatory hyperpigmentation from annular dermatoses such as tinea corporis and pityriasis rosea. Annular sarcoidosis may appear brown or red-brown. Annular plaques known as "nickels and dimes" are a manifestation of secondary syphilis that is typically seen on the face, usually in darker skin types. Tertiary syphilis presents as copper-colored coalescing papules and nodules that form annuli and arcuate and serpiginous configurations.

Linear brown macules may occur secondary to an "outside job," such as phytophotodermatitis, or an "inside job," such as macules that follow Blaschko lines. Phytophotodermatitis occurs after contact with plants or fruits that contain furocoumarins or psoralens. These chemicals act as photosensitizers and give rise to a phototoxic reactions in areas of contact. Linear and geometric red macules resolve with a prominent brown pigmentation. Linear and whorled hypermelanosis and the third stage of incontinentia pigmenti follow Blaschko lines (a whorled configuration is seen here, too). Flagellate erythema, caused by bleomycin, may present purely with hyperpigmented

TABLE 4.3. Brown, by Grouping or Configuration

LINEAR
- Phytophotodermatitis (also geometric)
- Serpentine supravenous hyperpigmentation from chemotherapy (also serpentine)
- Flagellate erythema
  - Flagellate erythema of chemotherapy
  - Adult-onset Still's disease
- Blaschko lines (also whorled)
  - Linear and whorled hypermelanosis
  - Third stage of incontinentia pigmenti
  - Epidermal nevi and systematized verrucous nevus (ichthyosis hystrix)

ANNULAR
- Postinflammatory following tinea corporis, pityriasis rosea, or urticarial vasculitis
- Annular sarcoidosis
- Secondary syphilis
- Tertiary syphilis

AGMINATE
- Lupus miliaria disseminata faciei (acne agminata)
- Agminated Spitz nevi
- Leiomyomas
- Melanoma metastases

RETICULATE
- Inherited
  - Dowling–Degos disease (reticulate pigmented anomaly of flexures)
  - Reticulate acropigmentation of Kitamura
  - Dermatopathia pigmentosa reticularis
  - Naegeli–Franceschetti–Jadassohn syndrome
  - Dyskeratosis congenita
  - Epidermolysis bullosa simplex with mottled pigmentation
- Acquired
  - Erythema ab igne
  - CARP
  - Prurigo pigmentosa
  - Reticulate hyperpigmentation from intravenous 5-fluorouracil

streaks, or a prolonged period of hyperpigmentation may follow the erythematous phase. The chronic skin findings in adult-onset Still's disease present as itchy, persistent, reddish-brown linear plaques on the trunk.

Agminated brown papules of lupus miliaris disseminata faciei are reddish brown or orange-brown. Clusters of Spitz nevi are not infrequently seen; these pink or brown papules develop early in life in a localized area or segment on the face or an upper limb. Leiomyomas are reddish-brown or flesh-colored elongated papules that may arise in clusters or within a Blaschko line. A "do not miss" diagnosis in agminated brown papules is local metastases of melanoma (satellitosis), where papules or nodules cluster around a melanoma or melanoma excision scar. These may also be amelanotic or black.

The differential diagnosis of the brown reticulate configuration houses many rare inherited conditions as can be seen in Table 4.3 and in further detail in Chapter 11, as well as some acquired conditions that are rare or uncommon. Of these, erythema ab igne and CARP are most rarely seen. In erythema ab igne, a livedoid lacy pattern of brown or red-brown macules can occur in areas of chronic heat or infrared exposure. Prurigo pigmentosa is a rare inflammatory disorder that presents with pruritic papules on the trunk and neck that coalesce and resolve, leaving reticulate hyperpigmentation.

Table 4.4 displays a differential diagnosis for brown by distribution. Hyperkeratosis of elbows and knees that occurs as part of a keratoderma appears dark brown, especially in darker skin types.

TABLE 4.4. Brown, by Distribution

PHOTOEXPOSED AREAS
- Pellagra
- Photoaccentuated drug pigmentation—antimalarials, minocycline
- Photoaccentuated systemic hyperpigmentation: chronic renal insufficiency, primary biliary cirrhosis
- Phytophotodermatitis
- Xeroderma pigmentosum

SEBORRHEIC
- Tinea versicolor
- CARP
- Darier disease

FLEXURES
- Postinflammatory hyperpigmentation from atopic or formaldehyde contact dermatitis
- Flexural pigmentation in vitamin B_{12} deficiency

FLEXURES AND INTERTRIGINOUS AREAS
- Erythrasma
- Dowling–Degos disease

INTERTRIGINOUS
- Acanthosis nigricans

PALMS AND SOLES
- Postinflammatory hyperpigmentation, seen especially in darker skin
- Vitamin B_{12} deficiency
- Tinea nigra
- Melanocytic nevi
- Melanoma

EXTENSORS
- Hyperkeratosis of elbows and knees as part of a keratoderma

DORSAL HANDS
- Acanthosis nigricans
- Vitamin B_{12} deficiency
- Photoinduced conditions; see "photoexposed areas," this table, above
- Keratodermas with transgrediens
- Reticulate acropigmentation of Kitamura
- Dyschromatosis symmetrica hereditaria

WHITE

White in the skin may be generalized or localized. Causes of a generalized white color will be considered with the causes of other white macules.

The differential diagnosis of white macules is broad. An etiologic classification may be used to create a differential diagnosis as seen in Table 4.5. Alternatively, a morphologic classification and creating differential diagnostic lists based on the primary lesion are valuable tools for clinicians (Table 4.6).

In appraising white macules on the skin, a convenient initial decision point is whether they are hypo- or depigmented. This decision may in most cases be made with the naked eye. In cases of doubt, Wood's lamp (see Chapter 14) may be employed for clarification. Depigmented macules appear bright white or milk-white under Wood's lamp, whereas hypopigmented macules are more of a yellow-white color. The differential diagnosis of depigmented macules is a fairly short and encapsulated list. Vitiligo is the most commonly encountered dermatosis that presents with white macules (Figure 1.2A). In albinism, there is global absence of pigment in the skin. Depigmented macules are also seen in chronic eczema, such as atopic dermatitis, secondary to disruption of the basement membrane zone from scratching. Chemical leukoderma is rare; it usually occurs as a result of cutaneous exposure to aromatic or aliphatic derivatives of phenols and catechols, such as monobenzyl ether of hydroquinone and chloroquine. Drug-induced vitiligo-like depigmentation should be considered for new-onset vitiligo in patients on immunotherapy. A "do not miss" diagnosis in new-onset vitiligo in a patient with a prior history of a melanoma is that of new-onset metastatic disease. The leukoderma of scleroderma (Figure 4.4A) may occur in normal or sclerotic skin. Perifollicular pigment retention is characteristic. Treponemal diseases may present with depigmented and hypopigmented macules. Pinta, for example, is a rare cause of depigmented macules and it also is a rare cause of hypopigmented macules. In the late stages of pinta, hypopigmented macules arise over bony prominences, and these become depigmented with time. It has been hypothesized, but never proven, that the causative organism has an inhibitory effect on the melanocyte. Yaws and bejel are also rare; similar changes to pinta are seen in tertiary yaws and bejel, but truncal sites such as the areolae and genitals may also be involved. In onchocerciasis, tiny hypopigmented macules on the shins enlarge, coalesce, and lighten, becoming depigmented. These spread to involve other areas of the legs and the lower abdomen. The etiopathogenesis is unclear. With appropriate treatment, hypopigmented, but not depigmented, macules resolve.

The differential diagnosis of hypopigmented macules is broad. It encompasses not only postinflammatory hypopigmentation from a variety of dermatoses but also a number or primary dermatoses. Common causes include postinflammatory hypopigmentation from a variety of causes, tinea versicolor, and flat warts (that may be so flat as to resemble macules). Pityriasis lichenoides chronica and seborrheic dermatitis (Figure 4.4B) commonly leave hypopigmentation in their wake, especially in darker skin types. Pityriasis alba, a form of eczema, is largely hypopigmented. Psoriasis can resolve with hypopigmentation. Nevus anemicus, which is not a pigmentary disorder per se but rather a localized area of sympathetic hyperactivity in the skin, leads to a hypopigmented macule because of relative vasoconstriction in the area (Figure 4.4C). *Progressive macular hypomelanosis* refers to the hypopigmented macules that are usually seen on the trunk of young women. They are not preceded by inflammation.

TABLE 4.5. White Macules, by Etiologic Classification

INHERITED

- Albinism
- Piebaldism
- Nevoid hypopigmentation (including hypomelanosis of Ito and nevus depigmentosus)
- Fourth stage of incontinentia pigmenti
- Tuberous sclerosis: segmental, oval, ash leaf, polygonal, confetti-like macules
- Albopapuloid (Pasini) variant of dominant dystrophic epidermolysis bullosa
- Keratosis follicularis (Darier disease): leukodermic macules
- Guttate macules with keratosis punctata
- Nevus anemicus

ACQUIRED

- Infectious
  - Tinea versicolor
  - Flat warts in a dark skin: may be so thin as to appear as macules.
  - Epidermodysplasia verruciformis
  - Pinta
  - Yaws, bejel
  - Secondary syphilis leukoderma syphiliticum
    - Leukoderma syphiliticum
    - "Necklace of Venus"
    - More generalized as a postinflammatory phenomenon
  - Leprosy: any subtype
  - Onchocerciasis
  - Progressive macular hypomelanosis
- Inflammatory
  - Vitiligo
  - Vitiligo-like leukoderma associated with scleroderma or metastatic melanoma
  - Neonatal lupus
  - Halo nevus
  - Pityriasis alba
  - Depigmentation associated with scratching from chronic eczema
  - Hypopigmented sarcoidosis: a rare variant of sarcoidosis
- Postinflammatory
  - Postinflammatory hypopigmentation
- Neoplastic
  - Hypopigmented mycosis fungoides
  - Seborrheic keratoses in a dark skin
  - Tumor of the follicular infundibulum
- Drug
  - Chemical leukoderma
  - Posttopical or intralesional/intraarticular steroids
  - Arsenic exposure: guttate macules
  - Vitiligo-like depigmentation
    - Tyrosine kinase inhibitors: imatinib, gefitinib
    - Programmed cell death 1 (PD1) inhibitors: nivolumab
    - BRAF inhibitors: vemurafenib, dabrafenib
    - Ipilimumab
    - Tumor necrosis factor α inhibitors: infliximab, adalimumab
- Idiopathic
  - Idiopathic guttate hypomelanosis

TABLE 4.6. White Macules, by Morphologic Classification

DEPIGMENTED MACULES
- Generalized
  - Albinism
- Segmental
  - Vitiligo
- Localized
  - Piebaldism
  - Vitiligo
  - Vitiligo-like leukoderma in scleroderma or metastatic melanoma
  - Chemical leukoderma
  - Vitiligo-like depigmentation from systemic drugs
  - Halo around halo nevus
  - Chronic eczema
  - Pinta, yaws, bejel
  - Onchocerciasis

HYPOPIGMENTED
- Blaschko lines
  - Nevoid hypopigmentation (hypomelanosis of Ito, nevus depigmentosus)
  - Fourth stage of incontinentia pigmenti
  - Lichen striatus
- Segmental
  - Tuberous sclerosis
  - Nevus depigmentosus
- Guttate
  - Confetti-like macules of tuberous sclerosis
  - Idiopathic guttate hypomelanosis
  - Darier disease: leukodermic macules
  - Multiple tumors of follicular infundibulum
  - Arsenic exposure
  - Seborrheic keratoses in a dark skin
  - Flat warts and epidermodysplasia verruciformis in a dark skin
  - Pinta
  - Pityriasis alba
  - In association with keratosis punctata
- Other: typically single macule
  - Nevus anemicus
- Other: typically multiple macules
  - Tinea versicolor
  - Pityriasis alba
  - Oval, ash leaf, polygonal macules of tuberous sclerosis
  - Neonatal lupus
  - Hypopigmented mycosis fungoides
  - Hypopigmented sarcoidosis
  - Leprosy; any subtype
  - Pinta, yaws, bejel
  - Onchocerciasis
  - Postinflammatory hypopigmentation

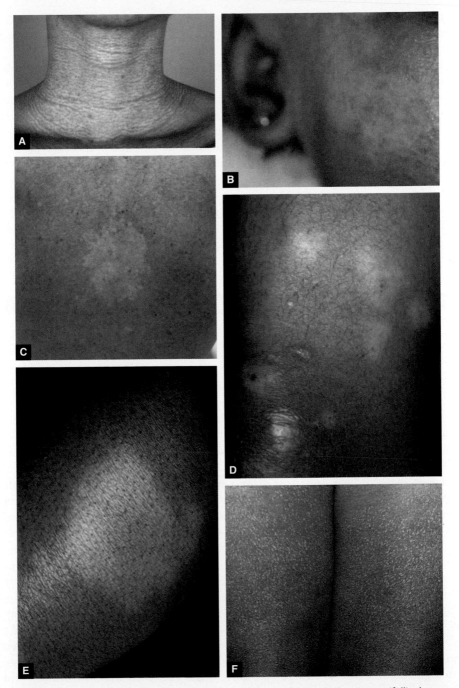

FIGURE 4.4 • Examples of white macules: (A) Leukoderma of scleroderma showing perifollicular retention of pigment; (B) seborrheic dermatitis with postinflammatory hypopigmentation; (C) nevus anemicus displaying a sizeable white macule on the back; (D) hypopigmented sarcoid with hypopigmented
macules on an extremity; (E) hypopigmented patches of borderline tuberculoid leprosy; (F) guttate leukodermic macules of Darier disease. (Image (B) used with permission from Dr. Deepak Modi, Department
of Dermatology, University of the Witwatersrand, Johannesburg, South Africa; Image (E) appears with
permission from VisualDx. Copyright VisualDx..)

They are nummular in shape and may be confluent centrally. It is thought that *Proprionebacterium acnes* plays a pathogenic role. The "do not miss" diagnostic tetrad in hypopigmented macules comprises the hypopigmented sarcoid (Figure 4.4D), hypopigmented mycosis fungoides, leprosy (Figure 4.4E), and secondary syphilis. These diagnoses may also be confirmed by the presence of thin white plaques. The hypopigmented form of sarcoid is a rare manifestation of sarcoid. Macules or thin plaques are present. Hypopigmented mycosis fungoides usually presents in younger individuals. It is more easily appreciated, and therefore more easily diagnosed, in individuals with darker skin phototypes. Scale may be minimal in this subtype. The indeterminate form of leprosy may be appreciated as a hypopigmented macule. This is the initial lesion that may then progress to either the tuberculoid or the lepromatous side of the leprosy spectrum, which may all occasionally present with hypopigmented macules. Secondary syphilis rarely presents with hypopigmented macules, known as *leukoderma syphiliticum*. The "necklace of Venus" is a finding that is seen on the lateral neck 3–4 months after infection; 1–2-mm hypomelanotic macules are seen within a larger hyperpigmented macule.

The "Do Not Miss" Diagnostic Tetrad of White Macules:

- Hypopigmented sarcoid
- Hypopigmented mycosis fungoides
- Leprosy
- Secondary syphilis

Conceptualizing macules as single or multiple, or as generalized or localized, may be advantageous in subcategorizing these dermatoses. The size of macules and their distribution may also assist in differentiating diseases; guttate white macules, or white macules in a segment or in Blaschko lines, can be valuable clinical pointers that can help to narrow diagnoses. The differential diagnosis of guttate white macules (small, raindrop-like) includes commonly encountered and rarer dermatoses. Flat warts or seborrheic keratosis in a darker skin phototype may appear white. *Idiopathic guttate hypomelanosis* refers to the presence of multiple small white macules in sun-damaged skin. Tuberous sclerosus may present with confetti-type white macules as well as the more typical larger ash-leaf macule or macules. Very rarely encountered guttate white macules include those seen in Darier disease (Figure 4.4F; onset of these leukodermic macules is in childhood, and they are appreciated more frequently in patients with darker skin phototypes), in arsenic exposure (raindrop-like hypopigmentation is seen on the trunk), and as a presentation of single or multiple tumors of the follicular infundibulum (seen on the neck and upper torso). Segmental white macules include segmental vitiligo (depigmented; a type of vitiligo with early onset that is treatment-resistant) and nevus depigmentosus (hypopigmented; a type of nevoid hypopigmentation involving a single segment).

Figure 4.5 summarizes the possible approaches to white macules. The initial decision point may be to determine whether there is depigmentation or hypopigmentation, as seen in Figure 4.5A. An alternative approach is to classify white macules initially by their pattern and then by whether they are de- or hypopigmented, as seen in

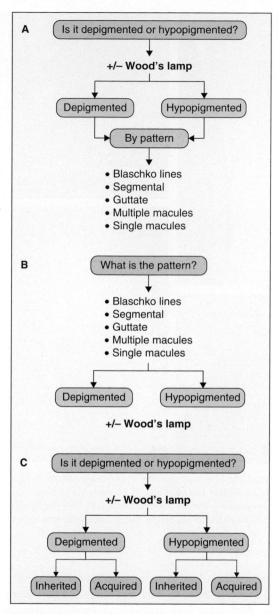

FIGURE 4.5 · Approaches to white macules.

Figure 4.5B. A third approach is to combine the etiologic and morphologic approaches together as seen in Figure 4.5C.

White plaques are usually atrophic, as seen in lichen sclerosus, morphea (Figure 4.6A), and scars. Late-stage pinta may also appear atrophic. A specific type of white ("porcelain-white") describes atrophic scars that appear bright white like porcelain. The end-stage scars of two diseases are classically porcelain-white: malignant atrophic papulosis (Degos disease) and livedoid vasculopathy (atrophie blanche; Figure 4.6B). Punctate red papules stippled over the plaque's surface are a feature of

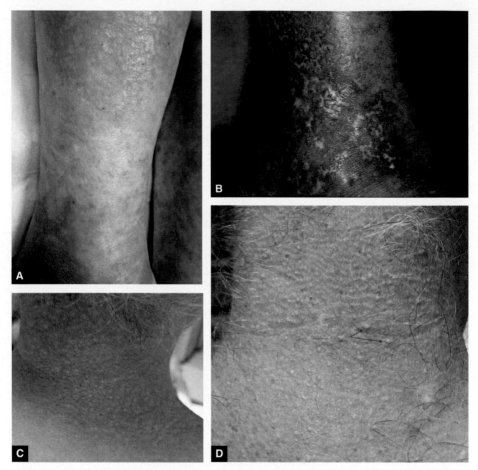

FIGURE 4.6 • Examples of white dermatoses other than macules: (A) White papules and plaques in a case of coexisting lichen sclerosus and morphea; (B) atrophie blanche with porcelain-white small depressed plaques on the medial ankle; (C) fibroelastolytic papulosis displaying 3–4-mm white papules on the posterior neck; (D) fibrofolliculomas of Birt–Hogg–Dube syndrome with 1-mm white papules on the posterior neck.

both. Malignant atrophic papulosis is a veno-occlusive systemic disease, although less malignant forms localized to the skin have also been reported. Dermatologically there are crops of papules that evolve into atrophic scars with a porcelain-white center and a telangiectatic rim. Livedoid vasculopathy is more usually seen in the setting of vari-cose veins on the medial ankle and lower medial calf. In those without varicose veins, hypercoagulable states, as outlined in Table 4.7, need to be excluded. Idiopathic cases may also occur.

Porcelain-White Depressed Papules and Small Plaques are Seen in:
• Malignant atrophic papulosis (Degos disease)
• Livedoid vasculopathy (atrophie blanche)

TABLE 4.7. Hypercoagulable States Reported with Livedoid Vasculopathy

- Antiphospholipid syndrome
- Factor V Leiden heterozygosity/homozygosity
- Protein C or protein S deficiency
- Hyperhomocysteinemia
- Methylenetetrahydrofolate reductase gene mutations
- Antithrombin III deficiency
- Prothrombin gene mutation
- Cryoglobulinemia, cryofibronogenemia

White papules are milia, tiny cysts, calcium deposits, tophi, extragenital lichen sclerosus, or rarely, fibroelastolytic papulosis (Figure 4.6C). Lichen sclerosus in extragenital sites presents with flat white papules with follicular prominence and scale (Figure 4.6A). *Fibroelastolytic papulosis* is a term that has been proposed to encompass the spectrum of histopathologic change that is seen in white fibrous papulosis of the neck (WFPN) and papillary dermal elastolysis (PDE). These conditions are overlapping disorders that are seen in middle-aged women on the posterior aspect of the neck. The antecubital fossae and the axillae may be involved. Clinically, there are discrete or confluent white or yellowish papules. Histologically, WFPN shows increased collagen (fibrosis) in the reticular dermis with early loss of elastic fibers, and PDE shows normal collagen, but a loss of elastic fibers in the dermis. Degenerative changes secondary to ultraviolet light have been proposed as the inciting cause.

Another rarely encountered disorder that presents with white papules is Birt–Hogg–Dube syndrome, in which fibrofolliculomas (Figure 4.6D) and trichodiscomas are seen. They are 1–2-mm white papules that arise on the face, neck, in the axillae and antecubital folds, and more generally.

Cysts, calcium deposits, or tophi may also be seen as white nodules.

White Papules and Nodules

Papules:
- Milia
- Extragenital lichen sclerosus
- Fibrofolliculomas, trichodiscomas
- Fibroelastolytic papulosis

Papules or nodules:
- Cysts
- Calcium deposits
- Tophi

The general approach to white in the skin can be consolidated with the wheel of diagnosis, as seen in Figure 4.7, and its associated tables (Tables 4.8 and 4.9). Table 4.8 enumerates the differential diagnosis of white lesions by grouping and distribution. White annuli are seen in psoriasis, active morphea, lichenoid melanodermatitis, and leprosy. Halo nevi are nevi with a surrounding ring of depigmentation. Woronoff ring is a poorly understood phenomenon where a psoriatic plaque is surrounded by a ring of hypopigmentation. It may occur in treated or untreated psoriasis. In active morphea, the center may be white and the active annular border may be pink or violaceous. Lichenoid melanodermatitis is rare; it is a variant of pityriasis alba that is seen in darker

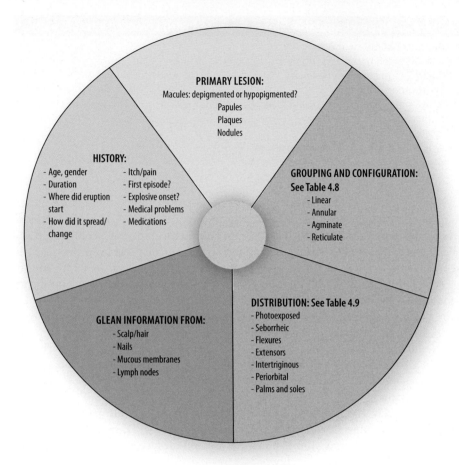

PRIMARY LESION:
Macules: depigmented or hypopigmented?
Papules
Plaques
Nodules

HISTORY:
- Age, gender   - Itch/pain
- Duration   - First episode?
- Where did eruption   - Explosive onset?
  start   - Medical problems
- How did it spread/   - Medications
  change

GROUPING AND CONFIGURATION:
See Table 4.8
   - Linear
   - Annular
   - Agminate
   - Reticulate

DISTRIBUTION: See Table 4.9
- Photoexposed
- Seborrheic
- Flexures
- Extensors
- Intertriginous
- Periorbital
- Palms and soles

GLEAN INFORMATION FROM:
   - Scalp/hair
   - Nails
   - Mucous membranes
   - Lymph nodes

FIGURE 4.7 • The wheel of diagnosis, customized to white.

skin phototypes. Centrally, in these thin plaques on the face, there is hyperpigmentation, which is surrounded by a ring of hypopigmentation. A "do not miss" diagnosis
in white annuli is leprosy, including tuberculoid, borderline tuberculoid (Figure 4.4F),
and borderline subtypes.

The distribution of white lesions is presented in Table 4.9. Regarding depigmented macules on the face, vitiligo is most frequent. A perioral and periorbital
distribution is common. Segmental vitiligo is also seen in this location. If vitiliginous macules are associated with hearing loss, two rare syndromes should
be considered. Alezzandrini syndrome is characterized by the presence of unilateral vitiligo on the face that may be accompanied by ipsilateral hearing and
visual loss and poliosis. Vogt–Koyanagi–Harada syndrome is a similar autoimmune phenomenon with bilateral involvement. Inherited diseases with vitiliginous macules should be considered in early-onset disease, and these include
piebaldism and Waardenburg syndrome. In piebaldism, the central parts of limbs
and trunk are depigmented. The central face may be similarly affected. Various
subtypes of Waardenburg syndrome have been identified. In general, these may

TABLE 4.8. White, by Grouping or Configuration

LINEAR
- Blaschko lines (also whorled)
  - Nevoid hypopigmentation (hypomelanosis of Ito, nevus depigmentosus)
  - Fourth stage of incontinentia pigmenti
  - Lichen striatus
- Segmental
  - Segmental vitiligo
  - Tuberous sclerosis
  - Nevus depigmentosus
- Koebner phenomenon
  - As seen in vitiligo
- Autoinoculation
  - Flat warts
- Striae, and other scars (secondary lesions)

ANNULAR
- Woronoff ring of psoriasis
- Halo nevus
- Active morphea
- Lichenoid melanodermatitis
- Leprosy

PHYLLOID
- Ash-leaf macules of tuberous sclerosis
- Trisomy 13

present with poliosis (white hair, including a white forelock), heterochromic irides, broad nasal bridge and dystopia canthorum, and depigmented piebaldism-like macules. For depigmented macules in this location in a newborn, consider neonatal lupus. For hypopigmented facial macules, consider postinflammatory change after seborrheic dermatitis. Pityriasis alba is also seen in this location, commonly in children. Regarding white papules on the face, consider milia, cysts, or benign adnexal tumors, such as fibrofolliculomas and trichodiscomas. Multiple 1–2-mm firm whitish papules may be seen in miliary osteoma cutis, a rarely encountered sequela of acne.

A common site for vitiligo is the extensor aspects of the extremities, including the elbows, knees, and over the joints of the hands and feet. For white papules or nodules over extensors, consider tophi. Scaly plaques with particularly white scales include psoriasis and keratoderma with transgrediens. The elbows, knees, and extensor extremities are sites of predilection for these dermatoses.

On the dorsal hands, white papules may be flat warts (including those of epidermodysplasia verruciformis), actinic keratosis (white, gritty-feeling scale), or milia (as may be seen secondary to deep blistering diseases such as porphyria cutanea tarda or epidermolysis bullosa acquisita). In dyschromatosis symmetrica hereditaria (reticulate acropigmentation of Dohi), a very rare inherited dermatosis, hypopigmented macules appear on dorsal hands in childhood. Hyperpigmented macules then appear in association.

TABLE 4.9. White, by Distribution

SEBORRHEIC
- Tinea versicolor
- Progressive macular hypomelanosis
- Postinflammatory hypopigmentation from seborrheic dermatitis

FACE
- Pityriasis alba (cheeks)
- Postinflammatory hypopigmentation from seborrheic dermatitis (nasolabial folds, beard area)
- Discoid lupus erythematosus: end stage
- Neonatal lupus
- Segmental vitiligo
- Alezzandrini syndrome
- Vogt–Koyanagi–Harada syndrome
- Piebaldism
- Wardenburg syndrome
- Fibrofolliculomas, trichodiscomas
- Milia, cysts
- Osteoma cutis

EXTENSORS
- Vitiligo: has a predilection for sites of trauma, including the bony prominences of the elbows and knees
- Psoriasis: silvery or white scales
- Keratoderma with transgrediens—scale may appear white
- Tophi ·

DORSAL HANDS
- Flat warts and epidermodysplasia verruciformis
- Actinic keratosis: scale appears white
- Vitiligo, especially over bony prominences
- Keratoderma with transgrediens
- Milia from porphyria cutanea tarda
- Dyschromatosis symmetrica hereditaria

YELLOW

Yellow in the skin may be generalized or localized. Diffuse yellowing of the skin is seen secondary to the deposition of bile pigments in jaundice, carotenoids in carotenemia, and lycopenes in lycopenemia (orange-yellow color). In carotenemia, palms, soles, the tip of the nose, and the nasolabial folds are preferentially affected as a result of carotenoids being excreted by sebaceous and sweat glands. In chronic renal insufficiency, urobilin (a breakdown product of heme that is normally excreted in the urine) confers a yellowish hue. A diffuse yellow discoloration of the skin has been reported from sorafenib, a multikinase inhibitor that is effective in advanced renal and pancreatic cancer. Here, a dye used in the formulation of the drug is thought to be responsible. The dye contained in mepacrine is also deposited in the skin. A bright yellow or greenish-yellow color is seen on the face, hands, and feet initially. This color then generalizes, and flexural areas may also be prominently involved.

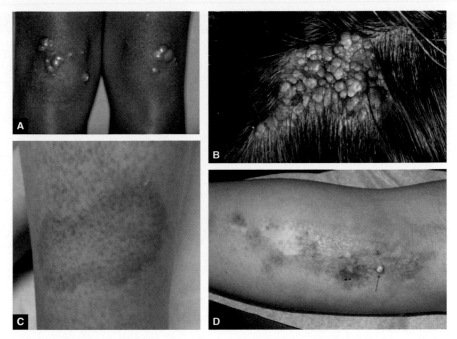

FIGURE 4.8 • Examples of yellow dermatoses: (A) Tuberous xanthomas displaying yellow papules and nodules over the knees; (B) nevus sebaceus showing a yellow papillated plaque on the scalp; (C) necrobiosis lipoidica showing yellow plaques on the shin; (D) calcinosis cutis arising within a plaque of linear morphea.

A localized yellow color in the skin may be from lipid deposition, either within macrophages, as seen in xanthomas except tendinous xanthomas, which are flesh-colored (Figure 4.8A), xanthogranulomas (which may appear yellow or orange), or within sebaceous structures. A comprehensive differential diagnosis of yellow by primary lesion is summarized in Table 4.10.

A complete list of the types of xanthomas, incuding their classic clinical appearance, sites of predilection, and associated conditions, may be found in Table 4.11. Table 4.12 lists the xanthogranulomatous conditions that typically appear as yellow papules, plaques, or nodules. These are non-Langerhans cell histiocytoses that infiltrate the skin and internal organs. Secondary lipid accumulation within histiocytoses renders lesions yellow. Sebaceous material in Fordyce spots, nevus sebaceus (Figure 4.8B), and sebaceous hyperplasia confers a yellow color to these lesions. Sebaceous adenomas, sebaceomas, and sebaceous carcinomas are also occasionally yellow. Juxtaclavicular beaded lines are the linear arrays of monomorphic yellow papules that are found on the neck and upper chest in sun-damaged skin. Histopathologically, these represent sebaceous glands.

The plaques of necrobiosis lipoidica appear yellow in later stages (Figure 4.8C). Histopathologically, there is extracellular lipid between collagen bundles in the superficial dermis, which confers the yellow color.

Lipid deposition is seen in:	
• Xanthomas	• Sebaceous structures
• Xanthogranulomas	• Necrobiosis lipoidica

TABLE 4.10. Differential Diagnosis of Yellow in the Skin by Primary Lesion

GENERALIZED, MACULAR
- Jaundice
- Carotenemia: predilection for palms, soles, nose, nasolabial folds
- Lycopenemia
- Drug-related pigmentation: sorafenib, mepacrine

PAPULES
- Fordyce spots
- Juxtaclavicular beaded lines
- Sebaceous hyperplasia
- Sebaceous adenoma
- Sebaceous carcinoma
- Eruptive xanthomas

PAPULES AND PLAQUES
- Xanthelasma
- Necrobiotic xanthogranuloma
- Orbital xanthogranuloma
- Xanthoma disseminatum
- Erdheim–Chester syndrome
- Pseudoxanthoma elasticum
- Fibroelastolytic papulosis

PLAQUES
- Palmar xanthoma
- Diffuse plane xanthoma
- Intertriginous xanthoma
- Nevus sebaceus
- Keratodermas
- Sclerodermoid conditions

PAPULES AND NODULES
- Gouty tophi
- Juvenile and adult xanthogranulomas
- Tuberous xanthomas

PAPULES, NODULES, OR PLAQUES
- Calcium deposits
- Connective tissue nevi
- Pustules (see Chapter 2 for a complete differential diagnosis)

Yellow also denotes the presence of pus. A complete discussion of the approach to pustules can be found in Chapter 2. Altered connective tissue may appear yellow. Examples include altered elastic tissue, such as pseudoxanthoma elasticum and fibroelastolytic papulosis (see section titled "White" above) and altered collagen, such as in morphea, scleroderma, and other sclerodermoid conditions. In perifollicular elastolysis, an anetodermatous form of scarring seen in acne, there is loss of elastin and collagen secondary to elastases and other proteases secreted by the neutrophils in acne. This appears as perifollicular yellow papules, usually on the back and sometimes seen on the chest. Connective tissue nevi may have excess collagen and/or elastin, and these appear yellow, too.

TABLE 4.11. Classification of Xanthomas, Their Predilection Sites, and Their Associated Systemic Conditions

PRIMARY LESION	TYPE OF XANTHOMA	SITES OF PREDILECTION	UNDERLYING SYSTEMIC DISORDER
Yellow or red-yellow papules with or without a red halo	Eruptive xanthoma	Extensor aspects of the extremities, including buttocks, shoulders, and thighs	Characteristic of pure hypertriglyceridemia, as seen in types I, IV, and V hyperlipoprotenemia, and in acquired causes, such as diabetes or from systemic retinoids
Yellow papules and nodules	Tuberous xanthoma	Elbows, knees, buttocks	Seen in patients with pure hypercholesterolemia, such as type IIA and mixed hyper-triglyceridemia and hypercholesterolemia, such as type III: acquired: nephrotic syndrome, hypothyroidism
Subcutaneous nodules, firm to hard, flesh-colored	Tendinous xanthoma	Extensor tendons of hands and feet; Achilles tendon	Seen in severe hypercholesterolemia, such as type IIA, or in cholestasis
Flat yellow papules, plaques	Xanthelasma (xanthelasma palpebrarum)	Superior and inferior eyelids	Normal lipid profile in up to half of patients. Any inherited hyperlipoproteinemia or acquired forms, such as cholestasis may be present
Flat yellow plaques	Palmar crease xanthomas (xanthoma striatum palmare) and palmar xanthomas	Palms and volar fingers	Mixed hypertriglycer-idemia and hyper-cholesterolemia, as seen in type III (familial dysbetalipoproteinemia); primary biliary cirrhosis; multiple myeloma
Widespread flat yellow plaques	Diffuse plane xanthomas	Trunk, neck, and face are classically involved	Type III hyperlipopro-teinemia, IgA monoclo-nal gammopathy, and myeloma
Yellow corrugated plaques	Intertriginous xanthomas	Finger webs, palmar creases, axillae, buttocks, and antecubital and popliteal fossae	Characteristic finding in type IIA

TABLE 4.12. Xanthogranulomatous Conditions Presenting with a Yellow Hue

CONDITION	SKIN FINDINGS	SYSTEMIC FINDINGS
Necrobiotic xanthogranuloma (NXG)	Yellow, orange, or yellow-red plaques, papules and nodules; occur initially periorbitally; face, trunk, and limbs may be involved; lesions may ulcerate	IgGκ gammopathy, IgGλ or IgA gammopathy more rarely seen; eye involvement (NXG extending intraocularly, conjunctivitis, keratitis, uveitis, corneal ulceration)
Orbital xanthogranuloma	Periorbital plaques, similar to NXG; slow extension over years	No systemic involvement
Xanthoma disseminatum	Red-brown papules and plaques become yellower with time; these involve the flexures, trunk, and proximal arms and legs	Infiltration of oral mucosa and respiratory tract, meninges, and bones; diabetes insipidus common
Erdheim–Chester disease	Xanthelasma and xanthoma disseminatum-like plaques and nodules are seen in the minority of cases	Sclerosis of long bones and infiltration of viscera, retroperitoneum, and the orbit occur

Calcium in the dermis may appear white or yellow. Calcium may be deposited in the skin in areas of local tissue damage (the dystrophic type) or in normal tissue in patients who have an underlying disorder of calcium metabolism (the metastatic type). Dystrophic calcification may be found in a broad range of diseases, including genetic, autoimmune, and iatrogenic types (Figure 4.8D). Panniculitis, neoplasms, and infections may also manifest secondary calcification. Metastatic calcification may be seen in primary or secondary hyperparathyroidism (as in chronic renal failure) and in hypervitaminosis D. Calcinosis cutis may also be idiopathic in some cases. Table 4.13 lists a comprehensive differential diagnosis of cutaneous calcification.

Urate deposition in gouty tophi may appear white, yellow, or orange. Finally, the thickened stratum corneum of palms and soles, as seen in inherited and acquired keratodermas, appears yellowish.

Yellowish greasy scales are typical of the papules and plaques of seborrheic dermatitis. Secondary lesions may also be yellow. Yellow crusting is seen in a wide variety of inflammatory conditions. Honey-colored crusts are typical of impetigo.

Differential Diagnosis of Yellow in the Skin: A Succinct View

Generalized
- Jaundice
- Chronic renal insufficiency
- Carotenemia
- Lycopenemia
- Medications: sorafenib, mepacrine

Localized
- Lipid deposition
- Pus
- Altered connective tissue
- Calcium
- Urate
- Keratodermas
- Yellow greasy scales of seborrheic dermatitis
- Crusts

TABLE 4.13. Clinical Variants of Cutaneous Calcification

DYSTROPHIC CALCIFICATION

- Inherited disorders
  - Pseudoxanthoma elasticum; there is secondary calcification of abnormal elastic fibers
  - Ehlers–Danlos syndrome; spherules are calcified herniated fat lobules that occur especially around joints
  - Werner syndrome
  - Rothmund–Thompson syndrome
  - Porphyria cutanea tarda: calcification of sclerodermoid plaques
- Acquired
  - Autoimmune connective tissue disease
    - Localized scleroderma: usually seen over bony prominences and tendons of hands and arms
    - Dermatomyositis: 4 common types exist:
      - Tumoral: subcutaneous, near joints
      - Popcorn-like: superficial deposits in skin
      - Along fascial planes and muscles
      - Severe "exoskeleton" pattern
    - Systemic lupus, discoid lupus, subacute cutaneous lupus, and scleroderma show dystrophic calcification within lesions less commonly
  - Panniculitis
    - Pancreatic panniculitis
    - Lupus profundus
    - Subcutaneous fat necrosis of the newborn
  - Iatrogenic
    - Calcified nodules on the heel of neonates from heel sticks
    - At extravasation sites of calcium-containing intravenous or intramuscular solutions
    - Trauma, surgical scars, keloids
    - Burn scars
  - Infections
    - Parasitic infections are the most common cause here, including calcified cysts around tapeworm larvae or filariae
  - Neoplasms
    - Benign: pilomatricomas, pilar and epidermal inclusion cysts, desmoplastic trichoepitheliomas, mixed tumors
    - Malignant: basal cell carcinomas, atypical fibroxanthomas

METASTATIC CALCIFICATION

- Papules and nodules that are in the deep dermis or subcutis occur in the intertriginous areas (axillae, inner thighs, vulva), the abdomen, and the flexures

IDIOPATHIC CALCIFICATION

- Subepidermal calcified nodule: solitary nodule on the head (especially the ear) or extremities of infants or children
- Scrotal calcinosis—usually numerous nodules are seen; these may represent the remnants of disintegrated calcified epidermal inclusion cysts
- Auricular calcinosis: involves cartilage of the ear as well as surrounding structures

TABLE 4.14. Yellow, by Grouping and Configuration

ANNULAR
- Pus
  - Subcorneal pustular dermatosis
  - IgA pemphigus
  - Dermatophytosis
  - Impetigo herpetiformis
  - Eosinophilic pustular folliculitis of Ofuji
- Lipid
  - Necrobiosis lipoidica
- Altered connective tissue
  - Active morphea

LINEAR
- Elastic tissue
  - Linear focal elastosis
  - Linear morphea
- Pus
  - Fire ant bites
  - Herpes zoster with pustules
- Lipid
  - Linear nevus sebaceus
  - Linear nevus sebaceous syndrome

HERPETIFORM
- Pus
  - Herpes simplex with pustules
  - Herpes zoster with pustules
  - Impetigo herpetiformis

"LAKES" OF PUS
- Generalized pustular psoriasis
- Acute generalized erythematous pustulosis
- Erosive pustular dermatosis of the scalp

Table 4.14 summarizes yellow groupings and configurations. Annular yellow lesions include the annular arrays of pustules that are typically seen in subcorneal pustular dermatosis, the intraepidermal neutrophilic type of IgA pemphigus, amicrobial pustulosis of the folds, and eosinophilic pustular folliculitis of Ofuji. Linear pustules connote fire ant bites or the pustular stage of zoster. Linear focal elastosis refers to the horizontal striae that occur on the lower back in teenagers undergoing a growth spurt. These may be yellow in color. Linear nevus sebaceous follows the lines of Blaschko and is typically located on the scalp or face. In the rarely encountered linear nevus sebaceous syndrome, a linear nevus sebaceous accompanies central nervous systemic, eye, and skeletal abnormalities. Herpetiform pustules are seen in the pustular stage of herpes and zoster, and in impetigo herpetiformis. Confluent superficial pustules form "lakes" of pus. This sign is seen in generalized pustular psoriasis, acute generalized exanthematous pustulosis (AGEP) and erosive pustular dermatosis of the scalp.

In Table 4.15, the characteristic distribution of yellow dermatoses is detailed. The periorbital location is a site of predilection for numerous yellow dermatoses as outlined in the table. The diagnostic wheel customized to yellow in seen in Figure 4.9.

TABLE 4.15. Yellow, by Distribution

FLEXURES
- Lipid
  - Xanthoma disseminatum
- Altered connective tissue
  - Pseudoxanthoma elasticum
  - Fibroelastolytic papulosis
- Calcium
  - Metastatic calcification

EXTENSORS
- Pus
  - Bowel-associated dermatosis–arthritis syndrome
  - Papulonecrotic tuberculide
- Lipid
  - Tuberous xanthomas
  - Eruptive xanthomas
  - Tendinous xanthomas
- Urate
  - Gouty tophi

INTERTRIGINOUS
- Pus
  - Bacterial folliculitis
  - Pseudofolliculitis
  - Candidiasis
  - Subcorneal pustular dermatosis
  - Eosinophilic pustular folliculitis of Ofuji
  - Amicrobial pustulosis of the folds
- Lipid
  - Xanthoma disseminatum
  - Intertriginous xanthomas
  - Erdheim–Chester disease
- Altered connective tissue
  - Pseudoxanthoma elasticum
  - Fibroelastolytic papulosis
- Calcium
  - Metastatic calcification

SEBORRHEIC
- Pus
  - Acne
  - *Pityrosporum* folliculitis
  - Eosinophilic pustular folliculitis of HIV
  - Neonatal cephalic pustulosis
  - Halogenodermas

(Continued)

TABLE 4.15. Yellow, by Distribution (continued)

SEBORRHEIC (CONT.)
- Altered connective tissue
  - Perifollicular elastolysis
- Yellow greasy scales
  - Seborrheic dermatitis

PALMS AND SOLES, INCLUDING DIGITS
- Carotenemia
- Pus
  - Infantile acropustulosis
  - Transient neonatal pustular melanosis—rare
  - Eosinophilic pustular folliculitis of infancy
  - Eosinophilic pustular folliculitis of Ofuji
  - Palmoplantar pustular psoriasis
  - Acrodermatitis continua of Hallopeau: can involve palmar aspects of fingers and plantar aspects of toes
  - SAPHO syndrome (synovitis, acne, pustulosis, hyperostosis, osteitis)
  - Papulonecrotic tuberculide
  - Longstanding eczema
  - Septic vasculitis: distal, acral, purpuric
  - Disseminated gonococcemia
  - Candidemia
  - Herpetic whitlow
  - Herpes simplex, zoster
  - Scabies: secondarily infected
  - Septic vasculitis: distal, acral, purpuric
  - Blistering distal dactylitis
  - Milker's nodule
- Lipid
  - Palmar crease and palmar xanthomas
  - Intertriginous xanthomas
- Keratodermas

PERIORBITAL
- Pus
  - Hordoleum
- Lipid
  - Xanthelasma
  - Plane xanthoma
  - Necrobiotic xanthogranuloma
  - Orbital xanthogranuloma
  - Erdheim–Chester disease
  - Sebaceous carcinoma
  - Steatoblepharon (eyelid fat prolapse)

RELATION TO APPENDAGES: FOLLICULAR
- See follicular pustule differential in Table 2.11

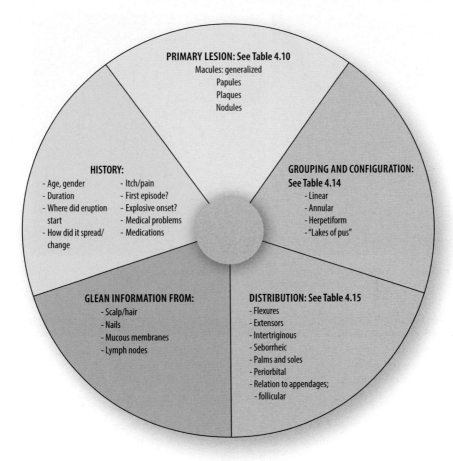

PRIMARY LESION: See Table 4.10
Macules: generalized
Papules
Plaques
Nodules

HISTORY:
- Age, gender   - Itch/pain
- Duration   - First episode?
- Where did eruption - Explosive onset?
  start   - Medical problems
- How did it spread/ - Medications
  change

GROUPING AND CONFIGURATION:
See Table 4.14
  - Linear
  - Annular
  - Herpetiform
  - "Lakes of pus"

GLEAN INFORMATION FROM:
  - Scalp/hair
  - Nails
  - Mucous membranes
  - Lymph nodes

DISTRIBUTION: See Table 4.15
- Flexures
- Extensors
- Intertriginous
- Seborrheic
- Palms and soles
- Periorbital
- Relation to appendages;
- follicular

FIGURE 4.9 · The wheel of diagnosis, customized to yellow.

ORANGE

The differential diagnosis of orange is a shorter list. As discussed above, tophi and xanthogranulomas, such as juvenile xanthogranuloma (Figure 4.10A), may appear orange. A list of the class II histiocytoses that classically present with an orange hue is found in Table 4.16. While the palmoplantar keratoderma of pityriasis rubra pilaris (PRP) is characteristically described as having an orange hue, the skin findings of PRP at large may also appear orange or red-orange. Zoon's plasma cell balanitis and plasma cell vulvitis may appear orange. This usually presents as one or more glistening plaques on the glans penis and prepuce. It may also be bright red, or rust-colored. Similarly, the benign pigmented purpuras may have a "cayenne pepper"-type appearance. Cayenne pepper is a deep rust color. Occasionally, shades of orange may be seen. In the Schamburg variant of pigmented purpura, showers of cayenne pepper-type macules may coalesce to form orange-brown macules. Lichen aureus is a subtype of benign pigmented purpura that presents with a solitary plaque on the leg. This may be yellow-brown or orange in color (Figure 4.10B).

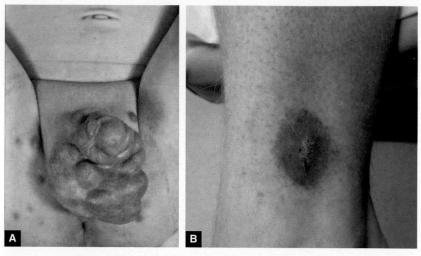

FIGURE 4.10 • Examples of orange dermatoses: (A) Juvenile xanthogranulomas on the scrotum of an infant; (B) lichen aureus showing an orange-brown plaque on the leg.

Differential Diagnosis of Orange

- Tophi
- Xanthogranuloma
- Pityriasis rubra pilaris
- Zoon's plasma cell balanitis/vulvitis
- Pigmented purpuras

Types II and II cryoglobulinema may present with a Schamburg appearance is association with tiny ulcers. Similarly, the rare purpuric variant of mycosis fungoides has been reported to resemble pigmented purpura.

> **Clinical Tip** Types II and III cryoglobulinemia and the purpuric form of mycosis fungoides may resemble pigmented purpura.

In terms of orange groupings and configurations, purpura annularis telangiectoides (of Majocchi) typically presents with cayenne pepper-type macules that are clustered

---

TABLE 4.16. Class II Histiocytoses That Commonly Present with an Orange Hue

CONDITION	SKIN FINDINGS	SYSTEMIC FINDINGS
Juvenile xanthogranuloma	Single or multiple orange or reddish-yellow papules or nodules; typically on the face, neck, scalp, and upper trunk	Eye, oral mucosal, visceral, and CNS involvement may occur
Benign progressive histiocytosis	Yellow-orange papules and red-orange nodules; may be diffuse	Conjunctivae, oral mucosa, and larynx may be involved

together to form annuli. Consider the diagnosis of PRP for any orangish keratoderma on palms and/or soles. PRP also presents with follicular papules. The orange color may or may not be discernible in these papules. Tophi are typically found on the ears (helix, anti-helix), hands, and feet (finger and toe pulps and over joints), and over the elbows and the Achilles tendons. Xanthogranulomas usually affect the face and other parts of the upper body. Pigmented purpuras classically involve the shins. They may spread to involve other parts of the lower extremities, and occasionally, truncal involvement is seen.

THE PURPLE SPECTRUM

A range of colors may be seen in the purple spectrum. *Purple, light purple, pinkish purple*, and *grayish purple* are on the blue side of the spectrum. This range of colors may be encountered in the conditions summarized in Table 4.17. These conditions are summarized in the textbox below.

Purple in the Skin is Caused by:

- Macules: fading erythema, incipient necrosis, interface dermatitides, drug pigmentation
- Papules, plaques: lichenoid dermatitides
- Plaques, nodules (the "purple plums"): benign and malignant vascular proliferations, cutaneous metastases, nonpigmented cutaneous tumors such as amelanotic melanoma and dermatofibrosarcoma protuberans

---

Maroon, plum, and *wine* colors are on the red side of the purple spectrum. Eccymoses, telangiectatic conditions, vasculitides, and vasculopathies may appear maroon or plum- or wine-colored. Granulomatous conditions, such as lupus vulgaris, may also have this color range, as may class II histiocytoses, such as cutaneous Rosai–Dorfman disease or generalized eruptive histiocytomas. The "purple plums" outlined above may also be in this color spectrum.

Clinical Tip Maroon signifies a vascular-related condition or granulomatous or histiocytic disease. The purple plums may also be a maroon color.

The word *violaceous* is sometimes used synonymously with *purple*. In terms of purple macules, *dusky* describes the grayish-purple color that is seen in the fading erythema of an exanthematous drug eruption, or in the beginnings of epidermal necrosis, as seen in toxic epidermal necrolysis or fixed drug eruption. Drug pigmentation may appear purple (as in the case of amiodarone or gold salts), or purple-brown (as with clofazimine).

With respect to papules and plaques, lichen planus is a light purple (Figure 4.11A; see also Figures 1.2E and 1.7). However, any shade of purple may be seen depending on the degree of inflammation and the background skin type. In fact, early papules, especially in a lighter skin types, may appear pink. Similarly, lichenoid drug eruptions, lichenoid graft versus host disease, and lichen planus/lupus erythematosus (LE/LP) overlap (plaques with lichen planus–like clinical and histopathological features occurring in a patient with lupus; Figure 4.11B) usually appear purple. Other dermatoses with a lichenoid histology that appear light purple or pinkish

---

TABLE 4.17. Purple Lesions

MACULES
- Dermatomyositis
  - Interphalangeal joint erythema of dermatomyositis
  - Linear macules over bony prominences
  - Flagellate erythema
  - "Shawl" sign
  - Photosensitive eruption that accompanies dermatomyositis
- Necrotic macules of SJS/TEN
- Fading erythema of an exanthematous drug eruption
- Drug-related pigmentation
  - Purple (as in the case of amiodarone or gold salts)
  - Purple-brown (as with clofazimine)

PAPULES AND PLAQUES
- Lichen planus
- Lichenoid drug eruption
- Lichenoid graft-versus-host disease
- Lichenoid benign pigmented purpura
- Lichenoid sarcoidosis
- Pityriasis lichenoides chronica
- Keratosis lichenoides chronica
- Any inflammation in dark skin

PAPULES OR NODULES "PURPLE PLUMS"
- Benign vascular proliferations
  - Pyogenic granuloma
  - Hemangioma
  - Glomeruloid and microvenular hemangioma
  - Bacillary angiomatosis
- Malignant neoplasms
  - Dermatofibrosarcoma protuberans
  - Amelanotic melanoma
  - Kaposi sarcoma
  - Lymphoma
  - Leukemia
  - Cutaneous metastases

---

purple include pityriasis lichenoides chronica (PLC; Figure 4.11C), lichenoid sarcoidosis, and lichenoid benign pigmented purpura (of Gougerot–Blum). Other conditions with a histopathologic interface dermatitis without a lymphocytic infiltrate may also be purple or pinkish-purple, such as dermatomyositis. Here, the superficial telangiectasias present are thought to be responsible for the color. Patterned macules, papules, or plaques, including those in the periorbital location (heliotrope rash), back of the neck and upper back ("shawl" sign), V of the neck ("V" sign; Figure 4.11D), lateral thighs ("holster" sign), interphalangeal joints [atrophic dermal papules of dermatomyositis (ADPDM), formerly known as Gottron papules; and the interphalangeal and metacarpophalangeal joint erythema of DM, formerly known as Gottron sign), linear erythema arising from elbows, knees, and the ulnar styloid, and flagellate erythema are seen. Patients with dermatomyositis may be photosensitive.

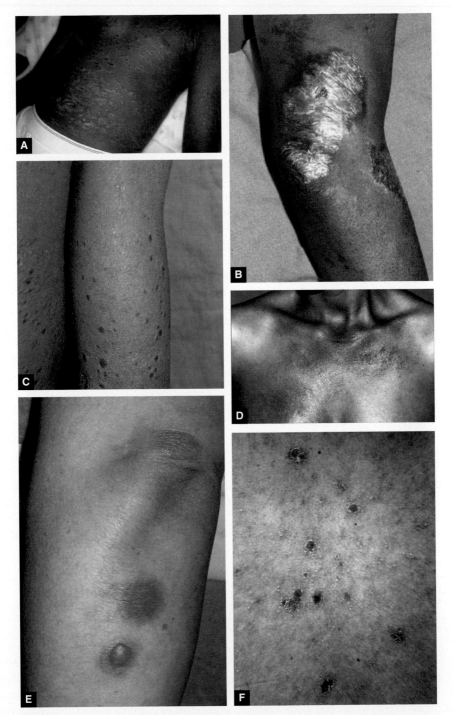

FIGURE 4.11 • (A) Violaceous plaques in lichen planus; (B) pink and purple plaque of LE/LP overlap on an extremity; (C) pityriasis lichenoides chronica with violaceous and flat-topped scaly papules; (D) dermatomyositis, showing a violaceous "V" sign; (E) early fixed drug eruption with a light purple appearance (Used with permission from Dr. Miguel Sanchez, New York University, New York, NY.); (F) pityriasis rosea with pityriasiform scale and a violaceous hue in a darker skin phototype.

The resultant photodistributed erythema may also have a violaceous hue. The eruption of dermatomyositis is described in general as being more violaceous and pruritic than that of systemic lupus erythematosus.

> **Clinical Tip** The dermatologic manifestations of dermatomyositis are protean. Consider this diagnosis in any patterned erythema with a violaceous hue.

Epidermal necrosis, such as that of early Stevens–Johnson syndrome/toxic epidermal necrolysis (SJS/TEN) and fixed drug eruption (Figure 4.11E), may appear dusky, violaceous, or gray.

As mentioned previously, any inflammation in a darker skin type may appear violaceous or purple, so the color loses its sensitivity in this setting. An example of this is seen in Figure 4.11F, which displays a case of pityriasis rosea in a darker skin phototype that presented with some violaceous papules and small plaques.

In generalized essential telangiectasia, engorged superficial telangiectasias may be appear red, maroon, or violaceous (Figure 4.12A). Angiokeratomas may appear purple, deep purple, or black (Figure 4.12B). In small and medium vessel vasculitis, a deep red, wine color or maroon color may eventuate from exuberant inflammation (Figure 4.12C) or from necrosis (Figure 4.12D). An ecchymotic appearance may occur in cases necrotizing vasculitis (Figure 4.12E). Deeper dermal necrosis in thrombotic vasculopathies, such as in calciphylaxis (Figure 4.12F) and warfarin necrosis, may also appear plum-colored, deep purple, livid, or gray-purple, before becoming black.

The differential diagnosis of purple nodules, also designated "purple plums," includes a range of vascular proliferations, as well as a range of nonbenign diagnoses. Purple plums may be pinkish-purple, maroon, or plum-colored. Hemangiomas, pyogenic granulomas, bacillary angiomatosis, and other benign vascular tumors may appear purple, maroon, or plum-colored. Kaposi sarcoma typically presents with purple or maroon macules, plaques, and nodules (Figure 4.13A). Other nonvascular malignancies may also present nodules in the purple color spectrum mentioned above, including lymphoma or leukemia in the skin, dermatofibrosarcoma protuberans (DFSP), amelanotic melanomas, and cutaneous metastases (Figure 4.13B).

> **Clinical Tip** Purple papules and nodules are colloquially known as "purple plums." These dermal papules and nodules fall into two broad categories: vascular in origin or malignant.

The groupings and configuration of purple are summarized in Table 4.18. A range of conditions may appear linear as a result of the Koebner phenomenon, occurrence of the dermatosis in Blaschko lines, or lymphatic spread of in-transit metastases. Angioma serpiginosum is a vascular malformation with onset in childhood that presents with telangiectasias or tiny vascular papules on a background of a pink vascular blush. Angioma serpiginosum may be linear in configuration or serpiginous.

Table 4.19 outlines characteristic distribution of purple lesions. Purple in the photoexposed distribution may signify dermatomyositis, a photolichenoid eruption,

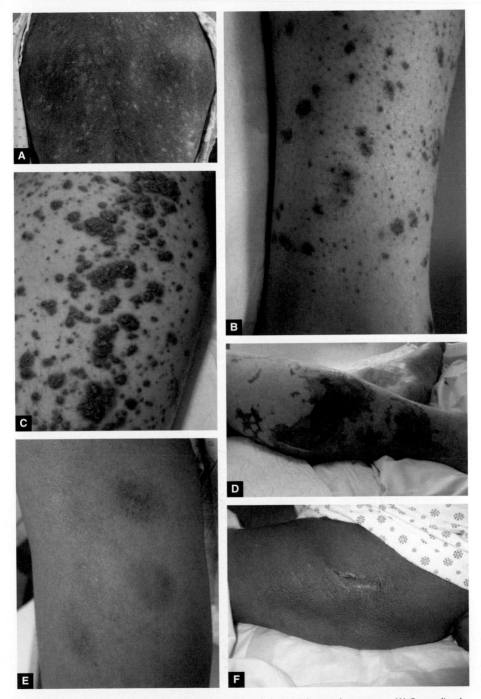

FIGURE 4.12 • Vascular conditions with a range of purple hues in the purple spectrum: (A) Generalized essential telangiectasia with maroon color; (B) leukocytoclastic vasculitis with a wine color secondary to robust inflammation; (C) small vessel vasculitis with purple color secondary to early necrosis; (D) cutaneous polyarteritis nodosa with bright purple retiform necrosis; (E) necrotizing vasculitis presenting with ecchymotic plaques as shown on the upper extremity; (F) depressed violaceous plaques of early calciphylaxis.

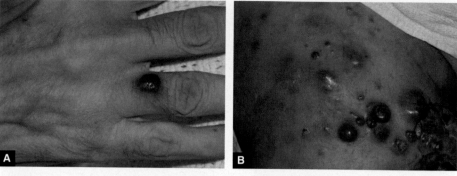

FIGURE 4.13 • Purple "plums": (A) Kaposi sarcoma with a deep purple nodule on the finger; (B) violacaeous and ulcerated nodules in a case of extensive melanoma metastases. (Image (A) used with permission from Dr. Miguel Sanchez, Bellevue Hospital, New York University School of Medicine, New York, NY.)

or drug-induced pigmentation. The palms and soles may house a range of conditions in the purple spectrum, including Kaposi sarcoma, vasculitides, and vasculopathies. The wheel of diagnosis customized to the purple spectrum is summarized in Figure 4.14.

TABLE 4.18. Groupings and Configuration of Purple Lesions

ANNULAR
• Lichen planus

LINEAR
• Koebner phenomenon
  • Lichen planus
  • Leukocytoclastic vasculitis
  • Kaposi sarcoma
• Blaschko lines
  • Linear lichen planus
• Along lymphatics
  • In-transit metastases of melanoma
• Other linear configuration
  • Angioma serpiginosum
  • Linear erythema over joints in dermatomyositis
  • Flagellate erythema of dermatomyositis

SERPIGINOUS
• Angioma serpiginosum

AGMINATED
• Pyogenic granulomas

RETICULATE
• Retiform purpura differential diagnosis (see Chapter 10)

TARGETOID
• SJS/TEN
• Early fixed drug eruption

TABLE 4.19. Distribution of Purple Lesions

PHOTOEXPOSED
- Photosensitive eruption in dermatomyositis
- Photolichenoid eruption
  - Tetracyclines
  - Thiazides
  - Antimalarials: quinine, quinidine
- Amiodarone pigmentation is photoaccentuated

EXTENSORS
- Dermatomyositis

PERIORBITAL
- Heliotrope of dermatomyositis

PALMS AND SOLES
- Kaposi sarcoma frequently occurs on soles
- Septic vasculitis
  - Asymmetric distal purpura
  - Janeway lesions
- Rocky Mountain spotted fever
- Leukocytoclastic vasculitis: rare location
- Thrombotic vasculopathies

RELATION TO APPENDAGES: FOLLICULAR
- Follicular lichen planus

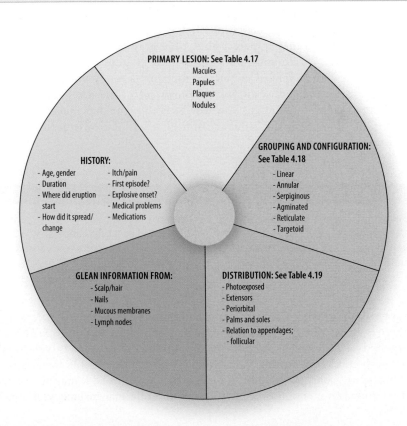

FIGURE 4.14 • The wheel of diagnosis, customized to the purple spectrum.

GRAY

Melanin in the superficial dermis may appear gray. Melanin-containing dermal melanocytes in conditions such as dermal melanocytosis (formerly known as *Mongolian spot*), nevus of Ito, and nevus of Ota are responsible of the gray and sometimes blue-gray color of these conditions. Acquired dermal melanocytosis refers to the onset in adulthood of gray macules that are typically seen on the lateral aspects of the forehead. Melanin in melanophages in the upper dermis also renders a gray color, such as may be seen in a regressing seborrheic keratosis or lentigo maligna and lentigo maligna melanoma. In burned-out interface dermatitides [such as lichen planus, fixed drug eruption (Figure 4.15A), erythema dyschromicum perstans, or Riehl's melanosis], it is the residual dermal melanophages that are responsible for this color. A gray color is also seen in incipient epidermal necrosis (such as active fixed drug eruption or SJS/TEN) or incipient dermal necrosis, such as in thrombotic vasculopathies. In disseminated intravascular coagulation from meningococcemia, plaques of retiform necrosis are classically described as having a "gunmetal gray" appearance (Figure 4.15B). A complete list of drug-related gray pigmentation is seen in Table 4.2. The color of drug pigmentation varies depending on the drug from slate-gray, blue-gray, brown-gray, purple-gray, purple, violet-brown, to a brownish hue. Some drugs, such as amiodarone, chlorpromazine, the tricyclic antidepressants, and minocycline (the type III pigmentary variety), produce pigmentation that is confined to photoexposed areas. Antimalarials induce brown-gray pigmentation that it typically localized to the shins (Figure 4.15C). Argyria may impart a blue, blue-gray or gray color to the skin. Pigmented basal cell carcinomas may appear gray (Figure 4.15D), brown-gray, or black. Patients with advanced metastatic melanoma rarely present with a diffuse gray-blue color, known as *diffuse melanosis cutis*. The mechanism driving this dyspigmentation is unknown; however, it is thought that melanogenesis is increased in the skin under the influence of high levels of growth factors such as α-MSH and endothelin 1.

Gray in the Skin is Caused by:	
• Melanin in the dermis in melanocytes or melanophages • Incipient necrosis of the epidermis or dermis	• Drug pigmentation • Pigmented basal cell cancer • Diffuse melanosis cutis in advanced metastatic melanoma

For gray configurations, fixed drug eruption may appear targetoid in early cases when there is an active red rim around a central round gray macule. SJS/TEN may have targetoid necrotic macules. Erythema dyschromicum perstans is typically distributed on the neck, upper torso, and proximal extremities. Riehl's melanosis is a form of pigmented contact dermatitis found on the face or neck. It may be reticulate in configuration. As mentioned previously, acquired dermal melanocytosis favors the temples.

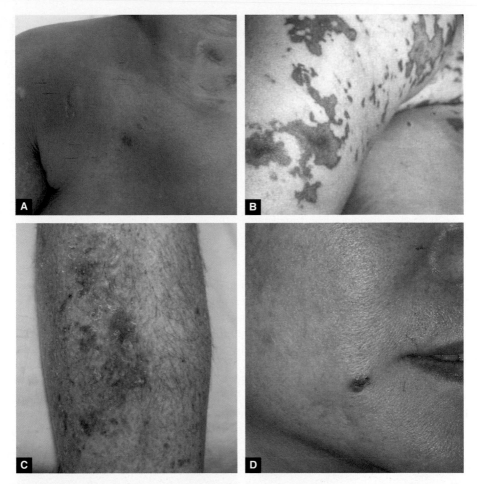

FIGURE 4.15 • Examples of gray dermatoses: (A) Fixed drug eruption with a gray color and surrounding erythema. (Reproduced with permission from Jameson J, Fauci AS, Kasper DL, et al: *Harrison's Principles of Internal Medicine*, 20th ed. New York, NY: McGraw Hill; 2018.) (B) retiform plaques of meningococcemia with a gunmetal gray appearance and a central bluish color; (C) hydroxychloroquine-induced brown-gray dyspigmentation on a shin; (D) a pigmented basal cell cancer with a gray hue.

BLUE

Blue in the skin may be generalized or localized, as is summarized in Table 4.20. A generalized bluish tinge may be seen in cyanosis and methemoglobinemia. Cyanosis occurs when there is increased deoxygenated hemoglobin in the small blood vessels of the skin and mucous membranes. In central cyanosis, the oxygen saturation is decreased, such as in states of respiratory failure. In peripheral cyanosis, the oxygen saturation is normal centrally, but there is a slowing in blood flow peripherally with consequent increased extraction of oxygen by the tissues, such as in low-cardiac-output states, or peripheral vasoconstriction from cold exposure. In peripheral cyanosis, the mucous membranes appear normal. In methemoglobinemia, there is an increased concentration of methemoglobin in the blood. Methemoglobin contains the ferric form of iron that has a greater

TABLE 4.20. Differential Diagnosis of Blue in the Skin

GENERALIZED
- Cyanosis
- Methemoglobinemia
- Argyria

LOCALIZED
- Macules
  - Dermal melanocytosis, nevus of Ito, nevus of Ota
  - Drug pigmentation
  - Maculae cerulae
  - Alkaptonuria
- Papules, nodules
  - Blue nevus, combined nevus, melanoma
  - Epidermal inclusion cyst, hidrocystomas

affinity for oxygen than the ferrous form of iron that hemoglobin usually contains. Therefore, oxygen is given up less readily in methemoglobinemia, resulting in a relative lack of oxygen in the tissues. This imparts a blue-gray color to the skin. Argyria is a third, rarer, cause of a generalized blue color. A blue-gray color may also be seen. Argyria is caused by ongoing exposure to silver-containing substances, such as in those who use silver salts for purported medicinal purposes.

The differential diagnosis of a localized blue color in the skin may also be succinctly summarized by primary lesion, as seen in Table 4.20. Melanin in the dermis appears blue or blue-gray, such as in blue nevi, combined nevi, melanoma, or metastatic melanoma (Figure 4.16A). Longer wavelengths of light (the red side of the color spectrum)

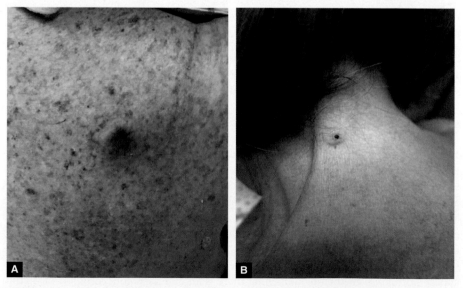

FIGURE 4.16 • Examples of blue dermatoses: (A) Metastatic melanoma presenting as a bluish and flesh-colored nodule; (B) an epidermal inclusion cyst with a blue hue and a central punctum with oxidized keratin that appears black.

are preferentially absorbed by melanin, whereas the shorter wavelengths of light (on the blue side of the spectrum) are reflected and scattered by collagen bundles in the dermis. This effect is related to the *Tyndall effect*, where longer wavelengths of light are transmitted through a colloidal substance, whereas shorter wavelengths of light are reflected via scattering. The Tyndall effect accounts for the occasional bluish appearance of epidermal inclusions cysts (Figure 4.16B) and hidrocystomas. Venous lakes appear blue secondary to pooling of blood within dilated superficial vessels. Tattoo ink and exogenous drug pigments may be blue. Minocycline is responsible for three types of dyspigmentation, as detailed in the section titled "Brown" above. Types I and II appear blue or blue-gray. Clofazimine, antimalarials, silver salts, amiodarone, and chlorpropramine may all cause a blue discoloration. Endogenous ochronosis is seen in alkaptonuria, an autosomal recessive condition where a deficiency of homogentisic acid oxidase leads to the accumulation of homogentisic acid in cartilage, including joints. Ear cartilage will appear blue. Skin may also be affected—sites of predilection include eyelids, forehead, cheeks, buccal mucosa, and intertriginous areas. Sclerae also appear blue. *Maculae ceruleae* are the transient pea-sized blue or blue-gray macules that accompany heavy pubic louse infestations. It is thought that the pubic louse injects this pigment, which has been found in its salivary glands, while feeding.

Blue in the Skin is Caused by:

- Deoxygenated blood
- Melanin in the dermis
- Light scatter through fluid-filled structures, such as cysts
- Venous blood pooling superficially
- Endogenous pigment, such as from homogentisic acid excess
- Exogenous pigments, such as from drugs or maculae ceruleae

Characteristic distribution of blue lesions may be seen in amiodarone pigmentation (photoaccentuated) or minocycline pigmentation (type I, acne scars; type II, shins and forearms). Apocrine hidrocystomas are typically single and occur on the eyelid margin, while eccrine hidrocystomas are usually multiple and these occur anywhere on the face.

GREEN

Green is a color that is rarely seen in the skin. The most common cause of a green color is the greenish pus that is seen in pseudomonal infections. *Pseudomonas aeruginosa* produces two pigments that impart the characteristic green color to the pus. Pyocyanins are blue-green, and pyoverdins are a yellow-green color. These pigments also impart a green or greenish-brown color to the nail in cases of pseudomonal nail infection.

A chloroma is a rare tumor that comprises precursor cells of the granulocytic lineage. Chloromas, also known as *granulocytic sarcomas* or *extramedullary myeloblastomas*, may occur in concert with acute myelogenous leukemia, or they may predate its development. In the skin, chloromas appear as solitary reddish or violaceous nodules. There is a high concentration of myeloperoxidase within its cells, and this imparts a greenish hue that is best appreciated when the lesions' vascularity is diminished via diascopy.

Eosinophilic cellulitis (Wells syndrome) presents with one or more edematous and erythematous plaques that may mimic bacterial cellulitis. As the plaques fade, they may become annular, and they are characteristically described as having a green color in this phase.

Green in the Skin is Seen in:	
• Pseudomonal infections • Chloroma	• Resolving eosinophilic cellulitis

BLACK

The differential diagnosis of black in the skin is a circumscribed list. Melanin, dermal and deeper necrosis, eschars, oxidized keratin, and foreign bodies or exogenous pigments appear black. A very deep purple color in the skin may also appear black, such as in talon noir (intraepidermal hemorrhage, usually seen on feet and hands, secondary to trauma) and angiokeratomas.

Black in the Skin is Caused by:	
• Melanin • Dermal and subcutaneous necrosis • Eschars • Oxidized keratin • Foreign bodies	• Exogenous pigments • Metallic particles, as in black dermographism • Talon noir and angiokeratomas (deep purple, indistinguishable from black)

Melanocytic neoplasms with heavy concentrations of melanin appear black (Figure 4.17A). Deep penetrating nevi and pigmented spindle cell tumors of Reed are classically very dark brown or black. An ink-spot lentigo is a variant of lentigo that measures up to 5 mm and appears black. Melanomas may be entirely or partially black (Figure 4.17B). Melanoma satellites and metastases may or may not be black (Figure 4.17C). Deeply pigmented basal cell cancers appear dark gray or black. Vascular lesions may also appear black. For example, the sclerosing hemangioma variant of dermatofibroma may appear deep gray or black (Figure 4.17D). Angiokeratomas and talon noir (a black macule seen typically on the heel or on other areas of the foot that represents heme in the epidermis secondary to trauma; Figure 4.17E) may have a deep purple color that appears black as it is so dark.

Necrosis of the epidermis usually appears dusky, purplish, or gray. Deeper necrosis of the dermis and subcutaneous tissue occurs as a result of ischemia, and this may render a black color. Vascular occlusion from vasculitis, thrombotic or embolic vasculopathies, or vascular compromise from intravascular calcium (as in calciphylaxis), cryoprecipitates (as in cryoglobulinemia), or other foreign material (cholesterol emboli, etc) may be responsible. Necrotizing fasciitis is a serious soft tissue infection that spreads rapidly and devitalizes tissue. Tissue inflammation and injury from a spider bite may be so severe as to cause necrosis. Brown recluse spider bites are classically necrotic. In general, necrotic plaques may appear purple or dusky initially and then progress to a black color as tissue is further devitalized. *Eschars*, discussed in further detail in Chapter 3, are black crusts that represent complete devitalization of tissue.

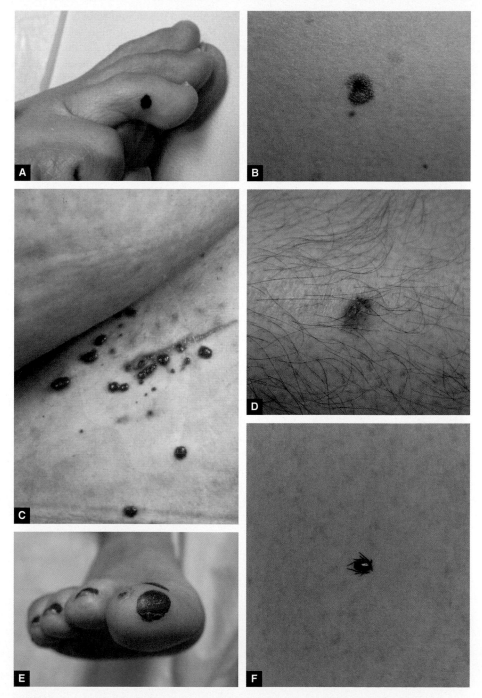

FIGURE 4.17 • Examples of black dermatoses: (A) A junctional dysplastic nevus with moderate atypia presenting as an acral black macule; (B) an early melanoma presenting as a brown plaque with an eccentric black papule; (C) melanoma satellitosis presenting with black papules; (D) a sclerosing hemangioma (variant of dermatofibroma) with a deep gray and black color; (E) talon noir with a deep purple color, almost indistinguishable from black; (F) a tick.

Oxidized keratin, as seen in open comedones, dilated pores, and puncta of epidermal inclusion cysts, appears black (see Figure 4.16B). A retained foreign body, such as a splinter, a tick (Figure 4.17F), or tick parts also looks black. Black dermographism occurs when pigmented metallic particles from jewelry or other metal objects containing gold and platinum, for example, are deposited on the skin. It is thought that these particles adhere to personal-care products that have been applied to the skin, with subsequent adherence to the epidermis.

For all colors, the remaining diagnostic boxes on the wheel of diagnosis (examining the scalp, hair, nails, mucous membranes, and lymph nodes for additional information, and garnering further relevant history) can also be leveraged to provide additional diagnostic information. Color changes or variances in hair and nails may render their own diagnostic clues. For example, the presence of silvery hair in infancy points to the diagnosis of a pigmentary dilution syndrome, such as Griscelli, Chediak-Higashi or Elejalde syndrome. Tar-containing products can turn gray hair yellow, and copper can give a green cast to the hair. The differential diagnosis of nail color changes is extensive and can be grouped by pattern of the abnormal color. For example, a longitudinal white streak might signify superficial white onychomycosis or Darier disease, whereas transverse white lines may be seen in trauma (these are short, and there may be more than one per nail) and asrsenic or heavy-metal poisoning (these are known as Mees' lines; a single white band spans the width of the nail). Hair and nail changes are discussed in more detail in Chapter 13 and are described in Tables 13.5. and 13.11.

SUMMARY

- A wide range of colors may be appreciable in the skin.
- Generalized color changes may be indicative of internal disease.
- For primary lesions, color is a diagnostic determinant and can be used to craft a differential diagnosis or hone a diagnosis.
- Background skin color influences the color of lesions.
- Color changes in hair and nails may render their own diagnostic clues.

An Introduction to Reaction Patterns

5

The term *reaction pattern* is used to describe a specific cluster of morphologic findings that groups of diseases have in common. This term is also used by dermatopathologists to describe histopathologically similar groups of disease, but this chapter will focus on clinical reaction patterns that are used to describe physical examination findings rather than histopathologic findings. Each of these reaction patterns will be discussed in more detail in subsequent chapters.

The clinical reaction patterns are an important constituent of the diagnostician's toolbox. An initial appraisal of the clinical features of a rash can guide a creation of a differential diagnosis based on reaction pattern. Five major clinical reaction patterns can be used to categorize dermatologic disease.

The Five Major Reaction Patterns are

- Papulosquamous
- Vesicobullous
- Eczematous
- Dermal
- Vascular/red

PAPULOSQUAMOUS

The *papulosquamous reaction pattern* encompasses those dermatoses that present with scaly papules, plaques, or nodules. This is a vast group of diseases that span infectious, inflammatory, neoplastic, and drug-induced disease. Examples include inflammatory diseases such as psoriasis and lichen planus, and neoplastic disease such as actinic keratosis and squamous cell cancer in situ. Papulosquamous diseases can be differentiated from each other by employing the diagnostic boxes of the wheel of diagnosis. An additional diagnostic clue for papulosquamous diseases is the quality and character of the scale present. For example, the scale of psoriasis may be silvery or micaceous (mica-like), and the scale of actinic keratoses is adherent and has a gritty feel. An in-depth description of the papulosquamous reaction pattern is found in Chapter 6.

VESICOBULLOUS

In the *vesicobullous reaction pattern,* the primary lesions are vesicles and bullae. Vesicobullous disease may also be accompanied by a host of secondary lesions (including collarettes of scale, erosions, ulcers, and crusts) and associated nonbullous primary lesions (such as urticarial plaques in bullous pemphigoid and erythematous papules and plaques in allergic contact dermatitis). These secondary and adjunctive primary lesions are replete with diagnostic clues and can help to create an approach. Additionally, clinical clues can guide an evaluation of the depth of the cleavage plane of vesicles or bullae and can therefore render important diagnostic information. Finally, elements of the wheel of diagnosis provide additional information, including grouping, configuration, and distribution of lesions. The vesicobullous reaction pattern will be explored in detail in Chapter 7.

ECZEMATOUS

The *eczematous reaction pattern* includes a constellation of findings, such as vesicles, bullae and erythema (of acute eczema), papules, scaling and erosions (of subacute eczema), and lichenification, scaling, and hyper- and hypopigmentation (of chronic eczema). The eczematous reaction pattern overlaps with the vesicobullous (acute eczema) and papulosquamous reaction patterns (chronic eczema). The eczematous reaction pattern is discussed in detail in Chapter 8.

DERMAL

The *dermal reaction pattern* refers to smooth papules, plaques, and nodules. There are no epidermal changes, such as scales. The substance of the primary lesions is inflammatory cells (such as lymphocytes in lymphocytoma cutis), granulomas (such as sarcoidosis), neoplastic cells (either benign or malignant), or substances that have been deposited in the dermis (e.g., urate, calcium, or bone). Even though this reaction pattern is termed *dermal*, these smooth lesions may occur as a result of subcutaneous disease as well (e.g., erythematous tender nodules in the panniculitides and smooth flesh-colored nodules from subcutaneous granulomas as in the Darier–Roussy form of sarcoid). Diseases that cause sclerosis of the dermis and/or subcutaneous fat are also included in this category. Examples include systemic sclerosis and morphea. These diseases produce sclerotic plaques, which may be elevated or depressed. A comprehensive approach to the dermal reaction pattern is found in Chapter 9.

VASCULAR/RED

The term *vascular reaction pattern* refers to lesions that are red, whether they are macules, papules, or plaques, rather than to vascular neoplasms. A more precise term for this reaction pattern therefore is the *red reaction pattern*. This reaction pattern houses a conglomeration of morphologic appearances that are unified by their red color. It covers an approach to generalized, localized, or patterned macular erythemas, urticaria and urticarial dermatoses, target and targetoid lesions, and purpuras. Chapter 10 is devoted to the vascular reaction pattern.

So, in summary, all those dermatoses presenting with similar clinical features can be grouped together. Reaction patterns are not characteristics of primary lesions, but rather each reaction pattern is defined by a set or subset of morphologic characteristics of primary or secondary lesions as is outlined above. In the wheel of diagnosis schema, *reaction pattern* can be layered onto the wheel. It is a branch point between the "Primary lesion" box and the "Grouping/configuration" box, as was seen in Figure 1.4 and as is summarized in Figure 5.1. It is a branch point and not an inherent part of the wheel because not all dermatologic disease falls into one of the reaction pattern categories (see the next page), and so a reaction pattern may not be applicable to all rashes. But sometimes it is the reaction pattern that is the most striking feature of a rash, and so considering these patterns in detail is important. Each reaction pattern will be covered in detail in the upcoming chapters.

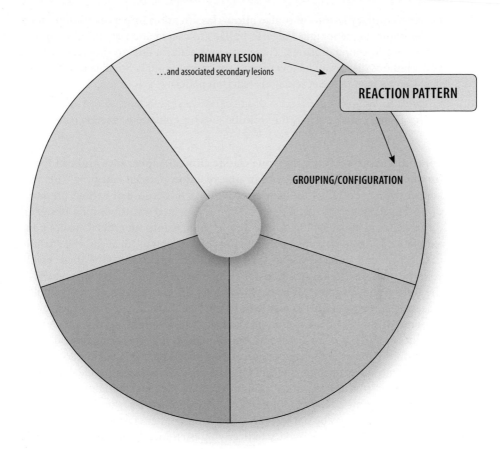

FIGURE 5.1 · Where reaction pattern fits into the wheel of diagnosis.

Clinical Tip Reaction pattern is layered onto the wheel of diagnosis between the "Primary lesion" and the "Grouping/configuration" boxes.

Further important considerations regarding reaction patterns include the following:

1. **The presence of scale is a major determinant of reaction pattern.** For example, scaly papules or plaques fall into the papulosquamous or eczematous reaction pattern categories, and smooth papules or plaques may fit into either the dermal or vascular reaction pattern.

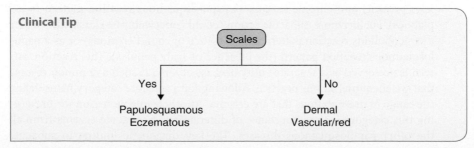

2. **Other secondary lesions may also allow classification into a reaction pattern.** For example, in pemphigus vulgaris, bullae are flaccid and may rapidly rupture, giving rise to round erosions. These erosions act as a clue to the presence of a vesicobullous disease and allow for categorization as such. Small round erosions may also be seen in the eczematous reaction pattern.

> **Clinical Tip** Round erosions signify the vesicobullous or eczematous reaction pattern.

3. **Some diseases have more than one classic clinical appearance and can therefore be categorized into more than one reaction pattern category.** This may happen either secondary to disease progression or because of variant presentations. For example, in pemphigus foliaceus, a primary autoimmune blistering disease, flaccid bullae rapidly rupture and eventuate into superficial erosions and exfoliative plaques. In certain presentations of pemphigus foliaceus, the erosions may be difficult to discern, and the predominant finding may be these exfoliative plaques—a papulosquamous presentation. So, pemphigus foliaceus is in the differential diagnosis of papulosquamous disease, as well as vesicobullous disease. Another example is pityriasis rosea. The classic type of pityriasis rosea presents with ovoid truncal scaly plaques—a papulosquamous disease. A rarer variant of pityriasis rosea has prominent spongiosis that is evident clinically with edematous papules and plaques and collarettes of scale. This could allow classification into the eczematous category. Finally, some primarily dermal conditions may present clinically as either smooth or scaly plaques or nodules. Granular cell tumors, some deep fungal infections (chromomycosis, sporotrichosis) and halogenodermas may be smooth (dermal reaction pattern) or scaly (papulosquamous reaction pattern secondary to overlying pseudoepitheliomatous hyperplasia as is seen on histopathology).

> **Clinical Tip** Some diseases may be categorized into more than one reaction pattern, depending on the following factors:
> - When in the time course of the disease you are seeing the patient
> - Whether there is a classic or variant presentation

4. **There is overlap between the reaction patterns themselves.** This is seen predominantly with the eczematous reaction pattern, which could conceivably be folded completely into the vesicobullous and papulosquamous reaction patterns. Acute eczema may also be classified as vesicobullous reaction pattern (vesicles present) and chronic eczema as papulosquamous reaction pattern (scaly plaques). Furthermore, subacute eczema could conceivably be classified as either a vesicobullous reaction pattern (the presence of round erosions) or as a papulosquamous reaction pattern (the presence of scaly papules). This reaction pattern is preserved as a separate entity because eczema is such a common disease that we encounter in our practice. Allowing for a separate category helps define the range of presentations that are eczema. Another notable reason for preserving this category is the importance of differentiating subacute eczema from all the other papulosquamous diseases. The key diagnostic finding in subacute

eczema is the presence of round erosions within scaly plaques. These represent intraepidermal vesicles that have "boiled over" and eroded. As discussed above, and in the chapter on secondary lesions (Chapter 3), round erosions connote vesicles that the body made, as opposed to the linear or angular erosions from scratching that the fingers made.

> **Clinical Tip** Reaction pattern categories may overlap. A notable example is the eczematous reaction pattern that overlaps with papulosquamous and vesicobullous reaction patterns.

5. **Papules may be too small to enable us to appreciate scale and thus may be difficult to classify.** For papules, additional diagnostic information can be garnered from their distribution (whether they are follicularly-based or not) and other diagnostic determinants, including color (see Chapter 2).

> **Clinical Tip** Reaction pattern may be difficult to discern, as in the case of papules.

6. **If the reaction pattern is in doubt, it is acceptable to render a "reaction pattern" differential diagnosis.** For example, sometimes it may be difficult to decide whether plaques are scaly (papulosquamous) or not (dermal). An example of this is plaques of seborrheic dermatitis on the face. These may appear minimally scaly, and so one might intuit a dermal process. Similarly, for dermal diseases such as granuloma annulare and sarcoid, overlying scale secondary to xerosis may occur. So, if the reaction pattern is in doubt, include all the possible reaction patterns in your differential diagnosis. For example, for the cases mentioned above, one could say for the differential diagnosis: "Papulosquamous versus dermal reaction pattern" and then list the possible diseases that are being considered in each reaction pattern.

> **Clinical Tip** In case of doubt, a differential diagnosis at the level of the reaction pattern can be rendered.

7. **Not all dermatoses fit into these five reaction patterns.** Notable exceptions include pustules and most macules (red macules fall into the vascular reaction pattern classification). An approach to pustules and macules is outlined in Chapter 2. While strictly speaking, pustules and macules are primary lesions, and reaction patterns are more than just primary lesions, to ensure completeness, some may argue for the inclusion of a pustular and a macular reaction pattern. From a purist's standpoint, I have limited the definition of reaction patterns for the reason outlined above. Another separate category that may not be classifiable in one of the reaction patterns above are the acanthotic conditions such as acanthosis nigricans, confluent and reticulated papillomatosis of Gougerot and Carteaud, and some warts. These conditions may be scaly, and if so, they can be classified as papulosquamous disease. But sometimes they are not scaly. If not, one could consider classifying them as dermal; however, their surfaces are rugose or ridged, and their substance

is in fact made up of epidermal thickening as opposed to dermal disease. So, if they are not scaly, they could be conceptualized as a separate group of diseases.

Clinical Tip Five reaction patterns + pustules + macules+ smooth acanthotic conditions = the breadth of dermatologic disease!

SUMMARY

- The reaction patterns are specific clusters of morphologic findings that groups of diseases have in common.
- Reaction pattern are useful descriptors of groups of diseases, and knowledge of them can help guide the creation of differential diagnoses.
- Not all dermatologic disease is classifiable by reaction pattern. The "Reaction pattern" box is therefore a branch point off the wheel of diagnosis.

The Papulosquamous Reaction Pattern

6

The primary lesions in this reaction pattern are scaly papules, plaques and nodules. A myriad of diseases display this reaction pattern. As mentioned in Chapter 5, some blistering diseases may have a papulosquamous presentation, such as pemphigus foliaceus, and some diseases that primarily have dermal inflammatory infiltrates or cells histopathologically may also be scaly, such as granular cell tumors, deep fungal infections, and plaques and nodules seen in halogenoderma.

> **Clinical Tip** Any primary lesion that is raised and scaly, no matter how it is formed, may be characterized as a papulosquamous lesion.

There is significant overlap between the papulosquamous and eczematous reaction patterns, as some forms of eczema fulfill the papulosquamous definition above. Examples include seborrheic dermatitis and lichen simplex chronicus. These diseases can fit into either reaction pattern.

> **Clinical Tip** Papulosquamous and eczematous reaction.patterns overlap; eczematous conditions such as seborrheic dermatitis and lichen simplex chronicus also fit into the papulosquamous reaction pattern.

Sometimes the scales of papulosquamous diseases are not conspicuous, in which case plaques can seem to fit into the dermal reaction pattern. An example here is any scaly dermatosis in an intertriginous area, where maceration of scales occurs. Another such example is the inflamed variant of seborrheic dermatitis that occurs on the face. Here, pink plaques have little scale and these plaques could be intuited as being dermal.

> **Clinical Tip** The papulosquamous reaction pattern may masquerade as dermal reaction pattern, when scales are not conspicuous.

The list of papulosquamous diseases is lengthy. As discussed in the introduction, it is useful to make one's own lists of diseases by diagnostic determinants, reaction pattern, grouping, configuration, and distribution when learning about each disease. It is also useful when encountering a patient with a papulosquamous disorder to have a ready-made differential diagnostic list that can be applied to the presenting dermatosis. Table 6.1 contains such a list, which is comprehensive, but by no means complete.

TABLE 6.1. Papulosquamous Diseases by Etiologic Classification

INHERITED
- Verrucous stage of incontinentia pigmenti
- Conradi–Hunermann–Happle syndrome
- Inherited ichthyoses
- Netherton syndrome
- Darier disease
- Hailey–Hailey disease
- Erythrokeratodermia variabilis (Mendes da Costa syndrome)
- Progressive symmetric erythrokeratoderma

ACQUIRED
- Infectious
  - Bacterial
    - Botryomycosis
    - Erythrasma
  - Mycobacterial
    - Tuberculoid and borderline tuberculoid leprosy
    - Tuberculosis verrucosa cutis
  - Viral
    - Verrucae
  - Fungal
    - Dermatophyte infection
    - Tinea versicolor
    - Chromomycosis
    - Sporotrichosis
    - Histoplasmosis
    - Primary cutaneous blastomycosis
  - Treponemal
    - Secondary syphilis
    - Tertiary syphilis
  - Parasitic
    - Crusted scabies
    - Leishmaniasis
- Inflammatory
  - Psoriasis
  - Lichen planus
  - Pityriasis rosea
  - Seborrheic dermatitis
  - Pityriasis rubra pilaris
  - Seborrheic dermatitis
  - Erythema annulare centrifugum
  - Discoid lupus erythematosus
  - Subacute cutaneous lupus erythematosus
  - Pityriasis lichenoides chronica
  - Lichenoid graft-versus-host disease
  - Lichenoid sarcoidosis
  - Keratosis lichenoides chronica
  - Frictional lichenoid dermatitis
  - Reactive arthritis
  - Flegel disease

(Continued)

TABLE 6.1. Papulosquamous Diseases by Etiologic Classification (continued)
ACQUIRED (CONT.)

- Degenerative
  - Perforating dermatoses
- Neoplastic
  - Actinic keratosis
  - Porokeratosis
  - Squamous cell carcinoma in situ
  - Squamous cell carcinoma
  - Keratoacanthoma
  - Verrucous carcinoma
  - Basal cell cancer
  - Mycosis fungoides
  - Pagetoid reticulosis
- Paraneoplastic
  - Bazex syndrome
- Drug
  - Lichenoid drug eruption
  - Mycosis fungoides–like drug eruption
  - Pityriasis rosea–like drug eruption
  - Psoriasis–like drug eruption
  - Drug-induced SCLE
  - INH or azathioprine-induced pellagra
- Nutritional
  - Vitamin B_3 deficiency (pellagra)
  - Vitamin B_2 or B_6 deficiency
  - Acrodermatitis enteropathica
  - Kwashiorkor

This list is subdivided into more digestible categories using the etiologic classification and a short description of these dermatoses follows here, including their morphologic features. Images of many of these conditions have been grouped together on the basis of morphologic grounds as outlined later in the chapter.

The inherited papulosquamous dermatoses are rarely encountered. Incontinentia pigmenti is inherited in an X-linked dominant fashion. The first stage is the vesicular stage. The second, the verrucous stage, can be classed as papulosquamous. Here, verrucous plaques are seen following Blaschko lines. In Conradi–Hunermann–Happle syndrome, linear and whorled hyperkeratotic plaques, also following Blaschko lines, are seen in early infancy. Netherton syndrome is an autosomal recessively inherited disease that presents with a scaly eruption (ichthyosis linearis circumflexa; plaques classically manifest a double-edged scale), hair abnormalities (trichorrhexis invaginata causes bamboo hairs), and atopy. Two autosomal dominant conditions that manifest in adolescence or after are keratosis follicularis (Darier disease) and benign familial pemphigus (Hailey–Hailey disease). In Darier disease, red-brown papules with dry or greasy scales develop in the second to third decades of life and involve the seborrheic and intertriginous areas (Figure 6.1). Hailey–Hailey disease presents with scaly, macerated, or eroded plaques in the same distribution, as well as the inframammary folds. It may also involve flexural skin or be more generalized. Linear erosions, or "rents"

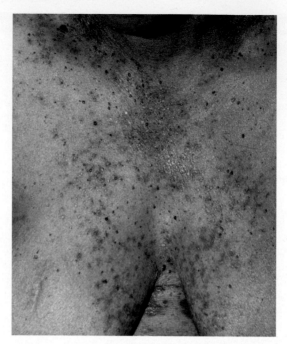

FIGURE 6.1 · Darier disease with scaly red and brown papules in a seborrheic distribution.

are a diagnostic hallmark (see Figure 1.7C). The inherited ichthyoses are a group of disorders that present with fine, lamellar, or coarse scales with or without erythroderma, depending on the ichthyosis. The erythrokeratodermas are very rarely encountered. In erythrokeratodermia variabilis (Mendes de Costa syndrome), fixed scaly plaques on the extensors coexist with migratory annular or arcuate plaques that may move over hours and fade slowly over days or weeks. Erythrokeratodermia variabilis starts in infancy and persists throughout life. In progressive symmetric erythrokeratoderma, fixed symmetric red scaly plaques that are well demarcated begin in early childhood. These involve the extremities, buttocks, and cheeks more often than the trunk.

The infectious category of acquired disease has many papulosquamous diseases. Thin scaly plaques are seen in dermatophyte infections, tinea versicolor, erythrasma, secondary syphilis, crusted scabies, and leprosy. While the first three diseases are frequently encountered, the last three are not and are important "do not miss" diseases in this category. In tinea corporis, tinea cruris, and tinea faciei, plaques are annular in configuration. Scales sit on top of the annuli. In tinea versicolor, caused by overgrowth of the commensal yeast, *Pityrosporum ovale*, brown, yellow-brown, or white macules are seen, typically in the seborrheic areas. Scales are fine or bran-like. Sometimes, scales are imperceptible, in which case they can be brought out by using one's thumbs to make the skin taut by applying lateral pressure. In erythrasma, caused by *Corynebacterium minutissimum*, brown scaly macules are seen that resemble tinea versicolor. Their distribution, however, is typically intertriginous and flexural. The three important "do not miss" diagnoses in this reaction pattern are secondary syphilis, crusted scabies, and leprosy. Secondary syphilis is one of the great mimickers of disease. Early on in the disease course, there are discrete macules and plaques that are nonscaly. Then, with time scales become more apparent. Palms and soles are areas of predilection (Figure 6.2). Secondary syphilis

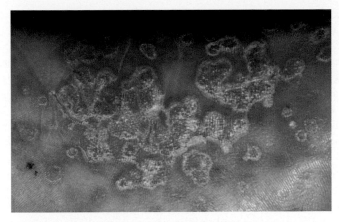

FIGURE 6.2 · Secondary syphilis with scaly papules and plaques on a sole.

may mimic a wide range of papulosquamous diseases. The diagnosis should therefore be considered for any unusual papulosquamous eruption. Crusted scabies (formerly known as Norwegian scabies) is a severe form of scabies that is usually seen in immunocompromised or elderly patients, or those with neurologic disorders. It may be pruritic or asymptomatic. Crusts are seen in areas with a high density of burrows, including wrists, webspaces, and around axillae. In more advanced cases, sheets of adherent powdery white scales develop, which may be generalized. The plaques of leprosy are more substantive than in those diseases mentioned above. Scaly plaques may be seen on the tuberculoid side of the leprosy spectrum, including the polar tuberculoid and borderline tuberculoid subtypes (Figure 6.3), whereas those on the lepromatous side of the spectrum are smooth (dermal reaction pattern). These plaques are typically annular as well.

Warts, commonly seen, can be classified as papulosquamous disease as well. The term *verrucous* means wart-like. Many chronic cutaneous infections present with wart-like plaques. The term *vegetative* means *vegetation-like*; this term is used to describe exophytic plaques with undulating surfaces. Some vegetative plaques are glistening, and some are dry. Most are also verrucous. The term *fungating* is used

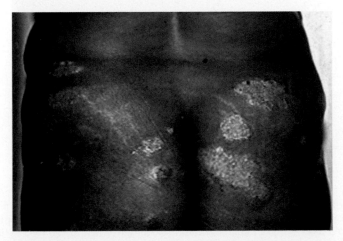

FIGURE 6.3 · Borderline tuberculoid leprosy, manifesting as scaly plaques on the buttocks.

interchangeably with *vegetative*. The likelihood of seeing one of these verrucous, sometimes vegetating, infections depends on geographic locale. Botryomycosis is globally a
rare disease. Botryomycosis is a chronic infection, usually from *Staphylococcus aureus*,
which presents with crusted ulcers, abscesses, or verrucous plaques. Tuberculosis verrucosa cutis results from direct inoculation of *Mycobacterium tuberculosis* bacilli into
the skin in an individual who has previously been infected by tuberculosis. It appears
as a slowly enlarging warty or vegetating plaque. In chromomycosis, a deep fungal
infection caused by a range of dematiaceous fungi, vegetating hyperkeratotic slowly
growing plaques are seen. In sporotrichosis, smooth nodules in a lymphocutaneous
pattern may ulcerate and crust. Chronic cases may become verrucous. Primary cutaneous blastomycosis, caused by *Blastomyces dermatitidis*, may be primarily pustular or
may present with verrucous plaques that may contain pustules and crust. In tertiary
syphilis, the superficial or noduloulcerative form may present as smooth or scaly dermal papules and plaques that tend to form arcs and annuli. Both forms may ulcerate,
forming crusts. Lesions spread slowly outward, leaving central wrinkled scarring. In
cutaneous and mucocutaneous leishamniasis, caused by a variety of *Leishmania* species, smooth papules, ulcerated plaques, and verrucous nodules may be seen.

The inflammatory category of papulosquamous disease includes some of the more
commonly encountered dermatoses in this reaction pattern. The following are descriptions of the classic appearance of each disease; variant presentations also occur. Psoriasis
classically presents with well-demarcated salmon-pink plaques with silvery, micaceous,
or ostraceous scale on the extensor aspects of the extremities and involving the scalp and
lower back (for scale definitions, see later on in the chapter). In lichen planus, flat-topped
polygonal violaceous papules and plaques with scant fine white scale are preferentially
located on the wrists, ankles, and lower back (Figure 6.4). Wickham's striae are white lines
that course across the top of lichen planus papules and plaques. These represent areas of
thickened stratum granulosum, a histopathologic feature of lichen planus. Wickham's striae

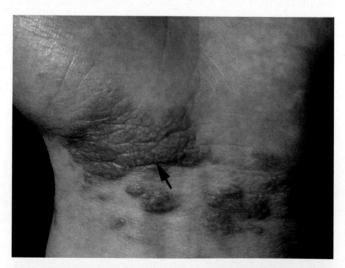

FIGURE 6.4 · Lichen planus with purplish polygonal papules becoming confluent to form a similar
plaque, with overlying fine white scale. (Reproduced with permission from Wolff K, Johnson RA, Saavedra
AP, et al: *Fitzpatrick's Color Atlas and Synopsis of Clinical Dermatology*, 8th ed. New York, NY: McGraw Hill; 2017.)

on the skin are rarely seen with the naked eye, but they can be rendered more prominent by applying mineral oil to the surface of lesions (see section titled "Bedside Diagnostics and Bloodwork" later in the chapter). Pityriasis rosea presents with ovoid medallions that follow cleavage lines of trunk and proximal limbs. A single scaly plaque, the *herald patch*, may erupt first and herald the disease. Branny scale overlies these plaques. Plaques may be annular, and if so, the branny scale is seen inside the annulus. Seborrheic dermatitis may be categorized as a papulosquamous or eczematous reaction pattern. It is a form of eczema but vesiculation is rarely seen, allowing categorization in this reaction pattern. Typical sites of involvement include the scalp, eyebrows, glabella, nasaolabial folds, beard area, in and behind ears, central chest, and intertriginous areas. Plaques may have greasy scale. In erythema annulare centrifugum, annular and arcuate plaques have scale that follows the leading erythematous edge of the plaque, a so-called trailing edge of scale. In pityriasis rubra pilaris, follicular scaly papules become confluent and form scaly well-demarcated plaques that are separated by "islands" of sparing. Two forms of cutaneous lupus are scaly; discoid lupus erythematosus (DLE) presents as hyperkeratotic well-demarcated papules or plaques, usually on the face (Figure 6.5), which resolve with atrophic, depigmented scars. In subacute cutaneous lupus erythematosus (SCLE), plaques may be psoriasiform or erythematous and annular without scale (vascular reaction pattern). A range of dermatoses with lichen planus-like features (the lichenoid dermatoses) is less commonly encountered; in pityriasis lichenoides chronica (PLC), crops of lichenoid scaly papules resolve with hypopigmentation. Lichenoid graft-versus-host disease (GVHD) is a subtype of chronic GVHD that presents with lichenoid papules. Lichenoid sarcoidosis, typically a dermal disease, is a rare subtype of sarcoid that presents with lichenoid papules that resemble lichen planus. Keratosis lichenoides chronica (Nekam disease) is an extremely rare dermatosis in which linear lichenoid plaques extend up the extremities slowly over time. Frictional lichenoid dermatitis is a form of subacute eczema that occurs over the extensors in childhood. It may have clinical features of lichen planus as well as eczema. Other rarely encountered scaly dermatoses include reactive arthritis, necrolytic migratory erythema, and Flegel disease. In reactive arthritis (formerly known as *Reiter syndrome*),

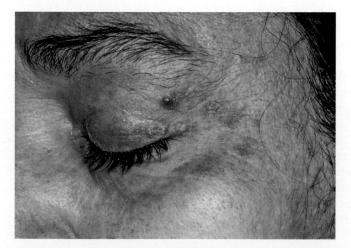

FIGURE 6.5 • Discoid lupus erythematosus, showing well-demarcated scaly papules on the eyelid.

the triad of arthritis, conjunctivitis, and urethritis can be accompanied by scaly, psoriasiform plaques. These plaques involve the penis (circinate balanitis) and palms and soles (keratoderma blennorhagicum) and may be more widespread. A geographic tongue is a frequent accompaniment. Necrolytic migratory erythema usually occurs secondary to an underlying glucagonoma. It may be classified as papulosquamous and vesicobullous disease. Periorificial small vesicles rupture early and form crusted and scaly annular and arcuate plaques. Hyperkeratosis lenticularis perstans Flegel disease is very rare. It presents with asymptomatic round or lens-shaped adherent scales that develop symmetrically over the distal extremities.

In the degenerative disease category, disorders that perforate present as papules with a central adherent core. On a histopathologic level, this core represents the dermal connective tissue that is undergoing transepidermal elimination. Perforating disorders are classified as primary (in the case of Kyrle disease, perforating folliculitis, reactive perforating collagenosis, and elastosis perforans serpiginosa). Secondary perforation may be seen in a wide variety of other dermatoses, including granuloma annulare, chondrodermatitis nodularis helicis, and pilomatricomas.

Neoplastic papulosquamous diseases are further "do not miss" entities. Those with premalignant potential include actinic keratoses and porokeratoses. Actinic keratosis are macules or very thin papules with overlying adherent scale that are seen in chronically sun-exposed areas. On palpation, this scale classically feels "gritty" or like sand or grit.

> **Clinical Tip** "Gritty" is a palpable, rather than a visual descriptor.

Porokeratoses are thin papules or plaques with a peripheral thread or thread-like scale. True carcinomas in this reaction pattern include squamous cell carcinoma in situ (SCCIS) and squamous cell carcinoma (SCC): SCCIS presents as a well-demarcated, sometimes psoriasiform-appearing scaly plaque. SCCs are scaly papules or nodules of varying sizes, although the very earliest lesions may not be scaly. A keratoacanthoma is a rapidly growing crateriform nodule with a central core of compact scale (Figure 6.6). Many believe that keratoacanthomas represent a variant of squamous cell carcinoma. Verrucous carcinoma is a variant of squamous cell cancer that is slowly growing. Verrucous carcinomas are related to the presence of human papilloma virus. Epithelioma cunniculatum is a type of verrucous carcinoma that arises from plantar warts and so, is seen on the sole. It presents as a verrucous or vegetating plaque that may be macerated or ulcerated. Buschke–Lowenstein tumor is a similar appearing verrucous carcinoma that arises on genital skin. Basal cell cancers, while rarely scaly, may have a variant presentation with scale. Finally, in this category is mycosis fungoides, a T-cell lymphoma. Scaly thin plaques with ill-defined "smudged" borders (patch stage) and thicker plaques with more clearly demarcated borders (plaque stage) have a predilection for sun-covered areas, including the posterior aspects of the axillae and the "bathing trunk" area. The third stage has smooth tumors, which can be classified in the dermal reaction pattern. Pagetoid reticulosis is a localized variant of mycosis fungoides that presents as a solitary scaly plaque on an extremity. It may be psoriasiform in appearance.

Acrokeratosis paraneoplastica (Bazex syndrome) is a paraneoplastic phenomenon that may accompany upper aerodigestive tract carcinomas. Psoriasiform or sometimes lichenoid papules appear acrally, including lateral aspects of the fingers, on the ears, and on the nose.

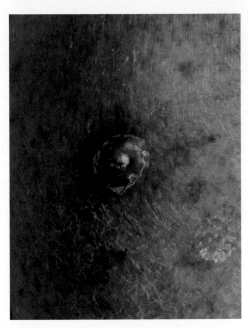

FIGURE 6.6 • A keratoacanthoma, showing the typical crateriform nodule with central compact scale.

In the papulosquamous reaction pattern, drug-induced disease always needs to be borne in mind. Lichenoid drug eruptions are fairly commonly seen. Angiotensin-converting enzyme (ACE) inhibitors; β-blockers; nonsteroidal anti-inflammatory drugs (NSAIDs); antimalarials, gold, lithium, penicillamine, ethambutol, and sulfonylurea agents are typical offenders. Lichenoid eruptions have also been described from newer agents, including ima-tinib mesylate, statins, tumor necrosis factor-α antagonists, sildenafil, and anti-PDI (pro-grammed death 1) drugs, such as nivolumab. A lichenoid drug eruption resembles lichen planus but is usually widespread. Pityriasis rosea–like drug eruptions are rare. ACE inhib-itors, terbinafine, imatinib, omeprazole, and gold have all been reported as culprits of this eruption. A mycosis fungoides–like eruption has been reported secondary to anticonvul-sant therapy, ACE inhibitors, or penicillamine. Psoriasis may be exacerbated by β-blockers and antimalarials, and induced by tumor necrosis factor-α (TNF-α) antagonists. Subacute cutaneous lupus erythematosus may be induced by calcium channel blockers, hydrochloro-thiazide, terbinafine, proton pump inhibitors (PPIs), and many chemotherapeutic drugs. Isonicotinylhydrazide (INH) and azathioprine can induce pellagra, as outlined below. INH binds vitamin B_6, a cofactor required in the endogenous synthesis of vitamin B_3 from tryp-tophan. Azathioprine also inhibits niacin metabolism.

Finally, nutritional deficiencies need to be considered in susceptible populations. Pellagra occurs as a result of vitamin B_3 deficiency, which may be a primary nutritional deficiency, or which may be seen in the setting of medications that inhibit niacin syn-thesis, in alcoholism, in carcinoid syndrome, or in Hartnup disease (an inherited disor-der where tryptophan is not absorbed). In pellagra, there are hyperpigmented plaques with varnish-like scale in the sun-exposed areas. Patients may have diarrhea and men-tal status changes as well. In vitamin B_2 and B_6 deficiency, there may be periorificial seborrheic-dermatitis-like eruption. Acrodermatitis enteropathica occurs as a result of hereditary or acquired zinc deficiency. There are perioral and acral erosions that become crusted and scaly. In kwashiorkor, superficial peeling scales resemble cracked paint. The findings may be flexural and intertriginous only or generalized.

As can be seen from the descriptions above, these diseases are variable in their morphology and their distribution. Applying the wheel of diagnosis to papulosquamous disease can help generate subcategories of differential diagnosis by the diagnostic box, including diagnostic determinants of the primary lesion; configuration and grouping; distribution; and whether scalp, hair, nails, mucous membranes, and lymph nodes are involved. Figure 6.7 shows the wheel that has been customized to the papulosquamous reaction pattern. Each diagnostic box contains a reference to the subsequent corresponding tabular differential diagnostic list.

The diagnostic determinants of the primary lesion are those features of a primary lesion that provide diagnostic information. The diagnostic determinants in this reaction pattern include color, the surface of the plaque and its border, and the type of scale present.

> **Clinical Tip** Color, the nature of the plaque's surface or border, and the type of scale present may hold the information needed to make a diagnosis.

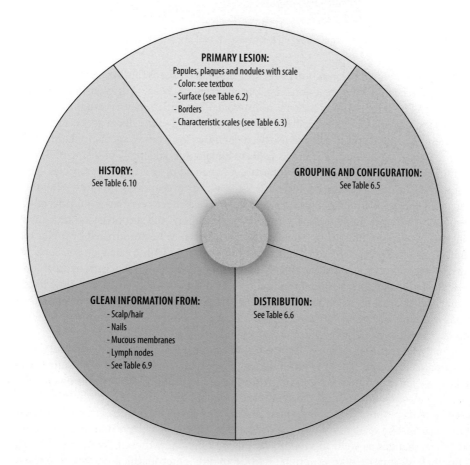

FIGURE 6.7 • The papulosquamous wheel of diagnosis.

Purple may signify lichen planus; psoriasis is classically described as having a "salmon-pink" color, and pityriasis rubra pilaris (PRP) may have an orange hue, especially the accompanying palmoplantar keratoderma.

Colors of Papulosquamous Disease

- Purple: lichen planus
- Salmon-pink: psoriasis
- Orange: pityriasis rubra pilaris, especially palms and soles

The surface of a plaque may be sufficiently distinctive as to suggest a diagnosis or a differential diagnosis. As mentioned above, verrucae and verrucous papules and plaques may be scaly as well and so may fit into this reaction pattern. A comprehensive differential diagnosis of verrucous papules and plaques is seen in Table 6.2, and some of these entities are represented in Figure 6.8. A rare finding of palmoplantar surfaces is that of acral verrucous keratosis. These are small scaly or verrucous plaques that also

TABLE 6.2. Differential Diagnosis of Verrucous Papules and Plaques

INHERITED
- Verrucous stage of incontinentia pigmenti
- Acrokeratosis verruciformis of Hopf
- Acrokeratosis verruciformis–like papules of Darier disease

ACQUIRED
- Infectious
  - Verrucae, including epidermodysplasia verruciformis
  - Botryomycosis
  - Blastomycosis
  - Chromomycosis
  - Histoplasmosis
  - Paracoccidiodomycosis
  - Sporotrichosis
  - Leishmaniasis
  - Tuberculosis verrucosa cutis
- Inflammatory
  - Pemphigus vegetans*
  - Superficial granulomatous pyoderma*
  - Halogenoderma*
  - Darier disease†
  - Hypertrophic lichen planus
- Neoplastic
  - Seborrheic keratosis
  - Granular cell tumor
  - Paget disease of the nipple and extramammary Paget disease*
  - Verrucous carcinomas
    - Epithelioma cuniculatum: arises from plantar warts and so, seen on the sole*
    - Buschke-Lowenstein tumor: arises on genital skin; HPV-related*

*May also be vegetative.
†Plaques in the folds may be vegetative.

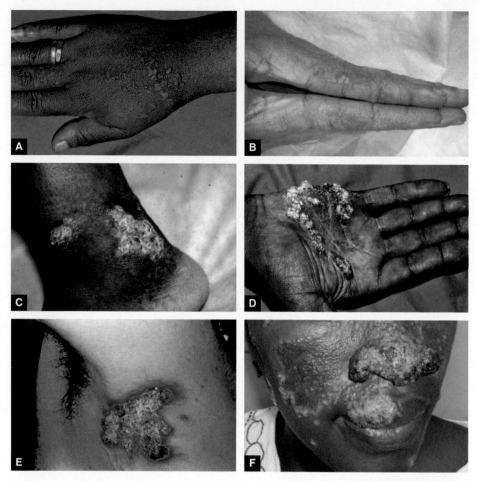

FIGURE 6.8 • Diseases that manifest with verrucous papules or plaques: (A) Darier disease with acro-keratosis verruciformis–like papules on distal arm and dorsal hand; (B) lipoid proteinosis, showing acral verrucous keratoses on lateral aspects of the fingers; (C) chromomycosis presenting as verrucous plaques on a lower extremity; (D) tuberculosis verrucosa cutis, presenting as a large warty plaque on the palm; (E) nodular tertiary syphilis with overlying verrucous changes; (F) histoplasmosis with verru-cous, crusted and vegetative plaques on the face. (Image (F) used with permission from Dr. Ncoza Dlova, University of KwaZulu-Natal, Durban, South Africa.)

occur on lateral aspects of palms and soles and of the digits. They are typically seen in three syndromes: Cowden syndrome, Rothmund–Thomson syndrome, and lipoid proteinosis. Table 6.2 highlights those verrucous plaques that are also vegetative.

The border of a plaque may be well demarcated, or clearly defined, as seen in psoriasis or PRP, or it may be ill-defined or "smudged" as is characteristic of the patch stage of mycosis fungoides (Figure 6.9).

> **Clinical Tip** The plaques of psoriasis and PRP have well-demarcated borders. Those of early mycosis fungoides are ill-defined or "smudged."

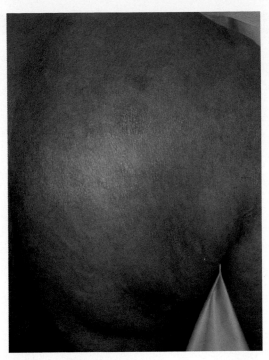

FIGURE 6.9 • Patch-stage mycosis fungoides showing ill-defined, "smudged" borders. (Used with permission from Dr. Miguel Sanchez, New York University, New York, NY.)

Another diagnostic determinant that is unique to this category is the type of scale seen. Scales in this reaction pattern category are usually primary and as such are part of the primary lesion. The type of scale can render important diagnostic information. Table 6.3 contains a complete list of scales and their associated dermatoses. Scale as a secondary lesion is discussed in Chapter 3.

Fine scale resembling bran is known as pityriasiform, bran-like, or furfuraceous scale. This is characteristic of the scale seen in pityriasis rosea (Figure 6.10) and in tinea versicolor (Figure 6.11). Powdery scales are even finer and resemble powder. Advanced cases of crusted scabies (Figure 6.12) and tinea pedis caused by *Trichophyton rubrum* (Figure 6.13) classically have powdery scales. The typical scale of seborrheic dermatitis is yellow and "greasy," as seen in Figure 6.14. Silvery scales are a hallmark of psoriasis. The silver color of these scales, as shown in Figure 6.15, is a bright shiny white color. These scales can be amplified by running the end of a cotton swab applicator over a psoriatic plaque. Other characteristic scales in psoriasis include *micaceous* and *ostraceous* scales. The term *mica* refers to a group of silica minerals with similar chemical structures that are naturally occurring in nature. The chemical structure leads to a laminated rock-like appearance, from which thin, shiny sheets can be cleaved. Micaceous scales in psoriasis resemble these sheets, as shown in Figure 6.16. *Rupioid* is a synonym for *ostraceous*. Both terms refer to an oyster shell-like appearance of scales. These are laminated adherent mounds of scale that resemble an oyster shell. Psoriasis, secondary syphilis, and reactive arthritis (Figure 6.17) may all present with ostraceous scales. A *limpet* is a marine snail that has a conical shell. The scales of reactive arthritis have also been

TABLE 6.3. Scale Types and Their Associated Dermatoses

TYPE OF SCALE	DISEASE
Pityriasiform, furfuraceous, bran-like	Pityriasis rosea Tinea versicolor
Powdery	Crusted scabies *Trichophyton rubrum* tinea pedis
Greasy	Seborrheic dermatitis
Silvery	Psoriasis
Micaceous	Psoriasis
Ostraceous, rupioid	Psoriasis Secondary syphilis Reactive arthritis
Limpet-like scale	Reactive arthritis
Ichthyotic, resembling fish scales	Inherited ichthyoses Acquired ichthyosis
Lamellar	Lamellar ichthyosis
Cracked, dry riverbed-like, cracked porcelain-like, crazy pavement appearance	Eczema craquele (asteatotic eczema)
Gritty	Actinic keratosis
Cutaneous horn	See Table 6.4
Thread-like, thready	Porokeratosis
Cornflake-like	Favus (scutula) Flegel disease
Double-edged	Ichthyosis linearis circumflexa of Netherton syndrome
Varnish-like or shellac-like	Pellagra Necrolytic acral erythema Acrodermatitis enteropathica Kwashiorkor
Cracked paint appearance	Kwashiorkor
Trailing edge of scale	Erythema annulare centrifugum
Follicular	Keratosis pilaris
Concretions around hair shafts	Pityriasis amiantacea
Peeling	Keratolysis exfoliativa Peeling skin syndrome Keratolytic winter erythema
Exfoliative scale	Pemphigus foliaceus
Collarettes of scale	Keratolysis exfoliativa Tinea pedis, manuum

described as limpet-like, also seen in Figure 6.18. Ichthyotic or ichthyosiform scales resemble those of a fish. They are thin, circumscribed, polygonal or diamond-shaped plates that are seen in inherited ichthyoses, such as ichthyosis vulgaris (Figure 6.19) and X-linked ichthyosis, and in the acquired forms of ichthyosis as well (such as the ichthyotic variant of sarcoidosis, or ichthyosis that is associated with underlying malignancy

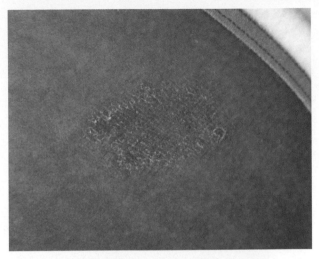

FIGURE 6.10 • Pityriasis rosea, displaying a herald patch with fine pityriasiform or bran-like scale.

or malnutrition). The term *lamellar* refers to scales that are arranged in large thin plates or shields. They are typically loose at the outer edges. The scales of lamellar ichthyosis, as those seen in Figure 6.20, embody this description. Asteatotic eczema, also known as *eczema craquele*, is a type of eczema that occurs in xerotic skin (see Chapter 8). Here, there are linear or polygonal superficial fissures that are bordered on both sides by fine dry scale. This leads to a cracked appearance of the skin that resembles a dry

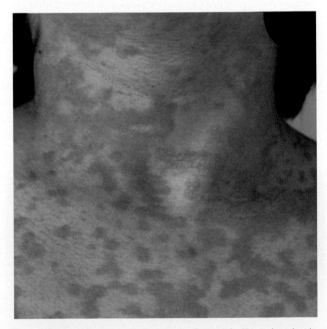

FIGURE 6.11 • Tinea versicolor, showing very fine pityriasiform scale. (Reproduced with permission from Wolff K, Johnson RA, Saavedra AP, et al: *Fitzpatrick's Color Atlas and Synopsis of Clinical Dermatology*, 8th ed. New York, NY: McGraw Hill; 2017.)

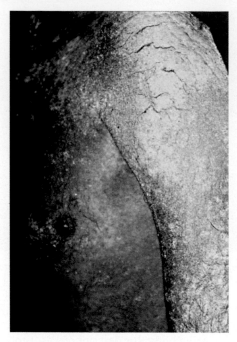

FIGURE 6.12 • Crusted scabies with "caked-on" powdery scales.

riverbed or "crazy paving", as is exemplified in Figure 6.21. ("Crazy paving" refers to the random placement of paving stones of varying sizes and shapes, such as on a walkway.) Actinic keratoses are surmounted by gritty scale (Figure 6.22). This term refers to a tactile rather than a visual finding; the characteristic adherent scale feels like sandpaper. A porokeratosis (Figure 6.23) has a border of extremely thin scale—as thin as thread, hence the threadlike or thread descriptor that is applied to this scale. A cutaneous horn is a compact conical or otherwise protuberant accumulation of scales that resembles a horn (Figure 6.24). A range of benign and malignant neoplasms may underlie a horn, including seborrheic keratoses, warts, trichilemmomas, actinic keratosis, keratoacanthomas, and squamous cell carcinoma. The full differential diagnosis of a cutaneous

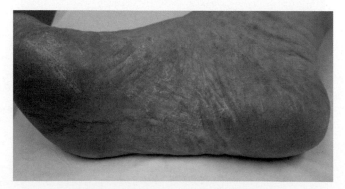

FIGURE 6.13 • *Trichophyton rubrum* tinea pedis with powdery scale.

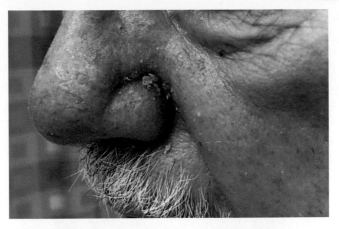

FIGURE 6.14 · Seborrheic dermatitis, displaying classic yellow, greasy scales.

horn is given in Table 6.4. The term *hyperkeratotic* refers to any compact accumulation of scales that is not conical or horn-like. This is a generic finding in many dermatoses, including hand eczema, hypertrophic actinic keratosis, and hypertrophic lichen planus, among others. An example of hyperkeratotic scale is seen in Figure 6.25 overlying an infiltrative basal cell cancer (a skin cancer that is rarely scaly). Some scales resemble cornflakes. As such, they are cup-shaped plates of scale. They are attached at their center and loose at the edge, which is also raised and undulating, like a cornflake. Flegel disease has small cornflake-like scales (Figure 6.26), as does favus (also known as *scutula*), a rarely encountered form of tinea capitis, caused by *Trichophyton*

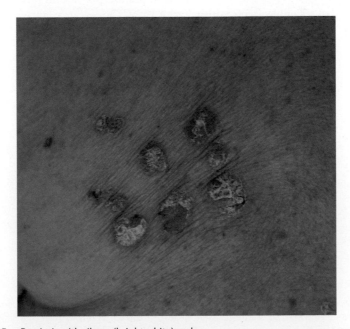

FIGURE 6.15 · Psoriasis with silvery (bright white) scales.

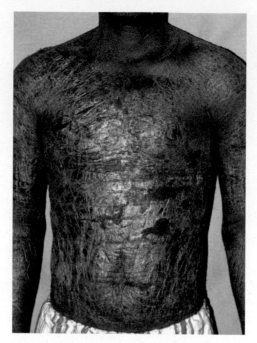

FIGURE 6.16 · Psoriatic erythroderma with typical micaceous scales.

schoenleinii. Double-edged scale is diagnostic of ichthyosis linearis circumflexa of Netherton syndrome. Here, plaques are oval, round, arcuate, annular, or serpiginous. The plaque edge is rimmed by two parallel rows of scales with erythema between them. Pellagra, as shown in Figure 6.27, presents with photoexposed thin plaques with thin shiny scales that resemble varnish or shellac. A similar appearance is seen in necrolytic

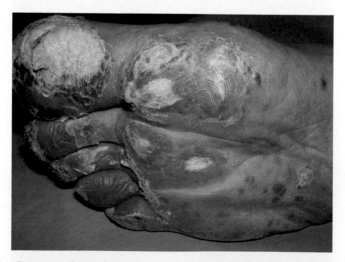

FIGURE 6.17 · Reactive arthritis, showing keratoderma blennorhagicum with ostraceous scales. (Used with permission from Dr. Miguel Sanchez, Bellevue Hospital, New York University School of Medicine, New York, NY.)

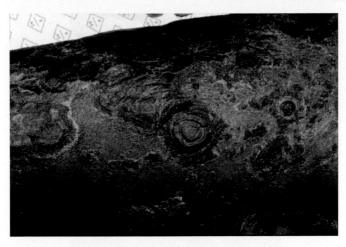

FIGURE 6.18 · Reactive arthritis with adherent scales resembling a limpet.

acral erythema on the distal extremities. The plaques of acrodermatitis enteropathica may also resemble varnish or shellac. In kwashiorkor, this varnish-like appearance is seen along with superficial cracking of these scales. The latter finding is known as the "cracked paint" appearance (Figure 6.28). A "trailing edge" of scale is a classic finding in erythema annulare centrifugum (Figure 6.29). Here, the scale trails the leading edge of the annular and arcuate plaques. This differs from the scales seen in tinea corporis, which sit atop the active annular rim, rather than trailing it.

Scales can accumulate in follicular ostia (see Chapter 2). Follicular scale may be indicative of keratosis pilaris and its variants. Other dermatoses with follicular scale include lichen spinulosis, pityriasis rubra pilaris (Figure 6.30), and phrynoderma. The papules of reactive perforating folliculitis each have a follicle-based central core of compact scale. In discoid lupus erythematosus and extragenital lichen sclerosus, scaly plaques or papules, respectively, with follicular prominence are seen.

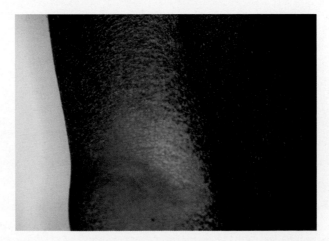

FIGURE 6.19 · Ichthyosis vulgaris showing ichthyotic (fish-like) scales and sparing of the antecubital fossa.

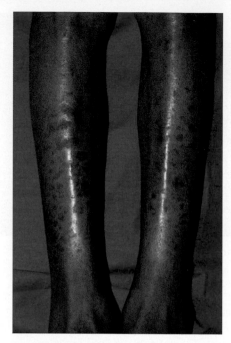

FIGURE 6.20 • Lamellar ichthyosis with classic lamellar scales.

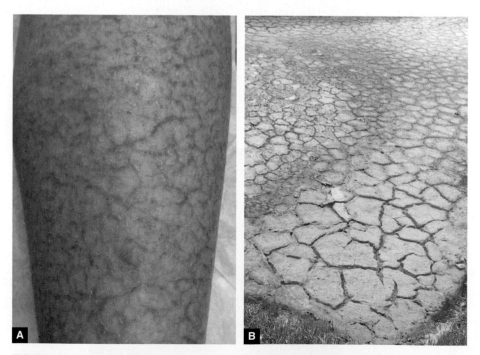

FIGURE 6.21 • (A) Asteatotic eczema (eczema craquele) with cracking that resembles a dry riverbed; (B) a dry riverbed with cracked earth that resembles eczema craquele.

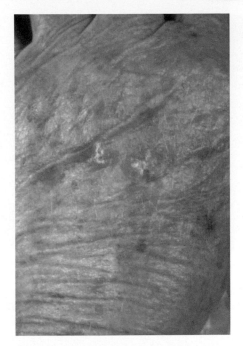

FIGURE 6.22 • Actinic keratoses on the dorsal hand with adherent scale that will on palpation have a gritty feel.

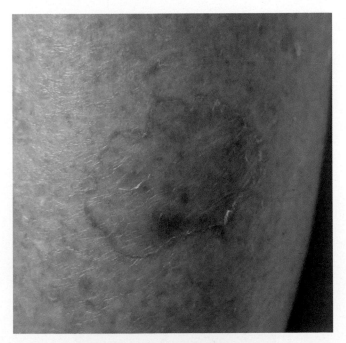

FIGURE 6.23 • Porokeratosis of Mibelli with a thread-like border.

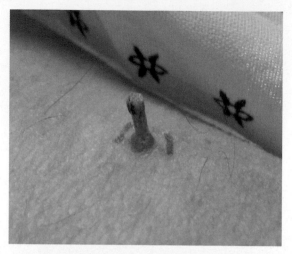

FIGURE 6.24 • A cutaneous horn: compact scales that resemble a horn.

TABLE 6.4. Differential Diagnosis of a Cutaneous Horn

- Hypertrophic actinic keratosis—most common
- Filiform wart
- Seborrheic keratosis
- Trichilemmoma
- Squamous cell cancer
- Keratoacanthoma
- Rarely reported
  - Metastatic renal cell cancer
  - Granular cell tumor
  - Sebaceous carcinoma
  - Kaposi sarcoma

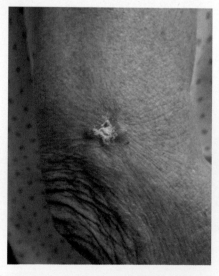

FIGURE 6.25 • A basal cell cancer with overlying hyperkeratotic scale.

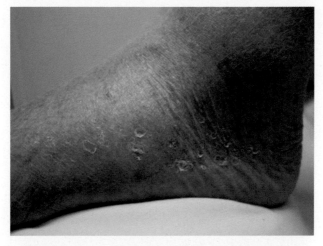

FIGURE 6.26 • Flegel disease with cup-shaped plates of scale resembling cornflakes.

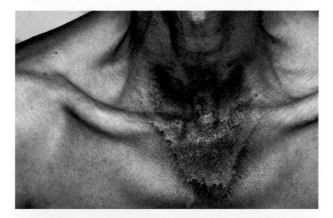

FIGURE 6.27 • Casal's necklace of pellagra: shellac-like scales on the V of the neck.

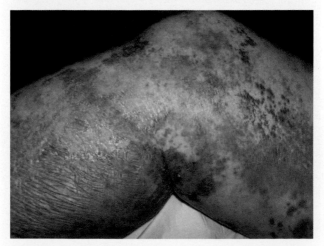

FIGURE 6.28 • Kwashiorkor, displaying a varnish-like and "cracked paint" appearance. (Used with permission from Dr. Miguel Sanchez, Bellevue Hospital, New York University School of Medicine, New York, NY.)

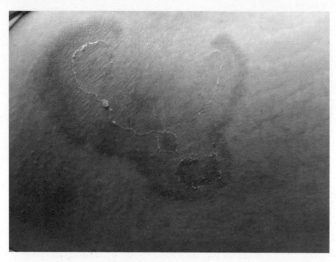

FIGURE 6.29 • Erythema annulare centrifugum with fine scales that trail the leading arcuate edge.

Scales may also accumulate around hair shafts, as is seen in pityriasis amiantacea (Figure 6.31). These are typically seen as adherent concretions around proximal hair shafts. This relatively rare condition may be associated with seborrheic dermatitis or psoriasis. A complete list of concretions around hair shafts is discussed later in the chapter and is summarized in Table 6.10.

As mentioned in Chapter 3, scale can accompany resolution of primary lesions. In this situation, scales are secondary. Desquamative scale (peeling), sheets of scale (exfoliative scale), and collarettes of scale are examples of these. But these scales may also be indicative of and characteristic for some disease states. For example, keratolysis exfoliativa presents predominantly with peeling scale and collarettes on the palms (Figure 6.32), and pemphigus foliaceus may present with exfoliative scale.

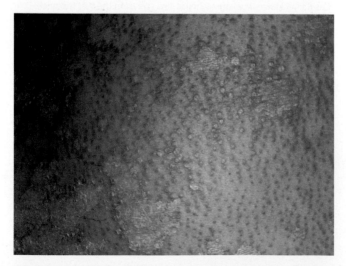

FIGURE 6.30 • Pityriasis rubra pilaris with follicle-based scaly papules. (Used with permission from Dr. Miguel Sanchez, Bellevue Hospital, New York University School of Medicine, New York, NY.)

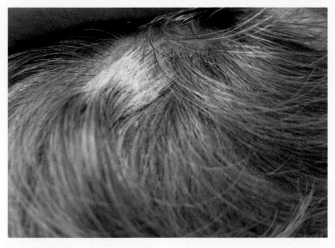

FIGURE 6.31 • Pityriasis amiantacea, showing concretions of scales surrounding a clump of hair.

It is useful to know that some diseases resemble psoriasis; these are termed *psoriasiform*. The eruption of reactive arthritis, Bazex syndrome, subacute lupus, squamous cell cancer in situ, and pagetoid reticulosis may all be psoriasiform.

Differential Diagnosis of Psoriasiform Plaques	
Single	Multiple
• Psoriasis	• Psoriasis
• Squamous cell cancer in situ (Figure 6.33A)	• Subacute lupus erythematosus
• Pagetoid reticulosis	• Reactive arthritis (Figure 6.33B)
	• Bazex syndrome (Figure 6.33C)
	• Multiple squamous cell cancers in situ
	• ILVEN (Figure 6.33D)

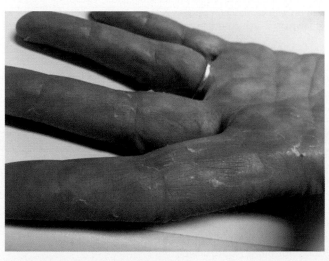

FIGURE 6.32 • Keratolysis exfoliativa, displaying peeling scale and collarettes.

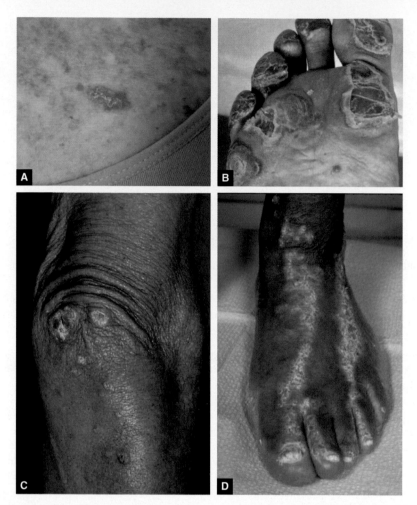

FIGURE 6.33 • Psoriasiform dermatoses: (A) squamous cell cancer in situ resembling a plaque of psoriasis; (B) reactive arthritis with psoriasiform plaques; (C) acrokeratosis paraneoplastica with psoriasiform plaques on the elbow; (D) inflammatory linear verrucous epidermal nevus (ILVEN) with linear psoriasiform plaques.

As outlined above, many dermatoses resemble lichen planus. Bazex syndrome may also be lichenoid. Lupus erythematosus/lichen planus (LE/LP) overlap is thought to be a presentation of lupus with lichenoid features.

Differential Diagnosis of Lichen Planus (Lichenoid Dermatoses)

- Lichenoid drug eruption
- LE/LP overlap (Figure 6.34A)
- Pityriasis lichenoides chronica (Figure 6.34B)
- Lichenoid sarcoidosis (Figure 6.34C)
- Lichenoid variant of benign pigmented purpura (Gougerot-Blum; Figure 6.34D)

- Lichenoid chronic graft-versus-host disease
- Keratosis lichenoides chronica
- Frictional lichenoid dermatitis
- Bazex syndrome

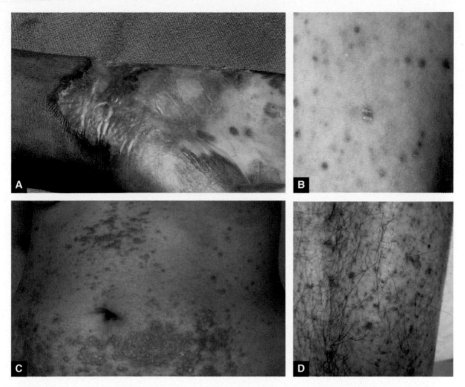

FIGURE 6.34 • Lichenoid dermatoses: (A) LE/LP overlap with a pink and violaceous plaque on the palm; (B) pityriasis lichenoides chronica with violaceous flat-topped papules (Reproduced with permission from Wolff K, Johnson RA, Saavedra AP, et al: *Fitzpatrick's Color Atlas and Synopsis of Clinical Dermatology*, 8th ed. New York, NY: McGraw Hill; 2017.); (C) lichenoid sarcoid, showing papules with lichenoid features on the abdomen; (D) lichenoid benign pigmented purpura, showing lichenoid papules.

Tables 6.5 and 6.6 summarize the differential diagnosis of papulosquamous lesions by configuration and distribution. The data in these lists are based on classic or common presentations of papulosquamous disease. In terms of configuration, most of the common papulosquamous diseases may present with annuli. If annuli are present in seborrheic dermatitis, they are found on the chest. The term *petaloid* has also been applied to these annuli because of their petal-like appearance. As mentioned previously, in tinea corporis, scales sit on top of the leading annular edge of the plaque (Figure 6.35), whereas in erythema annulare centrifugum, the scale trails the leading edge. Keratolytic winter erythema is a rare autosomal dominant condition that is seen in the Afrikaans population in South Africa. Cyclic peeling of palms and soles begins in infancy and becomes milder with age. It may be exacerbated by alcohol, cold, fevers, and menstruation. There is centrifugal peeling of skin that extends to the edge of the palms. Scaly annular plaques may occasionally be seen in association on the extremities.

Papulosquamous linear plaques may be secondary to the Koebner phenomenon or following Blaschko lines. Psoriasis and lichen planus both classically exhibit the Koebner phenomenon. Several papulosquamous dermatoses may be blaschkoid. Perhaps the most commonly encountered of these are lichen striatus, linear lichen planus, and ILVEN (as seen in Figure 6.33D). Lichen striatus is usually seen in children. *Blaschkitis* is the term used for lichen striatus in adults. Blaschkitis and lichen striatus may present

TABLE 6.5. Papulosquamous Differential Diagnosis by Configuration

ANNULAR
- Lichen planus
- Pityriasis rosea
- Psoriasis
- Seborrheic dermatitis
- Erythema annulare centrifugum
- Tinea corporis
- Secondary syphilis
- Tertiary syphilis
- Patch- and plaque-stage mycosis fungoides
- Necrolytic migratory erythema
- SCLE
- Ichthyosis linearis circumflexa
- Keratolytic winter erythema

ARCUATE
- Erythema annulare centrifugum
- Necrolytic migratory erythema

LINEAR
- Koebener phenomenon
  - Lichen planus
  - Psoriasis
- Blaschko lines
  - Linear lichen planus
  - Lichen striatus
  - ILVEN
  - Darier disease
  - Linear porokeratosis
  - Verrucous stage of incontinentia pigmenti
  - Conradi–Hunermann–Happle syndrome

RETICULATE
- Confluent and reticulated papillomatosis of Gougerot and Carteaud (CARP)

ROUND
- Pityriasis rotunda

with papulovesicles or fine scaly papules. ILVEN presents with erythematous and scaly plaques that follow Blaschko lines. As was mentioned above, ILVEN has a psoriasiform appearance. Rarely, true psoriasis may be Blaschkoid. Segmental Darier disease and linear porokeratosis are rare; they both follow Blaschko lines.

Confluent and reticulated papillomatosis of Gougerot and Carteaud (CARP) is a disorder of unknown etiology that manifests reticulate ridged and slightly scaly plaques. Finally, with respect to configuration, pityriasis rotunda is a rare dermatosis with scaly round flat plaques that resemble ichthyosis vulgaris. It has been associated with malnutrition, tuberculosis, hepatitis, and malignancy.

A unique configuration in this category is the so-called "islands of sparing" that are formed by widespread papulosquamous diseases that spare normal skin in small "islands." PRP and mycosis fungoides both leave islands where they do not involve the skin.

TABLE 6.6. Papulosquamous Differential Diagnosis by Distribution

PHOTOEXPOSED
- Discoid lupus erythematosus
- Subacute cutaneous lupus erythematosus
- Pellagra

SEBORRHEIC
- Seborrheic dermatitis
- Darier disease
- Pemphigus foliaceus
- Vitamin B_6 deficiency

FLEXURES
- Erythrasma
- Atopic dermatitis

EXTENSORS
- Psoriasis
- Frictional lichenoid dermatitis
- PRP, classic childhood form
- Palmoplantar keratodermas with transgrediens

INTERTRIGINOUS
- Intertrigo
- Inverse psoriasis
- Tinea cruris
- Erythrasma
- Pityriasis circinata et marginata of Vidal
- Acanthosis nigricans
- Hailey–Hailey disease
- Darier disease
- Pemphigus vegetans
- Extramammary Paget disease
- Granular parakeratosis

PALMS AND SOLES
- Tinea manuum, tinea pedis
- Inflammatory keratodermas
  - Psoriasis
  - Lichen planus
  - Discoid lupus
  - Lichen planus/lupus erythematosus overlap
  - Pityriasis rubra pilaris: orangey keratoderma
- Secondary syphilis
- Reactive arthritis
- Inherited palmoplantar keratodermas
  - Diffuse
  - Focal
  - Punctate
- Acquired palmoplantar keratodermas
  - Keratoderma climactericum

(Continued)

TABLE 6.6. Papulosquamous Differential Diagnosis by Distribution (continued)

PALMS AND SOLES (CONT.)
- Malignancy-associated
  - Tripe palms
- Porokeratosis palmaris et plantaris
- Palmar pits
  - Basal cell nevus syndrome
  - Cowden syndrome
- Acral verrucous keratoses
  - Cowden syndrome
  - Rothmund–Thompson syndrome
  - Lipoid proteinosis
- Neoplastic disease
  - Viral warts
  - Poroma
  - Porokeratosis
  - Epithelioma cuniculatum

Clinical Tip PRP and mycosis fungoides, when widespread, leave islands of normal skin. This phenomenon is known as "islands of sparing."

Many diseases in this category have favored sites of distribution. The intertriginous distribution has a broad differential diagnosis. In this location, scale may be attenuated

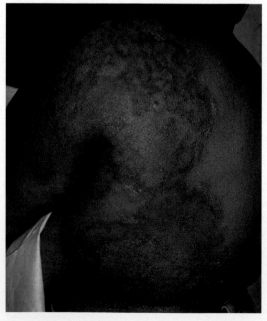

FIGURE 6.35 • Florid tinea corporis with an active scaly border and similar arcuate plaques centrally. (Used with permission from Dr. Miguel Sanchez, New York University, New York, NY.)

or secondarily macerated. Intertrigo (including that seen in seborrheic dermatitis) and inverse psoriasis are frequently seen here. Intertrigo has light pink, thin, ill-defined plaques, whereas inverse psoriasis displays the typical well-demarcated salmon-pink plaques. In the axillae, irritant or allergic contact dermatitis (Chapter 8) and acanthosis nigricans may be additional considerations. In the inguinal folds, tinea cruris is a "do not miss" diagnosis. While tinea cruris may be annular, it may also be secondarily lichenified owing to scratching from associated pruritus, and so the annular configuration may be masked. Other diseases in this location are rare. Thin plaques include erythrasma, granular parakeratosis, and pityriasis circinata et marginata of Vidal. The latter is a variant of pityriasis rosea in which large ovoid plaques preferentially cluster in and around the inguinal and axillary folds. Granular parakeratosis presents with well-demarcated plaques; scale may be superficial and peeling, or heaped up. This disease was initially identified in the axillae, but since then, cases in other folds as well as nonintertriginous skin have been reported. Extramammary Paget disease presents as a well-demarcated verrucous or vegetating plaque that is steroid-unresponsive. Pemphigus vegetans describes the vegetating subtype of pemphigus vulgaris that occurs in intertriginous areas. While this is an autoimmune blistering disease, it is this appearance that allows for classification in the papulosquamous category.

Many scaly conditions manifest on palms and soles. Asymmetric involvement is characteristic of tinea. The inflammatory keratodermas are a group of inflammatory dermatoses that occur on palms and soles. Psoriasis favors the central palm but may occur anywhere. Lichen planus and discoid lupus are rarely encountered on palms or soles. Lichen planus presents with a hyperkeratotic violaceous plaque, and discoid lupus may be annular. LE/LP overlap favors palms and soles. The keratoderma associated with pityriasis rubra pilaris is typically diffuse and classically is described as having an orange color. A "do not miss" diagnosis in this location is secondary syphilis (as seen in Figure 6.2). Early on, plaques and papules may be smooth, but they become scaly with time. Ollendorff sign is the presence of tenderness on applying pressure to secondary syphilis lesions in this location.

> **Clinical Tip** Ollendorff sign: presence of tenderness on applying pressure to palmoplantar papules and plaques of secondary syphilis.

Keratoderma blennorhagicum refers to the characteristic palmoplantar eruption of reactive arthritis (as seen in Figures 6.17 and 6.33B). Initially there may be vesicles or pustules that progress to brown scaly plaques. These are also tender. Ostraceous scale or scales resembling limpets may be seen. In the inherited keratoderma category, there may be diffuse, focal, or punctate patterns of involvement. For punctate keratodermas, it is useful to differentiate those diseases with keratoses (small keratin projections) from those with pits (or invaginations). Inherited punctate keratoderma is pitted. An autosomal variant occurs in the palmar creases. Pitted keratolysis is an infection caused by *Kytococcus sedentarius*. Small pits are seen in the thick stratum corneum of weight-bearing areas of the soles. A musty odor is a frequent accompaniment. Pits may be a sign of Darier disease (Figure 6.36). Other rarer causes of palmar pits are listed in Table 6.7. Spiny keratoderma presents with many keratotic protrusions that resemble music box spines (otherwise known as "music box spine dermatosis"). The differential diagnosis of keratosis on palms and soles in also listed in Table 6.7. Punctate

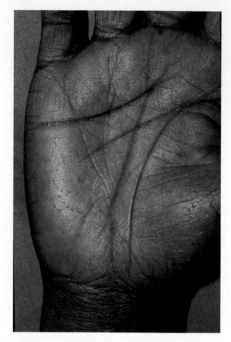

FIGURE 6.36 • Palmar pits of Darier disease.

porokeratosis of palms and soles may present with either pits or keratotic papules. Acquired keratodermas may be seen on the soles around midlife (keratoderma climactericum) or as a new finding in an underlying malignancy. "Tripe palms" is the name given to acanthosis nigricans on the palms. It is also known as *acanthosis palmaris*, and its appearance resembles the stomach lining of cows. A rare finding of palmoplantar surfaces is that of acral verrucous keratosis. These are small scaly or verrucous plaques

TABLE 6.7. Differential Diagnosis of Punctate Keratoderma

KERATOSES
- Spiny keratoderma
- Arsenical keratoses
- Porokeratosis of palms and soles
- Verrucae
- Cowden syndrome

PITS
- Punctate keratoderma
- Keratosis punctata of creases
- Pitted keratolysis
- Darier disease
- Hailey–Hailey disease
- Basal cell nevus syndrome
- Naegeli–Franceschetti–Jadassohn syndrome
- Dermatopathia pigmentosa reticularis

that occur on lateral aspects of palms and soles and of the digits. They are typically seen in three syndromes: Cowden syndrome, Rothmund–Thomson syndrome, and lipoid proteinosis. In terms of scaly neoplasms, viral warts are the most commonly seen in this location. Poroma is a benign growth of eccrine ductal cells. It is commonly located on the soles. It is characterized by a smooth pink papule or nodule with a collarette of scale. Besides the palmoplantar variant of porokeratosis, porokeratosis of Mibelli may be seen in this location. Also, as mentioned previously, verrucous carcinoma is a rarely encountered malignancy in this location.

The presence of superficial peeling scale on the palms invokes a broad differential diagnosis, which is encapsulated in a separate table, Table 6.8. Peeling of palmar surfaces can be divided into infectious and inflammatory causes. In practice, palmar peeling is most commonly encountered in keratolysis exfoliativa, also known as focal palmoplantar peeling (as seen in Figure 6.32). This condition is considered a mild form of dyshidrotic eczema where peeling rather than vesicles predominate. Some forms of tinea pedis may present with very superficial collarettes of scale, which resemble peeling. In the in-patient setting, palmar peeling may be seen after defervescence, called postinfectious desquamation. It may also be a part of more generalized peeling seen in a toxin-mediated erythema, such as staphylococcal scalded skin syndrome or toxic shock syndrome. It can be seen after scarlet fever resolves. In Kawasaki disease, fingertip peeling is one of the pathognomonic signs. Peeling skin syndrome is a very rare disorder with a heterogenous genotype and phenotype, including inflammatory and noninflammatory forms. Acral peeling skin syndrome is a subtype that is localized to the dorsal and volar surfaces of the hands and feet. In South Africans of Afrikaner descent, keratolytic winter erythema should be borne in mind.

Global or near-global involvement of the cutaneous surface is termed *erythroderma*. Erythrodermas may be scaly (papulosquamous or eczematous reaction pattern), in which case the term *exfoliative dermatitis* can be used, or they may be nonscaly (vascular reaction pattern).

> **Clinical Tip** Erythroderma may be scaly or nonscaly.

In the scaly category, it is psoriasis and eczema (atopic dermatitis, allergic contact dermatitis, and seborrheic dermatitis) that are most frequently seen. Mycosis fungoides

---

TABLE 6.8. Differential Diagnosis of Peeling Palms

INFECTIOUS
- Tinea manuum
- Kawasaki disease
- Post-scarlet fever
- Toxin-mediated processes
- Postinfectious desquamation

INFLAMMATORY
- Keratolysis exfoliativa
- Peeling skin syndrome
- Keratolytic winter erythema

may also become erythrodermic. Sezary syndrome is the presence of erythrodermic mycosis fungoides along with circulating atypical T cells. Internal lymphomas and leukemias can also cause a scaly erythroderma. Widespread drug eruptions may be nonscaly (diffuse exanthematous drug reaction, "red man syndrome") or scaly (any longstanding eruption). Rarer causes of scaly erythrodermas include pityriasis rubra pilaris, lichen planus, dermatomyositis, and nonbullous congenital ichthyosiform erythroderma. Very rarely, tinea corporis may become generalized.

> **Clinical Tip** Causes of erythroderma in the papulosquamous reaction pattern include psoriasis, pityriasis rubra pilaris, lichen planus, dermatomyositis, nonbullous congenital ichthyosiform erythroderma, and tinea corporis.

Table 6.9 focuses on information that can be gathered by searching the entire cutaneous surface. The scalp, hair, nails, mucous membranes, and lymph nodes may all reveal diagnostic clues. A systematic examination of these areas is therefore of vital importance. In erythroderma, specific morphologic features of the primary eruption may be difficult to discern and so, vital clues can be garnered in these locations.

Clues to papulosquamous disease in the scalp include the presence of alopecia as well as hair shaft abnormalities. Alopecia may be scarring or nonscarring. Lichen planopilaris is a scarring alopecia that typically presents over the anterior scalp and vertex with perifollicular erythema and scale that advances to scarred areas. Frontal fibrosing alopecia is a variant of lichen planus. It is usually seen in older women. The anterior and lateral hairline is preferentially involved with the same findings. Discoid lupus in the scalp presents with scaly plaques on the skin that eventuate into scarred atrophic plaques with color change. Kerion is an inflammatory response to the presence of a zoophilic tinea capitis. If untreated, it may lead to scarring. Scarring alopecia may be seen in the later stages of incontinentia pigmenti, usually after the verrucous stage. As mentioned above, favus is a form of tinea capitis caused by *Trichophyton schoenleinii*. It presents with cornflake-like scale and ultimately causes scarring. Nonscarring alopecia is seen in tinea capitis caused by *Microsporum canis* ("gray dot") or *Trichophyton tonsurans* ("black dot"). The gray-dot or black-dot appearance is caused by broken-off hairs. Follicular mucinosis may be seen in mycosis fungoides. There is hair loss in involved areas, which may appear as scaly plaques, boggy plaques, or close-to-normal skin. Secondary syphilis causes a patchy, so-called "moth-eaten" alopecia (Figure 6.37). Hair shaft abnormalities include those seen in Netherton syndrome and in tinea capitis, as alluded to above. In Netherton syndrome, trichorrhexis invaginata ("bamboo hair," which resembles a ball and socket) is the most frequent hair shaft abnormality encountered. Usually the frontal scalp hair and the eyebrows are affected. Other hair shaft abnormalities such as trichorrhexis nodosa (with breakage occurring at areas of weakness along the hair shaft) and pili torti (with hairs twisted around the long axis of the hair shaft) are also seen. There is a short list of conditions that cause grains or concretions of scale around hair shafts. Pityriasis amiantacea, as mentioned previously, is concretions of scale around shafts (as seen in Figure 6.31). In favus, the cornflake-like scale may trap hairs. In white piedra, loosely adherent powdery grains are found on pubic hair and on the face. *Trichosporon* species are responsible. In black piedra, firmly adherent small black grains are most commonly found on scalp hair. *Piedraia hortae* is the responsible organism. In trichomycosis axillaris, yellowish material surrounds

TABLE 6.9. Gathering Information from Scalp, Hair, Nails, Mucous Membranes, and Lymph Nodes for Papulosquamous Diseases

SCALP
- Scarring alopecia
  - Lichen planopilaris
  - DLE
  - Frontal fibrosing alopecia
  - Kerion
  - Incontinentia pigmenti
  - Favus
- Nonscarring alopecia
  - Tinea capitis
  - Follicular mucinosis
  - Secondary syphilis

HAIR
- Hair shaft abnormalities
  - Netherton syndrome
  - Tinea capitis
- Grains/concretions around the hair shaft
  - White piedra
  - Black piedra
  - Trichomycosis axillaris
  - Pityriasis amiantacea
  - Scutula
  - Nits

NAILS
- Psoriasis
  - Nail matrix disease: coarse, irregular pits
  - Nail bed disease: onycholysis, subungual hyperkeratosis, splinter hemorrhages, oil-drop sign
  - Acrodermatitis continua of Hallopeau
  - Psoriatic onychopachydermoperiostitis
- Lichen planus
  - Longitudinal ridging
  - Pterygium formation: nail fold carried forward on nail bed to form a triangular ridge
  - "Sandpapered" nail dystrophy: fine longitudinal lines
  - Twenty nail dystrophy: all nails display trachyonychia (a roughened surface)
  - Anonychia
- DLE, SCLE
  - Periungual erythema is a sign of SLE
  - Onycholysis, longitudinal ridging, red lunulae, leukonychia
- Onychomycosis
  - Distal lateral subungual onychomycosis
  - Superficial white onychomycosis
  - Total dystrophic onychomycosis
- Pityriasis rubra pilaris
  - Subungual hyperkeratosis
- Reactive arthritis
  - Pitting

(Continued)

TABLE 6.9. Gathering Information from Scalp, Hair, Nails, Mucous Membranes, and Lymph Nodes for Papulosquamous Diseases (continued)

NAILS (CONT.)
- Subungual hyperkeratosis
- Pustules
- Chronic graft-versus-host disease
  - Nail changes of lichen planus may be seen
- Darier disease
  - Distal V-shaped nick is characteristic
  - Longitudinal red lines
  - Longitudinal white lines
  - Alternating longitudinal red and white lines: known as the "sandwich sign" or "candy cane"
- Hailey–Hailey disease: longitudinal white lines
- ILVEN: trachyonychia (see Figure 6.33D)

MUCOUS MEMBRANES
- Lichen planus and lichenoid graft-versus-host disease
  - Reticulate white plaques on the buccal mucosa
  - Reticulate and confluent white plaques on the lips
  - Erosive oral disease: seen especially on the tongue
  - Violaceous plaques are also seen on the tongue
  - Penile involvement: annular form common on the penis
  - Vulvar involvement: whitish reticular plaques or erosive disease seen
- Secondary syphilis
  - Mucous patches
  - "Snail track" ulcers
- DLE
  - Plaques resemble those on the skin, typically found on the palate
  - Oral ulcers may also be seen in cases of systemic lupus erythematosus (SLE)
- Reactive arthritis
  - Geographic tongue
  - Circinate balanitis
- Vitamin B_2 or B_6 deficiency: glossitis
- SLE
  - Oral ulcers
  - Vulval ulcers resembling oral ulcers may also be seen
- Darier disease: "cobblestoning"—white corrugated plaques on the palate

LYMPH NODES
- Mycosis fungoides
- Erythroderma; reactive enlargement
- Tinea capitis: reactive occipital node enlargement

the axillary hair. Less frequently, pubic hair is involved. *Corynebacterium* species are responsible. Finally, nits are the egg casings of head lice that attach to the hair with a centimeter of the scalp.

Regarding nails, many papulosquamous diseases have characteristic nail findings that can provide clues to diagnosis, and these are detailed in Table 6.9. Typical nail findings in psoriasis include coarse irregular pits (nail matrix disease; Figure 6.38),

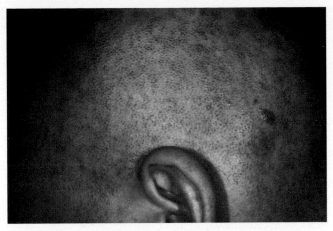

FIGURE 6.37 • Secondary syphilis, manifesting typical "moth-eaten" alopecia.

onycholysis, subungual hyperkeratosis, and the oil-drop sign (all signs of nail bed disease). The "oil-drop sign" refers to a light brown discoloration that is seen just proximal to the free edge of an affected nail, usually toward the side of the nail. It represents incipient onycholysis. Splinter hemorrhages are a further finding in nail psoriasis.

> **Clinical Tip** Oil-drop sign: light brown discoloration of distal nail in psoriasis.

Acrodermatitis continua of Hallopeau is a destructive form of pustular psoriasis in which painless pustules around and under the nail persist and recur and eventuate

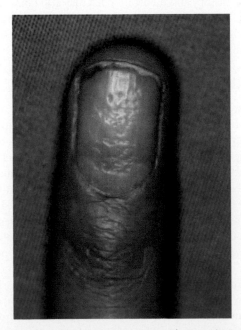

FIGURE 6.38 • Nail psoriasis: nail matrix disease presenting with coarse irregular nail pits.

> **TABLE 6.10. Important Pointers in History for Papulosquamous Diseases**
>
> **MEDICAL PROBLEMS**
> - DLE, SCLE: need to rule out SLE
> - Parkinson disease, HIV: associated with seborrheic dermatitis
> - Take a thorough nutrition history to rule out nutritional disorders
> - Is the patient a stem cell or bone marrow transplant recipient?
>
> **MEDICATION HISTORY**
> - Lichenoid drug eruption: ACE inhibitors, calcium channel blockers, β-blockers, HCTZ, NSAIDs, gold, anti-TB drugs, tumor necrosis factor-α antagonists, interferon
> - Psoriasis exacerbation: β-blockers, NSAIDs, lithium, antimalarials, tumor necrosis factor-α antagonists
> - Mycosis fungoides–like drug eruption: antihypertensive agents, antidepressants
> - Pityriasis rosea–like eruption: ACE inhibitors, terbinafine, imatinib, omeprazole, gold
> - INH, azathioprine can cause pellagra
> - Drug-induced SCLE: antihypertensives (HCTZ, calcium channel blockers, ACE inhibitors), terbinafine, proton pump inhibitors, taxanes

in scarring and anonychia. The condition typically initially involves the thumb. One or more nails may be involved. Psoriatic onychopachydermoperiostitis is a rarely encountered finding in psoriasis. Here, the terminal phalanges display a periostitis. The overlying nail manifests onycholysis and subungual hyperkeratosis, and the surrounding soft tissue is edematous and thickened. Table 6.9 also details the range of nail findings in lichen planus and Darier disease, among others. It goes on to summarize mucous membrane findings of papulosquamous disease, as well as lymph node findings.

A patient's medical history and medication list may also point toward a certain diagnosis, as seen in Table 6.10. Geographic locale is important when considering the diagnosis of a deep fungal infection, and knowledge of local prevalence of these diseases will also help guide differential diagnosis.

BEDSIDE DIAGNOSTICS AND BLOODWORK

Bedside diagnostics are tests that may be employed in the clinic to assist in diagnosis before performing a biopsy. Bloodwork may also assist with diagnosis and obviate the need for biopsy. Chapter 14 will cover the range of these tests in detail. For each reaction pattern, a subset of diagnostic tests can be useful. Table 6.11 lists those tests that are useful in formulating a definitive diagnosis among papulosquamous diseases.

The first set of tests for this reaction pattern aims to procure more information from scales. The fine white branny scales of tinea versicolor may not be immediately evident. If the skin around an affected plaque is stretched laterally, scales cleave and become more apparent. One of my teachers imparted the following global rule: "If it scales, scrape it." A simple microscopic examination of scales with potassium hydroxide (KOH) will allow for accurate diagnosis of dermatophytosis and tinea versicolor. This is especially important for nonclassic, nonannular dermatophytosis, the appearance of which may have been altered by topical steroid application, or by an immunocompromised host. So, for any scaly eruption in which the diagnosis is not clear, a scraping of scales for KOH examination should be performed.

TABLE 6.11 Bedside Diagnostics for Differentiating Papulosquamous Diseases

MORE DIAGNOSTIC INFORMATION FROM SCALES
- Apply gentle lateral pressure to the papules and plaques of suspected tinea versicolor
- Perform a skin scraping to look for fungal elements
- Examine suspected tinea versicolor, erythrasma, or tinea capitis under Wood's lamp
- Gently scrape a psoriatic plaque with the back of a cotton-tipped applicator

REMOVING SCALES FOR MORE DIAGNOSTIC INFORMATION
- Moisten scales with alcohol wipe
- Apply mineral oil to the plaques of suspected lichen planus
- Remove the thick scale of suspected discoid lupus

SEROLOGICAL TESTS
- RPR
- ANA
- Anti-Ro antibodies

Clinical Tip If it scales, scrape it.

Another tool for diagnosis of fungal disease is Wood's lamp. Tinea versicolor fluoresces a yellowish green color under Wood's lamp examination. It may be differentiated from erythrasma by the size of thin plaques (which tend to be larger in erythrasma), their location (tinea versicolor favors the seborrheic areas while erythrasma favors the intertriginous areas), and by the fact that erythrasma fluoresces a coral-pink color under Wood's lamp. A KOH preparation in erythrasma is also negative. Hairs affected by *Microsporum canis* and other zoophilic dermatophytes (ectothrix) fluoresce a bright green. Hairs involved by *Trichophyton schoenleinii* exhibit a blue-white fluorescence.

The Auspitz sign describes the bleeding points that eventuate when plaques of psoriasis are firmly scraped with the back of a cotton-tipped applicator. The bleeding points represent tips of the papillary dermis that are unroofed when the thinned rete ridges that are classic of psoriasis are removed. While I do not use this sign for diagnosis, I do modify the technique in cases where I suspect psoriasis but where the scales are adherent; lighter scraping will not cause bleeding, but it will detach diagnostic silvery scales.

While scales render a wealth of diagnostic information, removing the scales can reveal the morphology of their underlying papules and plaques more fully. An alcohol wipe can be used to accomplish this. Mineral oil application to a plaque of lichen planus will enhance the appearance of Wickham's striae. These are white lines that course along the surface of lesions of lichen planus. They represent areas of hypergranulosis that are characteristic of the disease histopathologically. Finally, lifting the sheet of hyperkeratotic scale from a plaque of discoid lupus will reveal widened follicular openings on the plaque and follicular plugs (the so-called carpet-tack sign) on the undersurface of the scaly sheet.

Clinical Tip Carpet-tack sign: follicular plugs on the underside of lifted scale in DLE.

This chapter would not be complete without mentioning serological tests. A high index of suspicion for syphilis should be held in this reaction pattern, and an RPR with serial dilution (so guard against a false negative result due to the prozone phenomenon) should be ordered for any unusual scaly eruption.

> **Clinical Tip** Perform an RPR with serial dilutions for any unusual papulosquamous eruption.

Antinuclear antibodies (ANA) and anti-Ro antibodies should be performed when subacute lupus is suspected and as part of systemic lupus screening in discoid lupus.

SUMMARY

- The papulosquamous reaction pattern includes a broad array of infectious, inflammatory, neoplastic, paraneoplastic, and drug-induced dermatoses.
- The diagnostic boxes of the wheel of diagnosis may assist in narrowing down a differential diagnosis.
- Scales are an important determinant that may hold diagnostic clues in this reaction pattern.
- Some "do not miss" diagnoses in this reaction pattern include the following:
  - Tinea
  - Crusted scabies
  - Secondary syphilis
  - Lupus
  - Mycosis fungoides
  - Other cancers: squamous cell cancer in situ, invasive squamous cell cancer, verrucous carcinoma
- Bedside diagnostics can be employed to narrow down a diagnosis. Serologic tests can also add diagnostic information.

The Vesicobullous Reaction Pattern

7

The vesicobullous reaction pattern includes those diseases that present with vesicles and bullae. These are both colloquially referred to as *blisters*. In this chapter, this term is used to imply a combination of vesicles and bullae. The vesicobullous reaction pattern overlaps with the eczematous reaction pattern, in that vesicles and bullae are seen in acute eczema. So, it would be accurate to categorize acute eczema as either eczematous or vesicobullous reaction pattern.

> **Clinical Tip** Vesicobullous and eczematous reaction patterns overlap; acute eczema, such as an allergic contact dermatitis due to poison ivy, also fits into the vesicobullous reaction pattern.

Some blistering diseases may have a papulosquamous presentation, as has been mentioned previously. Pemphigus foliaceus is a classic example of this. It frequently presents with exfoliative plaques and very few or indistinct erosions. Other blistering diseases, such as pemphigus vegetans, present as vegetating plaques.

> **Clinical Tip** A vesicobullous reaction pattern may have a papulosquamous presentation.

As with papulosquamous disease, it is useful when encountering a patient with vesicobullous disease to have a ready-made differential diagnostic list to be able to apply to the presenting dermatosis. Table 7.1 contains such a list for the vesicobullous reaction pattern, subdivided by the etiologic classification. Again, this list is comprehensive, but by no means complete. A description of the classic presentation of each disease follows:

All inherited blistering diseases are rarely encountered. The first stage of incontinentia pigmenti is the vesicobullous stage; vesicles and bullae are seen following Blaschko lines at birth or within the first few weeks of life (Figure 7.1). The inherited epidermolysis bullosa (EB) group is important to recognize. In EB simplex, blisters occur after minor trauma predominantly on the palms and soles. Onset is usually in childhood. There are four distinct subtypes. The Dowling–Meara variant may display herpetiform grouping of vesicles and bullae and an associated palmoplantar keratoderma. In EB simplex superficialis, skin peeling may occur without bona fide blisters. Scarring is uncommon. In junctional EB (JEB), severe skin fragility and widespread bulla formation and erosions appear shortly after birth (Figure 7.2). Tracheolaryngeal, corneal, and urogenital involvement may occur. Nails may be lost. Exuberant granulation tissue

TABLE 7.1. Vesicobullous Diseases by Etiologic Classification

INHERITED
- Vesicobullous stage of incontinentia pigmenti
- Epidermolysis bullosa simplex
- Junctional epidermolysis bullosa
- Dystrophic epidermolysis bullosa: recessive and dominant forms
- Bullous congenital ichthyosiform erythroderma
- Hailey–Hailey disease
- Darier disease

ACQUIRED
- Infectious
  - Bacterial
    - Bullous impetigo
    - Bullous erysipelas or cellulitis
    - Staphylococcal scalded skin syndrome
    - Blistering distal dactylitis
    - MIRM
  - Treponemal
    - Early congenital syphilis
  - Viral
    - HSV
      - Orolabial, genital HSV
      - Herpetic whitlow
      - Kaposi varicelliform eruption
      - Disseminated HSV
      - Neonatal HSV
    - VZV
      - Chickenpox
      - Herpes zoster
      - Disseminated zoster
    - Vesicular eruption of COVID-19 infection
    - Gianotti–Crosti syndrome
    - Hand–foot–mouth disease
    - Orf
    - Milker's nodule
  - Rickettsial
    - Rickettsialpox
  - Fungal
    - Bullous tinea pedis
- Inflammatory
  - Acute eczema
  - Bullous insect bites
  - Bullous erythema multiforme
  - Bullous Lyme
  - Bullous Sweet syndrome
  - Leukocytoclastic vasculitis
  - Bullae in septic vasculitis
  - Grover disease
  - Polymorphous light eruption
  - Prurigo pigmentosa

(Continued)

TABLE 7.1. Vesicobullous Diseases by Etiologic Classification (continued)

ACQUIRED (CONT.)

- Hydroa vacciniforme
- Autoimmune bullous disease
  - Intraepidermal group
    - Pemphigus folicaeous, fogo selvagem, pemphigus erythematosus
    - Pemphigus herpetiformis
    - IgA pemphigus
    - Pemphigus vulgaris, pemphigus vegetans
    - Paraneoplastic autoimmune mucosal syndrome
  - Subepidermal group
    - Bullous pemphigoid, pemphigoid gestationis
    - Anti-p200 pemphigoid
    - Lichen planus pemphigoides
    - Mucous membrane pemphigoid
    - Linear IgA disease and chronic bullous disease of childhood
    - Dermatitis herpetiformis
    - Epidermolysis bullosa acquisita
    - Bullous SLE
- Noninflammatory
  - Miliaria crystallina
  - Friction, suction, thermal
  - Phytophotodermatitis
  - Diabetic bulla
  - Coma bulla
  - Bullous amyloidosis
- Metabolic
  - Porphyrias
    - Porphyria cutanea tarda
    - Variegate porphyria
    - Erythropoietic protoporphyria
    - X-linked protoporphyria
    - Gunther disease
  - Necrolytic conditions
    - Necrolytic migratory erythema
    - Acrodermatitis enteropathica
    - Necrolytic acral erythema
- Drug-induced
  - Fixed drug eruption
  - SJS/TEN
  - Grover disease
  - Pseudoporphyria
  - Phototoxicity
  - Autoimmune bullous disease
    - Pemphigus vulgaris
    - Bullous pemphigoid
    - Linear IgA disease
    - Dermatitis herpetiformis

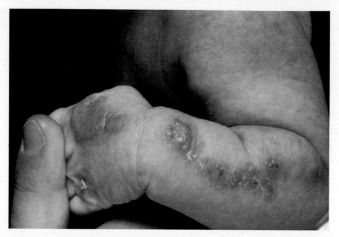

FIGURE 7.1 · The first stage of incontinentia pigmenti displaying vesicles, bullae, and crusting in Blaschko line.

is a feature in later childhood. Atrophic scarring is common. Generalized atrophic benign EB is a milder variant. Alopecia is common here. Localized and inverse types occur. In the recessive form of dystrophic EB (DEB), skin findings similar to those of JEB are seen. Scarring is common and severe. "Mitten" deformities of the hands may be seen. Milia are common. Squamous cell carcinomas arise in chronic wounds. Intraoral, esophageal, and other mucous membrane involvement may be seen. Milder, localized, and inverse variants occur. In autosomal dominantly inherited DEB, there

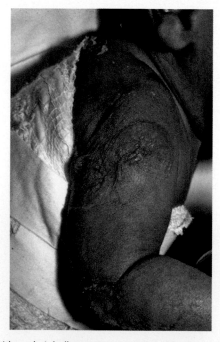

FIGURE 7.2 · Junctional epidermolysis bullosa presenting with bullae and erosions in the neonatal period.

is milder skin fragility, in general. Bullae, erosions and ulcers usually occur over bony prominences. White scarred papules and plaques dominate the clinical picture in the albopapuloid (Pasini) variant. Another inherited vesicobullous disease that appears at birth or shortly after is bullous congenital ichthyosiform erythroderma; blisters, erosions, and peeling with or without erythroderma are seen within hours of birth. These usually resolve in the first few months. While easy blistering may continue to be a feature until adolescence, widespread thick linear scales appear in early childhood and dominate the clinical picture thereafter. Two primarily vesicular inherited diseases that present later in life are Hailey–Hailey disease and Darier disease. As was seen in the papulosquamous reaction pattern chapter (Chapter 6), both may have a scaly presentation. In Hailey–Hailey disease, small flaccid vesicles rapidly become erosions in the intertriginous areas and other sites of friction. Macerated plaques with linear erosions ("rents") are seen in occluded areas (Figure 7.3). The rare vesicobullous variant of Darier disease presents with vesicles and bullae predominantly located on the upper half of the body.

In the infectious category of acquired disease, bacterial diseases including bullous impetigo, bullous erysipelas or cellulitis, staphylococcal scalded skin syndrome, and blistering distal dactylitis should be considered. In bullous impetigo, flaccid vesicles and bullae quickly eventuate into shallow erosions with collarettes of scale. Bullous forms of erysipelas or, more rarely, cellulitis may occur. A deep-seated tense bulla will eventuate within a preexisting warm, tender plaque in each case (Figure 7.4). In staphylococcal scalded skin syndrome, widespread flaccid blisters coalesce, producing sheets of superficial peeling, or exfoliation. It is caused by exfoliating toxin A- and B-producing strains of *Staphylococcus aureus*. Children are most frequently affected, and in adults with the disease, some degree of renal dysfunction is usually present and the toxin is not cleared. In blistering distal dactylitis, a tense cloudy bulla sits atop an erythematous plaque, characteristically on the finger or toe pad of the distal phalanx, usually in a child. Mycoplasma pneumoniae-induced rash and mucositis (MIRM) is a

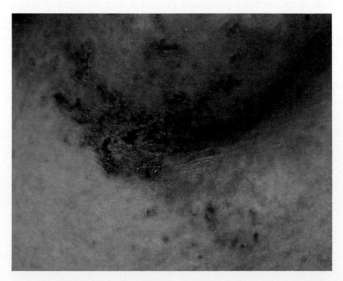

FIGURE 7.3 • Hailey–Hailey disease showing a macerated plaque and linear erosions in the fold.

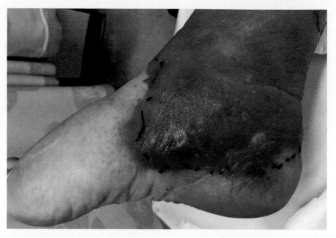

FIGURE 7.4 • Bullous erysipelas, demonstrating a well-demarcated brightly erythematous plaque with bulla formation, on an extremity.

recently recognized entity that likely accounts for most cases of erythema multiforme major. It is seen in children most frequently. *Mycoplasma pneumoniae* is the causative organism. There are prominent mucous membrane findings, including hemorrhagic crusting of lips and intraoral erosions. The associated cutaneous eruption is sparse and usually acrally located. Papular, vesicular, or targetoid morphologies may be seen. In early congenital syphilis, a treponemal disease, vesicles and bullae may be present. These may have a palmoplantar distribution or may be diffuse. The herpes virus family is a common cause of vesiculation in children and adults. In orolabial herpes simplex virus (HSV), the primary infection is a painful gingivostomatitis. Recurrent disease presents with groups of vesicles on an erythematous base (the herpetiform configuration), usually on or near the lip. These may become pustules before eroding (at which point the border appears scalloped) and crusting over. In genital HSV, the primary disease may manifest with single or grouped vesicles or erosions over genital skin. Recurrent disease resembles recurrent oral disease. The term *herpetic whitlow* refers to primary inoculation and recurrent disease of a digit, usually a finger (Figure 7.5). This may be vesicular or secondarily purulent. The herpetiform cluster of lesions can assist with diagnosis here. *Kaposi varicelliform eruption* refers to HSV that has become disseminated within an underlying dermatosis. Usually this is seen in atopic eczema, but other forms of eczema, Darier disease, burns, and autoimmune blistering diseases may be similarly infected. *Eczema herpeticum* is the term referring to HSV that disseminates in eczema. A diagnostic sign is the presence of monomorphic 1–2-mm vesicles, erosions or crusts (Figure 7.6).

> **Clinical Tip** The presence of monomorphic vesicles, erosions, or crusts is a clue to the presence of Kaposi varicelliform eruption.

In chickenpox, caused by varicella zoster virus (VZV), crops of macules, papules, vesicles, pustules, ulcers, and crusts erupt on the scalp, face, and chest and spread centrifugally (Figure 7.7). Reactivated VZV gives rise to zoster, in which grouped vesicles

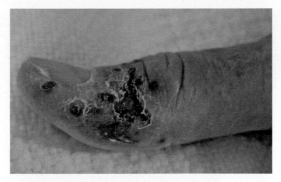

FIGURE 7.5 · Herpetic whitlow, showing grouped monomorphic crusts on a digit.

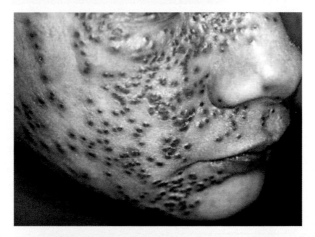

FIGURE 7.6 · Eczema herpeticum, demonstrating widespread, discrete monomorphic crusts.

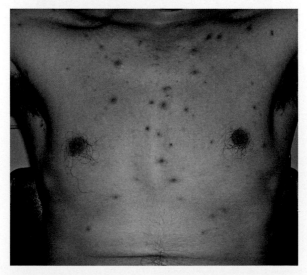

FIGURE 7.7 · Chickenpox with papules, vesicles, and pustules on the torso.

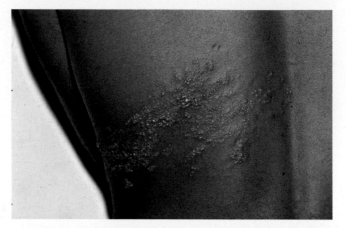

FIGURE 7.8 · Zoster with grouped vesicles on an erythematous base in a thoracic dermatome.

on an erythematous base are seen in a dermatomal distribution (Figure 7.8). Both HSV and zoster may become disseminated. This usually occurs in immunocompromised hosts. Necrotic, multidermatomal, or recurrent zoster is also seen in this population (Figure 7.9). Both HSV and chickenpox can be seen in the neonatal period, usually acquired from maternal disease. A monomporphic vesicular eruption has also been recognized as a manifestation of COVID-19 infection. Vesicles may coalesce to form bullae and hemorrrhagic bullae may occur. In papular acrodermatitis of childhood (Gianotti–Crosti syndrome), monomorphic papules or papulovesicles occur on the

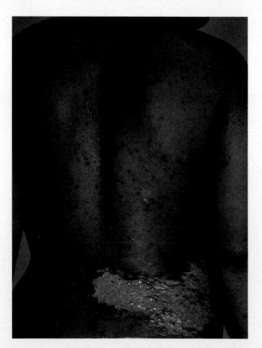

FIGURE 7.9 · Disseminated zoster with an eroded nonhealing primary dermatomal site and disseminated papules, in an HIV-positive patient.

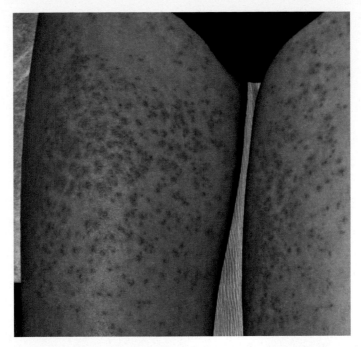

FIGURE 7.10 • Gianotti–Crosti syndrome with multiple, erythematous papulovesicles on the extremities. (Used with permission from Dr. Miguel Sanchez, Bellevue Hospital, New York University School of Medicine, New York, NY.)

extremities and face, and typically spare the trunk (Figure 7.10). This eruption has been associated with the Epstein–Barr virus, hepatitis B, cytomegalovirus, and some enteroviruses. Hand–foot–mouth disease is caused by coxsackie virus A16, but other strains and enteroviruses may be responsible. A high fever gives way to a vesicular eruption that is concentrated on the hands and feet. The vesicles may be oval-shaped, resembling a football, and a gray color. Enterovirus 71 infection gives rise to a more severe form of the disease with a more widespread exanthema. There are intraoral erosions, which cause pain on eating, and perioral vesicles may be seen. Young children are frequently affected. Orf and milker's nodule are two inoculation diseases caused by parapox viruses. A large vesicle may develop at the inoculation site, usually on the finger or hand, after contact with sheep or goats (orf) or cows (milker's nodule). Pustular or verrucous forms may occur.

Rickettsialpox is a rickettsial infection caused by *Rickettsia akari*. It is transmitted by the house mouse mite bite. A papulovesicular eruption of few to many lesions occurs in concert with systemic symptoms (malaise, fever, headache) following a primary eschar that is seen at the site of inoculation (Figure 7.11). Many cases have been reported in New York City. Finally, in the fungal category, is bullous tinea pedis, which is typically caused by *Trichophyton mentagrophytes*. Bullous tinea pedis is usually unilateral and is often itchy. Vesicles of varying sizes coalesce to form groups of bullae. The forefoot, central sole, and medial foot are most frequently affected.

In the inflammatory category, and as previously mentioned, vesicles and bullae with erythema are the hallmarks of acute eczema, such as an acute contact dermatitis (Figure 7.12). Eczemas will be covered in more detail in Chapter 8.

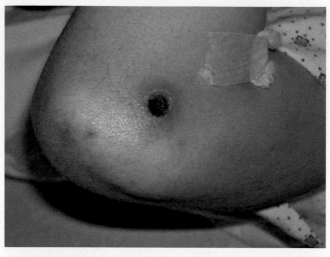

FIGURE 7.11 · Rickettsialpox displaying an eschar at the site of inoculation of *R. akari* and a couple of early papulovesicles over the elbow. (Used with permission from Dr. Miguel Sanchez, Bellevue Hospital, New York University School of Medicine, New York, NY.)

A robust arthropod assault will give rise to a bulla secondary to significant subepidermal edema (Figure 7.13). Bullous forms of erythema multiforme occur, especially when HSV is the inciting infection (Figure 7.14). Solitary mastocytomas are usually seen in childhood. Firmly stroking the surface of a mastocytoma will cause urtication

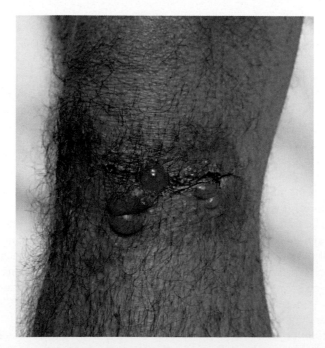

FIGURE 7.12 · Acute contact dermatitis due to poison ivy displaying vesicles and bullae superimposed on an erythematous plaque.

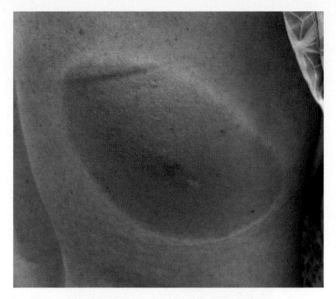

FIGURE 7.13 • A spider bite displaying central vesiculation.

(positive Darier sign). In severe cases, secondary bulla formation due to significant subepidermal edema is seen. Acute febrile neutrophilic dermatosis (Sweet syndrome) typically presents with juicy plaques with a pseudovesicular appearance (Figure 7.15). True bulla formation is rare, but grayish-blue bullae are seen in malignancy-associated cases.

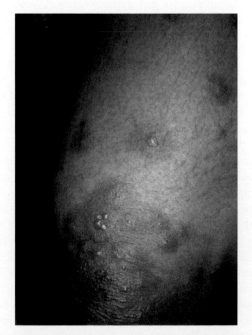

FIGURE 7.14 • Bullous erythema multiforme secondary to HSV infection with raised atypical target lesions on an elbow. (Used with permission from Dr. Miguel Sanchez, New York University, New York, NY.)

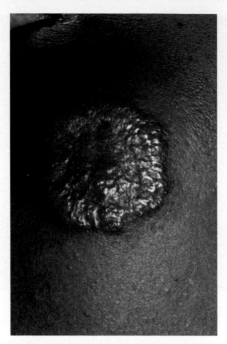

FIGURE 7.15 • Sweet syndrome showing a typical juicy plaque with a pseudovesicular appearance on the upper cheek.

Clinical Tip Very edematous plaques, such as those of Sweet syndrome, may appear vesicular when in actuality they are not. This phenomenon is termed a *pseudovesicular appearance*.

Erythema migrans of Lyme disease seldom blisters; however, cases of bullous erythema migrans occurring on flexural surfaces have been reported (Figure 7.16). Bullae may be secondary to robust inflammation and resultant tissue ischemia in small vessel vasculitis or septic vasculitis. Inflammatory diseases with vesicles include Grover disease, polymorphous light eruption, and prurigo pigmentosa. Grover disease (transient acantholytic dermatosis), usually presents with 2–3-mm scaly papules (a papulosquamous disease) on the trunk of middle-aged to elderly men. It is usually very pruritic, but asymptomatic cases also occur. Histopathologically, there are superficial clefts in the epidermis caused by acantholysis. These lead to tiny superficial vesicles that turn over rapidly given their superficial location. So, a true vesicular presentation is rare, and this has usually occurred in acute flares. In polymorphous light eruption, itchy papules, papulovesicles, vesicles, and/or plaques occur in the photoexposed distribution up to hours after sun exposure. Prurigo pigmentosa is a rare disorder that occurs predominantly in females in Japan. Ketosis associated with dieting has been implicated as a cause. Erythematous papules eventuate into papulovesicles (Figure 7.17). These ultimately crust and resolve, leaving reticulate brown macules. Hydroa vacciniforme is seen primarily in children (boys more frequently and severely affected than girls). Within hours of sun exposure, affected skin reddens and develops vesicles and bullae

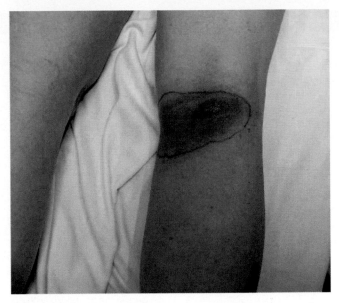

FIGURE 7.16 • Erythema migrans with a hemorrhagic and bullous appearance in the popliteal fossa.

that are typically umbilicated. These findings progress to hemorrhagic crusts and ultimately to depressed varioliform scarring. Chronic Epstein–Barr virus infection has been associated in some cases. Children usually outgrow the eruption by adolescence or early adulthood.

Of prime importance in this category is the consideration of primary autoimmune blistering diseases. A complete list of these diseases along with their target antigens appears in Table 7.2. The pemphigus group of diseases is considered to be superficial blistering diseases, given that they arise histopathologically above the basement membrane zone within the epidermis. In pemphigus foliaceus, fogo selvagem (the endemic

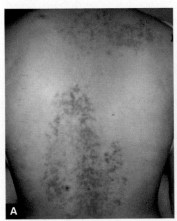

FIGURE 7.17 • (A) Prurigo pigmentosa—clusters of papulovesicles on the back with reticulated brown macules; (B) prurigo pigmentosa—a close-up of papulovesicles. (Used with permission from Dr. Miguel Sanchez, New York University, New York, NY.)

TABLE 7.2. Autoimmune Blistering Diseases and Their Target Antigens

DISEASE	TARGET ANTIGEN
Pemphigus foliaceus, fogo selvagem, pemphigus erythematosus	Dsg1
Pemphigus vulgaris, intraoral	Dsg3
Pemphigus vulgaris, pemphigus vegetans	Dsg3, Dsg1
Pemphigus herpetiformis	Dsg1, sometimes Dsg3 or Dsc1 or Dsg3
IgA pemphigus	
Subcorneal pustular dermatosis type	Dsc1
Intraepidermal neutrophilic type	Unknown
PAMS	Dsg3, Dsg1, envoplakin, periplakin, BPAG1, plectin, desmoplakins I and II
Bullous pemphigoid, pemphigoid gestationis	BP230, BP180
Lichen planus pemphigoides	BP230, BP180
Anti-p200 pemphigoid	200-kDa protein in the lamina lucida
	BP180, BP230, laminin 332 (previously known as *epiligrin* or *laminin 5*), α6β4 integrin, and type VII collagen
Linear IgA disease, chronic bullous disease of childhood	97- and 120-kDa antigens (part of the extracellular portion of BP180); or NC16a epitope of BP180
Dermatitis herpetiformis	Epidermal transglutaminase
Epidermolysis bullosa acquisita	Collagen VII, NC1 domain > NC2 domain
Bullous SLE	Collagen VII in some, others target antigen unknown

Abbreviations: Dsg = desmoglein, Dsc = desmocollin.

form of pemphigus foliaceus encountered in Brazil), and pemphigus erythematosus (a subtype of pemphigus foliaceus that involves the malar area), flaccid blisters are quickly superseded by superficial erosions and exfoliative plaques (Figure 7.18). Facial involvement with erythema and scale over the cheeks is classically seen in pemphigus erythematosus. This finding precedes involvement in other areas. In pemphigus herpetiformis, itchy herpetiform clusters of vesicles and round superficial erosions are seen (Figure 7.19). In IgA pemphigus, superficial vesicles and pustules, often in an annular configuration, are typical. Distribution is variable; predominant truncal, head and neck, or intertriginous presentations occur. Pemphigus vulgaris begins as a disease of mucous membranes, usually with painful oral erosions. It may progress to involve painful flaccid blisters and erosions on the skin (Figure 7.20). Pemphigus vegetans is a variant of pemphigus vulgaris in which vegetating plaques are seen in intertriginous areas and on the scalp (Figure 7.21). Paraneoplastic pemphigus (PNP) occurs in the setting of an underlying malignancy, typically non-Hodgkin lymphoma or Castleman disease. An intractable stomatitis is accompanied by a polymorphic skin eruption that may resemble pemphigus vulgaris, bullous pemphigoid, lichen planus, chronic graft-versus-host disease, or erythema multiforme. Other mucous membranes, including those of the conjunctivae, larynx, pharynx, esophagus, nasal mucosa, and anus, may be involved. PNP may involve respiratory mucosa and may

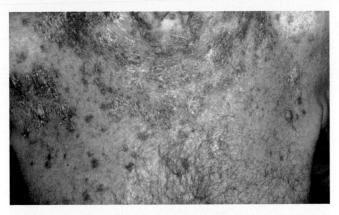

FIGURE 7.18 · Pemphigus foliaceus with few erosions around the neck and a predominance of scaly and exfoliative plaques.

cause an obliterating bronchiolitis in 20–40% of patients. Dyspnea is the first symptom here, and this may progress to respiratory failure. The term *paraneoplastic autoimmune multiorgan syndrome* (PAMS) has therefore been introduced to describe this disease more accurately, but both PNP and PAM.

The subepidermal autoimmune blistering diseases represent a heterogenous group. Bullous pemphigoid (BP) is the most frequently encountered entity in this category. A prebullous urticarial phase that manifests as urticarial plaques without bullae is

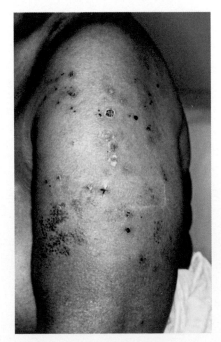

FIGURE 7.19 · Pemphigus herpetiformis with shallow erosions and crusts that are both clustered and discrete.

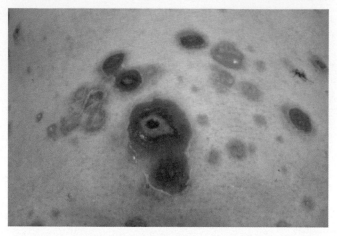

FIGURE 7.20 • Pemphigus vulgaris with a predominance of flaccid bullae and round erosions.

typical (Figure 7.22). It may last from weeks to months, and occasionally years. This is followed by the bullous phase with tense bullae arising in association (Figure 7.23). BP is most commonly generalized, but prsentations localized to legs or other sites have been reported. Variants include the pruriginous form, which resembles prurigo nodularis, and the dyshidrosiform variant, which occurs on palms and soles and may resemble dyshidrotic eczema (Figure 7.24). Further rarely encountered BP variants include pemphigoid vegetans (which resembles pemphigus vegetans) and a dermatitis

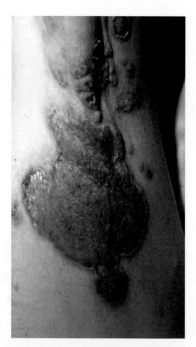

FIGURE 7.21 • Pemphigus vegetans, displaying a glistening vegetating plaque with a surrounding erosion, and many nearby eroded vesicles in the axilla.

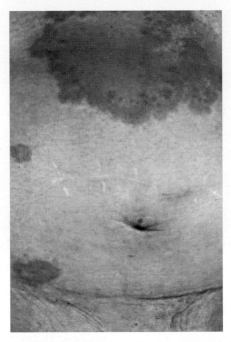

FIGURE 7.22 • Prebullous phase of bullous pemphigoid showing urticarial plaques.

herpetiformis–like vesicular variant. Bullous pemphigoid usually is seen in older individuals and may be drug-induced. Pemphigoid gestationis (herpes gestationis) is a bullous pemphigoid that arises in pregnancy. Annular plaques and arrays of bullae are typical. Anti-p200 pemphigoid is a more recently recognized entity that resembles dyshidrosiform bullous pemphigoid. The target antigen differs from the target antigens in bullous pemphigoid. Lichen planus pemphigoides is the coexistence of bullous pemphigoid and lichen planus. In mucous membrane pemphigoid (MMP; cicatricial pemphigoid), ocular, oral, and upper aerodigestive tract erosions dominate the clinical picture.

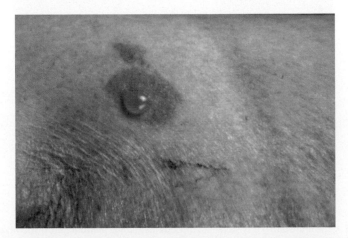

FIGURE 7.23 • Bullous pemphigoid, displaying a tense bulla arising from an urticarial plaque.

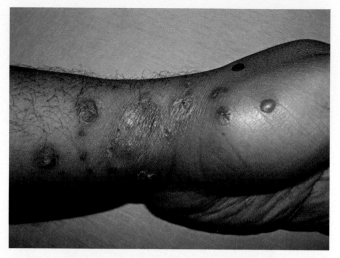

FIGURE 7.24 · Bullous pemphigioid with a resemblance to dyshidrotic eczema.

These may be accompanied by skin involvement with bullae, erosions, and prominent scarring. Many target antigens have been identified in MMP. An increased risk of malignancy is seen in those with antibodies to laminin 332. The Brunsting–Perry variant connotes isolated skin involvement, usually in the head-and-neck region (Figure 7.25). In linear IgA disease, annular arrays of tense vesicles on a background of erythema are

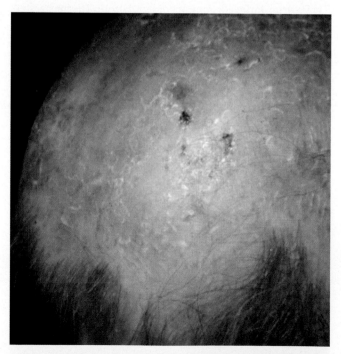

FIGURE 7.25 · The Brunsting–Perry variant of mucous membrane pemphigoid, displaying scattered crusting and scarring alopecia on the scalp.

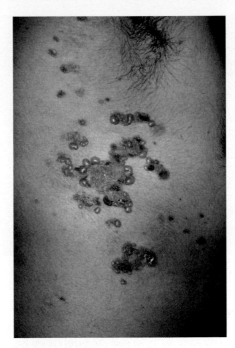

FIGURE 7.26 • Linear IgA disease, displaying annular and arcuate arrays of tense vesicles on the flank. (Image appears with permission from VisualDx. Copyright VisualDx.)

seen (Figure 7.26). Chronic bullous disease of childhood refers to linear IgA disease that occurs in childhood. In dermatitis herpetiformis, intensely itchy urticarial plaques surmounted by small tense vesicles, often in a herpetiform cluster, occur on the elbows, knees, and buttocks and in the scalp (Figure 7.27). Because of the intense associated pruritus, intact vesicles are rarely seen. In epidermolysis bullosa acquisita (EBA),

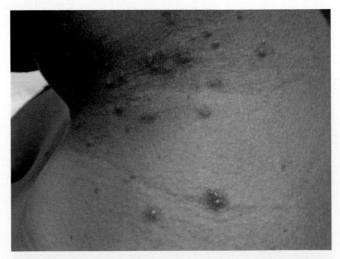

FIGURE 7.27 • Dermatitis herpetiformis, with tiny vesicles and papulovesicles surmounted on urticarial plaques. (Used with permission from Dr. Miguel Sanchez, Bellevue Hospital, New York University School of Medicine, New York, NY.)

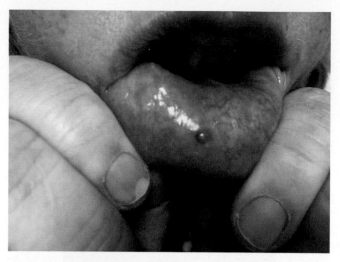

FIGURE 7.28 · Epidermolysis bullosa acquisita, displaying a tense vesicle on the buccal mucosa.

mechanobullous (deep-seated bullae on normal skin) and inflammatory (similar bullae on urticarial plaques) variants are seen. Scarring and milia formation accompany both types. The oral cavity may be involved (Figure 7.28). Bullous SLE is a primary autoimmune blistering disease that develops in patients with systemic lupus. These patients typically have major organ involvement from their lupus. Antibodies to the sublamina densa zone, including to collagen VII develop. Clinically, dermatitis herpetiformis- and bullous pemphigoid-like variants are reported. I have also seen a case that resembled linear IgA disease (Figure 7.29).

Noninflammatory vesicles and bullae are associated with a wide variety of physical stimuli. Miliaria crystallina are the fine, dewdrop-like vesicles that erupt secondary to blocked sweat ducts from increased heat and sweating, such as in a fever or in hot climates (Figure 7.30). Neonates and infants are most frequently affected. A sucking blister is seen at birth. It usually develops in a finger and is secondary to sucking of

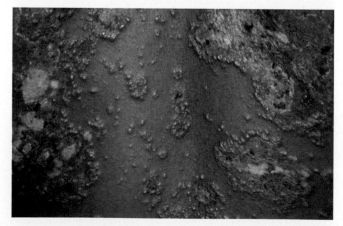

FIGURE 7.29 · Bullous SLE, resembling linear IgA disease with annular arrays of vesicles and central erosions.

FIGURE 7.30 · Miliaria crystallina with fine, dew drop-like vesicles. (Image appears with permission from VisualDx. Copyright VisualDx.)

that digit in utero. Thermal burns and friction also cause bullae. Friction bullae are seen most commonly on soles secondary to pressure from ill-fitting shoes, or on palms in athletes owing to repetitive pressure-inducing activities, such as gripping weights, gymnastic equipment or bats. Bullae are reported in bed-ridden people: these are termed coma bullae. They may be seen in the setting of fluid overload. Diabetic bullae are the noninflammatory bullae that occur on the distal lower extremities in a small proportion of longstanding diabetics. Phytophotodermatitis occurs after contact with botanicals that contain furocoumarins or psoralens. Examples include parsley, fennel, or limes. These chemicals photosensitize the skin, and acute blistering in a linear or geometric pattern may be seen. Bullous amyloidosis is a rare manifestation of primary systemic amyloidosis. Clinically, pinch purpura and a diffuse infiltration of skin with a doughy feel may be seen. Bullae may arise from minor trauma. A subepidermal split, likely arising above the lamina densa, is responsible.

The porphyrias are a group of inherited or acquired diseases that affect the heme biosynthetic pathway. Those that lead to cutaneous manifestations may all produce bullae. Erythropoietic protoporphyria (ferrochelastase deficiency) and X-linked protoporphyria (increased 5-aminolevulinate synthase activity) are marked by painful photosensitivity and edema of exposed areas. Onset is in infancy or childhood. Vesicles, bullae, and erosions are rare findings. Congenital erythropoietic porphyria (Gunther disease; uroporphyrinogen cosynthetase deficiency) is a severe disease of early onset that affects skin (photosensitivity, bullae, scarring, photomutilation of digits), teeth (erythrodontia), eyes (photosensitivity, keratoconjunctivitis, possible blindness), and red cells (hemolytic anemia). Porphyria cutanea tarda (PCT) typically has onset in adulthood. It may be inherited, with diminished uroporphyrinogen decarboxylase or acquired, in which liver disease such as from alcoholism, hepatitis C, or hemochromatosis diminishes the activity of uroporphyrinogen decarboxylase. Hepatoerythropoeitic porphyria (HEP) occur from homozygous loss of enzyme activity. It is a more severe disease with earlier onset. In both PCT and HEP, there are photosensitive bullae that lead to scarring and milia formation (Figures 7.31). Hypertrichosis and sclerodermoid changes are also seen. In porphyria variegata (variegate porphyria; protoporphyrinogen oxidase deficiency), there is photosensitivity and

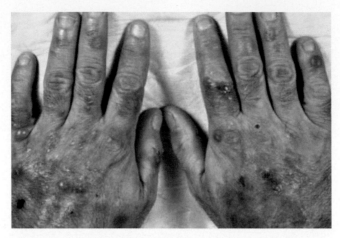

FIGURE 7.31 • Porphyria cutanea tarda, displaying tense bullae, erosions, crusts, and milia on dorsal hands.

acute neurovisceral involvement. Cutaneous findings are similar to those of PCT but may be more subtle.

The necrolytic conditions are a varied group of diseases that have a histopathologic finding in common: necrolysis. *Necrolysis* refers to necrosis of keratinocytes in the granular and upper spinous layers of the epidermis. These keratinocytes initially undergo vacuolar degeneration, where cells appear pale and large, and then these cells undergo necrosis. Underlying metabolic derangement is thought to be responsible. The necrolytic conditions include acrodermatitis enteropathica (ADE), necrolytic migratory erythema (NME), and necrolytic acral erythema (NAE). ADE is most commonly seen in infants who have been recently weaned. An inherited zinc transporter protein deficiency is responsible. Acquired forms may occur in adulthood, particularly in the setting of total parenteral nutrition that has not been supplemented with zinc. Clinically, there are eroded and crusted plaques in the periorificial location as well as on the hands and feet, including digits. Intact vesicles and bullae may be seen (Figure 7.32). A psoriasiform appearance with scaling (papulosquamous presentation) may also occur. These cutaneous findings are accompanied by stomatitis,

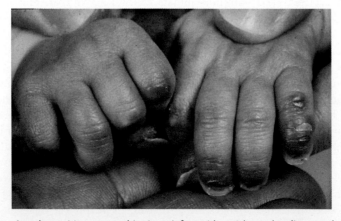

FIGURE 7.32 • Acrodermatitis enteropathica in an infant with vesicles and scaling on a hand.

glossitis, and alopecia. NME is rare. It begins with erythema in the perineal area. Bullae form and are superseded by erosions and crusting. Annular and polycyclic forms are seen. There are associated stomatitis, glossitis, and diarrhea. Most cases of NME are seen in association with an underlying glucagon-producing tumor of the α cells of the islets of Langerhans in the pancreas. However, cases associated with cirrhosis have been reported. NAE is very rarely seen. Eroded and crusted plaques occur in an acral location. Intact bullae may also be seen. All reported cases have occurred in the setting of hepatitis C infection.

A description of drug-related blistering disease, along with a short list of associated drug causes, are given in Table 7.2. In fixed drug eruption, one or more round pink macules become dusky and leave grayish postinflammatory hyperpigmentation when they resolve, only to become recrudescent on reingestion of the culprit drug. In Stevens-Johnson syndrome/toxic epidermal necrolysis (SJS/TEN), atypical target lesions and necrotic macules start on the upper chest and face and extend centrifugally. These may coalesce and rupture, resulting in widespread denudation of epidermis (Figures 7.33 and 7.34). Early SJS/TEN is a "do not miss" diagnosis. A PCT–like disease, but without abnormal porphyrins, has been induced by various drugs (pseudoporphyria), as has Grover disease and some of the autoimmune blistering diseases. Drugs may also induce phototoxicity, in which sunburn due to a lowered minimal erythema dose occurs.

These myriad diseases can be distinguished from each other on clinical grounds and by employing the wheel of diagnosis. Figure 7.35 shows the wheel that has been customized to this reaction pattern. As with all primary lesions, vesicles and bullae may manifest characteristics that may be harnessed to assist in diagnosis. An example is the size of the primary lesions. Some diseases preferentially create vesicles and in

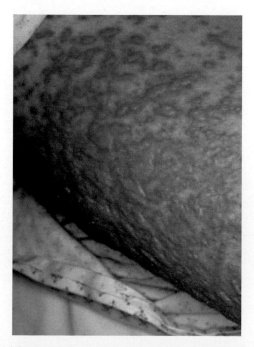

FIGURE 7.33 · Stevens–Johnson syndrome/toxic epidermal necrolysis with flaccid bullae arising in necrotic epidermis.

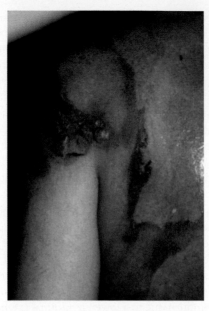

FIGURE 7.34 • Toxic epidermal necrolysis with full-thickness loss of epidermis. The necrotic epidermis appears darker than unaffected skin. There are flaccid vesicles arising in association.

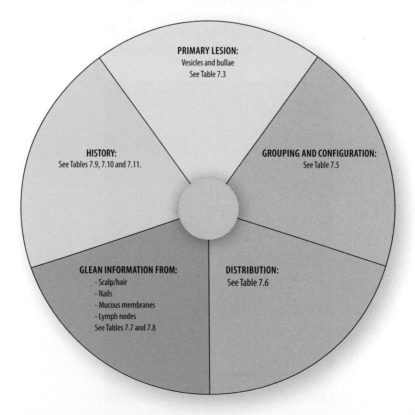

FIGURE 7.35 • The wheel of diagnosis customized to the vesicobullous reaction pattern.

TABLE 7.3. Vesicobullous Disease by Size of Primary Lesion	
DISEASES THAT USUALLY PRESENT WITH VESICLES	**DISEASES THAT USUALLY PRESENT WITH BULLAE**
HSV	Acute contact dermatitis
VZV: chickenpox and zoster	Coma bullae
Miliaria crystallina	Diabetic bullae
Dyshidrotic eczema	Bullous mastocytoma
Acute contact dermatitis	Bullous Lyme disease
HSV-associated bullous erythema multiforme	Bullous fixed drug eruption
Grover disease	Staphylococcal scalded skin syndrome
Pemphigus herpetiformis	Bullous erysipelas and cellulitis
Dyshidrosiform variant of bullous pemphigoid	Bullous Sweet syndrome
Dermatitis herpetiformis	Pemphigus vulgaris
Linear IgA disease	Bullous pemphigoid
Chronic bullous disease of childhood	Bullous SLE, BP-like variant
Bullous SLE, DH-like variant	JEB, DEB
Dowling–Meara EB simplex	EBA

others, bullae are classically seen. Table 7.3 displays a comprehensive list of vesicobullous diseases that usually present with vesicles and those that usually present with bullae. Regarding tenseness or flaccidity, this may help to determine the level of the blister cleavage plane, as is outlined in more detail below.

> **Clinical Tip**
> Diagnostic determinants of vesicles and bullae:
> • Size
> • Tense or flaccid?

In thinking more about the primary lesion (and the associated secondary lesions) diagnostic box on the wheel, there are three important points to consider:

1. **The diagnostic import of secondary lesions**: Sometimes only the "footprints" of vesicles and bullae are seen. These are the secondary lesions that follow vesicles and bullae. They are typically round erosions and round crusts. Collarettes of scale may also be seen as these lesions resolve. Figure 7.20 illustrates round erosions, early crusting, and collarettes of scale.

The Footprint of Vesicles and Bullae:
- Round erosions
- Round crusts
- Collarettes of scale

2. **Further diagnostic pointers: the company the blisters keep:** The presence of primary lesions other than vesicles and bullae can give clues to diagnosis. Furthermore, the secondary lesions present not only give clues to the presence of a

blistering disease as mentioned above but can also provide information about the location of the cleavage plane of the blister as will be seen, and sometimes can even narrow the differential diagnosis. Table 7.4 summarizes the diagnostic information proffered by the associated primary and accompanying secondary lesions. For diagnostically relevant associated primary lesions, examples include urticarial plaques in the presence of blisters pointing to a diagnosis of bullous pemphigoid (as is seen in Figures 7.22 and 7.23) and lichenoid plaques with blisters point to a diagnosis of lichen planus pemphigoides. Milia, as will be seen in the ensuing discussion about cleavage plane, are a feature of some of the deeper autoimmune blistering diseases, such as PCT (as is seen in Figure 7.31) and epidermolysis bullosa acquisita.

Further Clues to Diagnosis: The Company the Blisters Keep

- Are other primary lesions present?
- What are the secondary lesions?

3. **How to estimate depth of cleavage plane:** Figure 7.36 is a schematic representation of the skin and denotes where the blister cleavage plane lies for the diseases outlined above. Certain clinical clues can assist in an estimation of the depth of this split, as alluded to above. The first clue is the degree of tenseness or flaccidity that a bulla displays. In general, the presence of multiple flaccid bullae implies that the blister cleavage plane is superficially located [above the basement membrane zone (BMZ)], whereas the presence of multiple tense bullae implies a deeper split. There are some caveats to remember, however. Tense bullae may become flaccid over time, as serous blister fluid leaks, or is reabsorbed. Conversely, flaccid bullae may become tense, especially if serous fluid accumulates at their inferior poles secondary to gravity. Also, any bulla on acral skin may appear tense as a result of the overlying thick stratum corneum in these areas. An exception to the rule is dermatitis herpetiformis. It has a subepidermal cleavage plane, but the tense vesicles and bullae are rarely seen as this is an extremely pruritic condition and so blisters are manually disrupted by scratching. Additionally, this rule does not generally apply to small vesicles as they are all usually quite tense, given their size.

The Rule and Its Exceptions

Rule:
- The cleavage plane of a flaccid bulla is above the BMZ, and that of a tense bulla is within or below the BMZ.

Exceptions:
- With time, tense bullae become flaccid and flaccid bullae become tense.
- On acral sites with thick stratum corneum, all bullae tend to appear tense.
- Dermatitis herpetiformis is present.
- Most small vesicles are usually tense given their size.

Another clue to the depth of the cleavage plane lies in the company the vesicles and bullae keep. Flaccid bullae with many erosions or crusts reliably indicate the presence

TABLE 7.4. Making a Diagnosis by Associated Primary and Accompanying Secondary Lesions

INTRAEPIDERMAL CLEAVAGE
- Scaly or exfoliative plaques
  - Pemphigus foliaceus
  - Fogo selvagem
  - Pemphigus erythematosus
  - IgA pemphigus
  - Staphylococcal scalded skin syndrome
- Vegetating plaques
  - Pemphigus vegetans
  - Hailey–Hailey disease
  - Intertriginous Darier disease
  - Pemphigoid vegetans
- Lichenoid plaques
  - PNP/PAMS
- Targetoid plaques
  - PNP/PAMS
- Pustules
  - IgA pemphigus
- Scaly red papules
  - Grover disease

SUBEPIDERMAL CLEAVAGE: LAMINA LUCIDA
- Lichenoid plaques
  - Lichen planus pemphigoides
- Urticarial plaques
  - Bullous pemphigoid
  - Pemphigoid gestationis

DEEPER GROUP: SUBLAMINA DENSA ZONE OR DERMAL
- Ulcers with or without crusts
  - Dystrophic epidermolysis bullosa
- Milia
  - Porphyria cutanea tarda
  - Hepatoerythropoietic porphyria
  - Variegate porphyria
  - Epidermolysis bullosa acquisita
  - Less commonly in junctional and dystrophic epidermolysis bullosa
- Atrophic scars
  - All cutaneous porphyrias
  - Epidermolysis bullosa acquisita
  - Junctional and dystrophic EB
- Hyperkeratotic plaques
  - Squamous cell cancer arising in dystrophic epidermolysis bullosa
- Juicy plaques
  - Sweet syndrome

of a superficial split, such as in bullous impetigo or pemphigus vulgaris (as seen in Figures 7.20 and 7.37A). Diseases with deeper planes of cleavage will show proportionally more tense bullae and fewer erosions (Figure 7.37B). Another secondary lesion that may signal the depth of the primary split and thereby render important diagnostic

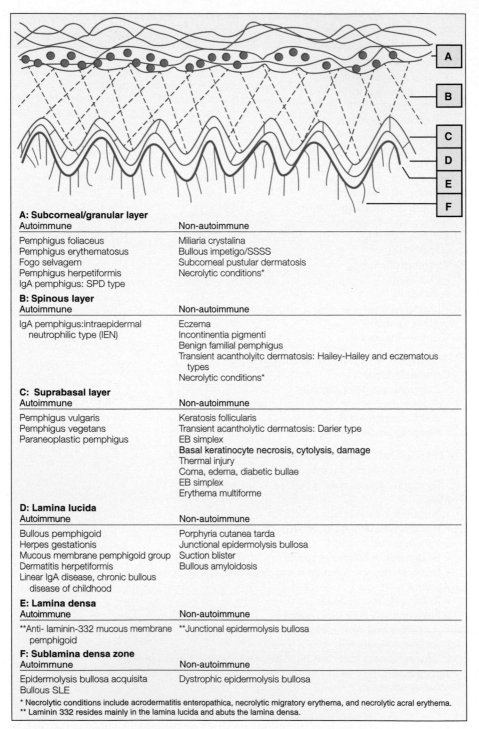

A: Subcorneal/granular layer

Autoimmune	Non-autoimmune
Pemphigus foliaceus	Miliaria crystalina
Pemphigus erythematosus	Bullous impetigo/SSSS
Fogo selvagem	Subcorneal pustular dermatosis
Pemphigus herpetiformis	Necrolytic conditions*
IgA pemphigus: SPD type	

B: Spinous layer

Autoimmune	Non-autoimmune
IgA pemphigus:intraepidermal	Eczema
neutrophilic type (IEN)	Incontinentia pigmenti
	Benign familial pemphigus
	Transient acantholyitc dermatosis: Hailey-Hailey and eczematous
	types
	Necrolytic conditions*

C: Suprabasal layer

Autoimmune	Non-autoimmune
Pemphigus vulgaris	Keratosis follicularis
Pemphigus vegetans	Transient acantholytic dermatosis: Darier type
Paraneoplastic pemphigus	EB simplex
	Basal keratinocyte necrosis, cytolysis, damage
	Thermal injury
	Coma, edema, diabetic bullae
	EB simplex
	Erythema multiforme

D: Lamina lucida

Autoimmune	Non-autoimmune
Bullous pemphigoid	Porphyria cutanea tarda
Herpes gestationis	Junctional epidermolysis bullosa
Mucous membrane pemphigoid group	Suction blister
Dermatitis herpetiformis	Bullous amyloidosis
Linear IgA disease, chronic bullous	
disease of childhood	

E: Lamina densa

Autoimmune	Non-autoimmune
**Anti- laminin-332 mucous membrane	**Junctional epidermolysis bullosa
pemphigoid	

F: Sublamina densa zone

Autoimmune	Non-autoimmune
Epidermolysis bullosa acquisita	Dystrophic epidermolysis bullosa
Bullous SLE	

* Necrolytic conditions include acrodermatitis enteropathica, necrolytic migratory erythema, and necrolytic acral erythema.
** Laminin 332 resides mainly in the lamina lucida and abuts the lamina densa.

FIGURE 7.36 • A schematic diagram showing the site of cleavage of each disease.

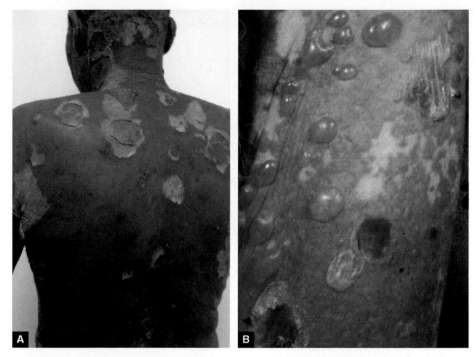

FIGURE 7.37 • (A) Pemphigus foliaceus (cleavage plane above the BMZ), demonstrating many erosions and few intact flaccid bullae; (B) bullous pemphigoid (cleavage plane in the BMZ), demonstrating many tense bullae, few flaccid bullae, and few erosions. (Image (A) used with permission from Dr. Ncoza Dlova, University of Kwa Zulu-Natal, Durban, South Africa.)

information is the scar. Diseases with primary intraepidermal cleavage planes do not scar, except if there has been a superimposed secondary infection, such as a bacterial infection of the erosions and crusts of chickenpox, for example. These diseases usually manifest postinflammatory pigmentary changes only. Diseases with a primary cleavage plane under the epidermis usually do heal with scarring. Milia are associated primary lesions that are seen after cleavage of the sublamina densa zone, such as in PCT and EBA.

Clinical Pointers to the Cleavage Plane in Blistering Diseases

The likelihood that the cleavage plane is above the basement membrane zone (BMZ) increases if
- There are flaccid bullae.
- There are more erosions than bullae.
- There is little scarring and no milia.
- Erosions are healing with postinflammatory hyperpigmentation.

The likelihood that the cleavage plane is in the BMZ or below increases if
- There are tense bullae.
- There are tense and flaccid bullae that are seen in concert with erosions.
- Erosions are healing with scarring.
- Milia are present.

> ### TABLE 7.5. Groupings and Configuration of Vesicles and Bullae
>
> **ANNULAR**
> - IgA pemphigus
> - Pemphigoid gestationis and bullous pemphigoid
> - Linear IgA disease and chronic bullous disease of childhood
>
> **LINEAR**
> - "Outside job" (eg, acute contact dermatitis due to poison ivy, bullous insect bites)
> - Blaschko lines: first stage of incontinentia pigmenti
> - Dermatomal: zoster
>
> **HERPETIFORM**
> - HSV and zoster
> - Dowling–Meara variant of EB simplex
> - Pemphigus herpetiformis
> - Dermatitis herpetiformis

The way that vesicles and bullae are grouped adds an extra layer of refinement to differential diagnostic lists, as seen in Table 7.5. Annular and arcuate arrays of vesicles are classically seen in linear IgA disease (Figure 7.26) and chronic bullous disease of childhood. They may be seen in bullous pemphigoid (Figure 7.38) and bullous SLE (Figure 7.29) as well. In the intraepidermal type of IgA pemphigus, the presence of a central crust with surrounding flaccid bullae or pustules is referred to as a "sunflower

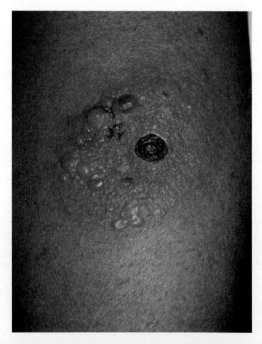

FIGURE 7.38 • Bullous pemphigoid showing an arcuate array of vesicles on an urticarial plaque.

configuration." Pemphigoid gestationis and bullous pemphigoid may present with annular urticarial plaques, as shown in Figure 7.22. Linear arrays of vesicles and bullae may occur secondary to an outside insult, such as acute eczema from contact with poison ivy (the lines are formed from the edges of leaves or stems brushing across the skin surface; see Figure 7.12) or arthropod bites; a dermatosis following Blaschko lines, such as the first stage of incontinentia pigmenti (Figure 7.1); or a dermatomal process, such as zoster (Figure 7.8). A fair number of conditions in this reaction pattern, besides HSV and zoster, form herpetiform clusters. Examples include pemphigus herpeti-formis (Figure 7.19), dermatitis herpetiformis (Figure 7.27), and the Dowling–Meara variant of EB simplex.

Regarding distribution, a myriad of conditions may give rise to vesicles and bullae in photoexposed areas (Table 7.6). These include sunburn and phototoxic conditions from topical or systemic drugs, as well as phytophotodermatitis. Furthermore, the presence of photodistributed blisters may point to the possibility of hydroa vacciniforme in children or the porphyrias in children and adults. Papulovesicles in sun-exposed areas may further connote the diagnosis of polymorphous light eruption. For exfoliative plaques in the seborrheic distribution with peripheral flaccid bullae or erosions, pemphigus folia-ceus should be considered (Figure 7.18). Sometimes the bullae and erosions are difficult to appreciate, and so pemphigus foliaceus should be in the differential diagnosis of any eruption resembling seborrheic dermatitis that is not responding to therapy.

> **Clinical Tip** Consider the diagnosis of pemphigus foliaceus for any eruption resembling seborrheic dermatitis that is therapy-resistant.

All blistering conditions are a rare finding in the intertriginous areas. IgA pem-phigus begins in intertriginous areas. Other blistering conditions with an intertrigi-nous distribution include pemphigus vegetans, Darier disease, Hailey–Hailey disease, and the very rarely encountered variant of bullous pemphigoid known as pemphigoid vegetans. Scaly and sometimes crusted plaques are seen in Darier disease and Hailey–Hailey disease (Figure 7.3). Vegetating plaques are seen in pemphigus vegetans and pemphigoid vegetans (Figure 7.21), and vegetating plaques are a variant presenta-tion of Darier diseases in this anatomic location. Flexural vesicles and bullae are also exceedingly rare. Hailey–Hailey disease can occur in this location. Eczema in the flex-ures usually displays a subacute (round erosions, papules, scaling) rather than an acute morphology (frank vesicles or bullae). Extensor aspects of the extremities are sites of predilection for dermatitis herpetiformis (along with scalp and buttocks). Similarly, the mechanobullous subtype of EBA favors elbows, knees, and joints of the hands and fingers, all of which are trauma-prone areas.

Many blistering diseases favor palms and/or soles. Dyshidrotic eczema (Figure 8.10), other acute eczemas, bullous erythema multiforme, hand–foot–mouth disease, and the more rarely encountered dyshidrosiform variant of bullous pemphigoid are typically bilateral, whereas bullous tinea pedis is usually unilateral. Bullous erythema multi-forme may classically manifest on either the palms and soles, or on the dorsal hands and feet, or both. Zoster is an important "do not miss" entity that may present with herpetiform clusters of vesicles on a palm or sole. Dermatomes C6, C7, or C8 involve the palm; dermatomes L4, L5, S1, and S2 involve the sole. While herpetic whitlow is usually seen on a digit, it may rarely occur on the palm.

TABLE 7.6. Vesicobullous Differential Diagnosis by Distribution

PHOTOEXPOSED
- Phytophotodermatitis
- Sunburn
- Phototoxic drug reaction
- Polymorphous light eruption
- Porphyria cutanea tarda, hepatoerythropoietic porphyria
- Variegate porphyria
- Gunther disease
- Erythropoietic protoporphyria
- Hydroa vacciniforme
- Pemphigus erythematosus

SEBORRHEIC
- Pemphigus foliaceus

INTERTRIGINOUS
- IgA pemphigus
- Pemphigus vegetans
- Pemphigoid vegetans
- Hailey–Hailey disease
- Darier disease

FLEXURES
- Atopic eczema
- Formaldehyde contact dermatitis
- Hailey–Hailey disease

EXTENSORS
- Dermatitis herpetiformis
- Epidermolysis bullosa acquisita; mechanical subtype

PALMS AND SOLES
- Typically bilateral
  - Dyshidrotic eczema
  - Friction bullae
  - Bullous erythema multiforme
  - Bullous pemphigoid, dyshidrosiform variant
  - Hand–foot–mouth disease
  - EB simplex
- Typically unilateral
  - Zoster
  - Herpetic whitlow
- Typically unilateral or asymmetric
  - Bullous tinea pedis

FINGERS, TOES
- Friction bullae
- Blistering distal dactylitis
- Herpetic whitlow
- Dyshidrotic eczema
- Hand, foot, and mouth disease
- Bullous fixed drug eruption
- Bullae in septic vasculitis
- Orf
- Milker's nodule

IN RELATION TO APPENDAGES
- Miliaria crystallina

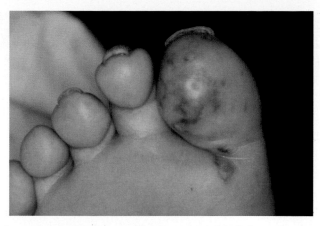

FIGURE 7.39 · Septic vasculitis displaying retiform purpura with bulla formation.

A single bulla on a finger may represent blistering distal dactylitis, a sucking blister, or a thermal burn. Orf and milker's nodule are rarer diagnoses to consider in the appropriate clinical context. A herpetiform cluster of vesicles or crusts on a finger represents herpetic whitlow (Figure 7.5). Zoster should also be considered for more extensive herpetiform clusters in a dermatome (Figure 7.8). The gray, oval vesicles of hand–foot–mouth disease involve the lateral aspects of fingers preferentially. Septic vasculitis may present with asymmetrically distributed angulated bullae on finger and toe pulps (Figure 7.39). Finally, bullous fixed drug eruption presents as a round bulla may extend over more than one finger.

For vesicobullous diseases, diagnostically important clues may be gleaned from a thorough examination of the scalp, hair, mucous membranes, nails, and lymph nodes (Table 7.7). With respect to mucous membranes, various morphologic patterns may hold diagnostic information. Hemorrhagic erosions and crusting of bilateral lips are characteristic of erythema multiforme major, MIRM, and SJS/TEN (Figure 7.40). PNP or PAMS is a fourth rare cause of this appearance.

> **Clinical Tip** Hemorrhagic erosions and crusting of both lips signify EM major, MIRM, SJS/TEN, or PNP/PAMS.

Stomatitis and glossitis may be seen in ADE and NME. In marginal gingivitis (also known as *desquamative gingivitis*), there are gingival erosions along the margins of the teeth. This is a classic finding in pemphigus vulgaris and MMP (as well as oral lichen planus). Laryngeal erosive disease may accompany pemphigus vulgaris, TEN, and PAMS. Conjunctivitis is an uncommon feature of Sweet syndrome. Table 7.8 details the range of mucous membrane findings of the autoimmune blistering diseases. Each has its own characteristic pattern of involvement (Figure 7.41).

The scalp is a site of predilection for pemphigus vegetans; crusts or vegetating plaques may be seen. It is also a site of predilection for dermatitis herpetiformis. Itching is a prominent symptom here. The Brunsting–Perry subtype of MMP leads to scarring alopecia (Figure 7.25). Nonscarring alopecia may be concomitant with ADE. Finally, with respect to hair, hypertrichosis is a finding in PCT.

TABLE 7.7. Gleaning Information from Scalp, Hair, Nails, Mucous Membranes, and Lymph Nodes for Vesicobullous Diseases

MUCOUS MEMBRANES
- Hemorrhagic crusts on lips
  - Erythema multiforme major
  - MIRM
  - SJS/TEN
  - PNP/PAMS
- Stomatitis/glossitis
  - ADE
  - NME
- Marginal gingivitis
  - Pemphigus vulgaris
  - MMP
- Laryngeal erosive disease
  - Pemphigus vulgaris
  - TEN
  - PNP/PAMS
- Conjunctivitis
  - Sweet syndrome
- Autoimmune vesicobullous disease findings: see Table 7.8.

SCALP/HAIR
- Pemphigus vegetans
- DH
- MMP: scarring alopecia
- PCT: hypertrichosis
- ADE: non scarring alopecia

NAILS
- Photoonycholysis: pseudoporphyria, PCT
- Epidermolysis bullosa acquisita
- Loss of nails with secondary scarring: JEB, DEB

LYMPH NODES
- PNP/PAMS

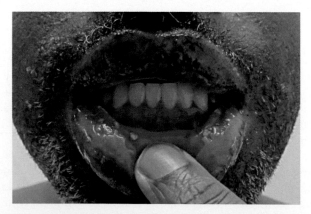

FIGURE 7.40 · Stevens–Johnson syndrome, displaying classic hemorrhagic erosions on bilateral lips, with intraoral erosions.

TABLE 7.8. Mucous Membrane Findings in Autoimmune Vesicobullous Diseases

DISEASE	ORAL INVOLVEMENT
Pemphigus foliaceus, fogo selvagem, pemphigus erythematosus	Rare
Pemphigus vulgaris	First presents with intraoral involvement: buccal mucosa and palate most commonly involved; nasal, ocular, anogenital mucosa can be involved; esopahageal, vaginal, and cervical involvement reported
Pemphigus herpetiformis	Rare
IgA pemphigus	
Subcorneal pustular dermatosis type	Rare
Intraepidermal neutrophilic type	Rare
PAMS	Intractable stomatitis characteristic; may resemble SJS with hemorrhagic crusting of lips and intraoral erosions; lichenoid features also seen intraorally
Bullous pemphigoid	Oral involvement is seen in ≤33.3% of patients; vesicles, bullae, or erosions seen
Anti-p200 pemphigoid	Oral, anogenital involvement reported
Mucous membrane pemphigoid	Oral mucosa is most frequently involved; desquamative gingivitis is a typical pattern; this is followed by conjunctival, skin, and pharyngeal involvement; anogenital, nasal mucosal, laryngeal, and esophageal involvement rare
Linear IgA disease	Seen in ≤80%; involvement of all mucosal sites has been reported; oral and conjunctival most frequent; erosions seen
Chronic bullous disease of childhood	Perineum is a predilection site; mucosal involvement reported; rates vary according to the study
Dermatitis herpetiformis	Rare, not well studied
Epidermolysis bullosa acquisita	Common, involvement of all mucosal surfaces has been reported; tense vesicles or erosions may be seen

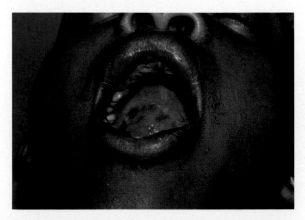

FIGURE 7.41 • Pemphigus vulgaris with a typical finding of erosions on the palate. (Used with permission from Dr. Deepak Modi, University of the Witwatersrand, Johannesburg, South Africa.)

With respect to nails, subungual vesicle formation may lead to painful onycholysis. This may be a feature of pseudoporphyria, PCT, or (rarely) epidermolysis bullosa acquisita.

> **Clinical Tip** Subungual blistering presents with painful onycholysis.

In junctional and dystrophic EB, repeated nail bed involvement leads to scarring and anonychia. Lymphadenopathy associated with the underlying malignancy may be found in cases of PAMS.

Important pointers in the history for vesicobullous diseases include the age of the patient (Table 7.9) and the patient's medication list (Table 7.10). Many bullous diseases are associated with underlying systemic involvement, including malignancy (Table 7.11), and so it is important to ask about clues to the presence of these and to investigate further if needed.

TABLE 7.9. Blistering Disease by Age

NEONATE
- Single
  - Sucking blister
- Multiple
  - Inherited epidermolysis bullosa group
  - Bullous congenital ichthyosiform erythroderma
  - Neonatal herpes simplex infection
  - Neonatal chickenpox
  - Miliaria crystallina
  - Neonatal pemphigus
  - Congenital syphilis

INFANT AND CHILD
- Single
  - Blistering distal dactylitis
  - Bullous insect bite
  - Thermal burn
  - Friction blister
  - Solitary mastocytoma
- Multiple
  - Bullous insect bites
  - Miliaria crystallina
  - Bullous impetigo
  - Orolabial HSV
  - Herpetic whitlow
  - Hand–foot–mouth disease
  - Gianotti–Crosti syndrome
  - Acute eczema: Chapter 8
  - Acrodermatitis enteropathica
  - Sunburn
  - Hydroa vacciniforme
  - Staphylococcal scalded skin syndrome
  - Chronic bullous disease of childhood
  - Bullae in septic vasculitis
  - SJS/TEN

(Continued)

TABLE 7.9. Blistering Disease by Age (continued)

INFANT AND CHILD (CONT.)
- Inherited epidermolysis bullosa group
- Bullous Lyme disease
- Chickenpox
- Zoster
- Porphyrias
  - Erythropoeitic protoporphyria
  - Congenital erythropoeitic porphyria

Adult
- Single
  - Friction blister
  - Bullous insect bite
  - Thermal burn
  - Coma blister
  - Diabetic bulla
  - Bullous tinea pedis
  - Bullous fixed drug eruption
  - Bullous erysipleas
  - Bullous cellulitis
- Multiple
  - Acute eczema: Chapter 8
  - Bullous tinea pedis
  - Sunburn
  - Multiple insect bites
  - Bullous impetigo
  - Bullous erysipleas
  - Bullous cellulitis
  - Zoster
  - Chickenpox
  - Polymorphous light eruption
  - Autoimmune blistering diseases
  - Porphyrias
  - Bullous leukocytoclastic vasculitis
  - Bullae in septic vasculitis
  - Bullous erythema multiforme
  - Bullous Lyme disease
  - Hailey–Hailey disease
  - Darier disease
  - Grover disease
  - Staphylococcal scalded skin syndrome
  - Phytophotodermatitis
  - Necrolytic migratory erythema
  - Necrolytic acral erythema
  - Bullous amyloidosis
  - Drug-induced bullae
    - Stevens–Johnson syndrome/toxic epidermal necrolysis
    - Drug-induced autoimmune blistering disease
    - Pseudoporphyria
    - Multiple bullous fixed drug eruption
    - Phototoxic eruption

TABLE 7.10. Blistering Diseases and Their Drug Associations

DISEASE	DRUG CAUSES
Pemphigus vulgaris	Penicillamine, captopril, rifampin
Bullous pemphigoid	Furosemide
Linear IgA disease	Vancomycin, lithium, diclofenac
Dermatitis herpetiformis	Iodides, indomethacin
Fixed drug eruption	Tetracyclines, sulfonamides, acetaminophen, NSAIDs, codeine, and derivatives
SJS/TEN	Allopurinol, sulfonamides, anticonvulsants (phenytoin, carbamazepine, phenobarbital, lamotrigine), oxicam NSAIDs, nevirapine
Grover disease	Interleukin 4, BRAF inhibitors
Pseudoporphyria	Furosemide, pyridoxine, tetracyclines, NSAIDs, especially propionic acid derivatives
Phototoxicity	Doxycycline, amiodarone, voriconazole, thiazides, quinolones, psoralens, tar preparations

TABLE 7.11. Blistering Diseases and Their Systemic Associations

DISEASE	SYSTEMIC ASSOCIATION
Pemphigus erythematosus	SLE in very few cases, myasthenia gravis, thymoma
IgA pemphigus, subcorneal pustular dermatosis type	IgA monoclonal gammopathy
PNP/PAMS	Non-Hodgkin lymphoma; CLL; Castleman disease; other carcinomas, sarcomas, thymoma; Waldenstrom macroglobulinemia
Bullous pemphigoid	Stroke, dementia, Parkinson disease, multiple sclerosis
Mucous membrane pemphigoid	Anti-laminin 332 subset associated with solid-organ malignancies
Linear IgA disease	Ulcerative colitis
Dermatitis herpetiformis	Celiac disease, non-Hodgkin lymphoma, autoimmune thyroid disease, type 1 diabetes, pernicious anemia
Epidermolysis bullosa acquisita	Inflammatory bowel disease
Bullous SLE	SLE
PCT	HIV disease, hepatitis C, hemochromatosis, alcoholic liver disease
NME	Glucagonoma, cirrhosis
NAE	Hepatitis C infection
Hydroa vacciniforme	Chronic EBV infection

BEDSIDE DIAGNOSTICS AND BLOODWORK

As discussed in Chapter 6, *bedside diagnostics* are tests that may be employed in the clinic to assist in diagnosis before performing a biopsy. Table 7.12 lists the tests that can provide diagnostic clues in this reaction pattern. Applying pressure to lesions may be useful, such as firmly stroking the surface of a plaque with the back of a cotton-tipped applicator. If this yields a wheal or a bulla, this is diagnostic of a mastocytoma. If exerting sideways/tangential pressure on tender red macules, flaccid bullae, or erosions results in a lateral extension of the bulla, or detachment of epidermis from dermis, this is a positive Nikolsky sign. This is seen in SJS/TEN and the pemphigus group of diseases. A positive Asboe–Hansen sign is lateral extension of a bulla or vesicle after applying downward pressure on its surface, also seen in SJS/TEN and the pemphigus group.

> **Clinical Tip**
> - Nikolsky sign: lateral extension of vesicle/bulla or detachable skin with lateral pressure.
> - Asboe-Hansen sign: lateral extension of a vesicle/bulla with downward pressure.

For infectious bullae, a further series of tests can be performed. Scrape the undersurface of the roof of a bulla and perform a potassium hydroxide (KOH) stain to diagnose bullous tinea pedis; scrape the base of an unroofed vesicle or bulla and perform a Tzanck smear to diagnose herpes simplex or varicella zoster viral infections; and examine bullae contents microscopically, including performing a Gram stain if the contents are too cloudy to rule out a secondary bacterial infection. Furthermore

TABLE 7.12. Bedside Diagnostics and Bloodwork for Vesicles and Bullae

APPLYING PRESSURE TO LESIONS
- Induce a bulla over a mastocytoma
- Induce lateral extension of a blister or detached epidermis
  - Press laterally: Nikolsky sign
  - Press down on the top of a blister: Asboe–Hansen sign

MORE DIAGNOSTIC INFORMATION FOR BLISTER
- Scrape undersurface of the roof of a bulla for KOH in suspected bullous tinea pedis
- Scrape base of an unroofed vesicle for a Tzanck smear and/or PCR in suspected HSV or VZV
- Examine the bulla contents microscopically:
  - Gram stain to rule out a secondary bacterial infection
  - Wright's stain to look for eosinophils in erythema toxicum neonatorum

SEROLOGICAL TESTS
- ANA, anti-dsDNA
- Zinc level
- Glucagon level
- Hepatitis C serology
- Lyme titers
- Mycoplasma serology
- Syphilis serology

regarding suspected HSV or VZV, viral PCR testing is so sensitive that a range of specimen types, including blister fluid, a moist erosion or a crust, may be used. Finally, perform a Wright's stain on vesicle fluid to look for eosinophils in erythema toxicum neonatorum.

For Best Yield:

- Scrape the inside of a bulla roof for fungus.
- Scrape the base of unroofed bulla for HSV/VZV.
- Collect cloudy bulla content for Gram stain and culture.

Serum zinc levels may be revealing in ADE, hepatitis C serologies in NAE, and high glucagon levels in NME. An autoimmune workup may assist in the diagnosis of bullous SLE. Lyme titers can be helpful when bullous Lyme disease is suspected, as may *Mycoplasma* serology in MIRM. In congenital syphilis, perform serologic tests for syphilis.

SUMMARY

- The vesciobullous reaction pattern includes a broad array of common and rare infectious, inflammatory, noninflammatory, metabolic, and drug-induced dermatoses.
- The diagnostic boxes of the wheel of diagnosis may assist with narrowing down a differential diagnosis.
- Diagnostically relevant information is obtained from
  - Looking for the footprint of vesicles and bullae
  - The company the blisters keep
- A determination of cleavage plane can be made:
  - By applying the "rule" and being aware of its exceptions
  - By looking at the company the blisters keep
- Bedside diagnostics can be employed to narrow down a diagnosis. Serologic tests can also add diagnostic information.

The Eczematous Reaction Pattern

8

The eczematous reaction pattern encompasses a wide variety of primary and associated secondary lesions. Eczema may be classified morphologically according to its chronicity. Table 8.1 lists the morphologic findings of acute, subacute, and chronic eczema. *Acute eczema* involves the constellation of vesicles and/or bullae, erythematous macules and/or plaques, oozing, and crusting (Figure 8.1). Early erosions may be seen. *Subacute eczema* is defined by the presence of scaly erythematous papules and/or plaques, along with round erosions and/or round crusts (Figure 8.2A,B). In *chronic eczema* there are scaly, lichenified plaques that may be hyper- and/or hypopigmented (Figure 8.3). Lichenification connotes thickened skin with increased skin markings and this finding occurs secondary to scratching and rubbing.

With the eczematous reaction pattern, we encounter, for the first time, a reaction pattern that comprises a single disease entity (albeit one with a wide variety of causes). From Table 8.1, and as discussed in Chapter 5, we see that, morphologically, there is significant overlap between acute eczema and the vesicobullous reaction pattern on one hand and chronic eczema and the papulosquamous reaction on the other. In fact, acute eczema may be classified with vesicobullous disease, and chronic eczema, with papulosquamous disease. Subacute ezema may also be categorized as a vesicobullous reaction pattern as the presence of round erosions infers preceding vesicles. It may additionally be classified as a papulosquamous reaction pattern if scaly plaques are the predominating clinical feature. It can therefore be argued that the eczematous reaction pattern can be folded completely into these two reaction patterns. The argument for keeping eczema as a separate reaction pattern rests on the fact that eczema is so commonly encountered that it is worthwhile to think about it separately. An additional reaction pattern that eczema can overlap with is the dermal reaction pattern. The earliest presentation of an acute contact dermatitis may be an edematous, erythematous plaque (Figure 8.4). This corresponds to early spongiosis on histopathologic examination.

> **Clinical Tip** The eczematous reaction pattern overlaps with papulosquamous, vesicobullous, and dermal reaction patterns.

A word about terminology. The term *eczema* is employed interchangeably with the term *dermatitis*, such as atopic eczema or atopic dermatitis, and contact eczema or contact dermatitis. However, the term *dermatitis* is used for other disease names also, so not all diseases with a *dermatitis* designation are *eczema*. An example here is the entity of palisaded and neutrophilic granulomatous dermatitis, a rare disease that usually

TABLE 8.1. Variants of Eczema by Chronicity and Their Morphologic Findings

TYPE	PRIMARY LESIONS	ASSOCIATED SECONDARY LESIONS
Acute	Vesicles and/or bullae	Early erosions
	Erythematous macules and plaques	Oozing, crusts
Subacute	Scaly red papules	Round erosions
	Scaly red plaques	Round crusts
Chronic	Scaly plaques	Lichenification
		Hyperpigmentation
		Hypopigmentation

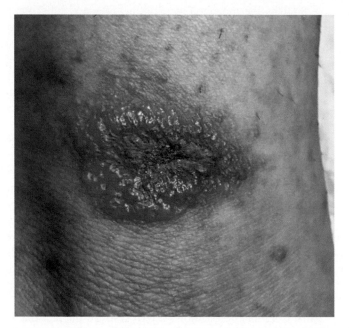

FIGURE 8.1 • Acute eczema with multiple vesicles that have coalesced to form a bulla, central crusting, and surrounding erythema.

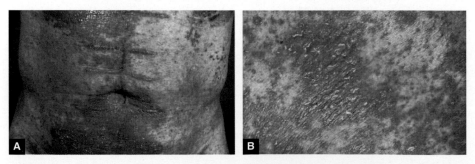

FIGURE 8.2 • (A) Subacute eczema showing widespread scaly plaques with small round erosions and crusts; (B) a close-up of subacute eczema showing the diagnostic small round erosions and crusts.

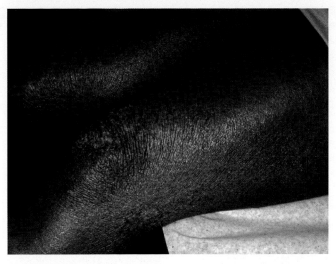

FIGURE 8.3 • Chronic eczema, displaying lichenification, scaling, and pigmentary changes.

occurs in the setting of connective tissue disease that presents with dermal reaction pattern morphology.

> **Clinical Tip** *Eczema* is synonymous with *dermatitis*; however, *dermatitis* is not always synonymous with *eczema*.

Eczema can also be categorized by etiology, as is seen in Table 8.2. Eczema may be a result of exogenous stimuli, such as is seen in irritant or allergic contact dermatitis; or it may arise secondary to endogenous factors—those inherent to the skin or individual,

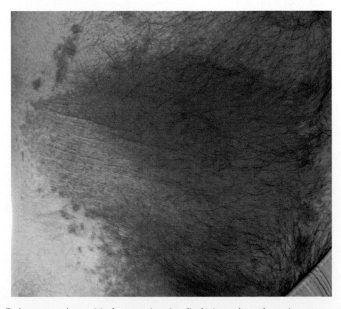

FIGURE 8.4 • Early contact dermatitis due to poison ivy displaying a dermal reaction pattern morphology.

TABLE 8.2. Etiologic Classification of Eczema

EXOGENOUS
- Irritant contact dermatitis
- Allergic contact dermatitis
  - Airborne contact dermatitis
- Infectious eczematoid dermatitis
- Id reaction/autosensitization
- Systematized contact dermatitis
- Eczematous drug eruption
  - Photoallergic drug eruption
- Actinic prurigo
- Frictional lichenoid dermatitis

ENDOGENOUS
- Atopic dermatitis
- Nummular dermatitis
- Dyshidrotic eczema
- Seborrheic dermatitis
- Asteatotic/xerotic eczema
- Stasis dermatitis
- Juvenile plantar dermatosis
- Prurigo nodularis
- Lichen simplex chronicus
- Follicular eczema
- Recurrent and disseminate infundibulofolliculitis
- Pityriasis alba

such as xerosis or an underlying atopic diathesis. An irritant contact dermatitis arises from chronic contact with a mild acid or alkali, or acute contact with a strong acid or alkali. The typical presentation is scaling on the hands, especially the fingertips (Figure 8.5). This is often seen in people who wash their hands frequently. In this setting, xerosis also contributes to the clinical picture. In the case of a stronger acid or

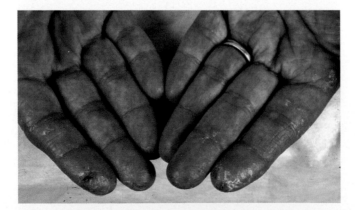

FIGURE 8.5 • Irritant contact dermatitis on the hands, displaying scaling, erosions, and crusting on the fingertips.

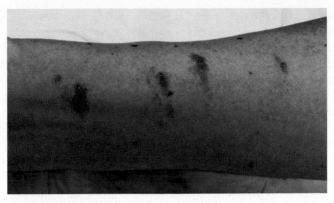

FIGURE 8.6 • Linear plaques with vesicles and early erosions in an allergic contact dermatitis due to poison ivy.

alkali contacting the skin, acute vesicle and bulla formation and widespread erosions, which are similar to those found in allergic contact dermatitis, may ensue. Allergic contact dermatitis most frequently presents with an acute or subacute morphology. The shape and configuration of lesions can provide clues to this diagnosis (such as the linear vesicular plaques that are seen after contact with the leaves and stems of poison ivy, for example, as is seen in Figure 8.6). Distribution of rash also renders vital clues as to the possible causative allergen. For example, nickel dermatitis classically is seen as a round or oval eczematous plaque in the belt-buckle area. It may also present with earlobe dermatitis in an individual with pierced ears, or as neck dermatitis in someone who has been wearing nickel earring hoops.

> **Clinical Tip**
> • Suspect allergic contact dermatitis in the case of linear eczematous plaques.
> • Note the distribution of findings that may point to a particular contact allergen.

Airborne allergens may cause airborne contact dermatitis. A common cause of airborne contact dermatitis is usnic acid in lichens found on wood, so this may be seen in people who saw wood. Exposed surfaces, such as the face and hands, are usually involved. Airborne contact dermatitis may be differentiated from photocontact (photoallergic) dermatitis and other photosensitive dermatitides by its involvement of, rather than sparing of photocovered areas. In photoinduced eruptions, the eyelid crease, the area in shadow under the central chin, and the skin behind the earlobe (known as Wilkinson's triangle) are spared, whereas in airborne contact dermatitis they are usually involved.

> **Clinical Tip** In photoinduced eruptions, the eyelid crease, the area in shadow under the central chin, and the skin behind the earlobe are spared, whereas in airborne contact dermatitis they are involved.

Photoallergic dermatitis usually occurs secondary to a topically applied product with photosensitizing properties, such as oxybenzone, a chemical contained in sunscreens.

Ingested drugs may also be responsible. In chronic actinic dermatitis, a photosensitive eczematous eruption is seen. It typically occurs in men over the age of 50. Eczematous plaques, usually with a chronic eczematous morphology occur in photodistributed areas. Many with chronic actinic dermatitis will have history of allergic contact dermatitis or other eczema. Photopatch tests are positive in most patients. Actinic prurigo may be classed with the exogenous causes of eczema, given the photosensitive nature of the disease. However, genetics are thought to be operable as well, and so, an interplay of exogenous and endogenous factors is a more accurate description of the pathogenesis of this disease. Onset is typically in childhood or at puberty. Eczematous plaques that become pruriginous (resembling the scaly nodules of prurigo nodularis) are initially seen in photoexposed areas. These may become more generalized in more advanced cases.

Infectious eczematoid dermatitis is the eczema that arises secondary to irritation from a purulent discharge such as in a draining otitis externa or a chronically draining wound. This usually has a subacute morphology. The term *id reaction* connotes the presence of a hypersensitivity reaction to either an infection or inflammation. Hypersensitivity reactions to tuberculosis (tuberculides) have a variable morphology and are not eczematous. The hypersensitivity reaction that occurs secondary to a very inflamed dermatophyte infection, such as a severe tinea capitis, kerion, or bullous tinea pedis, may have an eczematous morphology. Examples of the morphologic patterning of the id reaction to dermatophyte include the sago grain–type vesicles occurring on the lateral aspects of the fingers in the setting of a primary inflammatory tinea pedis, and the fine papules that occur on the neck and may be more widespread in a severe tinea capitis or kerion. Eczema itself may incite an id reaction. The term *autosensitization* can be used interchangeably with id reaction in this setting. A primary intensely inflammatory stasis dermatitis with or without a superimposed allergic contact dermatitis is a frequent cause of autosensitzation. The typical morphology seen is monomorphic widespread, evenly spaced, edematous papules occurring on limbs and torso (Figure 8.7). In a severe case of poison ivy, autosensitization may also occur. This may have an eczematous or an erythema multiforme–like appearance.

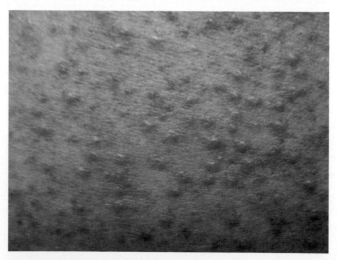

FIGURE 8.7 • A close-up of autosensitization displaying monomorphic widespread, evenly spaced, edematous papules.

An Id Reaction with Eczematous Morphology may be seen in:

- Inflammatory tinea capitis, such as severe tinea capitis or a kerion
- Inflammatory tinea pedis, such as bullous tinea pedis
- Very inflamed stasis dermatitis with or without superimposed contact dermatitis
- Severely inflamed poison ivy

The term *systematized contact dermatitis* implies a widespread eczematous reaction in a patient with a prior allergic contact dermatitis who ingests an allergen that s/he is allergic to. An example here is nickel. Nickel is ubiquitous and may be ingested after nickel contamination of food after cooking in nickel-containing cookware, for example. A widespread papular eruption is seen. Allergy to neomycin may result in a generalized eruption after intravenous neomycin is given. Cashew nuts or mangoes may incite a similar reaction in an individual who is allergic to poison ivy. The *baboon syndrome* describes the presence of confluent papules that form plaques in the intertriginous areas and around the buttocks. This presentation represents a systematized contact dermatitis. Eczematous drug eruptions have been reported in the setting of anti-TNFα therapy and ustekinumab (these eruptions resemble nummular eczema, dyshidrotic eczema, or a widespread eczematous eruption) and intravenous immunoglobulin (resembles dyshidrotic eczema that can be widespread). Hydrochlorothiazide may cause a photosensitive eruption with a variable, including an eczematous morphology. Other drug causes of a photoallergic dermatitis include quinine and sulfonylureas. Frictional lichenoid dermatitis describes the condition of scaly plaques, with a subacute to chronic morphology, that are typically seen on the elbows of children. Friction is considered to play a role in the pathogenesis.

The endogenous eczemas are a heterogenous group. *Endogenous* implies that the inciting factor is inherent or constitutive, and not a contactant or an ingestant. Atopic dermatitis is a frequent cause of eczema in childhood. The atopic diathesis is genetically inherited and may occur in concert with asthma and hayfever. Onset of atopic eczema is within the first few months of life. The face and extensors are involved in infancy and early childhood (Figure 8.8). As the child grows, flexural involvement becomes more common. Atopic dermatitis is adults may have a variable distribution. Subacute morphology is common. This may progress to lichenification in extremely pruritic cases. Atopic individuals are also predisposed to contracting dyshidrotic eczema, follicular eczema, pityriasis alba, and juvenile plantar dermatosis. These conditions are described below. Nummular dermatitis occurs in atopic individuals in around one-fourth of cases. Atopic individuals are also predisposed to acquiring allergic contact dermatitis, owing to skin barrier dysfunction.

Individuals with an Atopic Diathesis are Predisposed to Developing:

- Atopic dermatitis
- Dyshidrotic eczema
- Follicular eczema
- Pityriasis alba
- Juvenile plantar dermatosis
- Nummular eczema
- Allergic contact dermatitis

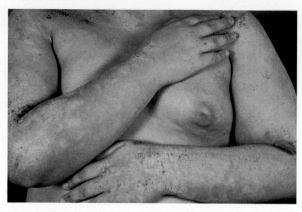

FIGURE 8.8 • Atopic dermatitis in a young child with scaly erythematous papules and plaques involving the extensors.

Nummular eczema is a morphologic entity of round eczematous plaques (Figure 8.9). These typically have subacute eczematous features. Occasionally, nummular eczema may be lichenified. The term *oid-oid disease* (exudative discoid and lichenoid chronic dermatosis of Sulzberger–Garbe) was initially described in elderly men of Jewish ancestry. It is currently thought that this disease represents a chronic form of nummular eczema. In dyshidrotic eczema, tiny vesicles that resemble tapioca pudding appear at the lateral aspects of digits. In more severe cases, palmar surfaces of fingers (Figure 8.10) and the palms themselves may be involved. In chronic cases, hyperkeratotic plaques are seen (Figure 8.11). It may be seen in the setting of atopy, and nickel allergy has been associated in a minority of patients in the literature. Keratolysis exfoliativa is a milder form of dyshidrotic eczema in which peeling and collarettes of scale rather than intact vesicles or bullae are seen (see Figure 6.32). Seborrheic dermatitis was discussed in Chapter 6. It is infrequently vesicular, and it therefore manifests as true papulosquamous disease in many instances. Sites of predilection include nasolabial folds (see Figure 6.14), glabella, eyebrows, scalp, behind and within the ears, the

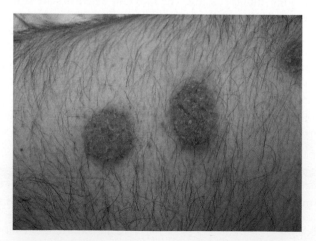

FIGURE 8.9 • Nummular eczema showing round plaques with a subacute eczema morphology. (Reproduced with permission from Soutor C, Hordinsky MK: *Clinical Dermatology.* New York, NY: McGraw Hill; 2013.)

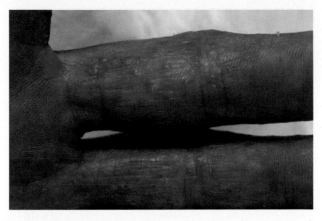

FIGURE 8.10 • Dyshidrotic eczema with tiny vesicles and brown incipient crusts on the fingers.

chest, and intertriginous areas. Occasionally the back is also involved. Seborrheic dermatitis on the back manifests with pink scaly somewhat ill-defined plaques (Figure 8.12).
Asteatotic or xerotic eczema occurs in areas of moderate to severe xerosis. The classic
site of involvement is the shins, which are predisposed to xerosis given the relatively low
concentration of eccrine glands in this location. The convex surfaces of the body, such
as the lower abdomen, may be a site as well given a possible secondary frictional component, but any other body site may be affected. Asteatotic eczema typically has a cracked
appearance that resembles a dry riverbed (as seen in Figures 6.21 and 8.13). There are
linear or angulated superficial fissures that are bordered on each side by fine scale. The
lower legs may also be affected by stasis dermatitis in the presence of varicose veins and
resulting edema. Stasis dermatitis frequently has a subacute morphology (Figure 8.14).
Juvenile plantar dermatosis is described almost exclusively in children. The balls of the
feet develop a shiny, cracked appearance. This entity may be associated with atopy and it
may be precipitated by prolonged wear of plastic or rubber shoes.

While all diseases in the eczematous reaction pattern are a type of eczema, not all
types of eczema present with acute, subacute, or chronic morphology. For example, the
hallmark of pityriasis alba is white macules that supersede a fleeting scaly stage. Pityriasis

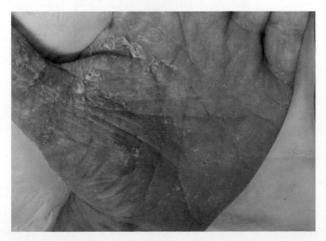

FIGURE 8.11 • Chronic dyshidrotic eczema displaying hyperkeratotic plaques on the palm.

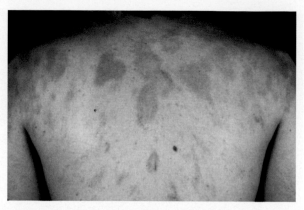

FIGURE 8.12 • Seborrheic dermatitis on the back displaying characteristic pink, scaly, ill-defined plaques.

alba may therefore be more readily classifiable with other white macules (see Chapter 2). Similarly, it is useful to categorize follicular eczema and recurrent and disseminate infundibulofolliculitis in the follicular differential diagnostic list (see Chapter 2). In follicular eczema, scaly papules sit atop follicular ostia (see Figure 2.23). Recurrent and disseminate infundibulofolliculitis describes itchy follicular papules that are commonly seen on the trunk of younger adults, especially males. The papules are more substantive than in follicular eczema (see Figure 2.24). Prurigo nodularis describes one or more papules or nodules that arise as a result from chronic scratching or picking. These are usually scaly and may be excoriated or crusted (Figure 8.15). Prurigo nodularis can also be classified as a papulosquamous reaction pattern. The differential diagnosis of prurigo nodularis is outlined in Table 8.3. In the case of a single nodule, the diagnosis of squamous cell cancer should be considered in the differential diagnosis; these frequently

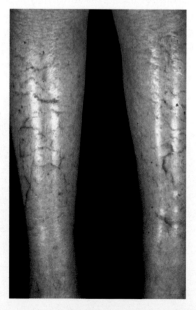

FIGURE 8.13 • Asteatotic eczema with a cracked appearance that resembles a dry riverbed.

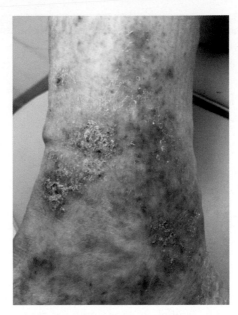

FIGURE 8.14 • Stasis eczema around the ankle showing morphologic features of subacute eczema and a background of varicose veins.

mimic each other (Figure 8.16). An evolving or resolving keratoacanthoma is another mimicker. The mimickers of multiple prurigo nodularis nodules are less frequently seen but should be borne in mind in atypical presentations. Hypertrophic lichen planus may resemble prurigo nodularis. Subtle clinical differentiators include an angulated rather than round outline in hypertrophic lichen planus and a violaceous color. In perforating diseases, papules with a central keratotic core are seen. Acquired perforating dermatosis is usually seen in the setting of diabetes or renal disease. Underlying itch is contributory. Other forms of perforating disease that may resemble prurigo papules include reactive perforating collagenosis and perforating folliculitis. Prurigo pemphigoides is an intensely itchy form of bullous pemphigoid in which prurigo nodules arise secondary

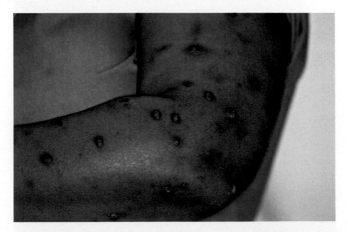

FIGURE 8.15 • Prurigo nodularis, displaying multiple scaly papules on the arm. (Used with permission from Dr. Deepak Modi, University of the Witwatersrand, Johannesburg, South Africa.)

> ### TABLE 8.3. Differential Diagnosis of Prurigo Nodularis
>
> **SINGLE PAPULE/NODULE**
> - Squamous cell cancer
> - Keratoacanthomas
>
> **MULTIPLE PAPULES/NODULES**
> - Hypertrophic lichen planus
> - Perforating disease
> - Prurigo pemphigoides
> - Actinic prurigo
> - Multiple keratoacanthomas
>   - Familial, Witten–Zak
>   - Familial, Ferguson–Smith
>   - Eruptive, Grzybowski
>   - Drug-induced
> - Nodular scabies

to repetitive scratching and dominate the clinic picture. Actinic prurigo should be considered in early onset cases. Multiple keratoacanthomas may be familial or acquired. Familial keratoacanthomas of Witten–Zak is an ill-defined entity in which multiple papular and nodular keratoacanthomas are found. The Ferguson–Smith type is autosomal dominant. Multiple keratoacanthomas erupt in a localized area and heal spontaneously with scarring. In eruptive keratoacanthomas of Grzybowski, hundreds of papular keratoacanthomas erupt in a widespread distribution. These also resolve spontaneously. Multiple keratoacanthomas that may occur in an eruptive fashion are reported secondary to the BRAF inhibitors (vemurafenib, dabrafenib), vismodegib, and sorafenib. Nodular scabies is a hypersensitivity reaction to the presence of the scabies mite or mite parts. While these papules and nodules are typically smooth (dermal reaction pattern), scaling may be seen, in which case prurigo may be mimicked.

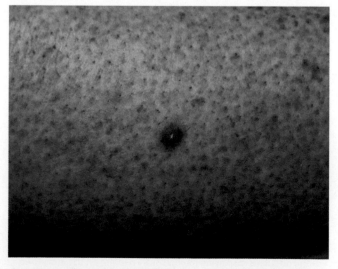

FIGURE 8.16 · Squamous cell carcinoma mimicking a papule of prurigo nodularis.

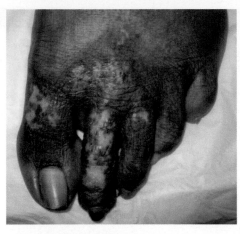

FIGURE 8.17 · Lichen simplex chronicus with lichenification and pigmentary changes on the forefoot.

While prurigo nodularis, as mentioned, is typically caused by chronic picking and scratching; lichen simplex chronicus, by contrast, is usually caused by chronic rubbing and scratching. Scratching or rubbing of an initially pruritic area may set up an itch–scratch cycle that eventuates in an isolated lichenified plaque. Pigmentary changes, including hyper- and hypopigmentation, may be seen. Classic sites of involvement include the distal, lateral shin, the nape of the neck, and the anogenital area but any area of the body may be affected (Figure 8.17).

Eczema may also be observed as a secondary phenomenon in a primary generalized pruritus. In this situation, underlying causes for pruritus (eg, thyroid, renal, or liver disease, or underlying HIV or lymphoma) should be looked for and treated. Eczema may accompany other pruritic dermatoses, such as scabies or bullous pemphigoid (prurigo pemphigoides). Lichenification may also be seen secondarily on any itchy dermatosis; lichenified psoriasis is an example of this phenomenon. Similarly, *Trichophyton rubrum* tinea corporis can be very pruritic, and so secondary lichenification can mask the classic annular morphology of an underlying tinea corporis or tinea cruris.

Some dermatoses that are not primarily eczema present with eczema-like morphology, including acute, subacute, and chronic types, and so these may be included in the differential diagnosis of eczematous reaction pattern. Table 8.4 provides a list of eczema mimickers.

All vesicobullous diseases are in the differential diagnosis for acute eczema, and all papulosquamous diseases are in the differential diagnosis of chronic eczema. Diseases that present with papules and papulovesicles (mimicking subacute eczema) include papular pityriasis rosea, miliaria rubra, pruritic urticarial papules and plaques of pregnancy (PUPPP), polymorphous light eruption, prurigo pigmentosa, Gianotti–Crosti syndrome, autoimmune blistering diseases, and autoimmune progesterone dermatitis. Pityriasis rosea and miliaria rubra are the most frequently encountered of this differential diagnostic group. A variant presentation of pityriasis rosea is the papular form. Papules and papulovesicles in a "Christmas tree" distribution on the trunk, and sparing distal extremities may be seen (Figure 8.18). Miliaria rubra is seen in hot climates or in febrile states secondary to sweating and occlusion of the eccrine ducts. Itchy red papules and/or papulovesicles are seen, especially in occluded areas, including the back in bed-bound patients or the intertriginous areas. In PUPPP, itchy papules and

TABLE 8.4. Conditions That May Mimic Eczema

ACUTE

Vesicobullous reaction pattern differential diagnosis

SUBACUTE

- Papules, papulovesicles
  - Papular pityriasis rosea
  - Miliaria rubra
  - Pruritic urticarial papules and plaques of pregnancy
  - Polymorphous light eruption
  - Prurigo pigmentosa
  - Gianotti–Crosti syndrome
  - Autoimmune progesterone dermatitis
  - Autoimmune blistering diseases
    - Dermatitis herpetiformis
    - Dyshidrosiform variant of bullous pemphigoid
- Scaly, eroded, and/or crusted plaques
  - Nutritional disorders
    - Pellagra
    - Acrodermatitis enteropathica
    - Necrolytic migratory erythema
    - Kwashiorkor
  - Crusted scabies
- Monomorphic papules, erosions, or crusts
  - Eczema herpeticum
  - Eczema coxsackium
  - Eczema vaccinatum

CHRONIC

- Papulosquamous reaction pattern differential diagnosis

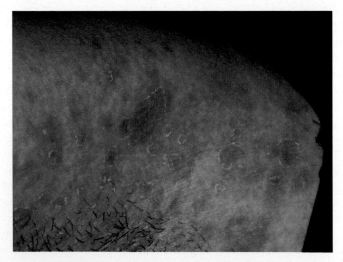

FIGURE 8.18 · Papular pityriasis rosea in the axilla resembling subacute eczema, with collarettes of scale.

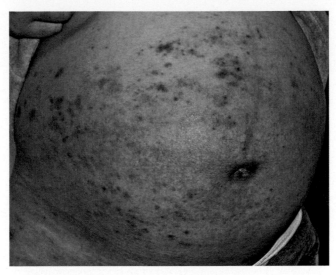

FIGURE 8.19 • PUPPP on the abdomen, displaying papules, round crusts, and round erosions that resemble subacute eczema.

plaques erupt in striae, typically in a nulliparous woman in the second or third trimester. This rash is very pruritic and may generalize (Figure 8.19). In polymorphous light eruption, itchy papules and/or papulovesicles erupt at the first sun exposure of the season, on the neck and other photoexposed areas, except the face (Figure 8.20). It is typically seen in women in the third or fourth decade of life, but both sexes can be affected. Prurigo pigmentosa is a very rare condition that is usually seen in adult females in Japan. Erythematous pruritic papules and papulovesicles that coalesce to produce reticular pattern and fade with reticular hyperpigmentation occur on the trunk and neck (see Figure 7.17A,B). Gianotti–Crosti syndrome is seen in childhood in association with a range of viruses or following immunization to influenza or diphtheria/pertussis/tetanus. A papular or papulovesicular eruption is most commonly seen on the face, buttocks, and extremities. The trunk is generally spared (see Figure 7.10 and Figure 8.21). In autoimmune progesterone dermatitis, the eruption may be polymorphic; red blanching papules, papulovesicles, a true eczematous appearance, targetoid plaques, or urticarial plaques are seen. The eruption worsens in the

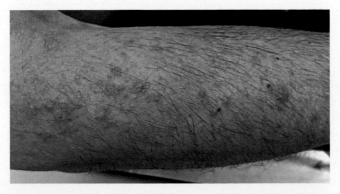

FIGURE 8.20 • Polymorphous light eruption with papules and papulovesicles on the forearm.

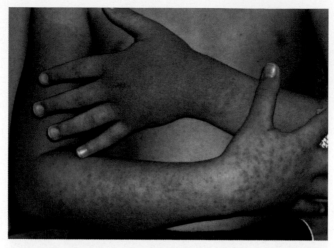

FIGURE 8.21 • Gianotti–Crosti syndrome with papulovesicles on the extremities. (Used with permission from Dr. Miguel Sanchez, Bellevue Hospital, New York University School of Medicine, New York, NY.)

second half of the menstrual cycle. Autoimmune blistering disease, including dermatitis herpetiformis and the dyshidrosiform variant of bullous pemphigoid may both mimic either acute or subacute eczema (see Figure 7.24). The differential diagnosis of scaly, eroded, and/or crusted plaques (another subacute eczema morphologic constellation) includes a variety of nutritional deficiency states, as detailed in Table 8.4 and outlined in the vesicobullous reaction pattern chapter (Chapter 7). Further "do not miss" diseases in this category include crusted scabies, which may have weeping, crusted and eroded plaques, and the disease entities of eczema herpeticum, eczema coxsackium, and eczema vaccinatum. These occur when herpes, coxsackie virus, or cowpox (from a smallpox vaccination) disseminate in a preexisting dermatosis. The most common dermatosis is atopic eczema, and here, eczema herpeticum is also known as *Kaposi varicelliform eruption*. Other dermatoses on which these viruses may disseminate include other forms of eczema (seborrheic dermatitis, irritant contact dermatitis), autoimmune bullous disease (such as pemphigus vulgaris and pemphigus foliaceus), mycosis fungoides, Darier disease, pityriasis rubra pilaris, and burns. The characteristic morphology of these entities is the presence of monomorphic erosions or crusts (Figure 8.22).

> **Clinical Tip** The finding of monomorphic erosions or crusts is a clue to the presence of eczema herpeticum, eczema coxsackium or eczema vaccinatum.

Elements of the diagnostic wheel can assist with the creation of differential diagnoses in this reaction pattern as seen in Figure 8.23. Acute, subacute, and chronic morphologies are a composite of the presence of various primary and secondary lesions, as discussed earlier. Shape and configuration may render additional diagnostic clues; nummular eczema has completely round plaques, and linear plaques are seen in some forms of allergic contact dermatitis as mentioned previously, such to poison ivy, oak, or sumac.

The site or distribution of eczema may yield useful diagnostic information, as is seen in Table 8.5. In allergic contact dermatitis, the site of involvement may offer clues

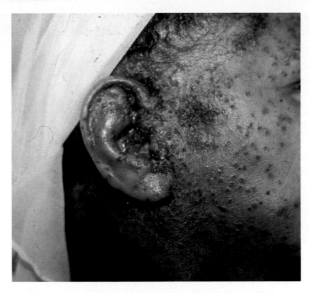

FIGURE 8.22 • Eczema herpeticum, displaying monomorphic erosions and crusts on the lateral face.

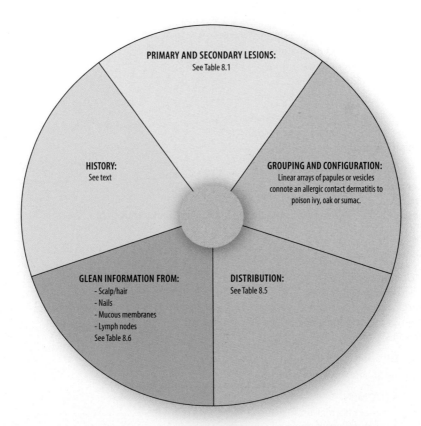

FIGURE 8.23 • The wheel of diagnosis customized to the eczematous reaction pattern.

TABLE 8.5. Eczematous Reaction Pattern by Distribution

PHOTODISTRIBUTED
- Photoallergic dermatitis
- Actinic prurigo
- Chronic actinic dermatitis

SEBORRHEIC
- Seborrheic dermatitis

ALONG HAIRLINE
- Seborrheic dermatitis
- Allergic contact dermatitis: hair products

CHEEKS
- Allergic contact dermatitis: personal-care products
- Irritant contact dermatitis
- Photoallergic dermatitis
- Chronic actinic dermatitis
- Pityriasis alba
- Seborrheic dermatitis: medial cheeks, including nasolabial folds

NECK
- Atopic dermatitis
- Irritant dermatitis
- Allergic contact dermatitis: fragrance, nickel
- Photoallergic contact dermatitis
- Chronic actinic dermatitis
- Lichen simplex chronicus

FLEXURES
- Atopic dermatitis
- Allergic contact dermatitis: formaldehyde
- Baboon syndrome

INTERTRIGINOUS
- Intertrigo
- Seborrheic dermatitis
- Allergic contact dermatitis: formaldehyde, azo dyes, flame retardants

BUTTOCKS
- Baboon syndrome

ANOGENITAL
- Irritant contact dermatitis
- Allergic contact dermatitis: preservatives in wipes, other personal-care products
- Lichen simplex chronicus
- Baboon syndrome

EXTENSORS
- Frictional lichenoid dermatitis

LOWER ABDOMEN
- Allergic contact dermatitis: nickel
- Allergic contact dermatitis: textile dyes (waistband)

(Continued)

TABLE 8.5. Eczematous Reaction Pattern by Distribution (continued)

EARLOBES
- Photoallergic contact dermatitis
- Chronic actinic dermatitis
- Airborne contact dermatitis
- Nickel dermatitis

HANDS
- Irritant contact dermatitis
- Allergic contact dermatitis
- Dyshidrotic eczema
- Chronic actinic dermatitis
- Atopic dermatitis
- ID reaction
- Keratolysis exfoliativa

FINGERTIPS
- Irritant dermatitis
- Allergic contact dermatitis: Alstroemeria plants: "tulip fingers"

REST OF THE FINGER
- Irritant dermatitis under ring
- Allergic contact dermatitis: nickel, gold in ring

FEET
- Rubber accelerators, dichromate, and dyes
- Dyshidrotic eczema
- Keratolysis exfoliativa
- Juvenile plantar dermatosis

EYELIDS
- Atopic dermatitis
- Allergic contact dermatitis
  - Fingertip-borne allergens (eg, toluene sulfonamide formaldehyde resin in nail varnish)
  - Hair dye and other hair product allergens
  - Allergens applied directly to eyelid or eye (eg, benzalkonium chloride in contact lens solution) or preservatives in personal-care products
- Airborne contact dermatitis
- Photoallergic dermatitis—spares eyelid crease

LEGS
- Stasis dermatitis
- Allergic contact dermatitis: bacitracin, neomycin
- Nummular dermatitis
- Asteatotic eczema
- Lichen simplex chronicus

RELATION TO APPENDAGEAL STRUCTURES: FOLLICULAR
- Follicular eczema
- Recurrent and disseminate infundibulofolliculitis

> **TABLE 8.6. Additional Diagnostic Clues That Can Be Found in the Eczematous Reaction Pattern**
>
> **SCALP**
> - Seborrheic dermatitis
> - Atopic dermatitis
> - Allergic contact dermatitis
>
> **NAILS**
> - Coarse pits and transverse ridging in nail fold eczema
>
> **LYMPH NODES**
> - Reactive enlargement in widespread eczema or erythroderma

to the causative allergen. Various important allergens and their typical sites of occurrence are included in Table 8.5. The differential diagnosis of peeling palms is covered in the papulosquamous reaction pattern chapter (Chapter 6). Keratolysis exfoliativa is a mild form of dyshidrotic eczema that classically presents with peeling only. Regarding a generalized distribution pattern, and as mentioned in Chapter 6, eczema is a frequent cause of erythroderma. Atopic dermatitis and allergic contact dermatitis are most commonly responsible. Seborrheic dermatitis may also become erythrodermic.

Examining the scalp, nails, and lymph nodes can provide key diagnostic clues, as summarized in Table 8.6. In seborrheic dermatitis, greasy scales and erythema are seen and itch is usually mild. This differs from atopic dermatitis, which is very itchy. Erythematous scaly plaques may become lichenified from scratching and rubbing. Allergic contact dermatitis is rarely encountered in the scalp; hair products that cause scalp dermatitis usually induce eczema on skin adjacent to the scalp first, such as the temples and the lateral aspects of the neck and ears. Only in longstanding or severe cases will the scalp be involved. Two itchy scalp dermatoses that may be mistaken for eczema are dermatomyositis of the scalp and crusted scabies. The former condition is not uncommon. Scalp dermatomyosistis may be pink, violaceous, or red. Scales may be seen. It is typically itchy. In contrast, crusted scabies is rarely seen in anatomic sites above the neck. Scalp scabies may, however, occur in immunocompromised individuals.

> **Clinical Tip** Differential diagnosis of itchy eczematous conditions of the scalp:
> - Dermatomyositis
> - Scabies

Regarding the nails, coarse pits and transverse ridging may be seen when eczema of the proximal nail folds is severe enough to interfere with keratinization in the nail matrix. The lymph nodes may be reactively enlarged in cases of widespread eczema, including erythroderma.

On taking the history, try to obtain a family history of atopy. A thorough history of possible contactant and ingestant allergens, including medications, should be elicited. In eczema that is secondary to generalized pruritus, try to elicit a cause for the pruritus through history, including attention to weight loss (hyperthyroidism, lymphoma) or other "B" symptoms (lymphoma), or weight gain (hypothyroidism). An important point of distinction in the history is to determine whether it is the itch or the rash that started first. Is it the rash that itches (eczema) or the itch that rashes (pruritus that will prompt a systemic workup if generalized)?

> **Clinical Tip** Is it a rash that itches or an itch that rashes?

BEDSIDE DIAGNOSTICS

Diagnostic tests for the papulosquamous (see Table 6.11) and vesicobullous (see Table 7.12) reaction patterns may apply to this reaction pattern as well, depending on the morphologic features of the presenting eruption. If it scales, scrape it! As mentioned earlier, some forms of dermatophytosis are extremely pruritic; tinea corporis or tinea cruris may be secondarily lichenified. Additionally, prior topical steroid application to a fungal rash may give rise to tinea incognito. Here, the tinea loses its typical annular morphology, and it may mimic eczema. Have a low threshold to perform a KOH preparation in this setting.

While honey-colored crusts may be seen in acute and subacute eczema as part of the inflammatory response, consider the diagnosis of a secondary bacterial infection in any case with tenderness, pustules, or purulent fluid, and perform a Gram stain and culture on the fluid in question. In suspected cases of eczema herpeticum, unroof a papule or papulovesicle and perform a scraping of the base or scrape the base of an erosion. Perform a Tzanck smear or send the specimen out for a viral PCR test. A viral culture can also be performed by rubbing a cotton swab over the base of the lesion types described above.

> **Clinical Tip** Do not miss a lichenified fungal infection and have a low threshold to perform a KOH on any scaly eruption.

SUMMARY

- The eczematous reaction pattern overlaps with both the papulosquamous and the vesicobullous reaction patterns.
- It encompasses all types of eczema, including acute, subacute and chronic forms, and eczemas of endogenous and exogenous origin.
- Some noneczematous eruptions can be included here, given their resemblance to eczema.
- The diagnostic boxes of the wheel of diagnosis may assist with narrowing down a differential diagnosis.
- Bedside diagnostics such as the tests for the papulosquamous reaction pattern when scales are present and for the vesicobullous reaction pattern when blisters are present can be employed to narrow down a diagnosis.

The Dermal Reaction Pattern 9

The *dermal reaction pattern* refers to those papules, plaques, and nodules that do not have epidermal changes, such as scales.

> **Clinical Tip** Smooth primary lesions (papules, nodules, plaques) = dermal reaction pattern.

The substance of dermal reaction pattern primary lesions may be made up of cells in the dermis or a dermal deposit. These cells may be inflammatory in nature (such as lymphocytes in lymphocytoma cutis or granulomas in sarcoidosis) or neoplastic, in which case they may be either benign (such as nevi or benign tumors arising from appendageal structures) or malignant (such as basal cell cancers, squamous cell cancers, melanomas, or cutaneous metastases). Dermal deposits, including urate, calcium, or mucin, may also give rise to these smooth primary lesions. Alterations in dermal collagen or elastic fibers, such as scleroderma or morphea, constitute a third category in this reaction pattern.

Papules, Nodules, and Plaques in the Dermal Reaction Pattern may be Composed of any or all of the Following Dermal Components:

- Inflammatory cells
- Neoplastic cells: benign or malignant
- Deposits
- Altered dermal connective tissue

The sclerotic plaques of scleroderma or morphea are firm to palpation and may be either slightly elevated or depressed.

> **Clinical Tip** Dermal plaques may be raised or depressed, as is seen in sclerotic conditions such as scleroderma and morphea.

A final group in this reaction pattern is diseases that are deep to the dermis. Subcutaneous disease, such as panniculitides and subcutaneous granulomatous disease or neoplasms, also gives rise to smooth nodules. Therefore, subcutaneous dermatoses can be categorized in the dermal reaction pattern. Conditions arising from other soft tissue structures may also present as smooth nodules without surface change.

Examples include nodular fasciitis that arises from the fascial plane, bursae, and giant cell tumor of the tendon sheath.

> **Clinical Tip** Subcutaneous diseases and conditions arising from other soft tissue structures are also classified as dermal reaction pattern as they manifest as smooth nodules.

Some dermal infiltrates are not classified in the dermal reaction pattern. Deep fungal infections, such as chromomycosis, may often have overlying epidermal changes, such as a hyperplastic epidermis and scale and, if so, present clinically as the papulosquamous reaction pattern. Some dermal infiltrates are so minimal as to create macules rather than papules, nodules, or plaques. An example here is telangiectasia macularis eruptiva perstans (TMEP), a form of cutaneous mastocytosis with minimal infiltration of the dermis by mast cells and lesions that appear as red macules. The macules of TMEP therefore may fall preferentially into the vascular (red) reaction pattern (see Chapter 10). Urticaria pigmentosa, another variant of cutaneous mastocytosis, may present as brownish smooth papules that allow it to be classified as dermal; however, sometimes the papular component is absent and the primary lesion therefore manifests as a macule. In this case, invoking the brown differential diagnosis will allow for the correct diagnosis.

Conversely, and as mentioned above, some conditions arise deep to the dermis and are classified as the dermal reaction pattern as they present as raised smooth papules, nodules, or plaques. The panniculitides manifest histopathologically as inflammation in the subcutaneous fat. Clinically, as a global rule, these present as tender, red, smooth nodules. Subcutaneous sarcoidosis presents as bland, skin-colored nodules usually on the lower extremities. Tumors arising from subcutaneous tissues, such as lipomas or liposarcomas, fit into this reaction pattern. Also as mentioned above, other soft tissue structures may give rise to dermal reaction pattern nodules.

Caveats

1. Some diseases that have dermal infiltrates are classified in other reaction patterns:
   a. Papulosquamous reaction pattern: chromomycosis presents as verrucous scaly plaques. Histopathologically, there are epidermal changes, including scale, overlying the dermal infiltrate.
   b. Vascular reaction pattern: red macules of TMEP. Even though there are mast cells that infiltrate the skin in TMEP, the infiltrate is slight and TMEP presents as red macules.
   c. Brown differential diagnosis: for urticaria pigmentosa that is macular.
2. Some dermatoses that fulfill criteria for classification into the dermal reaction pattern are not primarily in the dermis, such as the panniculitides, subcutaneous sarcoidosis, and subcutaneous and other soft tissue tumors and conditions.

The dermal reaction pattern overlaps most frequently with the vascular reaction pattern; some erythematous dermal papules, plaques, and nodules may be categorized as having an either dermal or vascular reaction pattern. These diseases will be discussed further in this chapter and in the vascular reaction pattern chapter (Chapter 10) as well.

TABLE 9.1. Erythematous Papules, Plaques, or Nodules That Can Be Classified as Vascular or Dermal Reaction Pattern

- Acute febrile neutrophilic dermatosis
- Arthropod assault
- Kikuchi disease
- Rheumatoid neutrophilic dermatosis
- Urticaria
- Urticarial vasculitis
- Urticarial phase of bullous pemphigoid
- Deep gyrate erythema
- Reticulate erythematous mucinosis
- Eosinophilic cellulitis
- Dermal hypersensitivity reaction
- Polymorphous light eruption
- Medium vessel vasculitides
  - Polyartertitis nodosa
  - Granulomatosis with polyangiitis

Table 9.1 displays those dermatoses that fit into both the dermal and vascular reaction patterns.

Clinical Tip Erythematous papules, plaques, and nodules may be classified as dermal or vascular reaction pattern.

Table 9.2 contains a comprehensive list of the range of dermatoses that fall into the dermal reaction pattern. Because of the relative lack of diagnostic features evident clinically as compared with the other reaction patterns (no scale, no vesicles, bullae, or erosions, etc), clinicians probably biopsy lesions in this reaction pattern most frequently for a definitive diagnosis. However, by harnessing elements of the wheel of diagnosis, a robust differential diagnosis can be created and then narrowed to provide a good pretest probability, or possibly to refute the need for a biopsy completely.

In the infectious category, furuncles and carbuncles are tender erythematous nodules. Secondary changes, such as erosion and crusting, may be seen (Figure 9.1). Botryomycosis may have a smooth dermal appearance or be verrucous, vegetating, or crusted. Erysipelas (see Figure 7.4) and erysipeloid are tender plaques. Erysipeloid (caused by *Erysipelothrix rhusiopathiae*) and *Vibrio vulnificus* infection may both resemble cellulitis.

Deep fungal infections, cutaneous tuberculosis, and atypical mycobacterial infections may present with smooth plaques and nodules. A verrucous (papulosquamous) presentation is also possible. *Mycobacterium marinum* presents as a solitary nodule at the site of inoculation of the organism, or as lymphocutaneous disease, in which multiple nodules that follow the lymphatics are seen. Lupus vulgaris is a form of cutaneous tuberculosis that typically presents around the nose or on other sites on the head and neck. There is typically an active focus of tuberculosis elsewhere, and skin involvement occurs secondary to hematogenous or lymphatic spread. Various morphologic types of lupus vulgaris have been described, including papulonodular (Figure 9.2), plaque, tumor-like, vegetating, and ulcerative or mutilating forms. Central atrophy causing an annular appearance may occur. In miliary tuberculosis, *Mycobacterium tuberculosis* seeds internal organs and

TABLE 9.2. The Dermal Differential Diagnosis

INFECTIOUS
- Bacterial
  - Furuncle
  - Carbuncle
  - Botryomycosis
  - Erysipelas
  - Cellulitis
  - Erysipeloid
  - *Vibrio* infection
- Treponemal
  - Early secondary syphilis
  - Tertiary syphilis
  - Borrelial lymphocytoma
- Mycobacterial
  - Atypical mycobacterial infections
  - Cutaneous tuberculosis
    - Lupus vulgaris
    - Miliary tuberculosis
  - Leprosy
    - Borderline, borderline lepromatous, and lepromatous subtypes
    - Histoid leprosy
    - Erythema nodosum leprosum
- Deep fungal
  - Histoplasmosis
  - Cryptococcosis
  - Coccidiodomycosis
  - Lobomycosis
- Parasitic
  - Nodular scabies

INFLAMMATORY
- Dermal lymphocytes
  - Tumid lupus
  - Subacute cutaneous lupus
  - Polymorphous light eruption
  - Pseudolymphom
  - Deep gyrate erythema
- Dermal neutrophils
  - Sweet syndrome
  - Rheumatoid neutrophilic dermatosis
  - Neutrophilic eccrine hidradenitis
  - Neutrophilic vasculitis such as is seen in polyarteritis nodosa
- Dermal eosinophils
  - Eosinophilic cellulitis
  - Eosinophilic fasciitis
  - Angiolymphoid hyperplasia with eosinophils
  - Dermal hypersensitivity reaction
- Mast cells
  - Mastocytoma

(Continued)

TABLE 9.2. The Dermal Differential Diagnosis (continued)

INFLAMMATORY (CONT.)
- Urticaria pigmentosa
- Diffuse cutaneous mastocytosis
- Mixed infiltrate
  - Granuloma faciale
  - Erythema elevatum diutinum
- Histiocytes: granulomatous disease
  - Granuloma annulare
  - Necrobiosis lipoidica
  - Sarcoidosis
  - Rheumatoid nodule
  - Palisaded and neutrophilic granulomatous dermatitis
  - Granulomatous rosacea
  - Granulomatous vasculitis
    - Granulomatosis with polyangiitis
    - Eosinophilic granulomatosis with polyangiitis
    - Sarcoidosis
- Panniculitis
  - Erythema nodosum
  - Erythema induratum
  - Lupus panniculitis
  - Pancreatic panniculitis
  - Cold panniculitis
  - Subcutaneous fat necrosis of the newborn
  - Sclerema

DEPOSITIONAL DISEASE
- Amyloid
- Urate: gouty tophi
- Calcium: calcinosis cutis
- Bone: osteoma cutis
- Lipid: xanthelasma; tuberous, tendon, plane, eruptive xanthomas
- Mucin
- Colloid in colloid milium
- "Hyalin material": lipoid proteinosis
- Mucopolysaccharides

NEOPLASTIC
- Benign
  - Arising from adnexal structures: hair, sebaceous, eccrine, apocrine
  - Fibroblast: keloid, dermatofibroma
  - Melanocytic: benign nevi
  - Neural: neurilemmona, neurofibroma, granular cell tumor, etc.
  - Smooth muscle: pilar leiomyoma, angioleiomyoma
  - Vascular: pyogenic granuloma, hemangioma, bacillary angiomatosis, etc.
  - Sebaceous: sebaceous hyperplasia, sebaceous adenoma
  - Lipocyte: lipoma, angiolipoma, spindle cell lipoma, hibernoma, etc.
  - Class II histiocytoses: benign cephalic histiocytosis, xanthoma disseminatum, necrobiotic xanthogranuloma, multicentric reticulohistiocytosis

(Continued)

the elbows and knees in rheumatoid arthritis. Palisaded and neutrophilic granuloma-tous dermatitis is a rarely encountered dermatosis that is seen usually in the setting of autoimmune disease. There are typically papules and plaques, usually on the extensor aspects of the extremities. Finally, in terms of granulomatous disease, two systemic granulomatous vasculitides should be considered. Granulomatosis with polyangiitis (formerly Wegener granulomatosis) may present with erythematous nodules, some-times ulcerated, and livedo reticularis. The dermatologic manifestations of eosinophilic granulomatosis with polyangiitis (formerly Churg–Strauss syndrome) are protean and include urticarial or purpuric plaques or nodules.

Subcutaneous disease presents as smooth nodules and less frequently papules. The panniculitides are a group of inflammatory dermatoses that occur in the fat. In general, they present as tender erythematous smooth nodules. Some types may ulcerate, and each type has its own typical presentation, including the site of predilection and associations. Table 9.3 outlines the differentiating features of some of the more commonly encountered panniculitides. Erythema nosoum is typified in Figure 9.16, and late-stage lupus pannic-ulitis is seen in Figure 9.17. Subcutaneous sarcoidosis, as mentioned above, presents as nontender flesh-colored papules and/or nodules, typically on an extremity. Lipomas and liposarcomas may also arise in this location. Lipomas are common and present as soft,

TABLE 9.3. Distinguishing Characteristics of Panniculitides

Erythema nodosum (erythema contusiforme)	Sudden onset, symmetric tender nodules and plaques Distribution: shins, knees, ankles (Figure 9.16) May be extensive and involve upper extremities May be associated with fever, malaise, and joint pain Bright red fading to purplish/bruise-like Never ulcerates or scars
Lupus panniculitis	Classic sites: upper arms, shoulders, cheeks, buttocks Heals with lipoatrophy (Figure 9.17) May ulcerate and discharge necrotic fat There may be overlying discoid lupus plaques
Lipodermatosclerosis	Acutely, there are tender firm plaques over the distal lower extremities with background varicosities Chronically, there are asymptomatic bound-down plaques Gives rise to a "champagne-bottle" appearance
Pancreatic panniculitis	Distribution: distal lower extremities around ankles and knees Ulcerate, discharge brownish material Only 1 nodule may be present.
Cold panniculitis	Distribution: cheeks of children who suck popsicles (popsicle panniculitis); buttocks of women who ride horses (equestrian panniculitis)
Erythema induratum	Nodules and plaques on posterior aspects of lower extremities Ulcerate; heal with scarring
Subcutaneous fat necrosis of the newborn	Occurs in the first few weeks of life Red nodules or plaques may be seen on trunk most frequently; these may ulcerate Affected newborns are generally healthy
Sclerema neonatorum	Usually seen in premature infants or those with low birth weight Skin is indurated and bound down Starts on thigh or buttock area and may involve wide areas

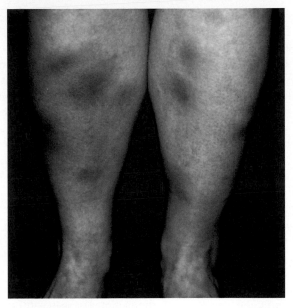

FIGURE 9.16 • Erythema nodosum, presenting as numerous erythematous nodules of varying sizes on the lower legs. (Reproduced with permission from Wolff K, Johnson RA, Saavedra AP, et al: *Fitzpatrick's Color Atlas and Synopsis of Clinical Dermatology*, 8th ed. New York, NY: McGraw Hill; 2017.)

well-demarcated nodules with a "rolling" edge (the edge seems to roll away from the fingertips on palpation). Lipomas are typically nontender and flesh-colored; however, the variant of angiolipoma may be spontaneously painful and tender to palpation, and this variant may also appear bluish secondary to the associated vascular component. Any rapid growth in a subcutaneous nodule should prompt consideration of biopsy to rule out malignancy. Of note, nodular fasciitis is a benign condition that presents as a rapidly enlarging nodule, typically on the arm of females.

> **Clinical Tip** Any rapid growth in a subcutaneous nodule should prompt consideration of biopsy to rule out malignancy.

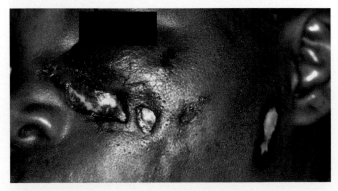

FIGURE 9.17 • Late stage of lupus panniculitis showing lipoatrophy on the central cheek. Note the overlying changes of burnt out discoid lupus.

In depositional disease, various substances are deposited in the dermis, including bone, calcium, urate, amyloid, lipid, mucopolysaccharides, mucin, colloid in colloid milium, and hyaline material in lipoid proteinosis. Primary osteomas are a finding in various rare inherited syndromes, including Albright hereditary osteodystrophy, progressive osseous heteroplasia, and congenital plate-like osteomatosis. Hard plaques, papules, or nodules are seen. An acquired papular form that follows severe acne is perhaps the form most frequently encountered in clinical practice. Hard 1–2-mm papules are seen scattered over the face. Calcium deposition in the skin also gives rise to hard papules, plaques, or nodules. A complete differential diagnosis of the causes of calcinosis cutis can be found in Table 4.13. Gouty tophi occur in uncontrolled gout and represent urate deposition in the skin. This is a very firm substance that may have a white, yellow, or yellow-orange hue. Tophi typically occur around joints and may also be seen on the pinna. Amyloid deposition in the skin is seen in a variety of conditions. Primary systemic amyloidosis (AL amyloidosis) occurs in the setting of a plasma cell dyscrasia. Light chains deposit in the skin and in internal organs. The skin may be diffusely infiltrated and prone to purpura, which occur secondary to minor trauma ("pinch purpura"). Infiltrated papules and plaques may also be seen on eyelid margins, around the nasal sill, and at other sites. These are termed "waxy papules" as they resemble wax because they are shiny and firm. Purpuric changes may be seen within these areas as well (Figure 9.18). Macroglossia is a further sign of primary systemic amyloidosis occurring secondary to amyloid infiltration of the tongue. Secondary systemic amyloidosis

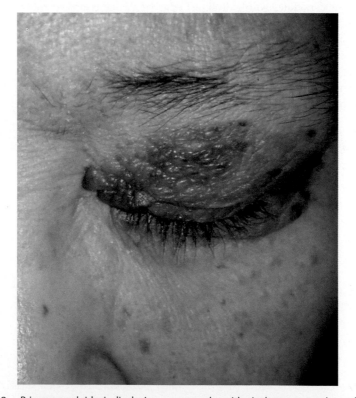

FIGURE 9.18 • Primary amyloidosis displaying waxy papules with pinch purpura at the eyelid margin.

(AA amyloidosis) does not typically lead to cutaneous manifestations. Localized forms of amyloid do occur in the skin, including macular and lichen amyloid, and nodular amyloid. Macular and lichen amyloid occur in the setting of pruritus. Cytokeratins make up the amyloid protein that deposits in the upper dermis. Clinically macular amyloid presents as brown reticulate and linear macules, usually on the back (classified with macules, not with a dermal reaction pattern). Lichen amyloid refers to small papules in this same configuration. These may be smooth (dermal reaction pattern) or scaly (papulosquamous reaction pattern). They occur on the back or legs most frequently. Macular and lichen amyloid are seen in the rare inherited multiple endocrine neoplasia type 2A (medullary thyroid cancer, pheochromocytoma, and parathyroid adenoma/ hyperplasia occur in this syndrome). Finally, nodular amyloid presents as a skin-colored or pink, reddish, or yellowish nodule on the face or acral areas (Figure 9.19). More than one lesion may be present. Nodular amyloid occurs secondary to a localized collection of plasma cells in the skin with secondary light-chain production.

Lipid deposition in the skin occurs in xanthomas and as a secondary phenomenon in class II histiocytoses, as histiocytes become lipidized. Xanthomas include tendinous, tuberous (see Figures 4.8A and 9.20) eruptive (Figure 9.20), palmar, planar, and intertriginous types, as well as xanthelasma (Figure 9.21). The clinical features of the xanthomas and xanthelasma are summarized in Table 4.11. The class II histiocytoses (discussed below) are a group of reactive proliferative diseases of histiocytes in the dermis. Some forms are preferentially secondarily lipidized. These entities are listed in Table 4.12.

The mucopolysaccharidoses are rarely encountered inherited group of diseases that affect the lysosomal enzymes responsible for mucopolysaccharide catabolism. Skin

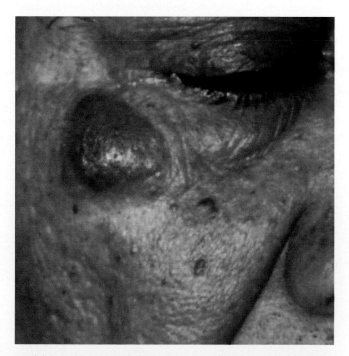

FIGURE 9.19 · Nodular amyloid presenting as a flesh-colored nodule on the cheek.

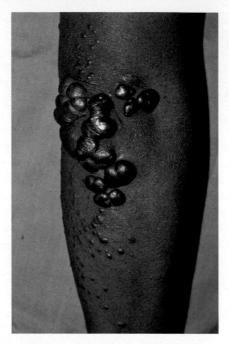

FIGURE 9.20 • Eruptive xanthomas presenting as small papules over the extensor forearm, with associated tuberous xanthomas on the elbow.

involvement is most prominent in Hunter's syndrome, where white papules and sometimes nodules are seen over the scapulae and more broadly over the back.

The mucinoses represent a heterogeneous group of diseases. Generalized myxedema is seen in longstanding hypothyroidism. The skin has a sallow, dry appearance. There is puffiness around the eyes and a waxy feel to the skin. Pretibial myxedema usually occurs in the setting of hyperthyroidism from Graves' disease; however, hypothyroidism is also a cause. Mucin deposition is localized to the pretibial area and may extend to the dorsal feet or even to the thighs in more severe cases. The typical appearance is that of edematous plaques that may be pink, red, yellowish, or flesh-colored. Variant presentations include the presence of nodules or tumors (Figure 9.22), a peau d'orange appearance, or a sclerotic appearance (Figures 9.23 and 9.24). Scleredema arises most

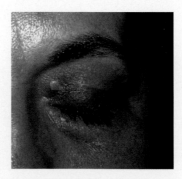

FIGURE 9.21 • Xanthelasma showing a thin yellow papule on the eyelid.

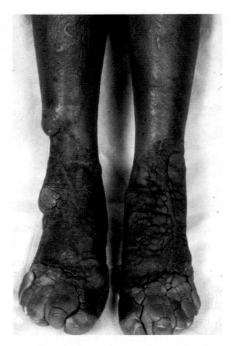

FIGURE 9.22 · Nodular variant of pretibial myxedema with overlying changes of elephantiasis nostras verrucosa.

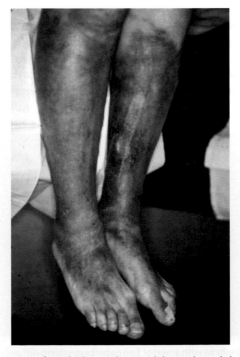

FIGURE 9.23 · Sclerotic variant of pretibial myxedema with brown bound-down plaques.

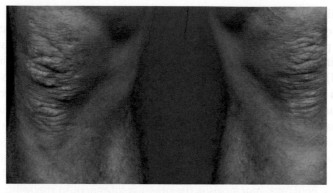

FIGURE 9.26 · Lipoid proteinosis displaying infiltrated plaques, some with overlying hyperkeratosis over the knees.

overlying scale. Nonscarring alopecia may be seen. Macroglossia is seen. Acral verrucous keratoses involve the lateral aspects of the fingers. Similar plaques with scale are seen on the knees and elbows (Figure 9.26). Laryngeal involvement may cause airway compromise in infants. Epilepsy may also occur.

A vast range of adnexal tumors occupies the benign neoplasm category, along with nevi and the class II histiocytoses. Benign nevi typically have one color, are small, and have regular borders and symmetry. Atypical nevi may have one or more of the clinical criteria for melanoma (see discussion of melanoma below). Adnexal tumors may be difficult to differentiate clinically. Table 9.4 lists the distinguishing clinical features of these neoplasms, including age and sex predilection and characteristic morphologic features and favored sites of distribution. The typical appearance of eruptive syringomas, an apocrine hidrocystoma, an eccrine poroma, a clear cell hidradenoma, and fibrofolliculomas is seen in Figures 9.27–9.32. Many adnexal tumors are clinical hallmarks of underlying syndromes. These associations are listed in Table 9.5. Any rapid growth may signify malignant degeneration, which is a rare phenomenon, generally speaking, for adnexal tumors.

The class II histiocytoses are very rarely encountered. As mentioned above, they are a group of reactive proliferative diseases of histiocytes in the dermis. Multicentric reticulohistiocytosis is a rare disorder of adults that presents with papules and nodules over the dorsal hands and fingers (Figure 9.33). The presence of confluent papules around the nail fold is referred to as a "coral bead" appearance. The face and other parts of the forearm may also be affected. An erosive arthropathy is usually present, and an association with solid-organ malignancies has been reported.

In the malignant category, basal cell cancer (BCC) and melanoma are usually smooth and therefore present with dermal reaction pattern morphology. While squamous cell cancers (SCCs) usually have a scaly or hyperkeratotic surface, they may be smooth, especially if early. Of these three cancers, SCC is the one that may be painful. Pain is not a global feature however, BCC is the most commonly encountered skin cancer. It occurs most frequently in older adults in areas that have been chronically exposed to the sun. BCCs may rarely arise in sun-covered areas. There are many clinical varieties of BCC. The earliest lesions of superficial BCC may be light pink. Well-developed superficial BCCs may be a pink or pink-red color ("ruby-red"), which is a strong diagnostic clue. Nodular basal cell cancers are pearly nodules with

TABLE 9.4. Distinguishing Characteristics of Adnexal Tumors

Syringomas	Onset in puberty
	Lower eyelids: 1–2 mm, firm, flesh-colored papules
	Enlarge with age and may be ≤5 mm in older adults
Eruptive syringomas	Arise in first decade
	Ventral surface of the body, especially upper body (Figure 9.27)
	Vulva may be involved
	Usually 1–3 mm, evenly spaced
	Some cases are inherited (familial variant)
Eccrine hidrocystoma	Single/few, sometimes many
	Translucent papules/papulonodules on face
	Number and size increase in hot weather
	Can be bluish
Apocrine hidrocystoma	Single, translucent papule/papulonodule
	Usually on the eyelid margin
	Can be bluish (Figure 9.28)
Poroma (previously eccrine poroma)	Palms and soles are sites of predilection
	May resemble firm pyogenic granuloma
	Can be surrounded by collarette of scale (Figure 9.29)
	Eccrine poromatosis: >100 lesions; may be associated with lymphoma
Eccrine spiradenoma	Solitary nodule, painful tumor, firm
Clear cell hidradenoma	Solitary nodule
	Some discharge serous material, or ulcerate, giving the appearance of a moist pyogenic granuloma (Figure 9.30)
	Size ranging within 0.5–2 cm
Mixed tumor (chondroid syringoma)	Predilection for head (including scalp) and neck
	Firm to hard
Papilliferum syringocystadenoma	Scalp or neck, can resemble nevus sebaceus (or arise within one)
	Verrucous, can be friable
Papilliferum hidradenoma	Postpubertal women, genitalia or surrounds
	Fleshy nodule
Cylindroma	Single or multiple (may be in association with multiple trichoepitheliomas and spiradenomas in Brooke–Spiegler syndrome)
	Dome-shaped, firm, may resemble BCC with telangiectasias, but firmer (Figure 9.31)
	Sites of predilection: scalp, face
Trichofolliculoma	Solitary papule, tuft of "cottony" white hairs from center.
Solitary trichoepithelioma	Face of adults, flesh- or brown-colored
Multiple trichoepithelioma	Predilection for centrofacial region, especially nasolabial folds
	Papules are larger than those of trililemmomas (≤5 mm).
	Familial
Desmoplastic trichoepithelioma	Firm papulonodule with central dell; resembles BCC, usually seen on the face of women
Pilomatricoma	Hard, craggy, may be bluish, children or adults
	May be multiple (if so, may be an association of myotonic dystrophy)
	0.5–5cm.

(Continued)

TABLE 9.4. Distinguishing Characteristics of Adnexal Tumors (continued)

Proliferating trichilemmal cyst	Elderly women most frequently affected
	Presents as an enlarging tumor on scalp that may resemble a pilar cyst
Trichilemmoma	Solitary or multiple (in Cowden syndrome), flesh-colored small papules on face
	Centrofacial, especially mouth, nose, and ears
	May be filiform or wart-like in appearance
Fibrofolliculoma	White 1–2-mm papules
	More than 5 signify a diagnosis of Birt–Hogg–Dube syndrome
	Sites of predilection: face, neck, axillae, and other folds (see Figures 4.6D and 9.32)
Familial multiple trichodiscomas (discoid fibromas)	Multiple 1–2-mm flesh-colored form papules on face and ears that arise in childhood or teenage years

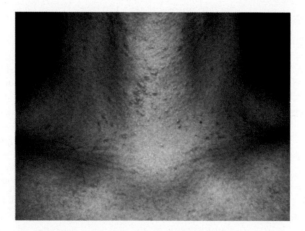

FIGURE 9.27 • Eruptive syringomas seen as flesh-colored, slightly shiny papules on the neck.

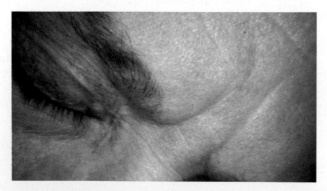

FIGURE 9.28 • An apocrine hidrocystoma presenting as a bluish translucent papule at the eyelid margin.

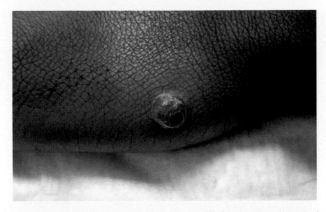

FIGURE 9.29 • A poroma displaying a reddish nodule with thin crust and scale at the lateral palm.

FIGURE 9.30 • A clear cell hidrocystoma with a pyogenic granuloma-like appearance on the scalp.

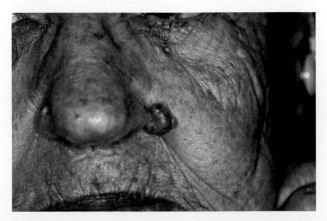

FIGURE 9.31 • A cylindroma displaying a pink centrofacial nodule with a central dell.

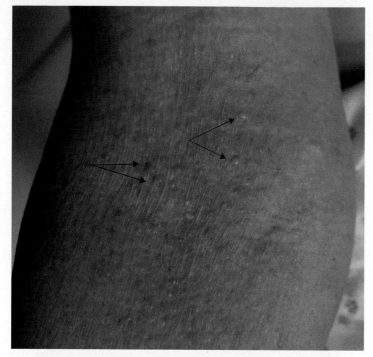

FIGURE 9.32 • Fibrofollicuomas (red arrows) at the antecubital fossa and skin tags (blue arrow), another feature of Birt–Hogg–Dube syndrome.

TABLE 9.5. Disease Associations of Adnexal Tumors

CUTANEOUS TUMOR	SYNDROME
Angiofibroma, Koenen tumor (periungual fibroma)	Tuberous sclerosis, multiple endocrine neoplasia (MEN) type 1
Koenen tumor (periungual fibroma)	Tuberous sclerosis
Collagenoma	Tuberous sclerosis, MEN type I
Mucosal neuroma	MEN type 2B
Trichilemmoma: ≥3	Cowden syndrome
Fibrofolliculoma: ≥6	Birt–Hogg–Dube syndrome
Trichodiscoma	Birt–Hogg–Dube syndrome, familial multiple discoid fibromas
Cylindroma	Brooke–Spiegler syndrome
Trichoepithelioma	Brooke–Spiegler syndrome
Spiradenoma	Brooke–Spiegler syndrome
Epithelioid blue nevi	Carney syndrome
Cutaneous myxoma	Carney syndrome
Psammomatous melanotic schwannoma	Carney syndrome
Plexiform neuroma	Neurofibromatosis type 1
Malignant peripheral nerve sheath tumor	Neurofibromatosis type 1
Rhabdomyosarcoma	Neurofibromatosis type 1, basal cell nevus syndrome
Pilomatricoma	Myotonic dystrophy

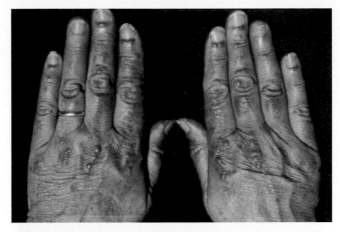

FIGURE 9.33 · Multicentric reticulohistiocytosis displaying reddish papules on dorsal hands and fingers and "coral beading" around the cuticles.

overlying telangiectasias (Figure 9.34). They may ulcerate centrally (a "rodent" ulcer). Morpheaform or infiltrative BCCs are firm and sclerotic. They may be depressed with respect to the surrounding skin, and they may resemble scars. Pigmented BCCs may be light or dark gray (as seen in Figure 4.15D), light brown, or even black. The nodular BCC in Figure 9.34 has some gray-brown punctate pigmentation.

Picking up an early melanoma is a diagnostic challenge and of vital importance prognostically; any history from the patient of a changing mole should be taken seriously by the diagnostician, and a careful, unhurried, complete skin examination, including a dermatoscopic study (see section titled "Bedside Diagnostics and Tests," below), should be undertaken. Invasive melanoma may present as a papule, plaque, or nodule. It may contain any shade of brown, or black, red, white, blue, or pink and is

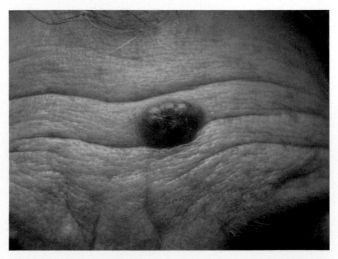

FIGURE 9.34 · A nodular pigmented BCC showing a shiny nodule with overlying telangiectasias and punctate gray-brown pigmentation within it.

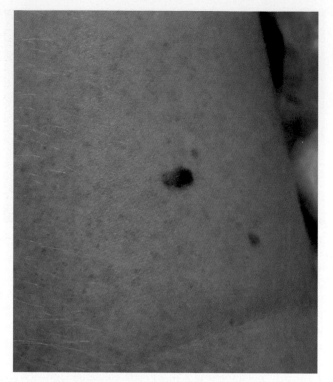

FIGURE 9.35 · A thin melanoma displaying a variegated brown plaque.

often variegated (Figures 9.35 and 9.36). Amelanotic melanoma may be skin-colored (Figure 9.37), pink, red, or violaceous. Ulceration is a poor prognostic sign. The ABCDE criteria as outlined in the textbox below are both sensitive and specific criteria for melanoma diagnosis. However, early melanomas or small nodular melanomas may

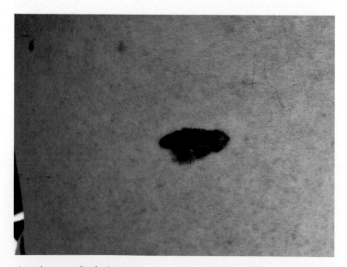

FIGURE 9.36 · A melanoma displaying a 2.5-cm variegated plaque with asymmetry, irregular borders, black, red, white, blue, and varying shades of brown.

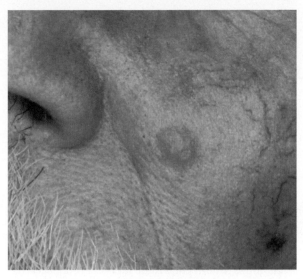

FIGURE 9.37 • An amelanotic melanoma displaying a flesh-colored papule on the cheek.

not have any of the ABCDE's, and so the "ugly duckling" sign (also defined in the text-box) is a useful sign to employ as well. Further caveats are that atypical nevi, which are benign, may have one or more of the ABCDEs. Similarly, congenital nevi are typically greater than 6 mm.

Clues to Melanoma Diagnosis

The ABCDEs
- A—Asymmetry: the two halves of the lesion differ from each other
- B—Border: irregular or ill-defined
- C—Color: variegated or not uniform throughout
- D—Diameter: more than 6 mm
- E—Evolution: change in any of the above criteria over a short time period, or development of symptoms, such as itch or bleeding
- Also pertinent here is the "ugly duckling" sign: any mole whose appearance is different from those of the surrounding mole population. It may be bigger or smaller; it may be more atypical or less atypical.
- Amelanotic melanoma may be skin-colored, pink, red or violaceous

---

True lymphomas in the skin that present with a dermal reaction pattern morphology include the tumor stage of mycosis fungoides, primary cutaneous anaplastic large cell lymphoma, and B-cell lymphomas. In the tumor stage of mycosis fungoides, tumors are usually seen in concert with patch and plaque stage disease. Ulceration may occur secondarily. In primary cutaneous anaplastic large cell lymphoma, a rare form of T-cell lymphoma, there is usually a solitary nodule or plaque. In cutaneous B-cell lymphoma, the skin may provide information on primary or systemic forms of the full moon. One or more smooth papules or nodules over plaques may occur.

In scleroderma, sclerosis starts distally on the fingers with edema and then eventuates to a bound-down appearance. It progresses proximally and symmetrically up the limbs to involve other body sites. An atypical form has been recognized where involvement of

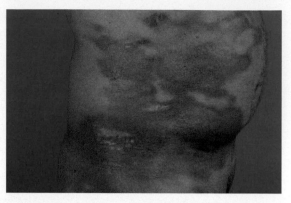

FIGURE 9.38 • Morphea presenting as yellow and brown plaques on the flank and abdomen. (Reproduced with permission from Wolff K, Johnson RA, Saavedra AP, et al: *Fitzpatrick's Color Atlas and Synopsis of Clinical Dermatology*, 8th ed. New York, NY: McGraw Hill; 2017.)

sclerosis does not follow this pattern but is more random. Esophageal dysmotility, interstitial fibrosis of the lungs, and renal involvement occur. In morphea, there are one or more sclerotic, indurated plaques. Active plaques have a pink to violaceous rim around them. Older plaques are softer and less indurated (Figure 9.38). In morphea, unlike scleroderma, there are no systemic manifestations. Atrophoderma of Pasini and Pierini is a variant of morphea in which soft light brown depressed plaques with a sharp cutoff from the normal surrounding skin (cliff-drop sign; see Figure 3.11). Sclerodermoid plaques accompany a broad array of rare inherited and acquired conditions as outlined in Table 9.6.

TABLE 9.6. Differential Diagnosis of Sclerodermoid Plaques

INHERITED
- Rothmund–Thomson syndrome
- Severe combined immunodeficiency (SCID)
- Progeria
- Werner disease
- Phenylketonuria

ACQUIRED
- Scleroderma
- Morphea
- Morpheaform sarcoidosis
- Porphyria cutanea tarda
- Carcinoid: lower extremities
- Primary amyloidosis: lower extremities
- POEMS (polyneuropathy, organomegaly, endocrinopathy, M protein, skin changes)
- Chronic graft-versus-host disease: sclerodermoid variant
- Scleremyxedema
- Sclerotic variant of pretibial myxedema
- Drugs:
  - Anticancer drugs (bleomycin, taxanes, gemcitabine)
  - Appetite suppressants
  - Texier's disease: sclerodermoid type of hypersensitivity reaction to vitamin K injection
- Environmental: rapeseed oil

Changes in dermal elastic fibers give rise to soft dermal papules, plaques, or nodules. In the case of pseudoxanthoma elasticum (PXE), the yellowish papules that are seen around the neck and in the folds are firm as the elastic fibers calcify. PXE has a "chicken skin" appearance. It is inherited in an autosomal recessive fashion. The elastic tissue in blood vessels is also affected. Involvement of arteries leads to hypertension and gastrointestinal hemorrhage. Retinal artery involvement gives rise to the classic angioid streaks that are seen on fundoscopy and can lead to blindness. *Fibroelastolytic papulosis* (FEP) (see Figure 4.6C) is a broad term that encompasses the conditions of white fibrous papulosis of the neck and PXE-like papillary dermal elastolysis. White or yellow small papules cluster on the neck, in folds, or in a more widespread fashion on the chest, abdomen, and thighs. FEP may resemble PXE, but onset is in later life and no systemic involvement is present. The cause is unknown. Anetoderma appears as soft papules or nodules, which may be wrinkled (Figure 9.39). There is loss of elastic fibers in the reticular dermis. In the primary type there is no obvious cause, but anetoderma may be seen secondary to a wide range of conditions, including syphilis, Lyme disease, HIV infection, or systemic lupus. The "button hole" sign refers to the sensation on palpation of one's finger going through a button hole. This occurs as the dermis is so soft. A similar sensation is felt when palpating neurofibromas.

> **Clinical Tip** A positive button hole sign is found on palpation of anetoderma and neurofibromas.

Mid-dermal elastolysis is another rare entity of loss of mid-dermal elastic fibers. Plaques are typically located over the upper torso and may be wrinkled or have a peau d'orange appearance.

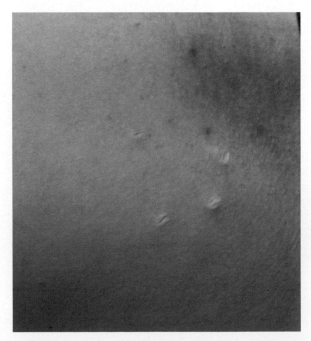

FIGURE 9.39 · Anetoderma arising from folliculitis, presenting as soft, wrinkled perifollicular papules on the inner upper thigh.

Drug-induced causes in the dermal reaction pattern category are all rarely encountered. Drug-induced interstitial granulomatous dermatitis presents as red-brown or brown dermal papules and/or plaques. Antihypertensive drugs (including angiotensin-converting enzyme inhibitors, calcium-channel blockers, β-blockers), lipid-lowering agents, antihistamines, anticonvulsants, and tumor necrosis factor-α blockers, have all been implicated. Morpheaform and sclerodermoid plaques have been reported from chemotherapy agents (including bleomycin, the taxanes, and gemcitabine), penicillamine, and appetite suppressants. *Texier's disease* refers to the sclerodermoid plaque that may develop at the site of a vitamin K injection.

As always, it is helpful to think through the wheel of diagnosis when creating a differential diagnosis of a dermal eruption. The wheel can help to generate subcategories of differential diagnosis by diagnostic determinants of the primary lesion, groupings or configuration, distribution, and whether scalp, hair, nails, mucous membranes, and lymph nodes are involved. Figure 9.40 shows the wheel that has been customized to the dermal reaction pattern. Each diagnostic box houses a reference to the subsequent corresponding tabular differential diagnostic list.

Regarding the visual diagnostic determinants of primary lesions in this reaction pattern, each dermatosis classically presents with papules, nodules, or plaques, or a combination. Color is another visual clue that assist in diagnosis. Table 9.7 displays the differential diagnosis for each color according to primary lesion. As discussed in

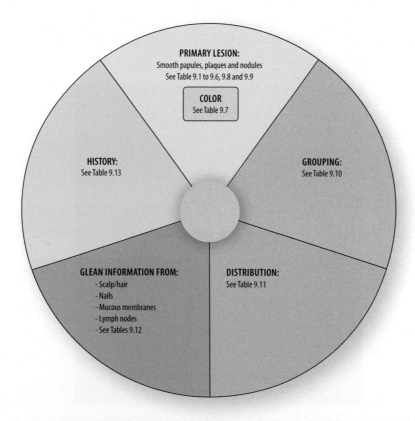

FIGURE 9.40 • The wheel of diagnosis, customized to the dermal reaction pattern.

TABLE 9.7. Dermal Disease by Color

PINK/RED

- Papules
  - Generalized eruptive histiocytosis
  - Neurofibromas
  - Compound nevi
  - Dermatofibromas
- Papules or nodules
  - Dermatofibrosarcoma protuberans (DFSP)
  - Merkel cell carcinoma
  - Amelanotic melanoma
  - Atypical fibroxanthoma
  - Lymphoma
  - Leukemia
  - Cutaneous metastases
  - Atypical mycobacterial infections
- Papules and plaques
  - Palisaded and neutrophilic granulomatous dermatitis
  - Rheumatoid nodules
- Nodules
  - Furuncle
  - Carbuncle
  - Majocchi granuloma
- Panniculitides
  - Nodules seen in medium vessel vasculitides

PURPLE/MAROON: "PURPLE PLUMS"

- Benign vascular proliferations
  - Hemangioma
  - Glomeruloid and microvenular hemangioma
  - Pyogenic granuloma (Figure 9.41)
  - Bacillary angiomatosis
- Malignant vascular proliferations
  - Angiosarcoma
  - Kaposi sarcoma (Figure 9.42)
  - Kaposiform hemangioendothelioma
  - Malignant hemangioendothelioma
- Malignant neoplasms
  - DFSP (Figure 9.43)
  - Amelanotic melanoma (Figure 9.37)
  - Atypical fibroxanthoma
  - Lymphoma (Figure 9.44)
  - Leukemia
  - Merkel cell cancer
  - Cutaneous metastases (Figure 9.46)

BROWN-GRAY

- Papules, plaques, and/or nodules
- Granuloma faciale is classically a brown-gray color, although variations of red and brown may be seen (see Figure 4.3c)

(Continued)

TABLE 9.7. Dermal Disease by Color (continued)

YELLOW
- Papules
  - Eruptive xanthomas (see Figures 4.8a and 9.20)
  - Fordyce spots
  - Sebaceous hyperplasia
  - Sebaceous adenoma
  - Juxtaclavicular beaded lines
- Papules and plaques
  - Xanthelasma (Figure 9.21)
  - Necrobiotic xanthogranuloma
  - Orbital xanthogranuloma
  - Xanthoma disseminatum
  - Erdheim–Chester syndrome
  - Pseudoxanthoma elasticum
  - Papillary dermal elastolysis/fibroelastolytic papulosis
  - Calcinosis cutis (see Figure 4.8d)
- Plaques
  - Palmar xanthoma
  - Diffuse plane xanthoma
  - Intertriginous xanthoma
  - Necrobiosis lipoidica (see Figure 4.8c)
- Nodules
  - Tuberous xanthomas (Figure 9.20)

ORANGE
- Papules and/or nodules
  - Juvenile/adult xanthogranuloma
  - Benign progressive histiocytosis
  - Gouty tophi

WHITE
- Papules
  - Milia
  - White fibrous papulosis of the neck
- Papules or nodules
  - Gouty tophi
  - Calcinosis cutis
  - Epidermal cyst
- Plaques
  - Morphea

BLUE
- Papules or nodules
  - Blue nevus
  - Venous lake
  - Epidermal cyst: may appear bluish
  - Pilomatricoma: may appear bluish
  - Apocrine hidrocystoma: may appear bluish (Figure 9.28)

(Continued)

TABLE 9.7. Dermal Disease by Color (continued)

BROWN
- Papules
  - Urticaria pigmentosa (see Figure 4.3a)
- Papules or nodules
  - Melanocytic nevi
  - Dermatofibromas
  - Melanoma
  - Granulomatous conditions such as sarcoidosis and granuloma annulare may appear light brown, yellow-brown, or orange-brown
- Plaques
  - Scleroderma

BLACK
- Papules
  - Heavily pigmented nevi such as spindle cell tumor of Reed and deep penetrating nevus
  - Papules or nodules
  - Melanoma metastasis

GREEN
- Plaques
  - Resolving eosinophilic cellulitis

NO COLOR (SKIN-COLORED)
- Papules
  - Many adnexal tumors
  - Dermal nevus
- Papules or nodules
  - Anetoderma
  - Subcutaneous sarcoid
  - Lipoma
  - Ganglion cyst, pilar cyst, epidermal cyst
  - Bursa
  - Giant cell tumor of the tendon sheath
  - Nodular fasciitis
  - Cutaneous metastases
  - Desmoplastic melanoma
  - Late-stage erythema elevatum diutinum
- Plaques
  - Mid-dermal elastolysis

Chapter 2, the term *purple plums* refers to the presence of purple or maroon nodules. These fall into three categories: (1,2) benign or malignant vascular neoplasms or (3) other malignant neoplasms (see Figures 9.41–9.45). In Table 9.7, the purple category has been divided up accordingly. Purple plums can sometimes also appear deep pink or just pink, as can be seen in some of the above images.

The term *juicy* can be applied to a plaque that appears to be fluid-filled. These conditions may have superficial dermal edema that leads to this appearance. Table 9.8 lists the conditions that present with juicy plaques. Sweet syndrome, as mentioned above, is a typical cause. Sweet-like conditions include rheumatoid neutrophilic dermatitis, and neutrophilic eccrine hidradenitis. Kikuchi disease (histiocytic necrotizing

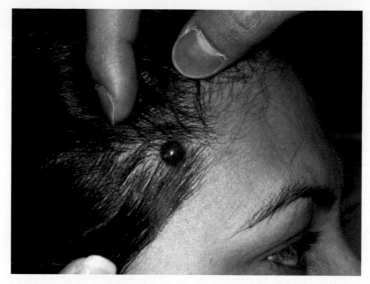

FIGURE 9.41 • Pyogenic granuloma: a benign "purple plum."

lymphadenitis) is a rare disease that has been reported mainly in Japan. Patients present with fever and lymphadenopathy that is accompanied by a rash in under half of cases. The rash may be polymorphic. A Sweet-like presentation of Kikuchi disease may occur (Figure 9.46). Exuberant arthropod bites, urticarial vasculitis, and

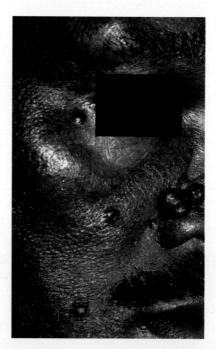

FIGURE 9.42 • Kaposi sarcoma with deep purple papules and nodules on the face.

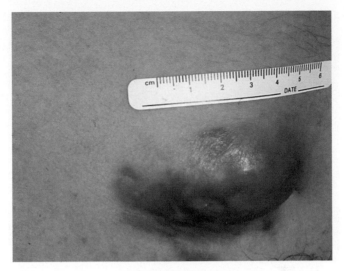

FIGURE 9.43 · Dermatofibrosarcoma protuberans showing a pink, violaceous, and brown tumor on the abdomen.

erythema elevatum diutinum may also appear juicy. A further visual clue relates to the surface contour.

A *peau d'orange* appearance refers to the surface of a plaque that resembles an orange peel. This appearance is seen in very few conditions, typically lymphedema of the breast secondary to lymphatic invasion in breast cancer. It may also be seen in

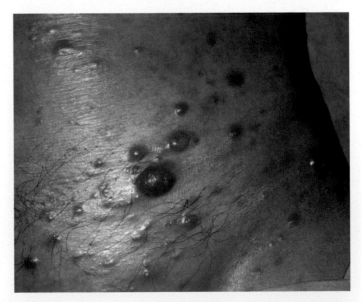

FIGURE 9.44 · Cutaneous involvement of a systemic lymphoma displaying deep pink papules and nodules on the abdomen.

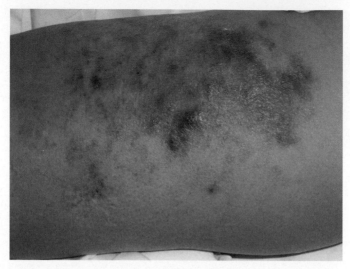

FIGURE 9.45 • Breast cancer metastasis showing an ill-defined violaceous plaque with more substantive papules within it.

TABLE 9.8. Differential Diagnosis of Juicy Plaques
• Sweet syndrome
• Rheumatoid neutrophilic dermatosis
• Neutrophilic eccrine hidradenitis
• Kikuchi disease
• Exuberant arthropod bites
• Urticarial vasculitis
• Erythema elevatum diutinum

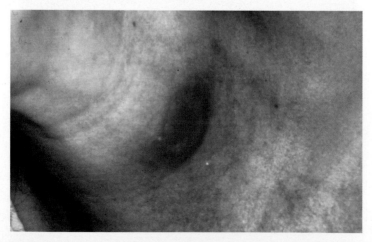

FIGURE 9.46 • Kikuchi disease presenting with a Sweet syndrome–like juicy plaque on the neck.

TABLE 9.9.   Differential Diagnosis of Keloidal Papules, Plaques, or Nodules
• Hypertrophic scar, keloid, acne keloidalis nuchae • Dermatofibroma • Dermatofibrosarcoma protuberans • Histoid leprosy • Chronic fibrotic stage of erythema elevatum diutinum • Mast cell leukemia • Lobomycosis

variant presentations of mid-dermal elastolysis, diffuse cutaneous mastocytosis, and pretibial myxedema.

A Peau D'orange Appearance may be Seen in:
• Breast cancer with lymphatic invasion • Middermal elastolysis • Diffuse cutaneous mastocytosis • Pretibial myxedema

In terms of secondary lesions, keloids may be mimicked by various primary dermatoses. The differential diagnosis of keloidal papules, plaques, or nodules is contained in Table 9.9. Figure 9.4 typifies histoid leprosy with keloidal papules. The chronic, fibrotic stage of erythema elevatum diutinum may also appear keloidal (as seen in Figure 9.8). Figure 9.47 shows a dermatofibrosarcoma protuberans with a keloidal appearance.

Palpation of lesions in this reaction pattern also renders vital diagnostic clues. The depth of a nodule may be ascertained in this way. Benign conditions, such as cysts, are freely mobile and not tethered to underlying structures, as opposed to malignant

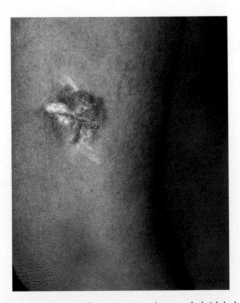

FIGURE 9.47 • Dermatofibrosarcoma protuberans presenting as a keloidal plaque.

nodules, or nodules that arise from deeper structures such as fascia. Furthermore, palpation allows for delineation of the borders of a deep nodule. As mentioned previously, the border of a lipoma rolls away from one's fingers. A pilomatricoma has a "craggy" border with hard, jutting-out edges. A well-demarcated border implies a benign process, as opposed to a border that is tethered to surrounding tissue.

Appreciation of the consistency of papules, plaques, and nodules may help immensely in narrowing down a differential diagnosis. Most conditions are firm. Each depositional disease has its own characteristic consistency, as is displayed graphically in Figure 9.48 along with examples of typical diseases in each category.

Tenderness is an additional diagnostic clue that can be gleaned through palpation. As mentioned above, plaques of Sweet syndrome, rheumatoid neutrophilic dermatosis, and neutrophilic eccrine hidradenitis are typically tender. Carbuncles and furuncles are infectious causes of tender dermal nodules or plaques. The panniculitides are also frequently tender.

Differential Diagnosis of Tender Dermal Papules, Plaques, and/or Nodules

- Infectious
  - Carbuncles
  - Furuncles
- Inflammatory
  - Sweet syndrome
  - Rheumatoid neutrophilic dermatosis
  - Neutrophilic eccrine hidradenitis
  - Panniculitides

The grouping and configuration diagnostic box renders further diagnostic clues as is outlined in Table 9.10. There are many dermatoses in this category that frequently present with annular plaques as is seen in Table 9.10 and typified in a number of the

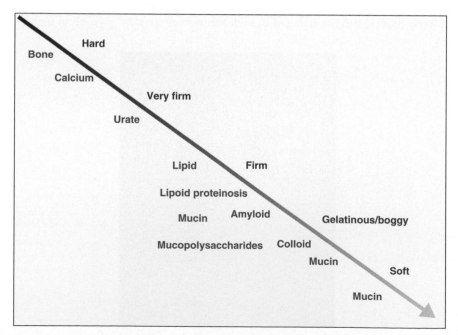

FIGURE 9.48 · The consistency spectrum of dermal depositional disease.

TABLE 9.10. Grouping and Configuration of Dermal Lesions

ANNULAR
- Granuloma annulare
- Necrobiosis lipoidica
- Tumid lupus
- Subacute cutaneous lupus
- Reticulate erythematous mucinosis
- Palisaded neutrophilic granulomatous dermatitis
- Erythema elevatum diutinum
- Lupus vulgaris
- Leprosy: BB subtype displays dermal annular plaques
- Sarcoidosis
- Eosinophilic cellulitis
- Deep gyrate erythema
- Equestrian perniosis
- Tertiary syphilis

LINEAR
- Following lymphatics
  - Infectious
    - *Mycobacterium marinum*
    - *Sporothrix schenckii*
    - *Francisella tularensis*
    - *Burkholderia mallei*: glanders; necrotic abscesses ("farcy buds")
    - Cat scratch disease: *Bartonella henselae*
    - Rarer: seldom seen:
      - Primary inoculation blastomycosis
      - Primary inoculation tuberculosis
      - Meliodosis
      - Sudoku
      - Nocardia
      - Leishmaniasis
  - Neoplastic
    - In-transit melanoma metastases
- Blaschkoid: benign adnexal tumors that have been reported in a blaschkoid distribution include:
  - Eccrine spiradenomas
  - Glomus tumors
  - Pilar leiomyomas
  - Segmental neurofibromas
- Koebner phenomenon
  - Kaposi sarcoma

AGMINATE
- Pyogenic granulomas
- Spitz nevi
- Melanoma satellitosis
- Leiomyomas

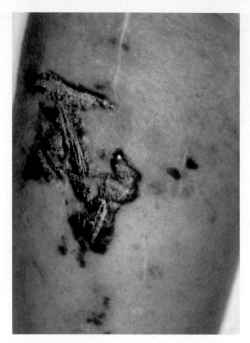

FIGURE 9.49 · Kaposi sarcoma displaying linear plaques as a result of the Koebner phenomenon.

images in this chapter (Figures 9.3, 9.6, 9.9, 9.11, 9.12, 9.14, 9.15, and 9.33). Equestrian perniosis is a rare cold-related condition that is typically seen on the outer thighs of female horseback riders and other sports enthusiasts who spend long periods outdoors in cold weather. Erythematous or violaceous plaques are seen on the outer thighs that may have an annular appearance. As opposed to equestrian panniculitis, equestrian perniosis shows a perniosis-like lymphocytic infiltrate in the dermis. Linear dermal dermatoses may follow lymphatics or Blaschko's lines, or they may arise as a result of the Koebner phenomenon. Kaposi sarcoma can Koebnerize and therefore may appear as linear purple plaques (Figure 9.49). Agminated or clustered dermal papules and/or nodules are typically seen in multiple Spitz nevi (Figure 9.50), pyogenic granulomas, leiomyomas (Figure 9.51), and melanoma satellitosis and metastases (see Figure 4.17C and Figure 9.52).

Regarding distribution, classic sites of dermal disease processes are listed in Table 9.11. Acrosclerosis, or sclerodactyly, is the presence of thickened skin involving the fingers (Figure 9.53). This may be seen in limited scleroderma [CREST (calcinosis, Raynaud phenomenon, esophageal dysmotility, sclerodactyly, and telangiectasia) syndrome], or it may occur as a result of physical trauma (use of jackhammers), chemical exposures [such as poly vinyl chloride or in miners with silicosis] or drug-induced disease. (Many of the drugs that cause sclerodermoid plaques also cause acrosclerosis, such as chemotherapy agents and appetite suppressants.) Dermal reaction pattern papules on the fingers include a range of common and rarer entities. A digital mucous cyst is a translucent papule that appears over the distal phalanx, usually in the setting of osteoarthritis of the distal interphalangeal joint. It is assumed to arise from a synovial

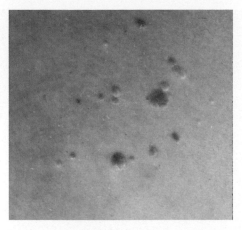

FIGURE 9.50 • Multiple Spitz nevi displaying a cluster of pink-brown papules.

outpouching, but the connection of the cyst to the joint is not always seen. A glomus tumor is a painful bluish papule that tends to arise on a finger and sometimes under a nail. It is a benign proliferation of glomus cells. The lateral aspect of the finger is not an uncommon site for a dermatofibroma to form, and cherry angiomas may also be seen around fingers. A Koenen tumor is a periungual fibroma that is commonly seen in tuberous sclerosis. Chilblains (also known as *perniosis*) are tender pink or red

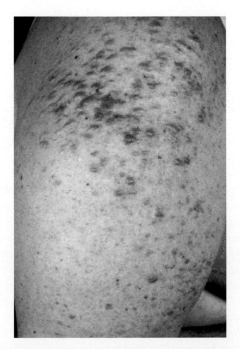

FIGURE 9.51 • Agminated leiomyomas displaying multiple red-brown elongated papules over the shoulder.

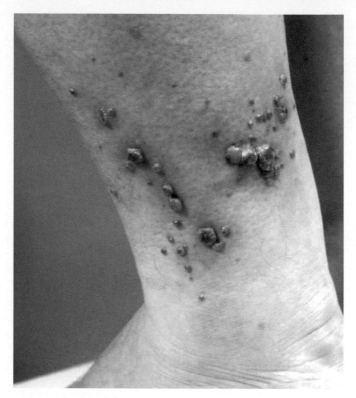

FIGURE 9.52 • Melanoma metastases, displaying clustered amelanotic smooth papules, of different sizes some with crust, on the leg.

papules that occur on the fingers, toes, palms, and soles in cold, damp conditions. Similar chilblain-like papules are seen in the setting of COVID-19 infection. Rarer entities include infantile digital fibromatosis, juvenile hyaline fibromatosis, and acquired digital fibrokeratoma. Infantile digital fibromatosis presents as a firm papule over a digit in a neonate or an infant. It is a benign proliferation of myofibroblasts that tend to resolve spontaneously. Juvenile hyaline fibromatosis is a rare autosomal recessive disorder of collagen syntheses that leads to deposition of hyaline material in the skin and around joints. There are flesh-colored or pink papules and nodules that occur over digits and around joints, along with joint contractures and gingival hyperplasia. It presents early in life. Acquired digital fibrokeratoma is a firm, small finger-like papule that arises in adulthood, usually around a distal digit. Trauma is thought to be an inciting factor to growth. There may be secondary hyperkeratosis over the distal portion.

Much information can be gleaned from examination of the scalp, hair, nails, mucous membranes, and lymph nodes in this category as is outlined in Table 9.12. Finally, on the wheel of diagnosis, we loop back around to history. Here, as mentioned, rapid growth of a nodule is important to assess as it may signify malignant degeneration. Similarly, any pigmented lesion that is evolving deserves careful clinical and dermatoscopic evaluation and consideration of biopsy. The presence of spontaneous pain is another key question on history. The tender processes mentioned above may also be spontaneously painful. Additionally, certain benign tumors are typically painful. These are listed in Table 9.13.

TABLE 9.11. Distribution of Dermal Papules, Plaques, and/or Nodules

PHOTOEXPOSED

- Tumid lupus
- Subacute cutaneous lupus
- Polymorphous light eruption

EXTENSORS

- Granuloma annulare
- Erythema elevatum diutinum
- Palisaded and neutrophilic granulomatous dermatitis
- Tuberous xanthomas
- Gouty tophi
- Rheumatoid nodules
- Olecranon burs

PERIORBITAL

- Xanthelasma
- Necrobiotic xanthogranuloma
- Orbital xanthogranuloma
- Granulomatous rosacea
- Apocrine hidrocystoma
- Eccrine hidrocystoma
- Syringomas
- Trichilemmoma
- Trichoepithelioma

EYELID MARGIN

- Lipoid proteinosis
- Primary amyloidosis

PALMS AND SOLES

- Poroma
- Pyogenic granuloma
- Kaposi sarcoma
- Intradermal nevi

DIGITS

- Digital mucous cyst
- Glomus tumor
- Dermatofibroma
- Periungual fibroma
- Acquired digital fibrokeratoma
- Chilblains
- Erythema elevatum diutinum
- Tuberous xanthomas
- Multicentric reticulohistiocytosis
- Giant cell tumor of the tendon sheath
- Infantile digital fibromatosis
- Juvenile hyaline fibromatosis

RELATION TO APPENDAGES

- Follicular: trichofolliculoma, trichodiscoma, trichilemmoma, trichoepithelioma
- Eccrine: poroma
- Sebaceous: sebaceous ademona, sebaceoma, sebaceous carcinoma

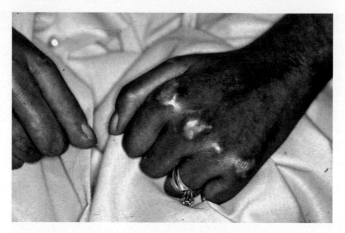

FIGURE 9.53 • Acrosclerosis in a patient with scleroderma showing shiny, taut skin over fingers and hands along with calcinosis cutis over the knuckles.

TABLE 9.12. Gleaning Information from Scalp, Hair, Nails, Mucous Membranes, and Lymph Nodes for Dermal Diseases

SCALP/HAIR
- Nonscarring or scarring alopecia: sarcoidosis
- Nonscarring alopecia: active systemic lupus
- Benign neoplasms seen on the scalp:
  - Cylindromas
  - Mixed tumor
  - Intradermal nevi
  - Pilar cyst
  - Proliferating trichilemmal cyst
  - Cherry angioma
  - Milia

NAILS
- Sarcoidosis: subungual hyperkeratosis, onycholysis, pterygium formation, painful clubbing, fusiform swelling of distal phalanx
- Amyloidosis: dense longitudinal ridging, anonychia
- Systemic lupus: periungual erythema, red lunulae, fine longitudinal lines, leukonychia
- Leprosy: dystrophic nails and loss of nails secondary to trauma related to neuropathy; leukonychia
- Multicentric reticulohistiocytosis: nail dystrophy secondary to nail fold involvement.

MUCOUS MEMBRANES
- Sweet syndrome: ocular involvement (conjunctivitis, episcleritis, limbal nodules, iridocyclitis)
- Primary amyloidosis: macroglossia
- Lipoid proteinosis: macroglossia
- Myxedema: macroglossia

LYMPH NODES
- Lymphoma
- Metastases

TABLE 9.13. Differential Diagnosis of Painful Tumors

- Angiolipoma
- Blue rubber bleb nevus syndrome
- Dercum's disease (adiposus dolorosa)
- Eccrine spiradenoma
- Endometrioma
- Glomus tumor
- Granular cell tumor
- Leiomyoma
- Neurilemmoma
- Neuroma

BEDSIDE DIAGNOSTICS AND TESTS

Dermoscopy (also known as epiluminescence microscopy) is the study of cutaneous lesions via a handheld microscopy device with a light source. It is extremely useful for evaluation of pigmented lesions and suspected skin cancers, including melanoma, prior to possible consideration of biopsy. The range of dermoscopic findings is detailed in textbooks devoted to the subject and is beyond the scope of this text. Suffice it to say that knowledge of classic patterns of benign and malignant neoplasms is an important facet of a clinician's diagnostic acumen.

As mentioned, in cases of suspected mastocytosis, firm stroking with the back of a cotton-tipped applicator may lead to urtication. This is known as a *positive Darier sign*. This phenomenon is frequently seen in solitary mastocytoma and urticaria pigmentosa in children, and in diffuse cutaneous mastocytosis, but is less frequently seen in adult urticaria pigmentosa (Figure 9.54). Squeezing the skin on either side of a dermatofibroma causes it to dimple; this is the *positive dimple sign* (Figure 9.55).

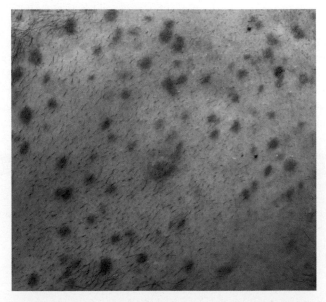

FIGURE 9.54 • A positive Darier sign with a wheal arising in a red macule of urticaria pigmentosa.

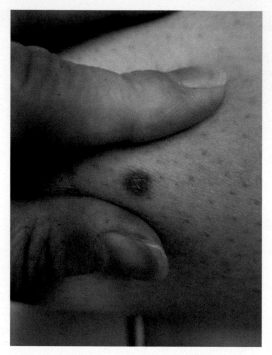

FIGURE 9.55 • A dermatofibroma displaying a positive dimple sign.

Diascopy with a microscope slide may be helpful for diagnosis in the dermal reaction pattern. Place a microscope slide on a plaque or nodule of suspected sarcoidosis to reveal an apple-jelly color that signifies granulomatous disease. This same color may be seen on diascopy of lupus vulgaris. While nodular scabies is usually seen after treatment of scabies, it may occur in concert with active scabies. In this situation, perform a mineral oil preparation of a suspected burrow to clinch the diagnosis of scabies. Mineral oil should be placed on the slide, on the blade, and on the burrow. Scrape firmly over the burrow, place specimen on the slide, cover with a coverslip, and examine under the microscope. Finally, in this reaction pattern, and in considering the possibility of infection, at the time of biopsy for histopathologic evaluation, perform an extra biopsy for tissue culture, including bacterial, mycobacterial, and fungal cultures, in the appropriate clinical setting. Table 9.14 summarizes this information.

TABLE 9.14. Bedside Diagnostics for the Dermal Reaction Pattern

- Dermoscopy to detect pigmented lesions and suspected skin cancers
- Diascopy looking for an apple-jelly color in granulomatous diseases
- Firm stroking with the back of a cotton-tipped applicator in suspected mastocytosis
- Lateral pressure applied to a suspected dermatofibroma
- Mineral oil evaluation in suspected scabies
- Biopsy for bacterial, mycobacterial, and fungal culture

SUMMARY

- The dermal reaction pattern includes a broad array of infectious, inflammatory, neoplastic, depositional, sclerotic, and drug-induced dermatoses that arise in the dermis and deep to the dermis.
- While there are no scales, vesicle, or bullae to guide differential diagnosis, employing the diagnostic boxes of the wheel of diagnosis may assist with narrowing down a differential diagnosis.
- Additional diagnostically relevant information is obtained from
  - Knowledge of how each panniculitis presents
  - Knowledge of clinical features of benign adnexal tumors
- Dermoscopy can add vital diagnostic information especially for pigmented lesions and suspected skin cancers. Bedside diagnostics can be employed to narrow down a diagnosis. Tissue cultures should be performed in cases of suspected infection.

The Vascular Reaction Pattern 10

The vascular reaction pattern comprises dermatoses that present with red, nonscaly macules, papules, or plaques. The term *vascular reaction pattern* may be misleading; it does not refer solely to vascular proliferations but rather to any red dermatosis without scale or blisters. Therefore, this reaction pattern can be synonymously referred to as the *red reaction pattern*. It is an important reaction pattern to be aware of as it houses a broad heterogeneous group of diseases that has, in common, their color.

> **The Primary Lesions in This Reaction Pattern:**
>
> - Red macules
> - Red papules
> - Red plaques

In contrast to the other reaction patterns, dermatoses in this reaction pattern display no scales, vesicles, or bullae, and there are no nodules, either, and so, to the novice clinician, these lesions may appear featureless. Therefore, and especially with red macules, there may be few diagnostic determinants to assist with making a diagnosis. So, it is useful to consider an approach to these lesions.

As mentioned in the previous chapter, the vascular reaction pattern overlaps with the dermal reaction pattern in that red plaques may fit into either of these reaction patterns. Dermatoses that may be classified as either a vascular or a dermal reaction pattern are listed in Table 9.1. Some vascular reaction pattern diseases may develop vesicles and bullae, such as erythema multiforme, Stevens–Johnson syndrome/toxic epidermal necrolysis (SJS/TEN), and fixed drug eruption. Also, bullous pemphigoid may begin with urticarial plaques only—the prebullous phase—and then progress to bulla formation (see Figure 7.22). The vascular reaction pattern may progress to the papulosquamous reaction pattern. An example here is secondary syphilis, which early on may have smooth red macules or thin papules, and later may develop scale. Early erythema annulare centrifugum may similarly lack scale. Early contact dermatitis (eczematous reaction pattern) may present as an edematous erythematous plaque (vascular reaction pattern; Figure 10.1). Langerhans cell histiocytosis spans many reaction patterns (Figure 10.2); there may be scale (papulosquamous reaction pattern), crusting (and so may connote vesicobullous reaction pattern), and purpuric macules (vascular reaction pattern).

An important diagnostic consideration in the initial approach to red macules, papules, and plaques is whether they blanch. To perform diascopy, a microscope slide is placed on top of the lesion in question. If the lesion blanches, then extravascular blood is absent. If it does not blanch, the diagnosis is usually extravascular blood, such as in petechiae or purpura.

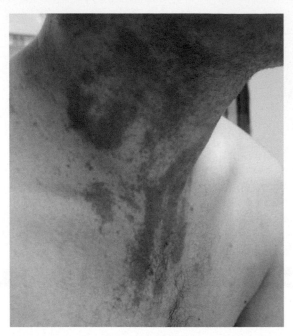

FIGURE 10.1 · Early acute contact dermatitis to poison ivy showing a broad edematous, erythematous plaque on the abdomen.

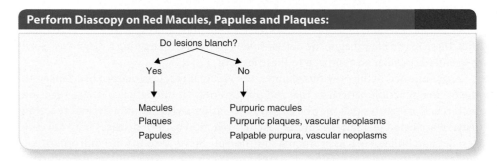

This rule is not entirely absolute. Thicker red papules and plaques, such as a port wine stain or a hemangioma, will not blanch owing to the depth of the lesion and the fact that not all vascular channels can be occluded by the superficial pressure of diascopy (rather than the presence of extravascular blood).

> **Clinical Tip** An exception to the nonblanching rule—vascular proliferations may not blanch.

In this chapter, each diagnostic box of the wheel of diagnosis will be divided into two sections. Blanching red lesions will be considered in the first and nonblanching lesions, in the second. Figure 10.3 displays the wheel that is customized to the vascular reaction pattern following this construct. The first consideration, as in all reaction patterns, is an assessment of the diagnostic determinants of the primary lesion(s) present. A useful approach is to group the entities in the blanching and the nonblanching categories

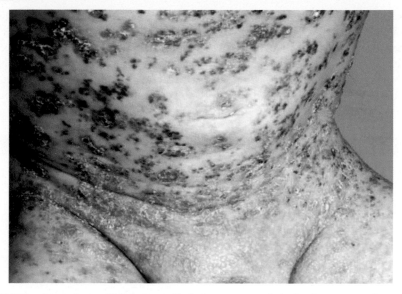

FIGURE 10.2 • Langerhans cell histiocytosis displaying many morphologies that span reaction patterns, including purpuric macules.

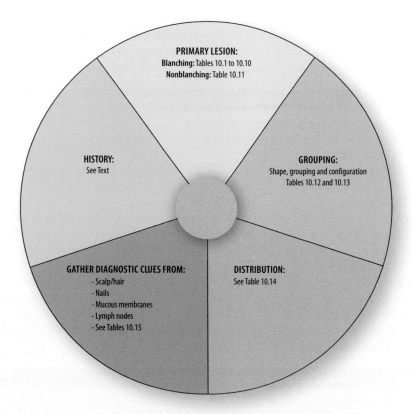

FIGURE 10.3 • The wheel of diagnosis, customized to the vascular reaction pattern.

according to their morphologic determinants. So, in the primary lesion diagnostic box, the following blanching entities will be considered: red macules and thin plaques (categorized together as they frequently coexist, and sometimes it is difficult to differentiate which of these is present); red, more substantive plaques; and red blanching papules. Red nodules are classified as having a dermal reaction pattern (see Chapter 9). Similarly, in the nonblanching category, we will consider macular and palpable purpura, as well as nonpurpuric entities that do not blanch, as alluded to above.

Red Lesions can be Classified as Follows:

- Blanching:
  - Red macules and thin plaques
  - Red more substantive plaques
  - Red blanching papules
- Nonblanching:
  - Macules
    - Macular purpura
  - Papules and plaques
    - Palpable purpura (purpuric papules and/or plaques)
  - Vascular proliferations/neoplasms

BLANCHING LESIONS

Red Macules and Thin Plaques

Blanching macules and thin plaques may be distinguished from each other by their appearance. Diagnostic determinants such as shape, and whether these primary lesions are fixed, expanding, migratory, or evanescent are important differentiators. The tactile clue of tenderness is a vital indicator in this reaction pattern of either infection or necrosis.

Diagnostic Determinants of Blanching Red Macules and Thin Plaques

- Diagnostic determinants of the primary lesions:
  - Visual: shape; fixed or moving (migratory, evanescent, expanding)?
  - Tactile: tender?

Shape

An important shape for this category is that of round macules or thin plaques. Macules (or thin plaques) of a fixed drug eruption are almost exclusively round (Figure 4.11E). A fixed drug eruption appears pink or red early on, and then may become violaceous or gray. The nonpigmenting variant of fixed drug eruption remains a pink or red color regardless of the stage. Erythema migrans of Lyme disease is the classic cutaneous manifestation of early Lyme disease. While erythema migrans is typically an annular, or a "bull's-eye" configuration, it can also present as a perfectly round macule in the early stages. Similarly, disseminated Lyme disease may have numerous shapes, including round macules (Figure 10.4).

Differential Diagnosis of Round Red Macules/ Thin Plaques

- Fixed drug eruption
- Erythema migrans

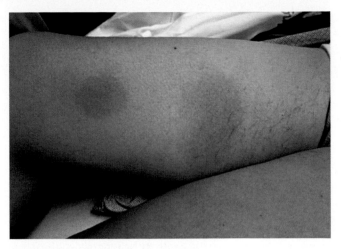

FIGURE 10.4 • Disseminated Lyme disease presenting with a round macule and an oval macule on the leg.

Two additional distinctive shapes of primary lesions in this category are target and target-like (targetoid) lesions. Target lesions may be macules or plaques and may have a central vesicle or bulla. If bullous, they may be categorized as vesicobullous reaction pattern as well. They are classically comprised of a central dusky macule or vesicle/ bulla surrounded by a lighter pink rim and a third darker red ring (Figure 10.5). The presence of target lesions connotes erythema multiforme. Targetoid macules and plaques contain two color zones rather than three (Figure 10.6). The central zone is usually dusky or darker than the surrounding zone.

> **Clinical Tip**
> • Target lesions have three color zones.
> • Targetoid lesions have two color zones.

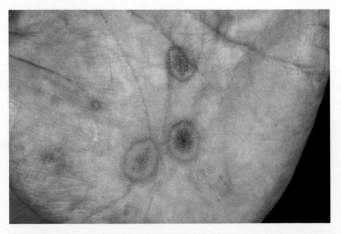

FIGURE 10.5 • **Target lesions with three zones of color.** (Reproduced with permission from Wolff K, Johnson RA, Saavedra AP, et al: *Fitzpatrick's Color Atlas and Synopsis of Clinical Dermatology*, 8th ed. New York, NY: McGraw Hill; 2017.)

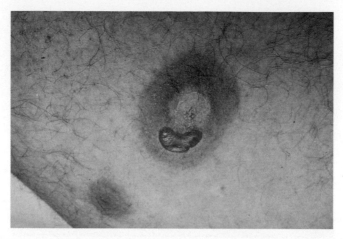

FIGURE 10.6 • A targetoid lesion showing two zones of color. Note the overlying small bulla inferiorly. (Reproduced with permission from Knoop KJ, Stack LB, Storrow AB, et al: *The Atlas of Emergency Medicine*, 4th ed. New York, NY: McGraw Hill; 2018. Photo contributor: J. Matthew Hardin, MD.)

Target lesions and targetoid macules and plaques are seen in erythema multiforme (EM), SJS and TEN. EM, SJS, and TEN may be distinguished on clinical grounds, especially in adults, based on the morphology and distribution of lesions present and the body surface area involved. EM typically displays acral target lesions and raised targetoid lesions. The patient feels well and is afebrile. The term *EM major* refers to the presence of mucous membrane involvement in EM, and EM minor has none. EM is frequently associated with herpes simplex virus as well as other viral, bacterial, and fungal diseases. SJS and TEN are adverse reactions to medications. More rarely, they are seen from radiation after intracranial surgery. In SJS and TEN, patients are ill-appearing, febrile, and in pain. SJS/TEN may be heralded by a prodromal period of malaise and fever that may be misconstrued as a viral prodrome. The classic flat targetoid lesions and necrotic macules occur centrally on the upper trunk and spread in a centrifugal pattern (Figure 10.7). SJS and TEN are differentiated by the body surface area involved with detached and detachable skin as is outlined in the textbox below. TEN may present with targetoid lesions ("spots") or without. Of note, the distinction between EM and SJS/TEN in children on the abovementioned clinical grounds is not so clear-cut, with clinically overlapping cases frequently reported.

Distinction between EM, SJS, and TEN	
EM	**SJS/TEN**
Morphology, Distribution	
Typical targets	Macules: purpuric, erythematous
Raised atypical targets	Flat atypical targets
Predominantly acral	Starts upper trunk → centripetal spread
Body Surface Area	
<10%	SJS :< 10%
	SJS/TEN: 10–30%
	TEN: >30%

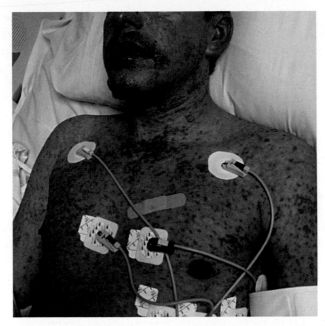

FIGURE 10.7 • Stevens–Johnson syndrome that evolved into toxic epidermal necrolysis with necrotic macules on the trunk and upper extremities. (Reproduced with permission from Usatine R: *The Color Atlas of Family Medicine*, 3rd ed. New York, NY: McGraw Hill; 2019. Photo contributor: Robert T. Gilson, MD.)

Targetoid lesions may also be seen in DRESS (drug reaction with eosinophilia and systemic symptoms) and in a variety of other inflammatory diseases (Table 10.1). Mycoplasma-induced rash and mucositis (MIRM) is a newly delineated entity that is characterized by prominent mucositis of two or more mucous membranes (usually oral and ocular) and a sparse eruption that may be targetoid, vesicobullous, or macular morphologically. MIRM occurs in the setting of *Mycoplasma pneumonia* infection that may be clinically evident as pneumonia or may be detected on X-ray or serologic testing.

TABLE 10.1. Differential Diagnosis of Targetoid Lesions
• Erythema multiforme: raised atypical targets
• SJS/TEN: flat atypical targets
• DRESS
• Mycoplasma-induced rash and mucositis (MIRM)
• Fixed drug eruption
• Erythema dyschromicum perstans
• Paraneoplastic pemphigus/paraneoplastic autoimmune multiorgan syndrome
• Urticaria multiforme
• Erythema migrans and disseminated Lyme disease
• Autoimmune progesterone dermatitis
• Pemphigoid gestationis
• Kawasaki syndrome
• Rowell syndrome
• COVID-19 infection

MIRM should be distinguished from EM major, and mucosal involvement is similar in these two entities, including a classic appearance of hemorrhagic crusting of the lips. It is possible that erstwhile cases of EM major represented MIRM instead. The lesions of fixed drug eruption are round. Active fixed drug eruption has a targetoid appearance with a pink border and a dusky center. Similarly, early erythema dyschronicum perstans (EDP) has an erythematous rim around dark gray or dusky macules. EDP is more common in darker skin phototypes and it has a predilection for the neck, trunk, and proximal extremities. Paraneoplastic pemphigus [also termed paraneoplastic autoimmune multi-organ syndrome (PAMS)] may have targetoid or lichenoid plaques on the skin and may also have oral findings that mimic erythema multiforme major or may resemble lichen planus. Urticaria multiforme is a subtype of urticarial with large polycyclic plaques that may have dusky centers and as such, may resemble erythema multiforme. This subtype of urticaria is more common in children than adults. Erythema migrans and disseminated Lyme disease may be targetoid (Figure 10.8). Targetoid presentations of autoimmune progesterone dermatitis and pemphigoid gestationis have also been reported. The rash of Kawasaki disease is polymorphic. Targetoid plaques may be seen. Rowell syndrome was initially described as the presence of targetoid lesions in discoid lupus erythematosus. This term has been loosely applied in cases of SLE as well. In recent years, the existence of Rowell syndrome as a true entity has been questioned. An erythema multiforme-like presentation of COVID-19 infection, with targetoid lesions, has been reported.

As stated previously regarding terminology, shape is the inherent property of one lesion whereas configuration is the shape formed by more than one primary lesion. Some macules or thin plaques may have a linear shape. Examples include the flagellate erythemas, the linear erythema that arises from joints in dermatomyositis and dermographism. Similarly, erythema migrans may present with an annular shape. These entities will also be considered later in the chapter for convenience.

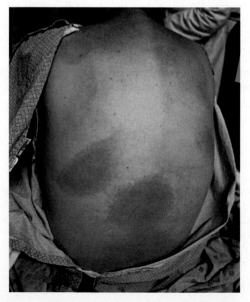

FIGURE 10.8 · Disseminated Lyme disease with large targetoid macules (dusky centers and erythematous borders) on the back.

> **TABLE 10.2. Differential Diagnosis of Migratory Erythemas**
>
> **INFECTIOUS**
> - Cutaneous larva migrans
> - Larva currens
>
> **INFLAMMATORY**
> - Erythrokeratoderma variabilis
> - Erythema marginatum
> - Annular erythema of infancy
> - Necrolytic migratory erythema
> - Tumor necrosis factor-α receptor-associated periodic syndrome
> - Annular epidermolytic ichthyosis
> - Epidermolysis bullosa simplex, migratory circinate type

Fixed or Migratory

Another diagnostic determinant of red macules and plaques is whether they are fixed. Primary lesions that are not "fixed" may migrate from one part of the skin to another, may be evanescent or fleeting, or may slowly enlarge over hours or days.

The migratory erythemas are a heterogenous group of diseases. They are, for the most part, rarely encountered. Table 10.2 provides a comprehensive differential diagnosis for migratory erythema. In the infectious category, there are two entities to consider:

1. In cutaneous larva migrans (also known as a "creeping eruption"), larvae of animal hookworms of the *Ancylostoma* species penetrate the epidermis and cause itchy linear and serpiginous tracks as they move (≤2 cm per day). A vesicle may occur at the leading edge.
2. In larva currens, larvae of *Strongyloides stercoralis* penetrate perianal skin and move at the rate of many centimeters a day in a subcutaneous locale. Clinically, there are urticarial linear tracks that migrate quickly and are evanescent.

The differential diagnostic list of inflammatory migratory erythemas is longer, and each entity is also rarely encountered. Erythrokeratoderma variabilis (also known as Mendes da Costa syndrome) is an autosomal dominant condition. Fixed hyperkeratotic plaques on the extensors coexist with migratory annular or arcuate plaques that may move over hours and fade slowly over days or weeks. It starts in infancy and persists throughout life. Erythema marginatum is seen in acute rheumatic fever. Macules and small annular, arcuate, and polycyclic thin plaques migrate up to a centimeter within hours. They may also be evanescent and last from hours to days. Annular erythema of infancy is a very rare disorder where erythematous macules or papules spread in a centrifugal fashion over weeks. In necrolytic migratory erythema (NME), erythematous macules occur on the lower abdomen, groin, and legs. They expand peripherally over 1–2 weeks, forming annular plaques and develop peripheral vesicles, crusting, and scaling. NME is associated with glucagonomas or chronic hepatic insufficiency. It may also be classified as vesicobullous reaction pattern (when vesicles or crusting seen) or papulosquamous (when scaling seen). In TRAPS (tumor necrosis factor-α receptor-associated periodic syndrome), periodic fevers, arthralgia, myalgia, serositis, and conjunctivitis are accompanied by migratory erythematous macules and plaques that usually overlie inflamed muscles. Attacks last about a week and occur cyclically every 6 weeks or so. Annular epidermolytic ichthyosis is rare variant of epidermolytic hyperkeratosis. Annular and polycyclic migratory plaques are seen on the trunk in patients with flexural hyperkeratotic epidermolytic plaques. Finally, the migratory circinate type of epidermolysis bullosa simplex is a rarely reported, autosomal dominant condition that presents early in life with generalized vesicles or bullae in association with migratory circinate erythema.

Gradual centrifugal enlargement of macules or plaques is a classic feature of erythema migrans. It is also seen in erythema annulare centrifugum, morphea, and annular erythema of infancy.

Gradual Centrifugal Enlargement is seen in:

- Erythema migrans
- Erythema annulare centrifugum
- Morphea
- Annular erythema of infancy

Erythema marginatum and larva currens are typically evanescent (fleeting, short-lived) as well as migratory. Adult-onset Still's disease is another cause of evanescent macules. It is an uncommon acute or subacute systemic illness that presents with a high spiking fever, a sore throat, and a rash. The characteristic associated eruption consists of salmon-pink macules that wax and wane with the fever. The eruption is usually more prominent in sites of pressure. Urticaria, as detailed in the section titled "Red, More Substantive Plaques" below, is evanescent with each hive lasting less than 24 hours.

Flushing can be regarded as an evanescent erythema and may occur with or without an underlying causative systemic disease.

Evanescent Erythema is seen in:

- Larva currens
- Erythema marginatum
- Adult-onset Still's disease
- Urticaria
- Flushing

Flushing typically involves the face, but the chest may also be affected. A patterned flush occurs in the auriculotemporal nerve syndrome and harlequin syndrome, (hemifacial flushing and sweating). The causes of flushing are detailed in Table 10.3. Emotional states, alcohol intake, menopause, and rosacea are common causes. Foods may also cause flushing. Monosodium glutamate and other food additives, such as nitrites and sulfites, may be causative. Scombroid food poisoning occurs secondary to ingestion of the scombroid group of fish (tuna and mackerel) and other nonscombroid fish (mahimahi, bluefish, sardines, amberjack, and abalone) that have been inadequately refrigerated. Contaminating *Enterobacteriaceae* multiply in this setting and degrade the fish's dark meat, causing decarboxylation of muscle histidine. Other histamine-related substances, such as urocanic acid, a mast cell degranulator, may augment the immune response. Even brief lapses in refrigeration are dangerous, and once toxins are formed, cooking or canning cannot destroy them. A pruritic erythematous rash, especially of the face and arms, appears 20–30 minutes after eating affected fish, which may have a bitter, metallic, or peppery taste. Flushing, throbbing headache,

TABLE 10.3. Causes of Flushing

NO UNDERLYING SYSTEMIC DISEASE
- Physiologic, in response to emotional states
- Menopause, associated with "hot flushes"
- Rosacea
- Alcohol
- Foods
  - Spicy foods
  - Monosodium glutamate and other additives
  - Scombroid
- Medications
  - Nicotinic acid
  - Calcium channel blockers
  - Opiates
  - Sildenafil
  - Tamoxifen
  - Metronidazole

UNDERLYING SYSTEMIC DISEASE
- Neurological disease
- Mastocytosis
- Carcinoid
- Pheochromocytoma
- Male hypogonadism pseudocarcinoid syndrome
- Medullary carcinoma of the thyroid
- Renal cell carcinoma
- VIPoma
- Horseshoe kidneys (Rovsing's syndrome)
- Basophilic granulocytic leukemia

palpitations, and gastrointestinal symptoms are common concomitants. Many medications are associated with flushing. Disulfiram inhibits aldehyde dehydrogenase, which is important in the catabolism of alcohol. In its presence, aldehyde builds up and causes an acute reaction in which flushing is accompanied by headache, nausea and vomiting, palpitations, dyspnea, and even syncope. Metronidazole produces a similar disulfiram-like effect. Neurologic disease such as Parkinson disease or spinal cord tumors can cause flushing. Localized nerve damage can occur also, such as the auriculotemporal nerve syndrome, where damage to the auriculotemporal nerve gives rise to localized flushing on the cheek, particularly after eating. Flushing occurs in mastocytosis after ingestion of alcohol or other mast cell degranulators. This is a bright red flush that may be accompanied by systemic signs including wheezing and diarrhea. It typically lasts for 30 minutes or longer. Carcinoid tumors cause two different types of flushing syndromes: (1) with pheochromocytoma, which is rarely associated with flushing, and (2) with medullary thyroid cancer, in which flushing and diarrhea may occur. In bronchial carcinoid, the flush is described as being bright red. In carcinoid of the foregut (including stomach and pancreas), the flush is a deeper red, violaceous color and it is longlasting. Ileal tumors that are metastatic to the liver give rise to dark red flush that is more patchy and less sustained. Other rare causes are detailed in Table 10.3.

Tenderness

An important tactile property of red macules and thin red plaques is whether they are tender. *Tenderness* in this context implies infection, sunburn, or active epidermal necrosis. Pain is a symptom, and tenderness is a sign. These tender dermatoses are also spontaneously painful. The constellation of erythema, edema, tenderness, and warmth connotes cellulitis or erysipelas. Many conditions may simulate cellulitis and present with red plaques that may be warm, edematous, and tender. These conditions are considered in Table 10.4 by etiology, along with a brief clinical description. The differential diagnosis of solitary (or few) nontender nonpatterned erythematous plaques is a shorter list (Table 10.5) and comprises dermatoses that are more rarely encountered. These may also mimic cellulitis because of their color and should be distinguished from it. Another way of examining the differential diagnosis of tender and nontender single (or few) nonpatterned erythematous plaques is by preferential body part. This information is given in Table 10.6.

Tender erythema also connotes sunburn. It is thought that chemokines, particularly CXL5, mediates this phenomenon. Predisposition to sunburn is seen in photosensitivity states, such as SLE, dermatomyositis, and the porphyrias. It may also be induced from medications. Tetracyclines (especially doxycycline), NSAIDs, retinoids, and voriconazole are some of the drugs and drug classes implicated in phototoxic drug reactions. Ultraviolet (UV) recall is a rare manifestation that is seen in the setting of chemotherapy. Methotrexate has been reported as a culprit, as has docetaxel, although less frequently. Prior areas of sunburn "light up" after drug exposure.

Epidermal necrosis is a third cause of tenderness in this category. SJS/TEN is an important "do not miss" diagnosis when encountering erythematous macules that are tender. SJS/TEN begins with a prodromal phase with upper respiratory tract infection symptoms such as fever, sore throat, and malaise. Painful macules occur on the upper chest and spread centripetally. Various other conditions that give rise to full-thickness necrosis should be considered in the differential diagnosis of TEN. Severe acute graft-versus-host disease may undergo full-thickness necrosis and thus present with painful and tender superficially detachable skin (Figure 10.9). A similar constellation of finding may be seen in severe cutaneous involvement in SLE. A TEN-like appearance may be seen in severe acute generalized exanthematous pustulosis; severe subepidermal edema may cause detachment of epidermis. Large bullae and large erosions that may resemble TEN are present; however, there is no epidermal necrosis, and this condition is not typically tender. Staphylococcal scalded skin syndrome is a TEN look-alike. Staphylococcal exotoxins cleave desmosomes in the granular layer of the epidermis. Initially there is intense pain and tenderness as this process unfolds; then superficial flaccid bullae and sheets of desquamation and crusting are seen. Staphylococcal scalded skin syndrome is usually seen in children, although adults with renal compromise (toxin cannot be cleared) may be affected. Epidermal necrosis also occurs in fixed drug eruption, so these plaques may be painful and tender.

Differential Diagnosis of Tender Erythematous Macules or Thin Plaques

- Cellulitis and its mimickers
- Sunburn

- Epidermal necrosis
  - TEN
  - TEN-like acute graft-versus-host disease
  - TEN-like SLE
  - Fixed drug eruption

TABLE 10.4. Cellulitis and Its Mimickers: Differential Diagnosis of Tender Erythematous Plaques

DISEASE	CLINICAL FINDINGS
Infectious	
Bacterial cellulitis	Typically involves the lower limb and is unilateral. Erythematous, edematous, warm, and tender plaque with ill-defined borders.
Erysipelas	Warm, well-demarcated erythematous and edematous plaque. Usually unilateral.
Fungal cellulitis	Similar findings to bacterial cellulitis, less likely to involve lower limb only. Usually seen in immunocompromised individuals.
Erysipeloid	Caused by *Erysipelothrix rhusiopathiae*, a Gram-positive bacillus that infects animals. A tender red to violaceous plaque appears at inoculation site, usually on the hand including in a finger webspace. Seen in butchers and fishermen.
Vibrio vulnificus infection	A Gram-negative bacillus that lives in seawater. It may enter abraded skin and cause a cellulitis-like plaque with bullae or necrosis.
Inflammatory	
Lymphedema	Edematous, nonpitting, sometimes woody plaques. Usually bilateral. Seldom tender, unless there is severe acute edema. Erythema may be well- or poorly demarcated.
Acute phase of lipo-dermatoclerosis	Tender erythematous and indurated plaques localized typically over central calf.
Panniculitis	Deep tender panniculitis nodules may coalesce to form plaques that are reminiscent of cellulitis.
Superficial thrombophlebitis	Linear tender cords represent inflamed superficial veins.
Chemical cellulitis	Extravasation of intravenous medication gives rise to tender red, infiltrated plaques that resemble cellulitis
Acute gouty arthritis	Redness and warmth arise over a tender, swollen joint. Exquisitely tender.
Erythromelalgia	Episodic occurrence of erythema and burning of bilateral feet, more frequently than hands. Worse at night.
Complex regional pain syndrome [reflex sympathetic dystrophy (RSD)]	Acute RSD comprises pain, edema, and erythema in the affected limb. Redness subsides in subacute and chronic cases.
Acrodynia (pink disease)	Painful erythema is seen over fingertips and palms, usually in a child, in the setting of mercury poisoning. Rarely encountered.
Neutrophilic eccrine hidradenitis	One or more erythematous plaques are seen in the setting of chemotherapy, usually of leukemia. These plaques may be tender. A case resembling facial cellulitis has been reported.
Neoplastic	
Inflammatory breast carcinoma	Usually nontender but may be tender. Rapid-onset breast erythema, warmth, and/or edema. There may or may not be an underlying palpable mass or a peau d'orange appearance. Represents an aggressive primary breast cancer with contiguous spread to the skin.
Carcinoma eryispeloides	Well-demarcated red, infiltrated plaque that denotes invasion of superficial lymphatics and the dermis with carcinomatous cells. May be tender or nontender (usually). Represents secondary invasion from a prior primary tumor, usually breast, but other primaries have been reported.

TABLE 10.5. Mimickers of Cellulitis, Except That They Are Not Tender

DISEASE	CLINICAL FINDINGS
Infectious	
Erythema migrans	Erythematous macule or plaque expands centrifugally over days. Sites of predilection include intertriginous areas.
Inflammatory	
Lymphedema	Edematous, nonpitting, sometimes woody plaques. Usually bilateral. Erythema may be well- or poorly demarcated.
Acute contact dermatitis	Erythematous and edematous plaques are seen early on prior to the development of vesicles.
Wells syndrome	One or more edematous erythematous plaques occur and may become annular with a greenish tinge as they resolve. Occasionally a single broad plaque resembling cellulitis may be seen. Plaques are itchy and may burn but are seldom tender to the touch.
Inflammatory phase of morphea	Early morphea presents with an expanding red edematous plaque.
Familial Mediterranean fever	Erysipelas-like plaques are seen over the shins during attacks.
TRAPS	Red plaques are seen over tender, involved muscles during acute attacks.
Dermatomyositis	"Shawl sign"—nonphotodistributed erythema that involves the upper back and chest; "holster sign"— erythema on upper outer thigh.
Early zoster	Early zoster, before vesiculation occurs, may be misdiagnosed as cellulitis, especially on the face. It is not tender to the touch but may burn.
Reactive	
Intralymphatic histiocytosis	An ill-defined solid or reticulate plaque appears on the extremity in association with disease of a nearby joint, such as rheumatoid arthritis, osteoarthritis, or a metallic implant. Etiology unclear; chronic inflammation and lymphatic stasis thought to play a role.
Neoplastic	
Inflammatory breast carcinoma	As detailed in Table 10.4.
Carcinoma eryispeloides	As detailed in Table 10.4.
Paraneoplastic	
AESOP [adenopathy extensive skin (patch) overlying plasmacytoma]	An erythematous or violaceous plaque is seen, usually in the thoracic area. It enlarges slowly or rapidly. It overlies the site of a plasmacytoma (these are usually in the vertebrae). The tumor is thought to cause cytokine-induced angiogenesis and treatment of the plasmacytoma will result in resolution of the plaque.
Drug-Related	
Radiation recall	A red macule or plaque develops in a previously irradiated site. Anthracyclines and taxanes most frequently implicated.
Ultraviolet recall	A red macule or plaque develops in a site of prior sunburn. Methotrexate most frequently implicated.

TABLE 10.6. Differential Diagnosis of Tender or Nontender Solitary (or Few) Erythematous Plaques

LEG
- Tender
  - Cellulitis: bacterial, fungal
  - Erysipelas
  - Lipodermatosclerosis
  - Panniculitis
  - Superficial thrombophlebitis
  - Erythromelalgia: feet involved
  - Acute complex regional pain syndrome
  - Acute gout
  - Acute severe lymphedema
  - Carcinoma erysipeloides
- Nontender
  - Intralymphatic histiocytosis
  - Erythema migrans
  - Lymphedema
  - Inflammatory phase of morphea
  - Carcinoma erysipeloides
  - Dermatomyositis: "holster sign" on the upper outer thigh
  - Familial Mediterranean fever
  - TRAPS
  - Radiation recall
  - Acute contact dermatitis
  - Wells syndrome

ARM
- Tender
  - Cellulitis: bacterial, fungal, chemical
  - Erysipelas
  - Superficial thrombophlebitis
  - Acute complex regional pain syndrome
  - Carcinoma erysipeloides
  - Sunburn
  - Phototoxic drug reaction
- Nontender
  - Intralymphatic histiocytosis
  - Erythema migrans
  - Inflammatory phase of morphea
  - Carcinoma erysipeloides
  - TRAPS
  - Radiation recall
  - UV recall
  - Acute contact dermatitis
  - Wells syndrome

(Continued)

TABLE 10.6. Differential Diagnosis of Tender or Nontender Solitary (or Few) Erythematous Plaques (continued)

PALMS
- Tender
  - Erythromelalgia
  - Complex regional pain syndrome
  - Acrodynia
- Nontender
  - Palmar erythema: inherited, or acquired secondary to liver disease etc.
  - Kawasaki disease
  - Serum sickness, serum sickness–like reactions
  - Urticaria

DORSAL HAND
- Tender
  - Cellulitis
  - Erysipelas
  - Erysipeloid
  - *Vibrio vulnificus* infection
  - Sunburn
  - Phototoxic drug reaction
- Nontender
  - Dermatomyositis
  - Acute contact dermatitis
  - Lymphedema
  - Wells syndrome
  - Kawasaki disease

TRUNK
- Tender
  - Cellulitis: bacterial, fungal, chemical
  - Thrombophlebitis; eg, Mondor disease (sclerosing thrombophlebitis of the anterior chest wall veins)
  - Inflammatory breast carcinoma
  - Carcinoma erysipeloides
  - Sunburn
  - Phototoxic drug reaction
- Nontender
  - Erythema migrans
  - Intralymphatic histiocytosis
  - AESOP
  - Radiation recall
  - UV recall: photodistributed
  - Dermatomyositis: "shawl sign," "V sign," "holster sign," or photodistributed
  - Inflammatory phase of morphea
  - Inflammatory breast carcinoma
  - Carcinoma erysipeloides
  - Wells syndrome

(Continued)

TABLE 10.6. Differential Diagnosis of Tender or Nontender Solitary (or Few) Erythematous Plaques (continued)

FACE
- Tender
  - Cellulitis: bacterial, fungal
  - Erysipelas
  - Neutrophilic eccrine hidradenitis
  - Sunburn
  - Phototoxic drug reaction
- Nontender
  - Dermatomyositis
  - SLE
  - Acute contact dermatitis
  - Rosacea
  - Flushing syndromes
  - Early zoster

Further elements of the wheel of diagnosis are also important differentiators, including grouping or configuration of lesions and their distribution. Regarding grouping and configuration of lesions (discussed in detail after all the primary lesion categories), the figurate erythemas and urticarial vasculitis form annular, arcuate, polycyclic, and serpiginous plaques. Reticulate macules are seen in livedo reticularis (the differential diagnosis of which is given in Chapter 11). As was alluded to in the section on cellulitis and mimickers above, distribution of blanching red macules and plaques can hold diagnostic information. More information on distribution is seen in Table 10.14.

In summary, for blanching red macules and thin plaques, differentiating features include shape, whether plaques are fixed, whether tenderness is present, their configuration, and their location or distribution.

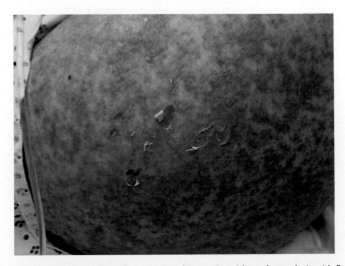

FIGURE 10.9 · Acute graft-versus-host disease mimicking toxic epidermal necrolysis with flaccid vesicles, small areas of full-thickness epidermal loss, and background erythema.

> **Summary: Distinguishing Characteristics of Blanching Red Macules and Thin Plaques**
>
> - What is their shape?
>   - Round?
>   - Target lesion or targetoid?
>   - Linear, annular, or retiform?
> - Do they move?
>   - Migratory erythemas
> - Do primary lesions slowly enlarge centrifugally?
>   - Are they evanescent?
> - Are they tender?
> - Configuration
> - Distribution

Red, More Substantive Plaques

The second group of primary lesions to consider in the blanching category is that of red, more substantive plaques. Urticaria and urticarial dermatoses make up this category. These red, smooth substantive plaques may also be regarded as being in the dermal reaction pattern, as discussed in Chapter 9. The subcategory of urticaria and urticarial plaques has dermal edema as its hallmark, and this should be differentiated from other dermal plaques with infiltration of cells or deposits. Edematous plaques are usually lighter pink and not as firm as infiltrated plaques. They may also be flesh-colored if edema is intense.

> **Clinical Tip** Urticaria and urticarial plaques can be classified as having an either vascular or dermal reaction pattern. They are edematous, not infiltrated with cells or deposits. Edema clinically appears subtly different from infiltration.

It is useful to be able to distinguish urticaria from similar-appearing urticarial eruptions. Table 10.7 presents a differential diagnostic list for urticarial plaques along with

TABLE 10.7. Differential Diagnosis of Urticarial Plaques and Their Associated Symptoms

DISEASE	SYMPTOMS
Urticaria	Itch; burning in chronic idiopathic urticaria
Schnitzler syndrome	Asymptomatic
Cryopyrin-associated periodic syndromes	Asymptomatic, pain
Urticarial vasculitis	Pain, burning
Serum sickness, serum sickness–like reactions	Itch
Urticaria of COVID-19 infection	Itch, burning
Arthropod reaction	Itch
Sweet syndrome	Pain
Rheumatoid neutrophilic dermatosis	Pain
Neutrophilic eccrine hidradenitis	Pain
Kikuchi disease	Itch, asymptomatic
Wells syndrome	Itch, burning
Urticarial phase of bullous pemphigoid, pemphigoid gestationis	Itch
Tumid lupus	Asymptomatic
Adult-onset Still's disease	Itch, burning
Acute hemorrhagic edema of infancy	Asymptomatic

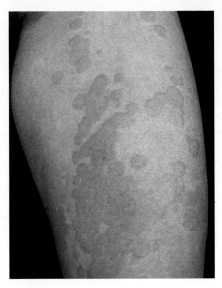

FIGURE 10.10 • A close-up of acute urticaria displaying edematous and erythematous papules and plaques. (Reproduced with permission from Wolff K, Johnson RA, Saavedra AP, et al: *Fitzpatrick's Color Atlas and Synopsis of Clinical Dermatology*, 8th ed. New York, NY: McGraw Hill; 2017.)

their typical accompanying symptomatology. The hives of urticaria are edematous papules and plaques that typically last less than 24 hours (see Figure 2.5 and Figure 10.10). They are itchy rather than painful and resolve without postinflammatory changes. Urticaria may be accompanied by angioedema, tongue edema, difficulty breathing or swallowing, or rarely, anaphylaxis. Urticarial vasculitis resembles urticaria clinically. The differences include plaques that last longer than 24 hours, a rash that is more painful than itchy, the presence of pinpoint petechiae seen within plaques on diascopy, and the presence of postinflammatory violaceous or brown discoloration when plaques resolve. Arthralgia or arthritis may be present.

Comparing Urticaria and Urticarial Vasculitis

URTICARIA	URTICARIAL VASCULITIS
<24 hours	>24 hours
Itch	Pain
Fade without PIH	Leave brown macules
Diascopy: blanch	Diascopy: pinpoint purpura
Associated Symptoms and Signs	
Angioedema	Arthralgia
Tongue edema	Arthritis
Difficulty swallowing	
Difficulty breathing	
Anaphylaxis	

An exception to this rule is that of chronic idiopathic urticaria, in which hives may last for more than 24 hours and these may also have a burning sensation rather than itch.

> **Clinical Tip** An exception: chronic idiopathic urticaria, even though a form of urticaria and not urticarial vasculitis, may burn, and hives may last longer than 24 hours.

Both urticaria and urticarial vasculitis may produce a range of shapes and configurations. Urticaria multiforme, as mentioned, may have large polycyclic plaques that may be targetoid in appearance. Urticarial presentations in COVID-19 infection have been reported. Rare causes of urticaria include Schnitzler syndrome (typically nonpruritic urticaria, bone pain, and a monoclonal gammopathy) and the cryopyrin-associated periodic syndromes (CAPS). These are a rarely encountered group of autoinflammatory syndromes in which cold-induced urticaria is accompanied by a range of systemic findings. In familial cold autonomic syndrome, skin findings predominate. In Muckle–Wells syndrome, urticarial plaques may be tender, and loss of hearing as well as renal amyloidosis may ensue. The most severe type of CAPS is neonatal-onset multisystemic inflammatory disease (also known as chronic infantile neurologic cutaneous and articular syndrome). Here, clinical features include fever, arthralgias, vision loss, aseptic meningitis, and the findings of Muckle–Wells syndrome. Urticarial vasculitis may produce annular, serpiginous, and polycyclic plaques (Figure 10.11). Other diseases with urticarial plaques are seen in Table 10.7. Serum sickness and serum sickness–like reactions from medications produce lesions that are similar to urticarial vasculitis. Bilateral symmetric palmar involvement and symmetric involvement of extremities in general may be additional features, as may joint involvement. Urticarial plaques may be seen in severe arthropod bite reactions, and in Sweet syndrome. The plaques of Sweet syndrome may then become very edematous, and pseudovesiculation may ensue (see Figure 9.7). Rheumatoid neutrophilic dermatosis resembles Sweet syndrome with tender edematous erythematous plaques. Neutrophilic eccrine hidradenitis occurs in the setting of chemotherapy. The manifestations of this disorder may vary and include a Sweet-like presentation. Kikuchi disease may present with a Sweet-like morphology (see Figure 9.41). In Wells syndrome (eosinophilic cellulitis), one or more itchy edematous plaques are seen. They may become annular and fade with a greenish or brown color. In bullous pemphigoid and pemphigoid gestationis,

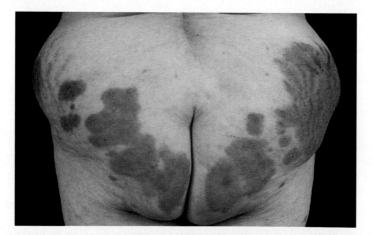

FIGURE 10.11 · Urticarial vasculitis: erythematous plaques and wheals on the buttocks. (Reproduced with permission from Wolff K, Johnson RA, Saavedra AP, et al: *Fitzpatrick's Color Atlas and Synopsis of Clinical Dermatology*, 8th ed. New York, NY: McGraw Hill; 2017.)

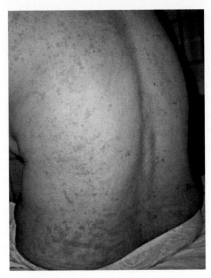

FIGURE 10.12 • Adult-onset Still's disease with urticarial plaques on the back and some linear plaques on the lower back (Koebner phenomenon).

urticarial plaques accompany tense vesicles and bullae. These plaques may also precede the development of blisters for many months (and sometimes longer), and so these blistering diseases may manifest with vascular reaction pattern morphology (see Figure 7.22, showing the urticarial phase of bullous pemphigoid). Tumid lupus may appear edematous. These plaques are usually annular in configuration. Adult-onset Still's disease may have light pink urticarial papules that wax and wane according to the patient's fever (Figure 10.12). In an infant or very young child, consider the diagnosis of mastocytoma. This presents as a single pink, red, or brown plaque that urticates with firm pressure (positive Darier sign). Also, in this age group, consider the diagnosis of acute hemorrhagic edema of infancy. This is a leukocytoclastic vasculitis that manifests initially with edematous, erythematous plaques that may simulate urticaria. These then progress to become purpuric.

For *tender*, more substantive plaques, consider the diagnosis of Sweet syndrome. The cause of tenderness in this condition is unclear. Rheumatoid neutrophilic dermatosis and neutrophilic eccrine hidradenitis may similarly be tender.

An appraisal of the distribution of plaques can provide additional diagnostically relevant information. As mentioned, in serum sickness and serum sickness–like reactions, urticarial plaques may involve palms and soles symmetrically, and Sweet syndrome favors the head, neck, and upper trunk.

Summary: Differentiating Features of Blanching Red Substantive Plaques

- How long do plaques last? (Urticaria vs urticarial processes.)
- Are there characteristic shapes/configurations—polycyclic, annular, serpiginous, targetoid? (Urticaria multiforme, urticarial vasculitis, serum sickness.)
- Are plaques tender, itchy, or asymptomatic? (See Table 10.7.)
- Discern edematous plaques from infiltrated plaques (dermal reaction pattern).
- Is there a particular distribution? (For example, serum sickness–like reactions and Sweet syndrome.)

Red Blanching Papules

The third group to consider in the blanching category is smooth red, blanching papules. Scaly red papules can be classified in the papulosquamous or eczematous reaction patterns. As was seen in chapters 6 and 8, respectively, diagnostic features of papules may not be so readily apparent, given their small size, and so the differentiation between scaly and nonscaly papules might be difficult. An alternative initial approach to red papules therefore is whether they arise in association with a hair follicle, as discussed in Chapter 2. Follicular processes have a hair egressing from each papule, and theoretically all lesions should have the same distance between them. The former property may be difficult to discern, especially in locations with fine vellus hairs. The latter sign of a uniform interfollicular distance may also not be sensitive, as some follicles may not be affected. In cases of doubt, dermoscopy can assist with this determination. Table 10.8 provides an overview of follicular and nonfollicular papules that fall into the vascular reaction pattern. This represents a heterogenous group. The follicular conditions are covered in Chapter 2. For the nonfollicular conditions, these may be diffusely

TABLE 10.8. Blanching Follicular and Nonfollicular Papules in the Vascular Reaction Pattern

FOLLICULAR
- Infection
  - Infectious folliculitides
- Infestation
  - Demodex folliculitis
- Inflammatory
  - Acne
  - Rosacea
  - Periorificial dermatitis
  - Pseudofolliuculitis barbae
  - Eosinophilic pustular folliculitis

NONFOLLICULAR
- Infection
  - Viral exanthems
  - HIV seroconversion disease
  - Early HSV or VZV infections, before vesiculation occurs
  - Early secondary syphilis, before scale is seen
  - Scarlet fever, before "sandpaper" scale appears
  - Some rickettsial infections
    - Early Rocky Mountain spotted fever, before purpura occurs
    - Endemic typhus
    - Scrub typhus
    - Epidemic typhus
    - Typhoid: "rose spots"
  - Scabies
- Toxin-mediated
  - Toxic shock syndrome
  - Streptococcal toxic shock–like syndrome

(Continued)

TABLE 10.8. Blanching Follicular and Nonfollicular Papules in the Vascular Reaction Pattern (continued)

NONFOLLICULAR (CONT.)
- Inflammatory
  - Papular urticaria
  - Arthropod bites
  - Other bite reactions: mites, body lice
  - Cercarial dermatitis
  - Seabather's eruption
  - Papular pityriasis rosea
  - Pruritic urticarial papules and plaques of pregnancy
  - Prurigo pigmentosa
  - Gianotti–Crosti syndrome
  - Early leukocytoclastic vasculitis, before purpura occurs
  - Acute graft-versus-host disease
  - Engraftment syndrome
  - Rash of lymphocyte recovery
  - Kawasaki disease
  - Kawasaki-like inflammatory syndrome of COVID-19 infection
  - Kikuchi disease
- Autoimmune
  - Autoimmune progesterone dermatitis
  - Lupus chilblains
- Hyperplasia
  - Urticaria pigmentosa
- Neoplasia
  - Basal cell cancer
  - Squamous cell cancer
  - Amelanotic melanoma
  - Merkel cell carcinoma
- Related to physical factors
  - Miliaria rubra
  - Cholinergic urticaria
  - Chilblains
  - Polymorphous light eruption
- Drug-related
  - Exanthematous drug eruption
  - DRESS
  - Dermal hypersensitivity reaction

distributed or focal. For diffuse papular dermatoses, viral and other infectious exanthems (early secondary syphilis, rickettsial dermatoses), exanthematous drug eruptions and DRESS, toxin-mediated erythemas, and eruptions in the setting of bone marrow or stem cell transplantation (acute graft-versus-host disease, engraftment syndrome, cutaneous eruption of lymphocyte recovery) should be considered. These eruptions may all display blanching macules in association. Many can become generalized, leading to erythroderma. The differential diagnosis of erythroderma without scale (vascular reaction pattern) is detailed in Table 10.9. This list differs from the scaly erythrodermas as were detailed in Chapter 6. Historically, diffuse macular and papular eruptions

TABLE 10.9. Differential Diagnosis of Widespread Erythema

- Widespread viral exanthems
  - Measles
  - Rubella
  - HIV seroconversion
- Exanthematous drug reaction
  - Morbilliform
  - Rubelliform
  - Scarlatiniform
- Drug reaction with eosinophilia and systemic symptoms (DRESS)
- Toxin-mediated erythema
  - Toxic shock syndrome
  - Streptococcal toxic shock–like syndrome
  - Staphylococcal scalded skin syndrome
  - Kawasaki disease
  - Scarlet fever
- Acute graft-versus-host disease
- Red man syndrome

have been described according to their resemblance to measles, rubella, or scarlet fever. *Morbilliform* connotes a measles-like eruption. The classic rash of measles starts behind ears and generalizes within 24 hours. Discrete macules coalesce to form irregularly patterned larger macules and may become raised. Individual macules are 3–4 mm or larger. Drug eruptions that were termed *morbilliform eruptions* are now referred to as *exanthematous drug eruptions* (Figure 10.13). Early toxin-mediated eruptions, such as

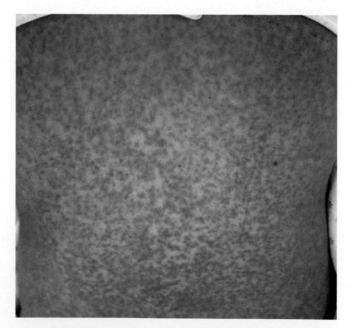

FIGURE 10.13 · A morbilliform drug eruption to amoxicillin, displaying confluent erythematous macules and papules on the back.

toxic shock syndrome or streptococcal toxic shock–like syndrome may resemble measles. The term *scarlatiniform* connotes a scarlet fever–like eruption. The rash consists of finely punctate generalized erythema, likened to "sunburn with goosebumps" or "rough sandpaper." Individual papules measure 1–2 mm. *Rubelliform* connotes a German measles–like eruption. Rubella itself starts on the face and progresses rapidly (<24 hours) downward to the trunk and limbs. The rash comprises discrete pink macules that are smaller than in measles and larger than in scarlet fever. Confluent erythema ensues, on the face first and then on the trunk and limbs. The rash of rubella is less persistent than measles, and it also fades downward. Early toxin-mediated eruptions can be rubelliform. A dermal hypersensitivity reaction occurs most frequently from a medication, or it may be idiopathic. Itchy erythematous papules occur in a symmetric distribution on the extremities and are seen on the trunk as well. Macules are rarely seen in this entity.

In scabies, pruritus is severe. Patients cannot help but scratch during the office visit. Itch is most severe when patients get in to bed at night (as opposed to bedbug bites, in which itch is most severe in the early hours of the morning, when the bugs are active, and will awaken patients from sleep).

> **Clinical Tip** The itch of scabies is worst just after getting into bed at night; the itch of bedbug bites is worst in the early hours of the morning.

The eruption of scabies comprises true burrows (small scaly lines that measure up to 3 mm that represent sites of mites tunneling into the epidermis) and a diffuse hypersensitivity reaction that comprises sparse or numerous nonfollicular vascular reaction pattern papules. Burrows are typically located in the webspaces of the hands and feet, especially in children. The wrist creases are also affected. In adults, periaxillary, suprapubic, genital, and breast papules may be seen. The hypersensitivity papules are randomly distributed. Mange or "animal scabies" is a mite infestation of dogs. Humans may develop a hypersensitivity reaction to this mite in sites of contact of the animal with the owner's body. A host of other mites that may infest animals, birds, or grain may cause a similar itchy eruption. Papular urticaria is a hypersensitivity reaction to insect bites (Figure 10.14). It is predominantly seen in children as a symmetrically

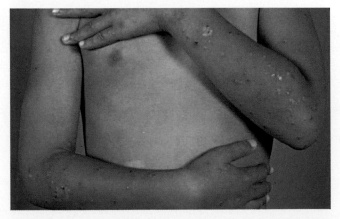

FIGURE 10.14 · Papular urticaria, displaying multiple erythematous papules, many excoriated and crusted, over the extensor forearms.

distributed papular eruption on the extensor aspects of the extremities. True insect bites may be papular or larger and are randomly distributed. Bedbug bites classically occur in sites that are not covered by nightwear, and these occur in rows ("breakfast–lunch–dinner" and sometimes some snacks in between!). Bedbug bites may give rise to urticarial reactions that are separate to the bites. Cercarial dermatitis and seabather's eruption are reactions to the cercariae of nonhuman schistosomes, and the larvae of sea creatures such as sea anemones and jellyfish, respectively. Cercarial dermatitis is common on the lower extremities (e.g., in clam diggers), whereas seabather's eruption occurs in areas of the body that are covered by swimwear (larvae get caught in clothing and release nematocysts that penetrate skin).

Pityriasis rosea may be papular or papulovesicular. Miliaria rubra, pruritic urticarial papules, and plaques of pregnancy (PUPPP), polymorphous light eruption, prurigo pigmentosa, and Gianotti–Crosti syndrome are detailed in Chapter 8. These diseases may have papulovesicles as well as papules, and if so, may be considered in the eczematous reaction pattern category also. Autoimmune progesterone dermatitis may similarly be considered in both reaction patterns. It has a multitude of morphologies (Table 10.10).

The Following Dermatoses may Present with Red, Blanching Papules (Vascular Reaction Pattern), or Papulovesicles (Eczematous Reaction Pattern):

- Papular pityriasis rosea
- Miliaria rubra
- PUPPP
- Polymorphous light eruption
- Prurigo pigmentosa
- Gianotti–Crosti syndrome
- Autoimmune progesterone dermatitis

Kawasaki disease, Kikuchi disease (histiocytic necrotizing lymphadenitis), autoimmune progesterone dermatitis, drug reaction with eosinophilia and systemic symptoms (DRESS)

TABLE 10.10. Dermatoses with a Variable Vascular Reaction Pattern Eruption

Kawasaki disease	Erythema, edema, and desquamation of hands, feet; desquamation of fingertips; diffuse morbilliform or scarlatiniform eruption; targetoid plaques, urticarial plaques
Kikuchi disease	Diffuse morbilliform, Sweet-like, erythematous macules, papules, plaques
Autoimmune progesterone dermatitis	Urticarial papules, papulovesicles, eczematous appearance, targetoid plaques, annular plaques
DRESS	Exanthematous, targetoid, resembling acute generalized exanthematous pustulosis(AGEP), TEN-like
COVID-19 infection	Macular erythema, exanthematous eruptions, urticarial plaques, vesicles, pseudo-chilblains, targetoid lesions, livedo reticularis, retiform purpura

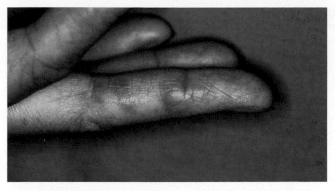

FIGURE 10.15 • Lupus chilblains with red-violaceous papules on the lateral finger.

and COVID-19 infection can present with a wide range of morphologies, including erythematous papules. This information is summarized in Table 10.10.

Urticaria pigmentosa is a form of cutaneous mastocytosis that presents with multiple red or red-brown macules and thin papules that may display a positive Darier sign (see Figure 9.54). Basal cell cancer (BCC) or squamous cell cancer (SCC) may present as a pink or red smooth papule. BCC may appear pearly or shiny, and SCC may be tender. Two important "do not miss" diagnoses in the red papule category are amelanotic melanoma and Merkel cell carcinoma. Chilblains are tender 3–5-mm papules that occur on the fingers and/or toes. These are typically seen in cold, moist climates. Lupus chilblains have a similar appearance. They are a form of chronic cutaneous lupus in the skin (Figure 10.15). Pseudo-chilblains of COVID-19 infection have a similar appearance.

Summary: Differentiating Features of Blanching Smooth Red Papules

- Follicular or nonfollicular?
- For generalized papular eruptions with macules: What size are they?
- Are they tender?
- Are there any groupings or configurations?
- Is there any distribution?

NONBLANCHING LESIONS

The second major category of primary lesion in this reaction pattern is the nonblanching category. If blood has egressed from vessels into the dermis, such as after trauma, from a bleeding diathesis, or from a vasculitis or vasculopathy, the lesion will not blanch. Macules, papules, and plaques may all be purpuric. An additional category to consider here is those papules or plaques that do not blanch given that all vascular channels cannot be compressed by diascopy. Examples here include vascular proliferations or neoplasms such as angiokeratomas, cherry angiomas, and hemangiomas.

Nonblanching Macules

The differential diagnosis for macular purpura is considered in Table 10.11. Solar purpura, also known as senile purpura or Bateman's purpura, is the phenomenon

---

TABLE 10.11. Differential Diagnosis of Macular Purpura

- Senile (Bateman's purpura), vibices
- Benign pigmented purpura
  - Purpura annularis telangiectodes of Majocci
  - Schamberg disease
  - Lichen aureus
  - Lichenoid type of Gougerot–Blum
  - Eczematous type of Doucas and Kapetanakis
  - Granulomatous variant
- Benign pigmented purpura-like
  - Hypergammaglobulinemic purpura of Waldenstrom
  - Purpuric form of mycosis fungoides
  - Type II or II cryoglobulinemia
- Langerhans cell histiocytosis
- Pityriasis rosea: rare finding
- Erythema annulare centrifugum: Rare finding
- Perifollicular: scurvy
- Underlying bleeding diathesis
  - Low platelets, abnormal clotting pathway
- Early rocky mountain spotted fever
- Early leukocytoclastic vasculitis

---

of easy bruising that occurs on chronically sun-damaged skin. It typically occurs on the forearms of older individuals who notice purpura and ecchymoses in this location after minor trauma. Geometric and angular shapes are seen given the initiating traumatic etiology. Linear forms are also seen and are referred to as *vibices*. Benign pigmented purpura (BPP) results from a capillaritis and typically occurs on the lower extremities. Table 10.11 details the different morphologic variants of BPP. Schamberg disease refers to the presence of pinpoint and slightly larger macules with a cayenne-pepper-type appearance (see Figure 2.2). This designation refers to the color of the macules, which may be red, deep red, orange-red, or brownish. Purpura annularis telangiectodes is the annular variant of BPP. Lichenoid papules coexist with cayenne pepper macules and also take on the color of BPP in the lichenoid variant (of Gougerot–Blum; Figure 10.16), and eczematous papules and plaques coexist in the eczematous variant (of Doucas and Kapetanakis). Lichen aureus refers to the presence of a typically single golden-brown plaque (see Figure 4.10B). The rarest variant of BPP is the granulomatous variant. Discrete and confluent papules with the range of colors detailed above are seen (Figure 10.17). Tiny granulomas are seen histopathologically in addition to pericapillary lymphocytes and extravasated red cells.

Three more rarely encountered entities may present with a benign pigmented purpura-like appearance: Hypergammaglobulinemic purpura of Waldenstrom usually presents with macular purpura that may resemble benign pigmented purpura, except that there are also larger purpura than are typically seen in BPP. Palpable purpura may develop later. Patients have an associated polyclonal gammopathy. The primary type occurs in isolation, but the condition may also be seen in association with a range of connective tissue diseases, including Sjogren syndrome, lupus, and rheumatoid arthritis. The second entity is the similarly rare purpuric variant of mycosis fungoides. It may be

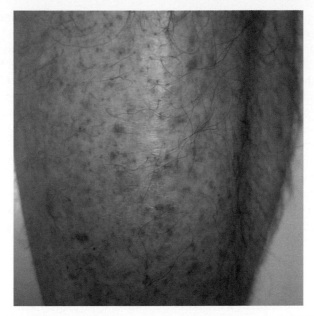

FIGURE 10.16 · Lichenoid variant of benign pigmented purpura, displaying pinkish lichenoid papules along with cayenne pepper-type macules.

seen on the lower extremities or may be in a more widespread distribution. The third entities are types II and II cryoglobulinemia, which may present with Schambergian purpura on the legs along with tiny ulcerations.

Rare Dermatoses That May Resemble Benign Pigmented Purpura
• Hypergammaglobulinemic purpura of Waldenstrom
• Purpuric mycosis fungoides
• Types II and II cryoglubulinemia

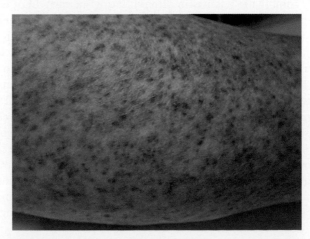

FIGURE 10.17 · Granulomatous variant of benign pigmented purpura, displaying brown, orange, and red macules and papules on the leg.

Langerhans cell histiocytosis is a rare histiocytic condition that most frequently occurs in infants and young children. There is a plethora of findings, including scaling, crusts, and purpuric macules, and so this disease spans many reaction patterns. The seborrheic areas, including intertriginous folds, are sites of predilection. Both pityriasis rosea and erythema annulare centrifugum may have extravasated red cells on histopathology. This phenomenon rarely translates into a clinical purpuric variant of each. In scurvy, vitamin C deficiency leads to diminished collagen formation and, in turn, to friable blood vessel walls. The classic cutaneous finding is perifollicular purpura, seen around corkscrew hairs. Ecchymoses and bleeding into muscles and joints may also occur. Gums are friable and bleed easily. Other bleeding diatheses also present with a range or petechiae, purpura, and ecchymoses on the skin.

A "do not miss" diagnosis in the category of macular purpura is Rocky Mountain spotted fever (RMSF). The causative organism is *Rickettsia rickettsiae*. Most RMSF cases are seen in five US states: Arkansas, Oklahoma, Missouri, Tennessee, and North Carolina; however, cases have been reported throughout the southern, southwestern, and northeastern states, as well as further afield. RMSF also occurs in Central and South America. Initial systemic symptoms (fever, nausea, vomiting, headache, and myalgias) may be accompanied by a blanching rash that becomes petechial and purpuric on around the fifth or sixth day of the illness. Classically, the distal extremities, including the palms and soles, are affected first, and then centripetal spread occurs. Palpable purpura also occurs. Histopathologically a lymphocytic vasculitis is seen. If the disease is not treated early enough, acute respiratory distress syndrome, organ failure, and rarely, disseminated intravascular coagulation with retiform purpura can occur.

Nonblanching Papules and Plaques

The term *palpable purpura* is synonymous with *purpuric papules* and is employed to specifically connote leukocytoclastic vasculitis (LCV), which is a type III hypersensitivity vasculitis with characteristic cutaneous findings. Initially there may be purpuric macules, which usually measure 2–3 mm in diameter and are round. This shape and size combination assists in differentiating an early LCV from petechiae from a bleeding disorder, for example. Purpuric macules are superseded by purpuric papules (*palpable purpura*), which is the hallmark cutaneous finding of LCV (Figure 10.18). Purpuric papules are symmetrically distributed over shins early on. Dorsal feet, forearms, and lower truncal involvement may also be seen. Occasionally palms may be involved symmetrically with purpuric macules. These macules need to be differentiated from those that occur in the setting of septic emboli (distal fingers and toes, asymmetric, purpuric, and sometimes stellate in shape; see text below). Necrosis and secondary bulla formation may be seen in late LCV owing to vascular occlusion from intense inflammation and resultant ischemia. LCV occurs in the setting of infections (such as streptococcal throat infection or a urinary tract infection), drugs (antibiotics, especially β-lactamases, nonsteroidal anti-inflammatory drugs, diuretics, tumor necrosis factor-α antagonists, allopurinol, etc), connective tissue disease, types II and II cryoglobulinemia, or sometimes in the setting of an associated medium-vessel vasculitis, such as microscopic polyangiitis or granulomatosis with polyangiitis. LCV may be idiopathic and recurrent in some. Henoch–Schoenlein purpura in adults may present as an LCV. Typically, these cases are extensive with

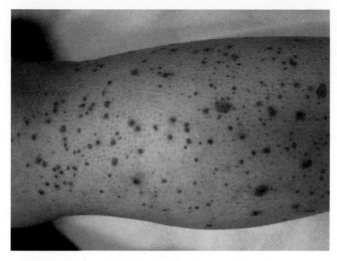

FIGURE 10.18 • Leukocytoclastic vasculitis displaying macular and palpable purpura on the leg.

symmetric involvement of buttocks, lower trunk, and forearms. Acute hemorrhagic edema of infancy is a leukocytoclastic vasculitis seen in this age group. One or more blanching plaques progress to become purpuric.

Septic embolic disease (such as in the setting of infectious endocarditis) may present with a septic vasculitis in the skin. Here, purpuric macules and papules are seen asymmetrically on distal acral sites, such as the fingertips, toes, ears, and the nasal tip. Osler nodes and Janeway lesions are two cutaneous hallmarks of infective endocarditis. *Osler nodes* refer to the tender violaceous papulonodules that occur on the fingers and toes. Longstanding lesions may be purpuric. Histopathologically, neutrophilic microabscesses are seen in early lesions; later a small vessel vasculitis can be found. *Janeway lesions* are asymptomatic purpuric macules on the palmar skin, usually on the thenar or hypothenar eminences.

> **Differentiating Osler Nodes from Janeway Lesions**
>
> • Osler nodes: tender, violaceous or purpuric papules on fingers and toes
> • Janeway lesions: purpuric macules on the palm

Pustules on a purpuric base may be seen in septic embolic disease, too; gonococcemia typically presents with sparse distal, asymmetric pustules on purpuric bases. Bowel-associated dermatosis arthritis syndrome occurs in the setting of inflammatory bowel disease or after bowel bypass surgery. Pustules may arise on purpuric bases on the extensor extremities. Ecthyma gangrenosum represents septic vasculitis from Gram-negative organisms, most frequently *Pseudomonas aeruginosa*. Primary tender erythematous macules become purpuric and then necrotic. Ecthyma gangrenosum differs clinically from other septic vasculitides in that a single or few plaques may be present, and plaques can measure 1–10 cm (Figure 10.19). The most commonly affected sites are the axillary and crural (inguinal) folds, followed by the lower extremities and abdomen. As discussed below, purpuric plaques of ecthyma

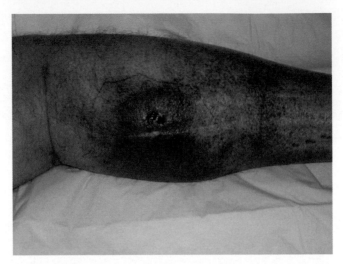

FIGURE 10.19 • Ecthyma gangrenosum showing a purpuric plaque with central necrosis on the calf. (Used with permission from Dr. Miguel Sanchez, Bellevue Hospital, New York University School of Medicine, New York, NY.)

gangrenosum may appear retiform. In general, the term *retiform purpura* refers to a lacy or reticulated pattern of confluent purpuric macules and plaques. Its presence connotes a subset of characteristic diseases that will be discussed later in the chapter with respect to configuration.

A group of papular diseases do not blanch, and yet they are not purpuric. This group falls into the exception category as defined above; blanching does not occur, given the depth of the lesion. Cherry angiomas and hemangiomas do not blanch. Angiokeratomas are a group of vascular anomalies comprising vascular ectasia with variable overlying hyperkeratosis. If there is clinically evident scale, these are classified as the papulosquamous reaction pattern. If not, they may be classified as the dermal or vascular reaction pattern. They present as deep red, violaceous, or almost black papules or plaques. Angiokeratomas of Fordyce are 2–3 mm nonblanching deep red or purplish papules that occur on the vulva or scrotum. In angiokeratoma corporis diffusum, hundreds of even smaller similar papules are seen over the lower trunk and thighs. It is associated with Fabry disease. Angiokeratoma of Mibelli may be associated with acrocyanosis. It occurs predominantly on the extremities of young women. Smooth papules may become scaly with time. Solitary angiokeratomas and angiokeratoma circumscriptum are more commonly plaques and are usually scaly. Port wine stains are smooth vascular plaques that do not blanch.

To summarize the primary lesion diagnostic box, red macules and plaques, whether blanching or nonblanching, manifest a wide array of diagnostic determinants that may be helpful in the creation of differential diagnoses. Distinctive red macules and plaques include round macules, target lesions, targetoid lesions, urticaria and urticarial plaques, red papules, and purpura, and the presence of each of these lesions invokes a unique differential diagnosis.

The grouping and configuration of red lesions, first the blanching entities and then the nonblanching dermatoses, is shown in Table 10.12. Grouping and configuration is lumped together with shape of red macules and thin plaques in that table for convenience. Annular erythema may connote the presence of infection, malignancy, autoimmune disease, vasculitis, the beginning of a vesicobullous disease, or it may be an isolated reactive phenomenon. The *figurate erythemas* are a group of diseases that typically form macules or thin erythematous plaques that have annular, arcuate,

TABLE 10.12. Approach to Vascular Reaction Pattern by Shape/Configuration

BLANCHING
- Annular
  - Erythema migrans
  - Erythema marginatum
  - Erythema gyratum repens
  - Early erythema annulare centrifugum
  - Deep gyrate erythema
  - Annular erythema of infancy
  - Urticarial vasculitis
  - Serum sickness and serum sickness–like reaction
  - Eosinophilic annular erythema
  - Subacute cutaneous LE: annular, polycyclic variant
  - Tumid lupus
  - Annular erythema of Sjogren syndrome
  - Urticarial phase of bullous pemphigoid
  - Pemphigoid gestationis
- Gyrate
  - Erythema gyratum repens
- Figurate
  - Erythema migrans
  - Erythema marginatum
  - Erythema gyratum repens
  - Early erythema annulare centrifugum
  - Deep gyrate erythema
  - Annular erythema of infancy
  - Urticarial vasculitis
  - Serum sickness and serum sickness–like reaction
  - Eosinophilic annular erythema
- Reticulate
  - Livedo reticularis; see differential diagnosis of causes, Table 11.11
  - Livedo racemosa
  - Erythema ab igne
  - Erythema infectiosum
  - Erythema marginatum
  - TRAPS: TNF-α receptor-associated periodic syndrome
  - Adult onset Still's disease
  - Reticulate erythematous mucinosis
  - Prurigo pigmentosa
  - Reticulate palmar erythema is seen in SLE

(Continued)

TABLE 10.12. Approach to Vascular Reaction Pattern by Shape/Configuration (continued)

BLANCHING (CONT.)
- Linear
  - Dermatomyositis: arising from bony prominences
  - Cutaneous larva migrans
  - Larva currens
  - Phytophotodermatitis
  - Koebner phenomenon
    - Adult-onset Still's disease
  - Flagellate erythema
    - Dermatomyositis
    - Adult-onset Still's disease
    - Shiitake mushroom-induced flagellate erythema
    - Chemotherapy-induced flagellate erythema
  - Dermographism
  - Red dermographism
  - Fire ant bites
  - Bedbug bites
  - Following lymphatics
    - Lymphangiitis
    - Lymphangitic spread of a carcinoma, such as carcinoma lymphangiectoides, carcinoma erysipeloides
  - Following Blaschko's lines
    - Angioma serpiginosum
- Targetoid: (see Table 10.1)

PURPURA
- Annular
  - Purpura annularis telangiectodes of Majocci
- Reticulate
  - Retiform purpura (see Table 10.13)
  - Livedoid vasculopathy
- Linear
  - Vibices
  - Koebner phenomenon
    - Leukocytoclastic vasculitis

polycyclic, and serpiginous and geographic shapes and configurations. Erythema annulare centrifugum (EAC) is a figurate erythema that may lack scale very early in the disease course but will develop scale soon afterward (and thus it fits into the papulosquamous category as well). Deep gyrate erythema is a deeper form of erythema annulare centrifugum without scale (Figure 10.20). It is a reactive process and a diagnosis of exclusion; all aforementioned entities should be excluded. Erythema migrans is an important "do not miss" diagnosis in this category. As alluded to earlier, erythema migrans is typically described as being annular or as having a "bull's-eye" appearance. However, variations in morphology are the norm. Perfectly round, oval (but not annular), and occasionally targetoid or bullous and hemorrhagic forms have been described. As mentioned earlier, slow centrifugal extension over days is classic.

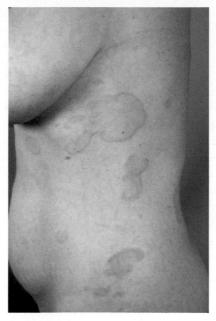

FIGURE 10.20 • Deep gyrate erythema showing annular, arcuate, and polycyclic plaques on the torso.

In disseminated Lyme disease, multiple erythematous macules or thin plaques with the aforementioned morphology, including annular shape or configuration, are seen (Figure 10.21). Variations in morphology across lesions in a single case may be seen. Erythema marginatum of rheumatic fever is a rare cause of annular erythema, as is erythema gyratum repens, an extremely rare paraneoplastic phenomenon that occurs in the setting of solid-organ malignancies, especially lung cancer. The term *gyrate* refers to lesions that spiral around each other. The presence of gyrate and concentric annular rings that have a wood-grain appearance is a typical finding. Eruptions have been reported

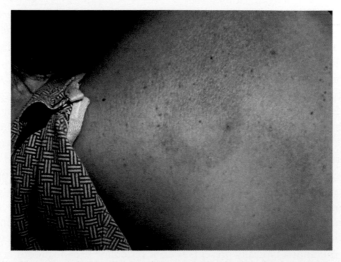

FIGURE 10.21 • Disseminated Lyme disease, showing an annular thin plaque on the shoulder.

as having a vascular reaction pattern, or as having minimal scale. Annular erythema in infancy is a rare, self-limited eruption that occurs in the first year of life. It may resemble EAC without scale. Annular and arcuate thin erythematous plaques resolve spontaneously after a few days.

Urticarial vasculitis, serum sickness and serum sickness–like reactions, and eosinophilic annular erythema are also figurate. These form edematous and erythematous plaques. Urticarial vasculitis is a type of small-vessel vasculitis that presents with urticarial plaques. As detailed previously, these plaques tend to persist for longer than 24 hours and then fade, leaving postinflammatory hyperpigmentation. Diascopy on a plaque of urticarial vasculitis reveals pinpoint petechiae within it. Urticarial vasculitis may also have annular, arcuate, polycylic, serpiginous, and otherwise patterned plaques (another figurate dermatosis). A similar eruption is seen in serum sickness and serum sickness–like reactions. Eosinophilic annular erythema is a rare dermatosis of unknown etiology seen in adults. Early on, it may resemble urticarial vasculitis with annular, arcuate, and serpiginous forms. In chronic cases, large annular plaques are seen. Some authors believe that it is a variant of eosinophilic cellulitis.

Figurate Dermatoses in the Vascular Reaction Pattern	
• Urticarial vasculitis	• Erythema gyratum repens
• Serum sickness and serum sickness-like reactions	• Erythema marginatum
	• Early erythema annulare centrifugum
• Eosinophilic annular erythema	• Deep gyrate erythema
• Erythema migrans	• Annular erythema of infancy

Annular erythema in autoimmune disease may signify tumid lupus (which also can be classified as having a dermal reaction pattern), the annular, polycyclic variant of subacute lupus erythematosus, and annular erythema of Sjogren disease. The latter finding is usually seen in photoexposed areas. The urticarial phase of bullous pemphigoid may have an annular morphology, and this is also true of pemphigoid gestationis.

Reticulate erythema may be blanching or nonblanching (retiform purpura). Blanching reticulate erythema is seen in livedo reticularis, livedo racemose, and erythema ab igne. The causes of livedo reticularis and livedo racemosa are detailed in Table 11.11. While livedo reticularis is seen in both physiologic and pathologic states, livedo racemosa (a broken-up lacy network) is always pathological (Figure 10.22). Erythema ab igne occurs from chronic application of heat. Initially it has a red lacy appearance (Figure 10.23). Later it may become brown. Chronically it may start to scale, and a rare complication in these cases is squamous cell carcinoma. The palmar erythema seen in SLE may have a reticulate appearance. Erythema infectiosum (fifth disease) is caused by parvovirus B19. It typically occurs in young children. A high fever is superseded by red cheeks ("slapped cheek" appearance) and a lacy, light pink rash on the body. These reticulate thin plaques and macules do not follow the cutaneous vasculature. They become more prominent with heat and may wax and wane for weeks. Erythema marginatum, as mentioned, has heterogeneous findings, including light pink reticulate plaques. The rash of Still's disease and TRAPS are similarly variable. Reticulate erythematous mucinosis typically presents with a reticulate broad smooth erythematous

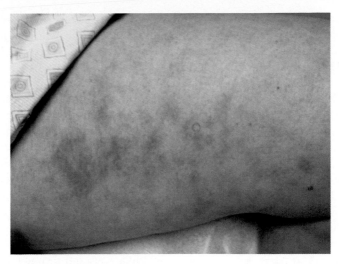

FIGURE 10.22 · Livedo racemosa showing branched incomplete reticular network on the thigh of a patient with systemic lupus erythematosus.

reticulate plaque on the chest of young women. It may be a marker of underlying systemic lupus. In prurigo pigmentosa, erythematous papules become confluent to form a reticulate pattern and fade with reticulate pigmentation. Retiform purpura is detailed in the discussion of purpura below.

Linear erythema has a broad differential diagnosis. The Koebner phenomenon is reported in adult Still's disease (see Figure 10.12). *Flagellate erythema* refers to the morphologic finding of linear red macules or thin plaques that resemble an imprint of a whip on the skin. The differential diagnosis of flagellate erythema comprises four entities. It is a rare dermatologic manifestation of dermatomyositis. In this setting, the linear erythematous streaks are pruritic and typically located on the trunk. They are erythematous or violaceous. As detailed above, the eruption of adult-onset Still's

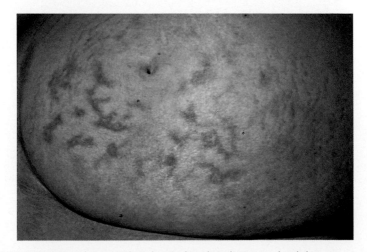

FIGURE 10.23 · Erythema ab igne with pink reticulate thin plaques on the abdomen.

disease is typically evanescent. A second type of adult Still's associated eruption has been characterized in recent decades, characterized by chronic persistent papules and plaques that are usually in a linear or flagellate configuration. There are linear itchy reddish and brownish plaques that occur on the trunk and are persistent. These may be scaly, in which case they would be classified with the papulosquamous reaction pattern. Shiitake mushroom dermatitis is most frequently seen in Japan. It typically occurs within a day or two of eating raw or partially cooked shiitake mushrooms. Erythematous pruritic papules coalesce to form linear plaques on the trunk, extremities, and sometimes, the face. The eruption spares areas that the patient cannot reach. Lentinan is a constituent of shiitake mushrooms that is believed to be responsible for this eruption. Finally, flagellate erythema may occur secondary to a drug eruption. Bleomycin is the most frequent inciting agent, but docetaxel, cisplatin, and peplomycin (a bleomycin derivative) have also been implicated. There is a variable time to onset of the eruption after drug administration; it may begin as early as the first day or as late as 6 months. Pruritic erythematous streaks occur on the chest, upper back, and shoulders, or extremities. As it resolves, it becomes more violaceous and secondary desquamative scale may be seen (Figure 10.24). Ultimately, prominent linear hyperpigmentation after complete resolution is a feature of this entity.

The Flagellate Erythemas
• Dermatomyositis • Chronic persistent papules and plaques of adult-onset Still's disease • Shiitake mushroom dermatitis • Induced by bleomycin and other chemotherapy drugs

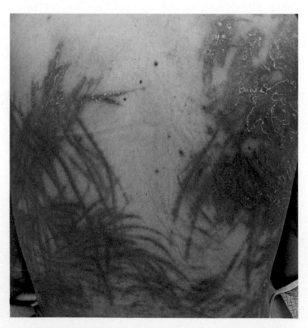

FIGURE 10.24 • Resolving flagellate erythema from bleomycin, displaying confluent linear plaques with secondary desquamative scale.

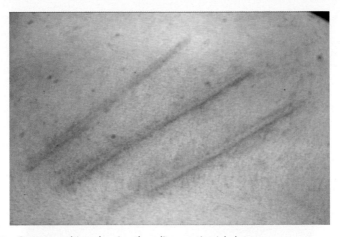

FIGURE 10.25 • Dermographism showing three linear urticarial plaques.

Linear erythema is also seen in dermatomyositis; linear erythematous or violaceous macules or thin plaques arise from joints and extend up or down an extremity. Examples include erythema from the ulnar styloid extending up the forearm, from the elbow extending distally and from the knee extending proximally. Cutaneous larva migrans and larva currens, as detailed earlier, also fit into this category. Linear erythema is seen in phytophotodermatitis (see Figure 1.6A). This is a phototoxic reaction that occurs after contact with plants or fruits of the Apiaceae and Rutaceae families that contain furocoumarins or psoralens. Examples include celery, fennel, and parsley (Apiaceae) and limes, lemons, and oranges (Rutaceae). These chemicals act as photosensitizers and give rise to a phototoxic reaction in areas of contact. There are linear and geometric vesicles, bullae, and red macules that leave behind prominent brown patterned pigmentation. *Dermographism* connotes the presence of linear hives that eventuate after superficial pressure, such as scratching, is applied to the skin (Figure 10.25). Dermographism may be seen in the presence of urticaria, or it may be an isolated finding. Testing for dermographism in the clinic involves applying firm pressure to the skin with the back of a cotton-tipped swab to obtain a sample of a linear thin red plaque. Red dermographism is the presence of red macules, rather than thin urticarial plaques, after firm stroking of the skin. Red dermographism may be seen in partially treated urticaria.

For the purpuric entities, *annular purpura* is seen in the Majocchi type of benign pigmented purpura. Showers of cayenne-pepper-type macules form annular shapes on the shins and other aspects of the lower extremities and occasionally the abdomen and buttocks. Vibices are a linear variant of solar purpura seen on chronically sun-damaged skin. Leukocytoclastic vasculitis may Koebnerize. Linear arrays of purpuric macules or papules are seen in Figure 10.26. A "do not miss" diagnosis is that of *retiform purpura;* this comprises purpuric and necrotic plaques that are characterized by angulated borders following a livedo pattern (Figure 10.27). Retiform purpura may be seen in the setting of infection, for example, sepsis or disseminated intravascular coagulation, or vasculitis, such as in medium-vessel vasculitides (see Figure 4.12D). In meningococcemia, plaques typically have a "gunmetal gray" appearance (Figure 10.28). Table 10.13 lists the causes of retiform purpura. Livedoid

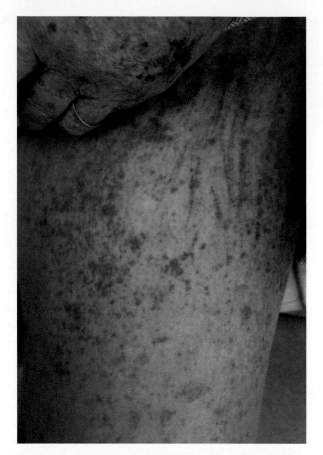

FIGURE 10.26 • Leukocytoclastic vasculitis displaying the Koebner phenomenon (numerous non-blanching linear macules on the thigh).

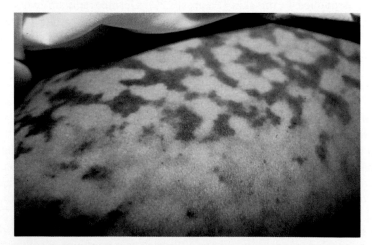

FIGURE 10.27 • Noninflammatory retiform purpura on the thigh in a patient with disseminated intravascular coagulation secondary to sepsis. (Reproduced with permission from Goldsmith LA, Katz SI, Gilchrest BA, et al: *Fitzpatrick's Dermatology in General Medicine*, 8th ed. New York, NY: McGraw Hill; 2012.)

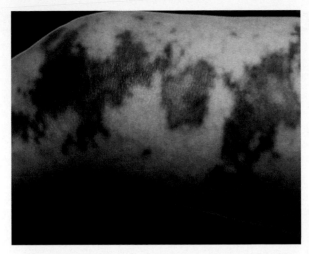

FIGURE 10.28 • Disseminated intravascular coagulopathy from meningococcemia with a typical gunmetal gray color. (Reproduced with permission from Wolff K, Johnson RA, Saavedra AP, et al: *Fitzpatrick's Color Atlas and Synopsis of Clinical Dermatology*, 8th ed. New York, NY: McGraw Hill; 2017.)

TABLE 10.13. Differential Diagnosis of Retiform Purpura

INFECTION
- Bacterial
  - Septic vasculopathy
  - Infective endocarditis
  - Ecthyma gangrenosum
- Viral
  - COVID-19 infection
- Mycobacterial
  - Lucio phenomenon in lepromatous leprosy
- Fungal
  - Mucor
  - Candidemia
  - Aspergillosis
- Rickettsial
  - Rocky Mountain spotted fever
- Parasitic
  - Disseminated strongyloidiasis

THROMBOTIC VASCULOPATHY
- Hypercoagulable states
  - Protein C or S deficiency
  - Factor V Leiden deficiency
  - Antiphospholipid syndrome
  - Hyperhomocysteinemia
  - Warfarin necrosis
  - Heparin necrosis
  - Cocaine levamisole toxicity
  - Disseminated intravascular coagulopathy

(Continued)

TABLE 10.13. Differential Diagnosis of Retiform Purpura (continued)

THROMBOTIC VASCULOPATHY (CONT.)
- Platelet plugs
  - Thrombocytosis

OCCLUSION OF VESSELS DUE TO OTHER INTRAVASCULAR SUBSTANCES
- Cholesterol: cholesterol emboli
- Calcium and thrombi: calciphylaxis
- Cryoproteins: cryoglobulinemias, cryofibrinogenemia
- Oxalate crystals: primary hyperoxaluria

VASCULITIS: MEDIUM-VESSEL
- Granulomatosis with polyangiitis
- Eosinophilic granulomatosis with polyangiitis
- Polyarteritis nodosa: cutaneous and systemic
- Vasculitis associated with lupus, rheumatoid arthritis
- Microscopic polyangiitis
- Macular lymphocytic arteritis

vasculopathy is a type of retiform purpura, which may be idiopathic or may occur in the setting of a prothrombotic state (similar causes as listed in the thrombotic vasculopathy section of Table 10.13). Fleeting painful retiform purpura break down rapidly to form tender stellate ulcerations, typically around the ankles, on the dorsal feet or elsewhere on the lower legs (Figure 10.29). The ulcers heal with classic porcelain-white atrophic scars.

Many diseases in this category have typical sites of distribution as is seen in Table 10.14. For photodistributed erythema that is painful, sunburn comes to mind. Photosensitivity

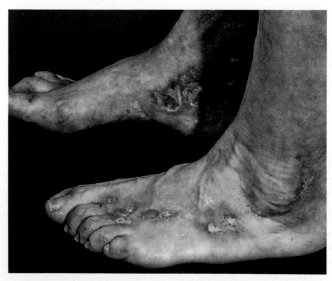

FIGURE 10.29 · Livedoid vasculopathy with recurrent, painful ulcers and livedo reticularis. (Reproduced with permission from Goldsmith LA, Katz SI, Gilchrest BA, et al: *Fitzpatrick's Dermatology in General Medicine*, 8th ed. New York, NY: McGraw Hill; 2012.)

TABLE 10.14. Vascular Reaction Pattern by Distribution

BLANCHING
- Photodistributed
  - Sunburn
  - SLE
  - Dermatomyositis
  - Porphyrias
  - Phototoxic drug reaction
  - UV recall
  - Tumid LE
  - SCLE
  - Polymorphous light eruption
- Extensors
  - Dermatomyositis
  - TRAPS
  - Erythema multiforme
  - Papular urticaria
- Intertriginous
  - Toxic erythema of chemotherapy
  - SDRIFE (symmetric drug-related intertriginous and flexural exanthem)
  - Miliaria rubra
- Buttocks
  - Baboon syndrome
  - Gianotti–Crosti syndrome
  - Henoch–Schonlein purpura
- Over bony prominences
  - Dermatomyositis
- Palms
  - Palmar erythema
    - Inherited
      - Erythema palmare hereditarium
    - Acquired
      - Physiologic in the setting of pregnancy
      - Smoking
      - Liver cirrhosis
      - Connective tissue disease, including SLE and rheumatoid arthritis
      - Thyrotoxicosis
      - Diabetes mellitus
  - Erythema multiforme
  - Urticaria
  - Urticarial vasculitis
  - Serum sickness
  - Rocky Mountain spotted fever
- Fingers and toes
  - Chilblains, lupus chilblains and pseudo-chilblains of COVID-19 infection
  - Kawasaki disease: fingertips
  - Scabies: webspaces
  - Dermatomyositis: over joints
  - Osler nodes: early blanching, later purpura

(Continued)

TABLE 10.14. Vascular Reaction Pattern by Distribution (continued)

PURPURA
- Extensors
  - Bowel-associated dermatosis arthritis syndrome
  - Leukocytoclastic vasculitis: starts on shins
  - BPP: shins
  - Hypergammaglobulinemic purpura of Waldenstrom: shins
  - Purpuric form of mycosis fungoides: shins
  - Type II or II cryoglobulinemia: shins
- Ankle
  - Livedoid vasculopathy
- Intertriginous
  - Langerhans cell histiocytosis
  - Ecthyma gangrenosum
- Seborrheic
  - Langerhans cell histiocytosis
- Buttocks
  - Widespread LCV
  - Henoch–Schonlein purpura
- Palms
  - Septic vasculitis
  - Janeway lesions
  - Rocky Mountain spotted fever
  - LCV: rare
- Fingers and toes
  - Septic vasculitis
  - Infective endocarditis
  - Disseminated gonococcemia
  - Osler nodes: early blanching, later purpura
  - Thrombotic vasculopathies: Table 10.13
  - Microvascular occlusion due to other intravascular substances: Table 10.13
  - Blue toe syndrome
    - Thrombotic vasculopathy
    - Septic and nonseptic emboli
    - Microvascular occlusion due to other intravascular substances
- Adipose-rich areas
  - Warfarin necrosis
- Ears, nose, cheeks
  - Cocaine levamisole toxicity
  - Disseminated intravascular coagulopathy

states, such as connective tissue diseases and phototoxic eruptions caused by medications, are important to consider in the appropriate clinical context as mentioned above. In dermatomyositis, photodistributed erythema may be violaceous (Figure 10.30).

For photodistributed erythematous papules, polymorphous light eruption should be borne in mind. Also, in dermatomyositis, besides linear macules or thin plaques arising from joints, localized erythema over the joint itself is also seen. Thin violaceous or erythematous plaques occurring over the interphalangeal joints are known as *atrophic dermal papules of dermatomyositis* (formerly known as Gottron papules). Violaceous or erythematous macules in this location are another diagnostic sign (formerly known as Gottron sign).

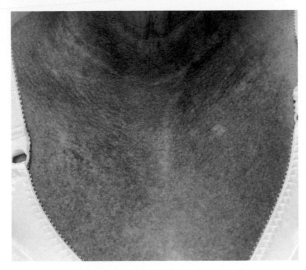

FIGURE 10.30 • Dermatomyositis, displaying violaceous erythema in a photoexposed distribution. (Reproduced with permission from Kang S, Amagai M, Bruckner AL, et al: *Fitzpatrick's Dermatology*, 9th ed. New York, NY: McGraw Hill; 2019.)

Palmar erythema may be inherited or acquired, as is detailed in Table 10.14. Erythema palmare hereditarium is the inherited form; onset is at birth, and erythema is present throughout life. Redness is constant and independent of temperature. In acquired palmar erythema, a host of reasons may be responsible, including physiologic and pathologic causes. As mentioned, the erythema may be reticulate in SLE. Palmar erythematous plaques may be seen in urticarial or urticarial vasculitis. Symmetric involvement is classically seen in serum sickness and serum sickness–like reactions. Acute graft-versus-host disease favors the palms and soles (Figure 10.31).

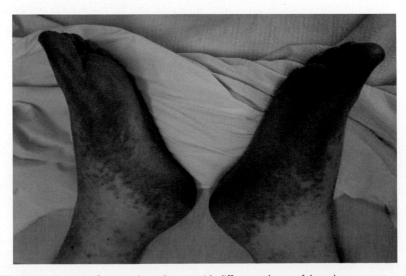

FIGURE 10.31 • Acute graft-versus-host disease with diffuse erythema of the soles.

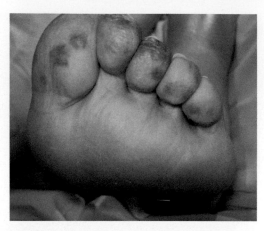

FIGURE 10.32 • Purplish discoloration of the toes secondary to type 1 cryoglobulinemia.

In the purpuric category, leukocytoclastic vasculitis typically occurs symmetrically on the shins in contrast to septic vasculitis, which presents with asymmetric purpura on the fingers, toes, and other acral sites. RMSF starts on the distal extremities and progresses proximally. The palms and soles are frequently involved. Blue toe syndrome (bluish or purplish toes) has a broad differential diagnosis, including vasoconstrictive states (acrocyanosis and Raynaud phenomenon and disease) and tissue ischemia caused by a thrombotic vasculopathy, embolic phenomena (such as cholesterol emboli after cardiac catheterization, septic emboli and nonseptic emboli such as from atrial myxoma or Libmann–Sacks endocarditis of SLE), or other intraluminal occlusion [such as cryoglobulins (Figure 10.32) and cryofibrinogens]. In disseminated intravascular coagulopathy, necrosis of digits may be seen in severe cases (Figure 10.33). Thrombotic vasculopathies may also involve the nasal tip and ears (other acral sites). The ears, nose, and cheeks are sites of predilection for cocaine levamisole toxicity—a newly recognized entity where vasculopathy and vasculitis occur in the setting of levamisole-adulterated cocaine use. These sites may also be involved in disseminated intravascular coagulopathy. Warfarin necrosis affects adipose-rich sites such as the

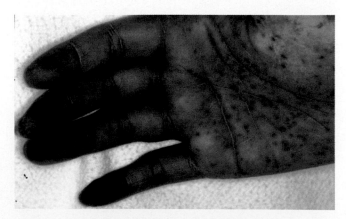

FIGURE 10.33 • Numerous purpuric macules on the palm and necrotic fingertips in disseminated intravascular coagulopathy.

breasts and thighs. It typically occurs symmetrically. Ecthyma gangrenosum affects the axillary and crural folds, the lower extremities, and the abdomen. Calciphylaxis usually involves the proximal thighs, but the abdomen and more rarely, the distal extremities may be involved. Calciphylaxis may also involve the distal penis. Livedoid vasculopathy favors the ankles and may involve the dorsal feet and other parts of the lower leg.

Table 10.15 provides a summary of the clinical signs that can be seen in the scalp, hair, nails, mucous membranes, and lymph nodes. In examining the entire skin and mucous membranes, many diagnostic clues can be gathered. Diffuse or patterned erythema is frequently seen in connective tissue disease, such as SLE or dermatomyositis, as discussed. In these conditions, there may be periungual erythema and nail fold changes (hyperkeratotic and "ragged" cuticles, nail fold infarcts, prominent nail fold capillary loops, and nail fold capillary dropout). In SLE, nails may exhibit onycholysis, longitudinal ridging, leukonychia, splinter hemorrhages, and red lunulae. Telogen effluvium may be seen in active SLE and dermatomyosiits. *Lupus hair* refers

---

TABLE 10.15. Gleaning Information from Scalp, Hair, Nails, Mucous Membranes, and Lymph Nodes for the Vascular Reaction Pattern

SCALP/HAIR
- Nonscarring alopecia, "lupus hair": active systemic lupus
- Crusting, scaling, purpura on the scalp: Langerhans cell histiocytosis
- Pruritic pink or violaceous plaques scalp: dermatomyositis

NAILS
- Systemic lupus: periungual erythema, red lunulae, fine longitudinal lines, leukonychia
- Dermatomyositis: ragged cuticles, nail fold capillary loop changes, nail fold infarcts
- Infective endocarditis and other septic vasculitis: splinter hemorrhages
- Kawasaki disease: periungual desquamation, a few weeks into the course; orange-brown or white discoloration of nails and Beau's lines in the convalescent phase

MUCOUS MEMBRANES
- Systemic lupus: oral ulcers, discoid lupus
- EM major, MIRM, SJS/TEN, PNP/PAMS: hemorrhagic crusting of lips and intraoral erosions; conjunctival injection, anogenital erosions
- SJS/TEN: esophageal and laryngeal involvement
- Fixed drug eruption: round macule involving lips, genital skin
- Measles: Koplik spots
- Rubella: Forschheimer spots
- Scarlet fever: strawberry tongue
- Kawasaki disease: strawberry tongue early and later, raspberry tongue; dry, red, and fissured lips and conjunctival injection
- Scurvy: gingival friability and bleeding
- Sweet syndrome: ocular involvement (conjunctivitis, episcleritis, limbal nodules, iridocyclitis)

LYMPH NODES
- Kikuchi disease
- Purpuric mycosis fungoides
- Amelanotic melanoma
- Merkel cell carcinoma

to shorter hairs seen at the frontal hair margin in active SLE. The length differential is thought to be due to slower anagen growth, rather than trichoschizia. Anagen effluvium may accompany radiation recall after chemotherapy. Scalp involvement in dermatomyositis is common. Pruritic erythematous plaques may be smooth or scaly and reminiscent of seborrheic dermatitis. Mucous membrane lesions are seen in approximately one-fourth of patients with SLE. Oral ulcers are 1 of the 11 American College of Rheumatology diagnostic criteria for SLE. These ulcers measure around 3–4 mm and are shallow and painful with surrounding red haloes. They occur not only on oral surfaces (palate, gums, buccal mucosa) but also within the nose and vulva and perianally. Plaques of discoid lupus may also be seen in the mouth, especially involving the palate and buccal mucosa.

Mucous membranes may be involved in EM, SJS, and TEN. Hemorrhagic erosions and crusting of both lips is a classic presenting feature of EM or SJS/TEN (Figure 10.34). MIRM manifests a similar picture. [Of note, this finding is also pathognomonic of paraneoplastic autoimmune multiorgan syndrome (PAMS).] Eyes, nasal mucosa, oral cavity, and the anogenital mucosa may all be involved. Skin involvement usually occurs prior to mucous membrane involvement, but this may be reversed in some cases. Symptoms and signs of mucous membrane involvement include a blood-streaked rhinorrhea, conjunctival injection, hemorrhagic crusting of the lips, burning on urination, pain on defecation, and oral and genital erosions. Erythema multiforme major connotes erythema multiforme in the presence of mucous membrane involvement. Mycoplasma mucositis is a subset of erythema multiforme, caused by *Mycoplasma pneumoniae*, which presents with mucosal findings without skin involvement. In SJS/TEN, the respiratory mucosa may also be involved, and patients with this disorder may be dyspneic and hypoxemic.

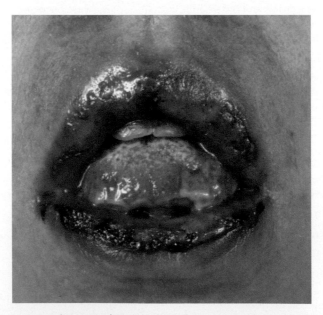

FIGURE 10.34 • Stevens–Johnson syndrome displaying hemorrhagic crusting of the lips. (Reproduced with permission from Wolff K, Johnson RA, Saavedra AP, et al: *Fitzpatrick's Color Atlas and Synopsis of Clinical Dermatology*, 8th ed. New York, NY: McGraw Hill; 2017.)

Fixed drug eruption may also involve the mucosa. Oral, lip margin, and genital cases have been reported. Measles may present with an enanthem prior to the exanthem: Koplik spots are pinpoint red papules with whitish centers on the buccal mucosa. Similarly, rubella may have pinpoint petechiae on the palate preceding or accompanying the exanthem (Forschheimer spots). In scarlet fever, the combination of inflammation of the tongue papillae and a white coating is known as a "strawberry tongue." This gives way to a "raspberry tongue" (prominent papillae without a coating) later in the course of the disease. A strawberry tongue is also seen in Kawasaki disease. Other mucosal manifestations of Kawasaki disease include dry, red, and fissured lips and conjunctival injection (a diagnostic criterion). Nail and periungual changes are also seen. Edema of the hands gives way to periungual desquamation, which is seen a few weeks into the course. Nail changes include an orange-brown or white discoloration and Beau lines in the convalescent phase. Eye involvement may be seen in Sweet syndrome.

Considering the purpuric entities, splinter hemorrhages are tiny linear hemorrhages under the nails. These may occur distally from trauma, but if seen under the proximal nail, they may be a sign of underlying septic vasculitis, such as infective endocarditis. In the antiphospholipid syndrome, nail and hair signs of lupus, as detailed above, may be seen. Gingival friability is a hallmark sign of scurvy. Gums are swollen and bleed easily.

Lymphadenopathy may be seen in Kikuchi disease, purpuric mycosis fungoides, amelanotic melanoma, and Merkel cell carcinoma (but usually in the latter two diagnoses, the disease that presents with lymphadenopathy is more advanced and nodules, rather than papules, will be present).

The final diagnostic box on the wheel of diagnosis is the history box. Age of onset and geographic locale are important diagnostic considerations. Also, as alluded to previously, associated symptomatology (itching, pain, burning, or no symptoms) and whether lesions are fixed, evanescent, migratory, or expanding can help guide diagnosis. Scabetic itch is worst at night just after getting into bed. Bedbug-bite-associated itch is worst in the early hours of the morning, when bedbugs are active. Patients with scabies commonly scratch in the clinic visit as the itch is so severe. Table 10.7 details these symptoms further. In urticaria, angioedema, tongue edema and difficulty swallowing or breathing may be a feature. Rarely, anaphylaxis is associated. In urticarial vasculitis, serum sickness and serum sickness–like eruptions, arthralgia, and arthritis may be a feature. In suspected thrombotic vasculopathy, ask about prior thrombotic episodes and family history. Associated connective tissue disease symptoms and signs may be present.

BEDSIDE DIAGNOSTICS AND BLOODWORK

As mentioned, diascopy is of prime importance in this reaction pattern to distinguish between blanching erythema and purpura. Diascopy may not effectively blanch out thicker vascular neoplasms such as a thicker port wine stain, so this rule is not absolute. As discussed in the vesicobullous reaction pattern chapter (Chapter 7), a positive Darier sign is the emergence of a wheal after application of firm pressure on the surface of a mastocytosis lesion, such as a mastocytoma or urticarial pigmentosa. A *positive Nikolsky sign* refers to detachment of epidermis from dermis when applying sideways/tangential pressure on tender red macules of SJS/TEN. For any pruritic papular dermatosis, consider scabies and perform a mineral oil preparation.

> **TABLE 10.16. Bedside Diagnostics and Blood work for the Vascular Reaction Patterne**
> - Helpful Diagnostic Tests for the Vascular Reaction Pattern
> - Diascopy: possible blanching
> - Firm stroking with the back of a cotton-tipped applicator in suspected mastocytosis
> - Lateral pressure on suspected early necrotic skin of SJS/TEN
> - Mineral oil evaluation in suspected scabies
> - Bloodwork: platelet count, PT, PTT, and infectious, coagulopathic, autoimmune disease, leukocytoclastic vasculitis and cryoglobulinemia work-up when appropriate
> - Lesional biopsy for direct immunofluorescence in suspected Henoch-Schonlein purpura

Regarding bloodwork, for any macular purpura without an obvious dermatologic cause, perform a platelet count, prothrombin time (PT) and partial thromboplastin time (PTT) to rule out an underlying bleeding diathesis. COVID-19 testing should be considered for pseudo-chilblains or in any ill patient with a new onset erythematous, urticarial, vesicular or livedo reticularis-like eruption, or with retiform purpura. The presence of retiform purpura may prompt consideration for further coagulation studies, an infectious disease work up including blood cultures, depending on the clinical setting. Many of the patterned erythemas mentioned above may signify autoimmune disease and so consider a laboratory work-up for SLE or dermatomyositis for any clinically suspicious cases. A laboratory workup to delineate possible etiologies (as mentioned above) and internal organ involvement should be considered in leukocytoclastic vasculitis and cryoglobulinemia. As always, skin biopsy provides additional diagnostic information. In suspected Henoch-Schonlein purpura, a second lesional biopsy for direct immunofluoresence may reveal IgA deposition in affected dermal vasculature. Table 10.16 summarizes this information.

> ## SUMMARY
> - The vascular reaction pattern includes a broad array of infectious, inflammatory, paraneoplastic, and drug-induced dermatoses that have in common their red color.
> - While there are no scales, vesicle, bullae, or nodules to guide differential diagnosis, employing the diagnostic boxes of the wheel of diagnosis will assist with narrowing down a differential diagnosis.
> - A useful starting point is to determine whether lesions blanch and to further subdivide differential diagnosis on the basis of the primary lesion present.
> - Distinctive shapes and configurations of lesions as well as their distribution further guide diagnosis.
> - Bedside diagnostics can be employed to help narrow down a diagnosis. A laboratory work up may be needed in many of the vascular reaction pattern conditions.

Shape, Configuration, and Grouping of Lesions

11

As we have seen in previous chapters, eruptions may manifest lesions with characteristic individual shapes, or characteristic configuration or arrangement of multiple lesions. These attributes of lesions and eruptions can be harnessed as diagnostic tools. As has been previously mentioned, *shape* is an inherent property of one individual lesion whereas *configuration* refers to the scheme or arrangement formed by confluent grouped lesions. Sometimes it is difficult to discern whether any given shape is made up of more than one lesion, and so, for convenience, the differential diagnoses of both shape and configuration are discussed in this chapter. For example, papules may be grouped together to form an annular configuration, as is seen in granuloma annulare. Or, a plaque of lichen planus may assume an annular shape if it is depressed in the center and raised at the periphery. Similarly, a line can be made up of a confluence of lesions (configuration), such as the confluent vesicles seen in poison ivy dermatitis, or of one lesion (a shape), such as in dermographism.

The terms *grouping* and *arrangement* may be used synonymously. These terms are applied to lesions that are closely related spatially to each other. Examples include a group of bedbug bites arranged in an annulus or a line.

An approach to the differential diagnoses of shape, grouping, and configuration was introduced in Chapter 1, including by etiologic classification and by primary lesion. This chapter will delve into these differential diagnoses in detail. This differential diagnostic approach will factor in diagnostic determinants such as reaction patterns and color. Each of the commonly encountered shapes, configurations, and groupings is listed in the textbox below and will be considered in turn. The textbox contains synonyms for each as well as a list of how each entity is formed.

Commonly Encountered Shapes, Configurations and Groupings

- *Round*—nummular, discoid (shape)
- *Annular*—ring-shaped (shape, configuration, grouping)
- *Arcuate*—part of a ring, arc-shaped (shape, configuration, grouping)
- *Concentric*—rings within rings (configuration)
- *Polycyclic*—formed from confluent annuli (configuration)
- *Gyrate*—forms spirals (configuration)
- *Figurate*—figure-forming (shape, configuration)
- *Linear*—forms a line (shape, configuration, grouping)
- *Serpiginous*—wavy, snake-like (shape, configuration, grouping)
- *Whorled*—forms swirls (shape, configuration)
- *Reticulate*—retiform, net-like, lacy (shape, configuration)
- *Herpetiform*—herpes-like (configuration, grouping)
- *Agminate*—clustered (grouping)

> **TABLE 11.1. Differential Diagnosis of Round, Flat Plaques and Macules by Reaction Pattern and Color**
>
> **PAPULOSQUAMOUS**
> • Pityriasis rotunda
>
> **ECZEMATOUS**
> • Nummular eczema
>
> **VASCULAR**
> • Blanching
>   • Fixed drug eruption
>   • Erythema migrans
> • Nonblanching
>   • Cupping
>
> **BROWN**
> • Fixed drug eruption

ROUND

The physical finding of macules or plaques that are completely round is very rare. Those dermatoses that are completely round are listed in Table 11.1 by reaction pattern and color. Pityriasis rotunda is a very rare dermatosis that may run in families or may be acquired. The acquired form has been associated with malnutrition, tuberculosis, and hepatocellular carcinoma. Plaques of pityriasis rotunda are very thin, are light brown, and have fine scales. The inherited type may resemble ichthyosis. Nummular eczema usually appears with a subacute morphology (scaly erythematous papules and/or plaques, along with round erosions and/or round crusts; see Figure 8.2A,B), but chronic forms also occur. Fixed drug eruption is usually pigmented. When active, directly following culprit drug exposure, it may blister. Inactive fixed drug eruption appears brown or gray-brown. Nonpigmented fixed drug eruption is a variant that appears pink and does not pigment. Fixed drug eruption may also appear oval. This is usually seen where the skin tension lines have relaxed along the mid- and lower back. Round variants of erythema migrans may occur and are a "do not miss" diagnosis (Figure 11.1). Cupping can cause circles of petechiae or purpura (Figure 11.2).

Vesicles and bullae are also round, unless confluent, or if induced by an "outside job," such as allergic contact dermatitis to poison ivy, in which case they can form linear and geometric shapes. Most papules, nodules and tumors are round.

ANNULAR

Annuli, or rings, are usually composed of grouped primary lesions. However, annuli may also be formed by a plaque with either a raised border or a depressed center, such as in the "nickels and dimes" of secondary syphilis, or in lichen planus as mentioned above. Similarly, with respect to macules, an annulus may be a single primary lesion rather than a confluence of separate macules. An example here is erythema migrans. Annuli may occasionally be formed by a grouping, such as may be seen in a series of bug bites. Some disorders of keratinization may also present with annuli so that scale is the primary lesion. Examples include the porokeratoses and ichthyosis linearis circumflexa of Netherton syndrome.

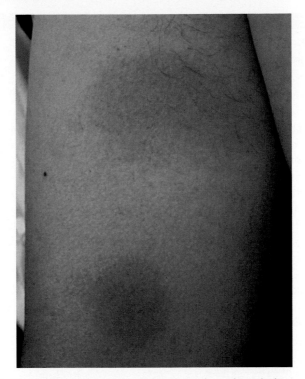

FIGURE 11.1 • Erythema migrans, displaying a light red round macule on the leg.

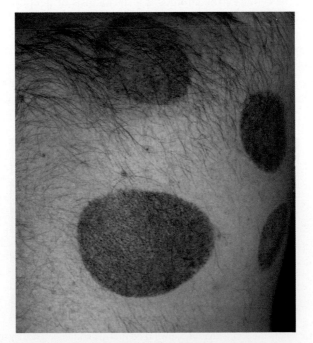

FIGURE 11.2 • A close-up of round purpuric macules following cupping.

Annuli Can Be	
• A shape, such as erythema migrans	• A grouping, such as bedbug bites
• A configuration, such as granuloma annulare	• Made from scale, such as porokeratosis

The center of annular lesions may be clear, or it may have a color. For example, a light brown color may appear as a postinflammatory phenomenon in the center of a plaque of tinea corporis. A dark brown color may be seen in the center of the annuli of "nickels and dimes" of secondary syphilis or in the entity known as lichenoid melanodermatitis. This is a variant of pityriasis alba that may occur in darker skin phototypes. Centrally, in these thin plaques on the face, there is hyperpigmentation, which is surrounded by a ring of hypopigmentation (Figure 11.3). The term *targetoid* implies the presence of two zones of color: a central dusky zone and an outer pink or red zone. Targetoid macules are annular because of their ring-shaped appearance. The presence of the central dusky zone clinches the diagnosis of a targetoid lesion. "Dusky" implies a violaceous color, and this is seen as an interface dermatitis under the microscope. Conceptually, therefore, targetoid lesions can be regarded as a subset of annular lesions.

Clinical Tip
• Annular: all ring-shaped lesions
• Targetoid: a ring-shaped lesion with a central dusky zone

Occasionally, the center of the annulus is a dermatosis or neoplasm and the outer ring is a color change. Examples here include *Woronoff ring*—the finding of hypopigmentation around a plaque of psoriasis (thought to occur in the clearing phase; see Figure 11.4)—and a halo nevus, where a ring of vitiligo-like depigmentation is seen around a regressing nevus.

An etiologic classification of annuli is given in Chapter 1. A useful way to create a morphologic classification is to employ the reaction patterns as seen in Table 11.2.

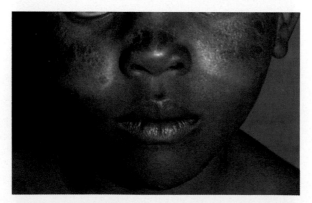

FIGURE 11.3 • Lichenoid melanodermatitis, showing central hyperpigmented scaly thin plaques on the cheeks, each surrounded by a hypopigmented annulus.

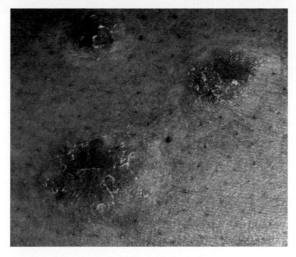

FIGURE 11.4 • Clearing plaque psoriasis, manifesting Woronoff ring.

TABLE 11.2. A Morphologic Classification of Annuli by Reaction Pattern and Pustules

PAPULOSQUAMOUS

- Psoriasis
- Pityriasis rosea
- Lichen planus
- Secondary syphilis
- Tinea corporis
- Candidiasis in chronic mucocutaneous candidiasis
- Porokeratosis
- Erythema annulare centrifugum
- Lichenoid melanodermatitis
- Elastosis perforans serpiginosa
- Keratoacanthoma centrifugum marginatum
- Lupus erythematosus
  - Discoid lupus
  - Subacute cutaneous lupus erythematosus
- Mycosis fungoides
- Leprosy: polar tuberculoid and borderline tuberculoid
- Necrolytic migratory erythema
- Ichthyosis linearis circumflexa
- Erythema gyratum repens
- Tinea imbricata

VESICOBULLOUS

- Linear IgA disease/chronic bullous disease of childhood
- IgA pemphigus
- Bullous pemphigoid, pemphigoid gestationis
- Bullous SLE

ECZEMATOUS

- Seborrheic dermatitis

(Continued)

DERMAL
- Granuloma annulare
  - Annular elastolytic granuloma, granuloma multiforme
- Necrobiosis lipoidica diabeticorum
- Tumid LE
- Morphea
- Tuberculosis: lupus vulgaris
- Leprosy: borderline, borderline lepromatous, lepromatous
- Tertiary syphilis: "nodular syphilide"
- Sarcoid
- Eosinophilic cellulitis

PUSTULES
- Candidal intertrigo
- Tinea corporis
- Majocchi granuloma
- Subcorneal pustular dermatosis
- IgA pemphigus
- Pustular psoriasis:
  - Recurrent circinate erythema of Bloch–Lapiere
  - Impetigo herpetiformis
- Eosinophilic pustular folliculitis of Ofuji

VASCULAR
- Blanching
  - Figurate erythemas
    - Erythema migrans
    - Deep gyrate erythema
    - Erythema marginatum
    - Erythema gyratum repens (in some cases, scale is not a feature)
    - Annular erythema of infancy
  - Annular urticaria, urticaria multiforme
  - Urticarial vasculitis
  - Serum sickness and serum sickness–like reactions
  - Eosinophilic annular erythema
  - Urticarial phase of bullous pemphigoid
  - Pemphigoid gestationis
  - Subacute cutaneous lupus erythematosus: annular, polycyclic variant
  - Eosinophilic cellulitis
- Targetoid
  - Erythema multiforme
  - SJS/TEN
  - DRESS
  - MIRM
  - Active fixed drug eruption
  - Erythema dyschromicum perstans
  - Paraneoplastic pemphigus/paraneoplastic autoimmune multiorgan syndrome
  - Urticaria multiforme
  - Erythema migrans and disseminated Lyme disease
  - Autoimmune progesterone dermatitis
  - Pemphigoid gestationis
  - Kawasaki syndrome
  - Rowell syndrome
- COVID-19 infection
- Nonblanching
  - Purpura annularis telangiectoides (benign pigmented purpura of Majocchi)

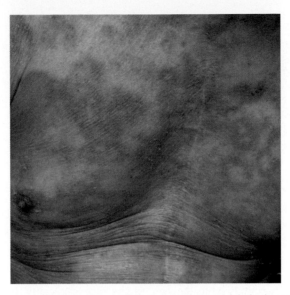

FIGURE 11.5 • Recurrent circinate erythema of Bloch–Lapiere in an adult displaying annular plaques on the chest after resolution of pustules.

The list of papulosquamous diseases that tend to form annuli is lengthy. Plaque psoriasis may form annular shapes (Figure 1.5C). Pustular psoriasis may also be annular. Here, a pustular morphology or a vascular reaction pattern morphology may be seen; the latter occurs when pustules have resolved. This subtype is usually, but not always, seen only in childhood and is known as *recurrent circinate erythema of Bloch–Lapiere* (Figure 11.5). Impetigo herpetiformis, or pustular psoriasis in pregnancy, also tends to form annular arrays of pustules (Figure 11.6). In pityriasis rosea, oval plaques are described as "ovoid medallions." In lichen planus, as mentioned, annular plaques may be composed of papules (a configuration), or they may be de facto plaques with depressed, atrophic centers (a shape; Figure 1.5F). Secondary syphilis is one of the great mimickers, and many morphologic variants are seen.

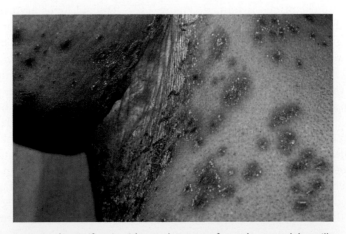

FIGURE 11.6 • Impetigo herpetiformis with annular arrays of pustules around the axilla.

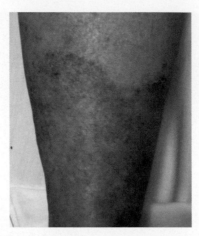

FIGURE 11.7 · Tinea corporis on the leg displaying an active annular border with a superimposed scale.

An annular morphology is typically seen on the face, especially in individuals with darker skin phototypes. These annular plaques typically have an active raised edge and central hyperpigmentation (Figure 1.5B). The *nodular syphilide* of tertiary syphilis presents as pink or red nodules. An annular form with ulceration and crusting of the border has been described. Tinea corporis is classically annular, with scale occurring on top of the annulus (Figures 1.5A and 11.7). There may be concentric annuli centrally representing prior "waves" of active edges as the infection has expanded. In contrast to tinea corporis, the scale of erythema annulare centrifugum "trails" the annular or arcuate rim, so-called "trailing edge" of scale (Figures 1.5E and 6.29). Cutaneous candidiasis in chronic mucocutaneous candidiasis may resemble tinea corporis (Figure 11.8). In porokeratoses, the annulus is formed primarily by scale. This scale has been described as being "thready" or "thread-like" (Figure 6.23). Similarly, in ichthyosis linearis circumflexa, scale is a dominant feature, Here it is a double-edged scale. Plaques may be annular, arcuate, or serpiginous. In elastosis perforans serpiginosa, transepidermal elimination of altered elastic tissue gives rise to compact tiny cores of dried scale. Papules group together to form annuli. In keratoacanthoma centrifugum marginatum, a rare type of keratoacanthoma, the center involutes as the keratoacanthoma enlarges and so an annular plaque is formed (Figure 11.9). Discoid lupus erythematosus is uncommonly annular, but tumid lupus (another form of chronic cutaneous lupus) is typically annular (Figure 9.6). As plaques are smooth, they are classified as being in the dermal reaction pattern. Subacute cutaneous lupus erythematosus is typically annular. It may be a papulosquamous (Figure 1.5D) or vascular reaction pattern (the annular, polycyclic variant). Mycosis fungoides may present with annular, arcuate, polycyclic, and bizarre shapes. Polar tuberculoid and borderline tuberculoid leprosy have one or more scaly, annular plaques. On the lepromatous side of the spectrum, a dermal reaction pattern morphology of annular plaques is seen. In borderline leprosy, plaques have a "swiss cheese" appearance: this implies a sharp cutoff at the inner edge of the annulus that is perpendicular to the cutaneous surface, as seen in Figure 11.10. In necrolytic migratory erythema, plaques are arcuate, annular, serpiginous, and geographic. They are scaly and may display erosions (thus making them classifiable as having a vesicobullous reaction pattern, too). In erythema gyratum repens (EGR) and tinea imbricata

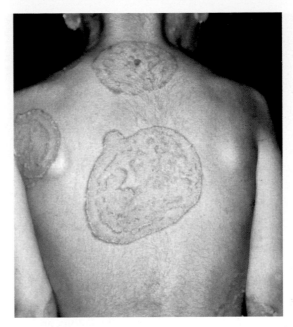

FIGURE 11.8 • Chronic mucocutaneous candidiasis resembling tinea corporis with annular scaly plaques on the back.

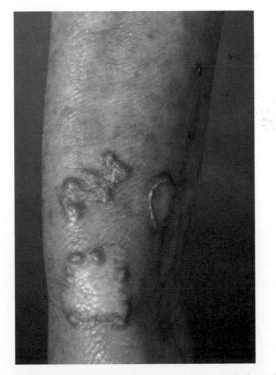

FIGURE 11.9 • Keratoacanthoma centrifugum marginatum with an annular hyperkeratotic plaque on the arm and outlying similar papules, grouped and arranged in an arcuate array.

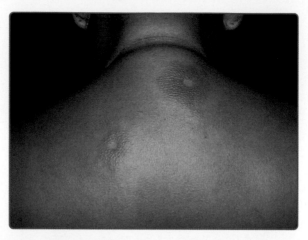

FIGURE 11.10 • Borderline leprosy displaying annular plaques with sharp central borders on the back. (Reproduced with permission from Kang S, Amagai M, Bruckner AL, et al: *Fitzpatrick's Dermatology*, 9th ed. New York, NY: McGraw Hill; 2019.)

(two very rarely encountered dermatoses), concentric annular plaques give rise to a "wood grain" appearance. In EGR, plaques are erythematous, and they may or may not have scale. In tinea imbricata, scale is the predominant feature.

With regard to annular autoimmune vesicobullous disorders, linear IgA disease (also known as chronic bullous disease of childhood) classically presents with annuli of vesicles, termed "clusters of jewels" or "strings of beads" (Figure 7.26). In both the subcorneal pustular dermatosis (SPD) and the intraepidermal neutrophilic (IEN) types of IgA pemphigus, annular configurations are seen. In the SPD type, annular arrays of pustules are seen that resemble subcorneal pustular dermatosis and in the IEN type, resolving lesions with a collarette of scale and the presence of tiny crusts central to the collarette is known as the "sunflower-like" configuration. However, a range of other autoimmune bullous diseases may have annular arrays of vesicles, including bullous pemphigoid, pemphigoid gestationis, and bullous SLE (Figure 7.29). Furthermore, the urticarial plaques seen in the pre-bullous phase of bullous pemphigoid may be annular (Figure 7.22). In the eczematous reaction pattern category, seborrheic dermatitis may appear annular on face or chest, or "petaloid" (like a flower), especially on the central chest.

The classic example of an annular dermatosis in the dermal reaction pattern is granuloma annulare. Smooth papules and plaques of granuloma annulare are typically seen on the extensor extremities (Figure 1.10). Atrophic forms do occur (Figure 9.9). Annular elastolytic granuloma is a subtype of granuloma annulare that occurs on chronically sun-exposed skin (Figures 9.11 and 11.11). Granuloma multiforme is a similar rarer eruption of fewer, larger annuli that occurs on sun-exposed skin. Older lesions of necrobiosis lipoidica typically have yellow centers and reddish borders and therefore can be classified as being annular (Figures 9.12 and 11.12). In active morphea, the center of the plaque may be white, yellow-white, or yellow-brown, and the active annular border is pink or violaceous. Cutaneous infections may form annuli, including lupus vulgaris (a subtype of cutaneous tuberculosis), leprosy, and tertiary syphilis (as detailed above). Sarcoid is another great mimicker of disease, and many subtypes have been recognized, including an annular variant. Finally, in the dermal

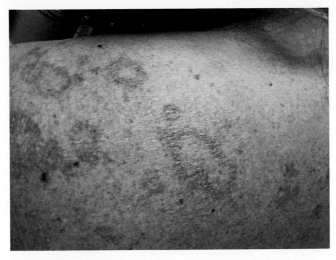

FIGURE 11.11 • A close-up of annular elastolytic giant cell granuloma showing smooth erythematous annular plaques with slight central hypopigmentation.

category is eosinophilic cellulitis (also known as Wells syndrome). This may appear annular and at times, greenish, as it resolves. Eosinophilic cellulitis can also be classified as vascular reaction pattern, depending on its appearance.

The list of pustular dermatoses that typically have annuli is shorter and is seen in Table 11.2. Intertriginous candidiasis characteristically presents with beefy red plaques in the folds with outlying satellite papules and pustules, which, if numerous, form

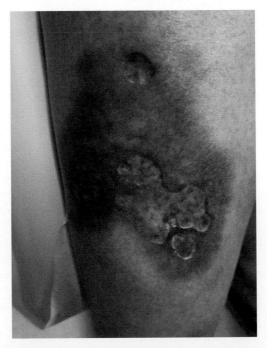

FIGURE 11.12 • Necrobiosis lipoidica with a central yellowish plaque surrounded by a light red rim.

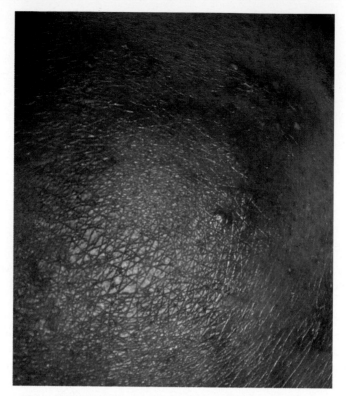

FIGURE 11.13 • Tinea corporis with an annular array of pustules at its border. (Used with permission from Dr. Barry L. Smith, Mount Sinai Beth Israel Medical Center, New York, NY.)

an annular grouping. Tinea corporis may rarely exhibit tiny pustules on its border (Figure 11.13). Majocchi granuloma, a dermatophytic folliculitis, also can present as an annular grouping of pustules and papules, usually on an extremity. In subcorneal pustular dermatosis of Sneddon–Wilkinson, annular arrays of superficial pustules may be seen. This condition affects the folds preferentially. Crops of pustules occur on a base of erythema. A classic finding in this disease is the presence of a "half-and-half" blister— this contains pus on the lower portion and fluid on the upper portion, with a sharp cutoff in between: a pus-fluid line. Eosinophilic pustular folliculitis of Ofuji is a rare dermatosis, most frequently encountered in Japan. Annular arrays of pustules are typical.

In the vascular reaction pattern, the figurate erythemas, urticarial vasculitis, serum sickness and serum sickness–like reactions, and eosinophilic annular erythema all have annuli as a part of their presentation. Erythema migrans typically has an annular (Figure 10.22) or "bull's-eye" appearance, but round, oval, and targetoid plaques, and bullous and hemorrhagic forms are also seen. Urticaria can appear both annular (Figure 10.10) and targetoid. Urticaria multiforme is the designation given to urticaria with this predominant morphology. The urticarial phases of bullous pemphigoid and pemphigoid gestationis commonly have annular shapes. In the nonblanching category, consider the diagnosis of purpura annularis telangiectoides—an annular variant of benign pigmented purpura.

Another useful classification of annular is by color, as is seen in Table 11.3. As discussed in Chapter 3, differentiating between brown and gray for postinflammatory

TABLE 11.3. Annuli by Color

PINK OR RED
- Most conditions listed in Table 11.1

BROWN
- Postinflammatory change from annular dermatoses such as tinea corporis and pityriasis rosea
- Annular sarcoidosis may appear brown or red-brown
- Granuloma annulare may be pink, red, or red-brown
- Secondary syphilis: includes "nickels and dimes" appearance on the face
- Tertiary syphilis: presents as copper-colored coalescing papules and nodules that form annuli and arcuate and serpiginous configurations

WHITE
- Tuberculoid, borderline tuberculoid, and borderline leprosy
- Morphea
- Lichenoid melanodermatitis
- Woronoff ring of psoriasis
- Halo nevus

YELLOW
- Pus
  - Candida intertrigo
  - Tinea corporis, cruris
  - Majocchi granuloma
  - Subcorneal pustular dermatosis
  - IgA pemphigus, SPD type
  - Pustular psoriasis
    - Recurrent circinate erythema of Bloch–Lapiere
    - Impetigo herpetiformis
  - Eosinophilic pustular folliculitis of Ofuji
- Lipid
  - Necrobiosis lipoidica
- Altered connective tissue
  - Active morphea

PURPLE
- Lichen planus—papules may coalesce to form annular plaques, or plaques may be depressed centrally, which renders an annular appearance
- Targetoid lesions—see differential diagnosis in Table 11.2

GRAY
- Targetoid lesions—see differential diagnosis in Table 11.2
- Postinflammatory annular macules that follow the resolution of an interface dermatitis, such as lichen planus, take on a gray color
  - Lichen planus

GREEN
- Eosinophilic cellulitis—fading plaques may have an annular and a greenish appearance

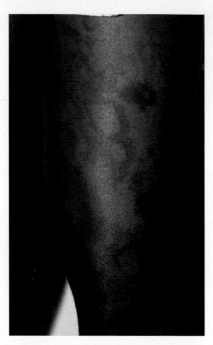

FIGURE 11.14 · Annular and other figurate hyperpigmented macules after resolution of urticarial vasculitis.

macules is a useful distinction that holds diagnostic information. Annular plaques may leave postinflammatory brown annular macules in their wake. Examples include tinea corporis, pityriasis rosea, or urticarial vasculitis (Figure 11.14). The presence of postinflammatory gray macules implies the presence of a preceding interface dermatitis, such as lichen platevnus.

The list of *tender* annuli is shorter and comprises two targetoid entities: Stevens–Johnson syndrome (SJS) and toxic epidermal necrolysis (TEN). The atypical targets of SJS/TEN are tender. Active fixed drug eruption may be tender.

> **Clinical Tip** If an annular eruption is tender, think SJS/TEN or fixed drug eruption.

ARCUATE

The term *arcuate* means an incomplete ring, or arc. The term *arciform* can be used synonymously. Arcuate plaques usually accompany annuli. Examples of eruptions that frequently manifest an arcuate morphology are detailed in Table 11.4. These include erythema annulare centrifugum and deep gyrate erythema (Figure 10.21), urticaria multiforme, urticarial vasculitis, serum sickness/serum sickness–like reactions, erythema marginatum, erythema gyratum repens, eosinophilic annular erythema, annular erythema of infancy, and necrolytic migratory erythema. All these entities fall into the vascular reaction pattern, except for necrolytic migratory erythema, which can be classified with a papulosquamous or vesicobullous reaction pattern. Tumid lupus (Figure 11.15) and the annular polycyclic variant of subacute cutaneous lupus also may have arcuate plaques. Early erythema annulare centrifugum has a vascular reaction

TABLE 11.4. Arcuate Dermatoses by Reaction Pattern and Pustules

PAPULOSQUAMOUS
- Erythema annulare centrifugum
- Tinea corporis
- Necrolytic migratory erythema

VESICOBULLOUS
- Necrolytic migratory erythema

DERMAL
- Tumid lupus
- Subacute cutaneous lupus

VASCULAR
- Erythema annulare centrifugum
- Deep gyrate erythema
- Urticaria multiforme
- Urticarial vasculitis
- Serum sickness/serum sickness–like reactions
- Erythema maginatum
- Erythema gyratum repens
- Eosinophilic annular erythema
- Annular erythema of infancy
- Bedbug bites

PUSTULES
- Candidal intertrigo
- Tinea corporis
- Majocchi granuloma
- Subcorneal pustular dermatosis
- IgA pemphigus
- Pustular psoriasis:
  - Recurrent circinate erythema of Bloch–Lapiere
  - Impetigo herpetiformis
- Eosinophilic pustular folliculitis of Ofuji

pattern, but when the trailing edge of scale develops, it can be classified as a papulosquamous reaction pattern. Erythema gyratum repens may or may not have scale (vascular or papulosquamous reaction pattern). In the center of a large plaque of tinea corporis, arcuate scaly plaques may be seen (papulosquamous; see Figure 1.5A). Finally, arcuate groupings of insect bites may also be classified as a vascular reaction pattern.

> **Clinical Tip** Many annular dermatoses have arcuate shapes and configurations as part of their presentation.

CONCENTRIC

The term *concentric* implies the presence of one ring inside another. Dermatoses that classically have concentric rings include tinea corporis (or there may be arcuate plaques centrally; this would be a papulosquamous reaction pattern), erythema gyratum repens, and tinea imbricata. Erythema gyratum repens and tinea imbricata are very rare

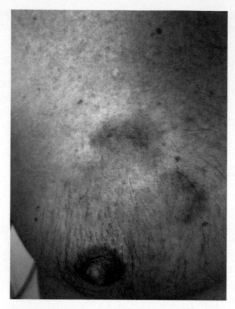

FIGURE 11.15 • Tumid lupus displaying an arcuate erythematous plaque on the chest.

but important "do not miss" dermatoses. Erythema annulare centrifugum will exhibit a concentric configuration more rarely.

Concentric:

- Tinea corporis: papulosquamous
- Tinea imbricata: papulosquamous
- Erythema annulare centrifugum: vascular, papulosquamous
- Erythema gyratum repens: vascular, papulosquamous

POLYCYCLIC

Polycyclic or "many rings" refers to the shape formed by a confluence of annuli. Many of the same dermatoses mentioned under the "Arcuate" heading form polycyclic rings. Examples include urticaria multiforme, urticarial vasculitis, serum sickness and serum sickness–like reactions, deep gyrate erythema (Figure 10.22), and necrolytic migratory erythema. The annular and polycyclic variants of subacute cutaneous lupus erythematosus (SCLE) present with annular and polycyclic vascular reaction pattern plaques.

Polycyclic:

- Vascular reaction pattern
  - Urticaria multiforme
  - Urticarial vasculitis
  - Serum sickness and serum sickness–like reactions
  - Deep gyrate erythema
  - SCLE: annular and polycyclic variant
- Papulosquamous or vesicobullous
  - Necrolytic migratory erythema

GYRATE

Gyrate refers to lesions that spiral around each other. Erythema gyratum repens and tinea imbricata classically exhibit this phenomenon. As mentioned previously, erythema gyratum repens may have a vascular or papulosquamous reaction pattern. For example, tinea imbricata has a papulosquamous reaction pattern.

> **Gyrate:**
>
> - Erythema gyratum repens: vascular or papulosquamous
> - Tinea imbricata: papulosquamous

FIGURATE

Figurate, or "figure-forming," refers to eruptions that form more than one shape or configuration simultaneously. The figurate erythemas, urticarial vasculitis, serum sickness and serum sickness–like reactions, eosinophilic annular erythema, mycosis fungoides, and necrolytic migratory erythema, fall into this category.

> **Figurate:**
>
> - Figurate erythemas:
>   - Erythema migrans
>   - Erythema annulare centrifugum
>   - Erythema marginatum
>   - Erythema gyratum repens
> - Annular erythema of infancy
> - Urticarial vasculitis
> - Eosinophilic annular erythema
> - Necrolytic migratory erythema
> - Mycosis fungoides

LINEAR

Many inherited and acquired diseases may present with a linear morphology. Lines may be a shape (such as in red dermographism; see Figure 10.26), a configuration (such as in confluent eczematous papules forming a line in poison ivy), or a grouping (as is seen in lymphocutaneous spread in sporotrichosis, for example).

> **Lines Can Be:**
>
> - A shape, such as red dermographism
> - A configuration, such as confluent papules of poison ivy
> - A grouping, such as lymphocutaneous spread, as in sporotrichosis

There are numerous approaches that can assist in creating differential diagnoses of linear lesions. A useful starting point is to determine whether the lines are created by external factors (so-called "outside job") or whether they follow inherent anatomic structures or embryonal developmental lines (so-called "inside job").

How Linear Lesions Are Created

- "Outside job"—lines are created by external factors
- "Inside job"—lines follow inherent anatomic structures or embryonal developmental lines

Table 11.5 classifies linear lesions in the above fashion. Of note, some conditions have components of both "outside" and "inside jobs". Examples include when external

TABLE 11.5. An Approach to Linear Lesions

"OUTSIDE JOB"
- Trauma, chemical exposure
  - Dermatitis artefacta
  - Vibices
  - Black dermographism
  - Berloque dermatitis/phytophotodermatitis
- Infestation
  - Scabies: burrows
  - Cutaneous larva migrans
  - Larva currens
  - Bug bites ("breakfast–lunch–dinner")
- Trauma and preexisting or new rash infection
  - Dermographism
  - Red dermographism
  - Allergic contact dermatitis: poison ivy
  - Koebner phenomenon
    - Psoriasis
    - Lichen planus
    - Vitiligo
    - Leukocytoclastic vasculitis
    - Kaposi sarcoma
  - Autoinnoculation
    - Mollusca
    - Flat warts
  - Flagellate erythemas
    - Flagellate erythema of chemotherapy
    - Dermatomyositis
    - Adult-onset Still's disease
    - Shiitake mushroom dermatitis

"INSIDE JOB" *
- Veins
  - Thrombophlebitis
  - Mondor Syndrome
  - DVT: linear cord
- Lymphatics
  - Lymphangitis
  - Lymphangitic spread of metastases (eg, carcinoma erysipeloides)
  - Lymphocutaneous (sporotrichoid) spread
    - Infectious
      - *Mycobacterium marinum*

(Continued)

TABLE 11.5. An Approach to Linear Lesions (continued)

"INSIDE JOB" (CONT.)

- *Sporothrix schenckii*
- *Francisella tularensis*
- *Leishmania peruvii*
- *Burkholderia mallei*: glanders: necrotic abscesses
- Cat scratch disease: *Bartonella henselae*
- Rarer; seldom seen:
  - Primary inoculation blastomycosis
  - Primary inoculation TB
  - Meliodosis
  - Soduku
  - Nocardia
- Neoplastic
  - Malignant melanoma: in-transit metastases
- Cutaneous sensory nerves
  - Dermatomal: zoster
  - Pseudodermatomal: zosteriform metastases
- Futcher lines
- Linea nigra
- Following Blaschko lines
  - X-linked dominant disease
    - Incontinentia pigmenti
    - Focal dermal hypoplasia (Goltz)
    - Chondrodysplasia punctata
    - CHILD
    - Oral–facial–digital syndrome type I (whorled alopecia)
  - X-linked recessive disease
    - Anhidrotic ectodermal dysplasia
    - Familial cutaneous amyloidosis, Partington type—here, streaks of hyperpigmentation resembling incontinentia pigmenti are seen, but with amyloid deposition
- Autosomal mosaicism
  - Hypomelanosis of Ito
  - Linear and whorled hypermelanosis
  - Ichthyosis hystrix, epidermal nevus syndrome
- Localized
  - Nevus depigmentosus
  - Segmental vitiligo
  - Segmental neurofibromatosis (type 5)
  - Nevus of Ito, nevus of Ota
  - Segmental Darier disease, Hailey–Hailey
  - Linear verrucous epidermal nevus, ILVEN
  - Nevus sebaceous
  - Lichen striatus
  - Linear lichen planus
  - Linear porokeratosis
  - Linear Darier disease
  - Linear morphea
  - Lymphangioma circumscriptum/angiokeratoma circumscriptum
  - Angioma serpiginosum
  - Benign tumors: glomus, trichoepitheliomas, pilar leiomyomas, eccrine spiradenomas

*Following anatomic structures or developmental lines.

trauma induces an internal disease (like the Koebner phenomenon in psoriasis), or when an infection is inoculated from the outside environment and follows an inherent anatomic structure (the lymphocutaneous spread pattern of sporotrichosis and sporotrichoid conditions). These conditions have been classified as "outside job" and "inside job" respectively in this classification scheme, as per the definitions provided here.

"Outside jobs" can be conceptualized as being created in three ways:

1. They may result from scratching, from trauma of any kind, or from chemical reactions (such as phytophotodermatitis or black dermographism). In these situations, lines are induced purely by mechanical or chemical trauma without any contribution of an inherent or induced dermatosis. Striae can also be classified in this category; mechanical stretching of skin gives rise to the linear (and curvilinear) dermal scars seen (Figure 11.16). In phytophotodermatitis, contact of the skin with furocoumarins induces phototoxicity that mainfests as erythematous and brown linear and geometric macules and thin plaques (Figures 1.6A and 11.17). In black dermographism, pigmented metallic particles from jewelry or other metal objects adhere to personal-care products on the epidermis and impart a black or gray color.

2. Superficial infestations, such as cutaneous larva migrans (CLM), larva currens, or scabies may produce lines as they migrate through the epidermis (CLM) or dermis (larva currens), or create burrows (scabies; see Figure 1.6B). Linear arrays of bug bites, such as bedbug bites, are also included in this category.

3. External trauma can induce an inherent dermatosis (such as that seen in the Koebner phenomenon or dermatographism) or a new dermatosis (such as inoculation of urushiol from poison ivy causing allergic contact dermatitis; see Figures 8.4 and 8.6). In the Koebner phenomenon, a preexisting dermatosis appears in sites of trauma on the skin. A handful of dermatoses have such a propensity, including psoriasis (Figure 11.18), lichen planus (Figure 1.9), vitiligo (Figure 11.19), leukocytoclastic vasculitis (Figure 10.27), and Kaposi sarcoma (Figure 11.20).

The Koebner Phenomenon May Be Seen In:

- Psoriasis
- Lichen planus
- Vitiligo
- Leukocytoclastic vasculitis
- Kaposi sarcoma

Dermographism is the induction of linear urticarial plaques at sites of scratching or superficial trauma to the skin. It is a type of superficial pressure urticaria and may occur with or without regular hives. Autoinoculation of viral papules, such as molluscum contagiosum (Figure 11.21) or warts, through shaving, for example, may cause linear groupings. Red dermographism is the formation of linear macules at sites of superficial trauma. This is seen in partially treated urticaria or dermographism. Flagellate dermatoses are an interesting category. The term *flagellate* means "whip-like." Although not conclusively proven, it is thought that scratching is instrumental in the pathogenesis of this group of diseases as these dermatoses display linear plaques that are usually itchy in areas that the patient can reach. Therefore, the flagellate erythemas can also be conceived of as an "outside job" with an underlying inherent dermatosis. Flagellate erythema may be seen in four situations:

i. **Flagellate erythema of chemotherapy** (Figure 10.25): The diagnosis of flagellate drug eruption is usually made in the context of a patient receiving chemotherapeutic agents. Bleomycin is most commonly implicated, but peplomycin (a bleomycin derivative) and docetaxel have also been reported as causes. The causative medication may have been administered intravenously or intramuscularly. Flagellate erythema has also been reported after intralesional bleomycin injections for plantar warts or after intrapleural or intraperitoneal instillation. Flagellate erythema is usually itchy. It may begin within 12–24 hours of medication administration, or its onset may be delayed for up to 6 months. Initially there are erythematous, or occasionally violaceous, linear streaks that may give the skin the appearance of having been whipped. These linear streaks may be urticarial or papulovesicular. The eruption classically occurs on the chest, upper back, and shoulders, and is also reported to occur on the arms and legs. When the erythema fades, it leaves hyperpigmentation in the same configuration that may persist for months. In some patients, the pruritus and erythema are minimal, and hyperpigmentation is the predominant presenting sign.

ii. **Dermatomyositis:** Flagellate erythema is a rare dermatologic manifestation in dermatomyositis. In one series, it was present in 5% of 84 patients. The linear streaks are more erythematous and violaceous, and less brown than those in bleomycin-induced flagellate erythema. They are also pruritic and are usually raised. They are typically located on the trunk.

iii. **Adult-onset Still's disease:** This is an uncommon acute or subacute systemic illness that presents with a high spiking fever, a sore throat, and a rash. The characteristic eruption consists of salmon-pink macules that wax and wane with the fever. The eruption is usually more prominent in sites of pressure. The Koebner phenomenon may be a feature. More rarely, a chronic eruption eventuates. This may resemble flagellate erythema. There are linear itchy reddish and brownish plaques that occur truncally and are persistent.

iv. **Shiitake-mushroom dermatitis:** This is most frequently seen in Japan and displays flagellate erythema. The typical eruption occurs 24–48 hours after eating raw or partially cooked shiitake mushrooms. Clinically, there are erythematous pruritic papules that coalesce to form linear plaques on the trunk, on the extremities, and sometimes on the face. Areas that the patient cannot reach are spared. The associated hyperpigmentation is short-lived. The eruption is thought to occur secondarily to a reaction to lentinan, which is a polysaccharide with antitumor properties that is found in the mushroom.

Differential Diagnosis of Flagellate Erythema

- Flagellate erythema of chemotherapy
- Dermatomyositis
- Adult-onset Still's disease
- Shiitake mushroom dermatitis

"Inside jobs" are those that follow anatomic structures (such as veins, lymphatics, and cutaneous sensory nerves) or embryonal developmental lines (such as pigmentary demarcation lines and Blaschko lines). Thrombophlebitis is inflammation of superficial veins and may manifest with a linear palpable or visible cord or a linear array of plaques if more

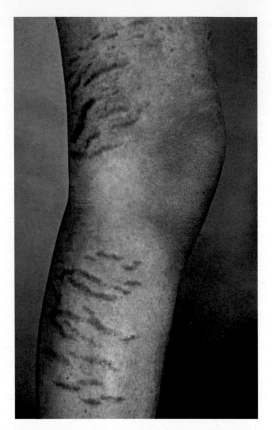

FIGURE 11.16 • Striae displaying linear and wavy reddish atrophic plaques on the leg.

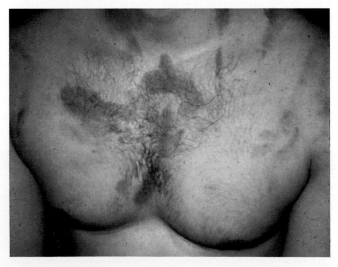

FIGURE 11.17 • Berloque dermatitis displaying linear and geometric erythematous plaques on the upper chest.

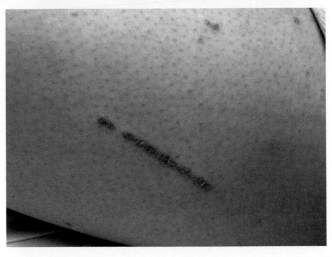

FIGURE 11.18 · Koebner phenomenon in psoriasis, showing a pink scaly linear plaque on the lateral thigh.

extensive (Figure 11.22). Mondor syndrome is superficial thrombophlebitis of the anterior chest wall. Deep-vein thrombosis may sometimes be palpated as a deep linear cord on the calf. Lymphangitis is a red streak emanating from a site of infection, such as cellulitis, usually on a limb. Lymphatic infiltration by malignant cells may cause an erysipelas-like appearance (carcinoma erysipeloides in the case of breast cancer, for example). When this phenomenon occurs off the breast, a broad pink and violaceous plaque with linear borders may be seen (Figure 11.23). Some infections, such as sporotrichosis and *Mycobacterium marinum*, may spread along lymphatics after their initial inoculation. Dermal or crusted nodules are seen in a linear array that follows lymphatics. Lymphatics run in a loose spiral around the limbs and this morphology may therefore seen (Figure 11.24).

During embryonal development, cutaneous sensory nerves migrate separately to supply so-called "dermatomes." A dermatomal map is shown in Figure 11.25. It is thought that cutaneous blood vessels develop in the same manner.

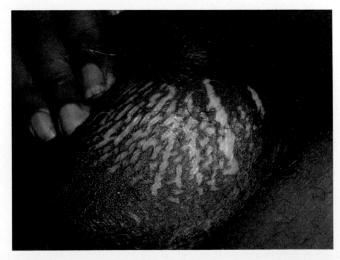

FIGURE 11.19 · Koebner phenomenon in vitiligo, displaying linear white and pinkish macules on the scrotum.

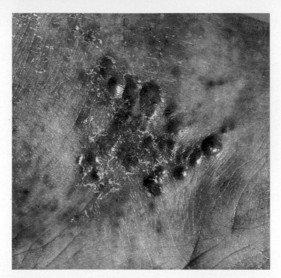

FIGURE 11.20 • Koebner phenomenon in Kaposi sarcoma, displaying linear and geometric purple plaques on the calf. (Reproduced with permission from Goldsmith LA, Katz SI, Gilchrest BA, et al: *Fitzpatrick's Dermatology in General Medicine*, 8th ed. New York, NY: McGraw Hill; 2012.)

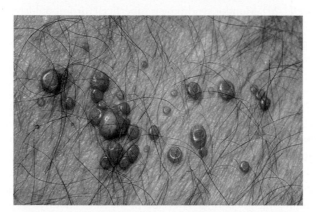

FIGURE 11.21 • A close-up of a linear groupings and clusters of mollusca from autoinoculation. (Image appears with permission from VisualDx. Copyright VisualDx.)

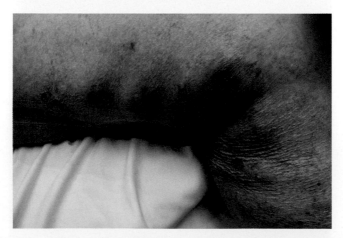

FIGURE 11.22 • Superficial thrombophlebitis displaying a linear array of erythematous nodules on the leg.

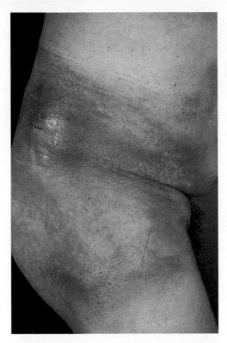

FIGURE 11.23 • Lymphatic infiltration of colon cancer, showing deep pink and somewhat violaceous plaques on the flank and upper thigh.

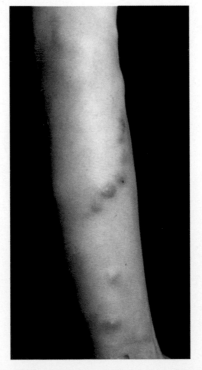

FIGURE 11.24 • Sporotrichosis displaying a loose spiral of nodules on the arm.

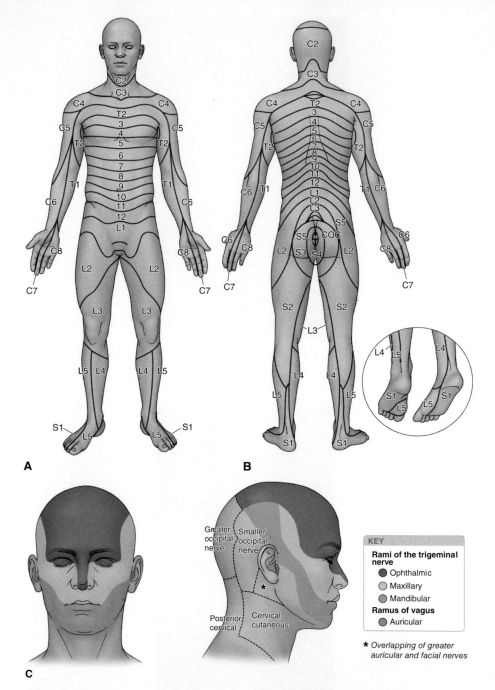

FIGURE 11.25 • Schematic diagrams of the dermatomes. (Reproduced with pemission from Wolff K, Johnson RA, Saavedra AP, et al: *Fitzpatrick's Color Atlas and Synopsis of Clinical Dermatology*, 8th ed. New York, NY: McGraw Hill; 2017.)

The dorsal aspect of the body generally is more pigmented than the ventral surface, and the difference between the two areas is more noticeable in darker skin phototypes. Lines of demarcation that mark pigmentary differences between dorsal and ventral surfaces of the body, are known as *Futcher lines* or *Voigt lines* (Figure 1.6D.). These may be appreciated on the anterior surface of the arms extending horizontally onto the medial chest, or on the posterior aspect of the thighs curving superiorly toward the perineal region and stopping inferiorly at the knee, or sometimes the ankle. Less commonly, vertical lines may be seen paraspinally and hypopigmented lines or patches parasternally.

Dermatoses following Blaschko lines (Figure 11.26A,B) are termed *blaschkoid*. These lines are S-shaped on the ventral surface of the body and V-shaped near the spine. They are linear and whorled. In the developing embryo, keratinocytes proliferate

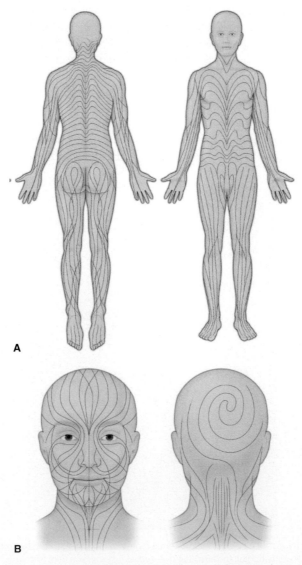

FIGURE 11.26 · Schematic representations of Blaschko lines on (A) the body and (B) the face and scalp.

directionally along Blaschko lines. A note about Blaschko lines and segments: Mela-noblasts migrate from the neural crest as single cells and then proliferate and reach the epidermis. Many developmental hyper- and hypopigmented conditions such as hypomelanosis of Ito and linear and whorled hyperpmelanosis follow Blaschko lines. In inherited pigmentary conditions, a block (segmental) pattern is sometimes seen. It is believed that the stage of development of any abnormality is important in this regard and perhaps the block pattern occurs if the aberrant development is prior to melanocyte migration to the epidermis. An example here is segmental vitiligo, which may adopt a block pattern or may look more blaschkoid. As mentioned previously, cutaneous nerves migrate separately in dermatomes during embryonal development. It is thought that cutaneous blood vessels develop in the same manner.

In blaschkoid dermatoses, one or many Blaschko lines may be involved. In X-linked dominant and recessive diseases, functional or actual mosaicism imparts the appearance of alternating Blaschko lines. Incontinentia pigmenti is an example of an X-linked dominant disease. Initially, there is a vesicular stage, where linear configurations of vesicles on erythematous bases are seen in the first few months of life, especially on the limbs (Figure 11.27). This is superseded by the second stage, known as the verrucous stage, where verrucous papules and plaques are seen on the limbs and trunk (Figure 11.28). Ultimately, in childhood, these flatten and the hyperpigmented stage occurs (third stage; Figure 11.28). In some patients, a fourth hypopigmented stage is seen in later childhood and beyond.

Autosomes may also exhibit mosaicism and autosomal dominantly inherited conditions and therefore also exhibit blaschkoid configurations. Ichthyosis

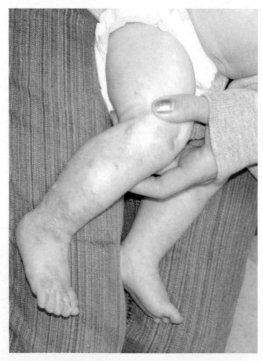

FIGURE 11.27 · The vesicular stage of incontinentia pigmenti displaying a blaschkoid configuration of vesicles, bullae, and crusting on the arm. (Reproduced with permission from Rimoin D, Pyeritz R, Korf B: *Emery and Rimoin's Principles and Practice of Medical Genetics*, 6th ed. Oxford, UK: Elsevier/Academic Press; 2013.)

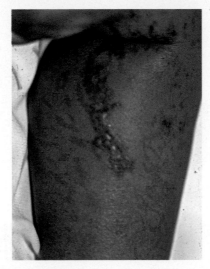

FIGURE 11.28 • The verrucous and hyperpigmented stages of incontinentia pigmenti, with a resolving verrucous plaque and linear hyperpigmentation in Blaschko lines on the leg.

hystrix is a widespread epidermal nevus. Patterning follows a blaschkoid configuration (Figure 11.29). Linear Darier disease, linear Hailey–Hailey disease, and linear porokeratosis are further examples of this phenomenon. Postzygotic mutations in one or more Blaschko lines may occur, giving rise to a more limited picture. Examples include lichen striatus (Figure 11.30), linear psoriasis (Figures 11.31 and 11.32), linear lichen planus (Figure 11.33), and inflammatory linear verrucous epidermal nevus (ILVEN;

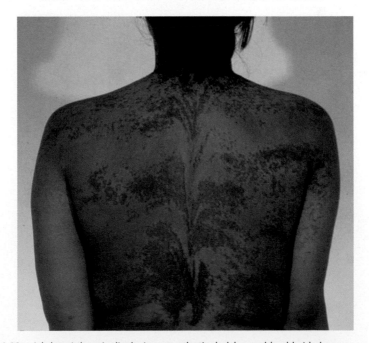

FIGURE 11.29 • Ichthyosis hystrix displaying acanthotic dark brown blaschkoid plaques.

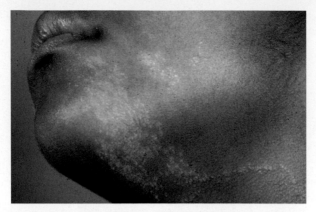

FIGURE 11.30 • Lichen striatus showing a blaschkoid configuration of hypopigmented fine papules on the neck and chin.

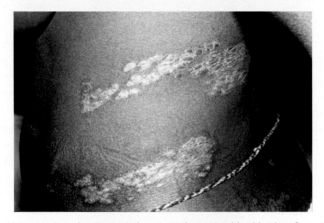

FIGURE 11.31 • Linear psoriasis showing typical psoriatic plaques in a blaschkoid configuration on the flank.

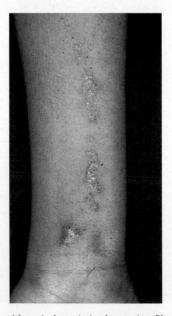

FIGURE 11.32 • Linear psoriasis with typical psoriatic plaques in a Blaschko line on the arm.

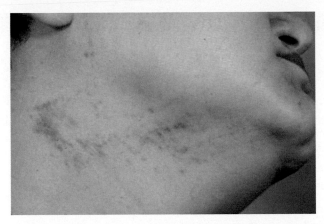

FIGURE 11.33 • Resolving linear lichen planus showing a blaschkoid configuration of brown and grayish macules on the neck.

see Figure 11.34). Linear morphea (Figure 4.8D) and linear atrophoderma of Moulin are two further examples here; the latter appears as a linear arrangement of slightly depressed plaques that resemble atrophoderma of Pasini and Pierini.

A note about terminology: Blaschkoid conditions are sometimes referred to as having a blaschkoid *distribution*. In this context, *distribution* refers to the body location of an eruption, and so the term blaschkoid *configuration* is arguably the more accurate term, except perhaps when the dermatosis is widespread and involves many Blaschko lines. Similarly, eruptions that follow dermatomes have been designated as having a dermatomal *distribution*, whereas, strictly speaking, this is a *configuration*.

The more traditional etiologic or morphologic classifications to the linear differential diagnosis are also useful. An etiologic approach is displayed in Table 11.6. Morphologically speaking, primary lesions can be used as the diagnostic determinant (Table 11.7), as can color (Table 11.8) and the reaction patterns (Table 11.9).

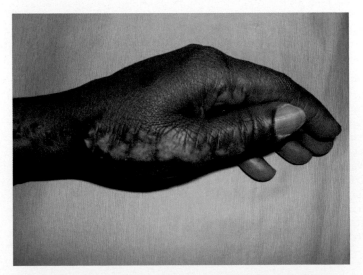

FIGURE 11.34 • Lichenified ILVEN, showing a linear lichenified plaque on the hand.

The Linear Differential Diagnosis

The linear differential diagnosis

"Outside job"   "Inside job"

Trauma/chemical   Infestation   Trauma + rash/infection   Following anatomic lines:

Dermographism ◄──────────────────┐   Veins

Koebner   Lymphatics
phenomenon ◄──────────────────────┤   Cutaneous sensory nerves

                                                              Embryonal developmental lines
Plant and
other contact   Flagellate
dermatitis   Autoinoculation   erythemas

TABLE 11.6. Linear Dermatoses by Etiologic Classification

INHERITED

- Futcher lines
- Incontinentia pigmenti
- Focal dermal hypoplasia
- Chondrodysplasia punctata
- CHILD
- Oral–facial–digital syndrome type I
- Anhidrotic ectodermal dysplasia
- Familial cutaneous amyloidosis, Partington type
- Nevus depigmentosus
- Hypomelanosis of Ito
- Angioma serpiginosum
- Any disorder in Blaschko lines implies an underlying inherited disorder/susceptibility of the clones within the affected line (eg, linear lichen planus)

ACQUIRED

- Infectious
  - Bacterial
    - Glanders
    - Meliodosis
    - Nocardia
    - Tularemia
- Mycobacterial
  - *Mycobacterium marinum*
  - Primary inoculation TB
- Rickettsial
  - *Bartonella henselae*

(Continued)

TABLE 11.6. Linear Dermatoses by Etiologic Classification (continued)

ACQUIRED (CONT.)
- Spirochetal
  - Soduku
- Viral
  - Herpes zoster
  - Flat warts
  - Molluscum
- Fungal
  - *Sporothrix schenckii*
  - Primary inoculation blastomycosis
- Protozoal
  - *Leishmania peruvii*
- Parasitic
  - Scabetic burrows
  - Cutaneous larva migrans
  - Larva currens
- Inflammatory
- Allergic contact dermatitis, such as to poison ivy
- Phytophotodermatitis
- Dermographism
- Koebner phenomenon in psoriasis, lichen planus, leukocytoclastic vasculitis, and vitiligo
- Flagellate erythemas: dermatomyositis, shiitake mushroom dermatitis, adult-onset Still's disease
- Segmental vitiligo
- Linear array of bites from an arthropod
- Linear morphea
- Dermatomyositis: arising from elbows or knees
- Neoplastic
- Segmental: neurofibromatosis, cutaneous leiomyomas
- Koebner phenomenon in Kaposi sarcoma
- Benign tumors in Blaschko lines: glomus, trichoepitheliomas, pilar leiomyomas
- Lymphangitic metastases: carcinoma lymphangiectoides, carcinoma erysipeloides
- Zosteriform metastases
- Lymphatic spread of melanoma metastases
- Drug-Related
- Flagellate erythema of chemotherapy
- Chemical
- Black dermographism
- Hormonal
- Linea nigra
- Self-Induced
- Dermatitis artefacta

TABLE 11.7. A Morphologic Classification of Linear Dermatoses by Primary Lesion

MACULES
- Vitiligo: Koebner phenomenon, or the segmental variant
- Nevus depigmentosus
- Hypomelanosis of Ito
- Incontinentia pigmenti: fourth stage
- Futcher lines
- Linea nigra
- Incontinentia pigmenti: third stage
- Familial cutaneous amyloidosis, Partington type
- Linear and whorled hypermelanosis
- Nevus of Ito
- Nevus of Ota
- Black dermographism
- Angioma serpiginosum
- Phytophotodermatitis
- Vibices

PAPULES
- Flat warts
- Molluscum
- Scabies
- Lichen striatus
- Linear Darier disease
- Glomus tumors
- Trichoepitheliomas
- Eccrine spiradenomas
- Arthropod assault
- Leukocytoclastic vasculitis

PAPULES AND PLAQUES
- Lichen planus
- Psoriasis
- Incontinentia pigmenti: verrucous stage
- Lymphangioma circumscriptum
- Kaposi sarcoma

PLAQUES
- Dermographism
- Cutaneous larva migrans
- Larva currens
- Thrombophlebitis, Mondor disease, deep venous thrombosis
- Lymphangitis
- Lymphangitic spread of a carcinoma, such as carcinoma lymphangiectoides, carcinoma erysipeloides
- Chondrodysplasia punctata, CHILD
- Ichthyosis hystrix
- Linear porokeratosis
- Angiokeratoma circumscriptum

NODULES
- *Mycobacterium marinum*
- *Sporothrix schenckii*

(Continued)

TABLE 11.7. A Morphologic Classification of Linear Dermatoses by Primary Lesion (continued)

NODULES (CONT.)

- *Francisella tularensis*
- Cat scratch disease: *Bartonella henselae*
- Neurofibromas
- Eccrine spiradenomas
- Metastases: lymphangitic spread
- Focal dermal hypoplasia
- Kaposi sarcoma

VESICLES

- Allergic contact dermatitis
- Incontinentia pigmenti: first phase
- Herpes zoster

PUSTULES

- Fire ant bites

TABLE 11.8. Linear Dermatoses by Color

PINK AND RED

- Phytophotodermatitis (also geometric)
- Allergic contact dermatitis to poison ivy
- Dermatitis artefacta
- Vibices
- Koebner phenomenon
  - Psoriasis
  - Lichen planus: pink in lighter skin phototypes
  - Leukocytoclastic vasculitis
- Bug bites ("breakfast–lunch–dinner")
- Scabies: burrows
- Cutaneous larva migrans
- Larva currens
- Flagellate erythemas
  - Dermatomyositis
  - Adult Still's disease
  - Shiitake mushroom dermatitis
  - Bleomycin-induced flagellate erythema
- Along blood vessels, lymphatics
  - Thrombophlebitis, Mondor disease
  - Lymphangitis
  - Lymphocutaneous spread (see list in Table 11.5)
- Cutaneous sensory nerves
  - Dermatomal: zoster
  - Pseudodermatomal: zosteriform metastases
- Following Blaschko lines
  - First and second stages of incontinentia pigmenti
- Segmental
  - Segmental Darier disease, Hailey–Hailey disease

(Continued)

TABLE 11.8. Linear Dermatoses by Color (continued)

BROWN
- Phytophotodermatitis (also geometric)
- Serpentine supravenous hyperpigmentation from chemotherapy (also serpentine)
- Futcher's lines
- Linea nigra
- Black dermographism
- Flagellate erythema
  - Flagellate erythema of chemotherapy
  - Adult-onset Still's disease
- Blaschko lines (also whorled)
  - Linear and whorled hypermelanosis
  - Third stage of incontinentia pigmenti
  - Epidermal nevi and systematized verrucous nevus (ichthyosis hystrix)
  - Familial cutaneous amyloidosis, Partington type
- Segmental
  - Nevus of Ito
  - Nevus of Ota

WHITE
- Blaschko lines (also whorled)
  - Nevoid hypopigmentation (hypomelanosis of Ito, nevus depigmentosus)
  - Fourth stage of incontinentia pigmenti
  - Lichen striatus
- Segmental
  - Segmental vitiligo
  - Tuberous sclerosis
  - Nevus depigmentosus
- Koebner phenomenon
  - As seen in vitiligo
- Autoinoculation
  - Flat warts
- Striae, and other scars (secondary lesions)

YELLOW
- Elastic tissue
  - Linear focal elastosis
  - Linear morphea
- Pus
  - Fire ant bites
  - Herpes zoster with pustules
- Lipid
  - Linear nevus sebaceus
  - Linear nevus sebaceous syndrome

PURPLE SPECTRUM
- Koebner phenomenon
  - Lichen planus
  - Leukocytoclastic vasculitis
  - Kaposi sarcoma
- Blaschko lines
  - Linear lichen planus

(Continued)

TABLE 11.8. Linear Dermatoses by Color (continued)

PURPLE SPECTRUM (CONT.)
- Along lymphatics
  - In-transit metastases of melanoma
- Other linear configurations
  - Angioma serpiginosum
  - Linear erythema over joints in dermatomyositis
  - Flagellate erythema of dermatomyositis

BLACK
- Black dermographism
- In-transit metastases of melanoma

TABLE 11.9. Linear Dermatoses by Reaction Pattern

PAPULOSQUAMOUS
- "Outside job"
  - Dermatitis artefacta
- Autoinoculation
  - Flat warts
- Koebner phenomenon
  - Psoriasis
  - Lichen planus
- Blaschko lines
  - Incontinentia pigmenti: verrucous stage
  - Chondrodysplasia punctata, CHILD
  - Ichthyosis hystrix, epidermal nevus syndrome
  - Lichen striatus
  - ILVEN
  - Linear psoriasis
  - Linear lichen planus
  - Linear porokeratosis
  - Linear Darier disease
  - Angiokeratoma circumscriptum
- Scabies: burrows

VESICOBULLOUS
- "Outside job"
  - Acute contact dermatitis due to poison ivy
  - Bullous insect bites
  - Dermatitis artefacta
- Dermatomal
  - Herpes zoster
- Blaschko lines
  - Incontinentia pigmenti: vesicular stage

ECZEMATOUS
- "Outside job"
  - Allergic contact dermatitis: poison ivy

(Continued)

TABLE 11.9. Linear Dermatoses by Reaction Pattern (continued)

DERMAL
- Autoinoculation
  - Molluscum contagiosum
- Koebner phenomenon
  - Kaposi sarcoma
- Lymphocutaneous spread
  - Infectious
    - *Mycobacterium marinum*
    - *Sporothrix schenckii*
    - *Francisella tularensis*
    - *Leishmania peruvii*
    - *Burkholderia mallei*: glanders: necrotic abcesses
    - Cat scratch disease: *Bartonella henselae*
  - Neoplastic
    - Malignant melanoma: in-transit metastases
    - Zosteriform metastases
- Blaschko lines
  - Focal dermal hypoplasia
  - Nevus sebaceous
  - Segmental neurofibromatosis
  - Benign tumors in Blaschko lines
  - Lymphangioma circumscriptum
  - Linear morphea
- Following veins
  - Thrombophlebitis
  - Mondor disease
  - Deep venous thrombosis

VASCULAR
- "Outside job"
  - Vibices
  - Linear arthropod assault
- Koebner phenomenon
  - Leukocytoclastic vasculitis
  - Adult-onset Still's disease
- Dermographism and red dermographism
- Dermatomyositis- arising from bony prominences
- Phytophotodermatitis
- Cutaneous larva migrans
- Larva currens
- Following lymphatics
  - Lymphangitis
  - Lymphangitic spread of a carcinoma, such as carcinoma lymphangiectoides, carcinoma erysipeloides
- Blaschko lines
  - Angioma serpiginosum

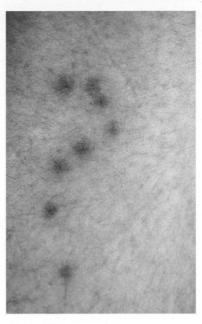

FIGURE 11.35 • Bedbug bites in a serpiginous grouping.

SERPIGINOUS

Serpiginous, or "snake-like" lines may be formed by interconnecting arcs, as is seen in erythema gyratum repens, erythema marginatum, urticarial vasculitis, serum sickness, and serum sickness–like reactions. They may also be evident in dermatoses that follow Blaschko lines (Figure 11.29). Finally, serpiginous eruptions may be secondary to "outside insults," such as larva currens, cutaneous larva migrans, and jellyfish stings. A grouping of bedbug bites can form a serpiginous outline (Figure 11.35). All dermatoses here, save for blaschkoid dermatoses, have a vascular reaction pattern. Cutaneous larva migrans may present with bullae (vesicobullous). Blaschkoid dermatoses may be papulosquamous, vesicobullous, dermal, or macular (see section titled "Whorled" below).

Serpiginous:	
• Vascular reaction pattern • Erythema gyratum repens • Erythema marginatum • Urticarial vasculitis • Serum sickness and serum sickness–like reactions	• Outside insults: larva currens, cutaneous larva migrans, and jellyfish stings • Papulosquamous, vesicobullous, dermal, macular • Blaschkoid dermatoses

WHORLED

Whorled means "spiraled" or "swirled." Whorls of color are seen in blaschkoid dermatoses such as linear and whorled hypermelanosis and hypomelanosis of Ito. Whorls may also be classified by reaction pattern as seen in Table 11.10. Epidermal nevi display lines,

TABLE 11.10. Whorled by Reaction Pattern

PAPULOSQUAMOUS
- Verrucous stage of incontinentia pigmenti
- ILVEN
- Linear psoriasis
- Linear lichen planus
- Chondrodysplasia punctata, CHILD
- Ichthyosis hystrix, epidermal nevus syndrome
- Lichen striatus
- Linear porokeratosis
- Linear Darier disease

VESICOBULLOUS
- First stage of incontinentia pigmenti

DERMAL
- Focal dermal hypoplasia
- Nevus sebaceous
- Segmental neurofibromatosis
- Benign tumors in Blaschko lines

VASCULAR
- Angioma serpiginosum

whorls, and serpiginous shapes and configurations (as seen in Figures 11.29 and 11.30, as well as in Figure 11.36).

RETICULATE

Many eruptions appear as lacy or reticular networks on the skin. Networks may comprise linear macules, such as in livedo reticularis; linear and angulated plaques, such as in retiform purpura; or papules as in confluent and reticulated papillomatosis of Gougerot and Carteaud (CARP).

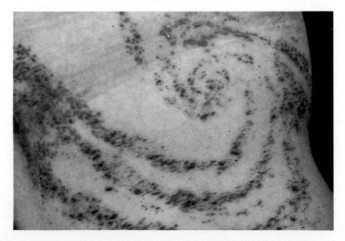

FIGURE 11.36 • An epidermal nevus showing a whorled configuration.

Many reticulate eruptions arise from abnormalities in flow to or from the microvasculature of the skin. The dermis and epidermis receive blood via perforating arterioles. Each arteriole supplies a small cone of skin that drains at its periphery into the subpapillary plexus of venules. These cones are not round at their edges, but rather have a stellate appearance. They vary in size from around 0.5 to 2 cm depending on body site. Figure 11.37A is a schematic representation of skin microvasculature in cross section, and Figure 11.37B is a view from above the skin's surface. The periphery of each "cone" is an area of lower oxygen tension. Livedo reticularis arises if blood flow to the microvasculature is diminished, or if venous drainage from the subpapillary plexus

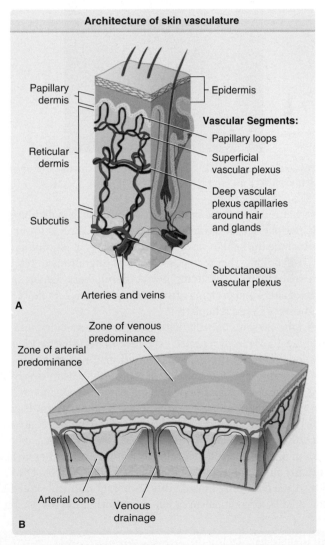

FIGURE 11.37 • Schematic representations of cutaneous microvasculature in cross section (A) and from above (B). As shown in image (B), each arteriole supplies circulation for a cone of skin. (Image (A) reproduced with permission from Goldsmith LA, Katz SI, Gilchrest BA, et al: *Fitzpatrick's Dermatology in General Medicine*, 8th ed. New York, NY: McGraw Hill; 2012.)

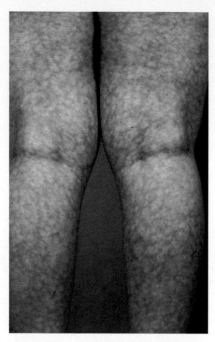

FIGURE 11.38 • Physiologic livedo reticularis showing a reticulate pattern corresponding to the cutaneous microvasculature on the legs.

is impaired. The net result of these is an increase in deoxygenated blood in the skin, especially at the periphery of the cones where oxygen tension is lower to begin with. Some examples include the benign vasospasm that occurs in physiologic livedo reticularis (Figure 11.38) and flow that is compromised by alterations in blood constituents leading to increased viscosity (including polycythemia vera, hypercoagulable states, and the presence of abnormal proteins such as cryoglobulins). Table 11.11 displays the differential diagnosis of livedo reticularis.

Erythema ab igne presents initially with pink to red macules in a livedo reticularis pattern (Figure 10.24) from repeated exposure to heat that is not in the temperature range to cause a burn. This is due to vasodilation. Ongoing exposure will cause a brownish color that represents induction of dyskeratotic cells in overlying epidermis, as is seen after a sunburn. Cutis marmorata telangiectatica congenita (CMTC) is a vascular neoplasm that presents with a livedo reticularis–like pattern. It usually presents shortly after birth and involves the lower extremities most frequently. Associated abnormalities (orthopedic, ocular, neurologic, and other vascular abnormalities) are seen in around half of diffuse cases. In localized cases, there is either no abnormality or hypotrophy (usually girth, not length) of the affected limb. Adams–Oliver syndrome is characterized by distal transverse limb defects and scalp skin and skull defects (aplasia cutis congenita). CMTC or a reticulate capillary malformation may be present.

Two Livedo Reticularis-Like Dermatoses:

- Erythema ab igne
- Cutis marmorata telangiectatica congenita

TABLE 11.11. Differential Diagnosis of Livedo Reticularis

PHYSIOLOGIC
- Cutis marmorata

PATHOLOGIC
- Factors inside vessel
  - Stasis
    - Cardiac failure
    - Paralysis
  - Viscosity
    - Polycythemia vera
    - Thrombocytosis
  - Other intraluminal factors
    - Cryoglobulins
    - Primary hyperoxaluria
    - Antiphospholipid syndrome
  - Embolic
    - Cholesterol emboli
- Within vessel wall
  - Calciphylaxis
  - Arteritis
    - SLE
    - Dermatomyositis
    - Rheumatoid arthritis
    - PAN
    - Cutaneous PAN
    - Granulomatous polyangiitis
    - Tuberculosis
    - Syphilis
- Drugs
  - Amantidine
  - Quinine
  - Quinidine

Abnormalities in the vessel walls and obstruction to vascular lumina may cause livedo reticularis, livedo racemosa, or retiform purpura (Figures 10.28 and 10.29). Vasculitides affecting the midsized vessels that supply the deep dermis and subcutis may give rise to livedo reticularis, owing to a diminished flow to the more superficial vessels. Livedo racemosa is a discontinuous, branching form of livedo reticularis. It results from irregular, focal, persistent, and usually physical impairment of the blood flow. Retiform purpura refers to the purpuric and necrotic stellate plaques that are common to a wide array of vasculitides and microvascular occlusion syndromes (Table 10.13). Finally, in this category, livedoid vasculopathy is the term given to a distinctive constellation of reticulated, stellate ulcerations that heal with small, punched-out, hypopigmented scars (Figure 10.30). Livedoid vasculopathy is classically seen on the lower extremities. It is usually the result of an underlying thrombophilic disorder such as factor V Leiden mutation, protein C or S deficiency, hyperhomocysteinemia, prothrombin gene mutation (G20210A), methylenetetrahydrofolate reductase C677T mutation, or antithrombin III deficiency.

Cryoglobulinemia and cryofibrinogenemia have also been associated. Livedoid vasculopathy can, however, also be idiopathic.

Reticulate Dermatoses that Follow Skin Microvasculature	
• Livedo reticularis	• Retiform purpura
• Livedo racemosa	• Livedoid vasculopathy

Reticulate dermatoses that do not follow skin microvasculature are listed in Table 11.12 by reaction pattern and reticulate dermatoses, including those that follow the skin microvasculature, are listed in Table 11.13 by color. In CARP, ridged brown thin discrete and confluent papules occur on the central chest and back and less frequently on the neck (Figure 11.27) and in the axillae. Atrophic CARP displays similar wrinkled and sometimes, nonpigmented plaques (Figure 11.28). Prurigo pigmentosa (Nagashima disease) is very rarely encountered outside Japan. Initially, there are erythematous papules, papulovesicles, and vesicles that are very itchy. These may form a reticulate pattern and are usually seen on the trunk or neck. As the disease progresses, the inflammatory stage resolves, leaving reticulate hyperpigmentation. Reticular erythematous mucinosis is usually seen in young women on the chest. Light pink or light brown smooth plaques with a reticular configuration are seen. Erythema infectiosum (fifth disease) manifests fever, followed by wispy reticulate macules and thin plaques on the body (Figure 11.39) along with a "slapped cheek" appearance on the face. The reticulate appearance may persist for weeks and be worsened by heat. Erythema marginatum is seen in rheumatic fever. Evanescent pink figurate macules and thin plaques, including reticulate forms, are seen. In Still's disease, evanescent erythema that follows the temperature curve is seen. Wispy and reticulate macules and thin plaques may be a part of the presentation. In TNF-α receptor-associated periodic syndrome (TRAPS), an autosomal dominantly inherited condition, periodic fever is associated with migratory reticulate macules on the extremities.

There are certain very rare inherited dermatoses that present with reticulate hyperpigmentation. Dowling–Degos disease, also known as a reticulate pigmented anomaly of the

---

TABLE 11.12. Differential Diagnosis of the Reticulate Configuration for Dermatoses Not Following the Livedo Reticularis Pattern, by Reaction Pattern

PAPULOSQUAMOUS
• Confluent and reticulated papillomatosis of Gougerot and Carteaud

VESICOBULLOUS
• Prurigo pigmentosa

DERMAL
• Reticulate erythematous mucinosis

VASCULAR
• Erythema infectiosum
• Erythema marginatum
• Juvenile and adult-onset Still's disease
• TNF-α receptor-associated periodic syndrome
• Prurigo pigmentosa

TABLE 11.13. Reticulate, by Color

PINK OR RED

- Livedo reticularis differential (see Table 11.11)
- Livedo racemosa
- Erythema ab igne
- Erythema infectiosum
- Erythema marginatum
- TRAPS
- Prurigo pigmentosa
- Adult-onset Still's disease
- Reticulate erythematous mucinosis
- Retiform purpura differential: (see Table 10.13)

BROWN

- Inherited
  - Dowling–Degos disease (reticulate pigmented anomaly of the flexures)
  - Reticulate acropigmentation of Kitamura
  - Dermatopathia pigmentosa reticularis
  - Naegeli–Franceschetti–Jadassohn syndrome
  - Dyskeratosis congenita
  - Epidermolysis bullosa simplex with mottled pigmentation
  - Prurigo pigmentosa
  - X-linked reticulate pigmentary disorder
  - Dyschromatosis universalis hereditaria
  - Dyschromatosis symmetrica hereditaria (acropigmentation of Dohi)
- Acquired
  - Erythema ab igne
  - CARP
  - Prurigo pigmentosa
  - Reticulate hyperpigmentation from intravenous 5-fluorouracil

PURPLE SPECTRUM

- Retiform purpura (see Table 10.13)
- Livedoid vasculopathy

flexures, or "dark dot disease," is an autosomal dominant dermatosis with onset in adulthood. Numerous small round brown freckle-like macules are seen in the folds, including the axillae, the inguinal area, inframammary and intergluteal areas, the neck, and the trunk. Macules become confluent, giving rise to a reticulate configuration. Comedo-like openings may also be seen in these areas along with pitted acneiform scars near angles of the mouth. Reticulate acropigmentation of Kitamura is also autosomal dominant. It was originally reported in Japan. Onset is in the first two decades of life. Freckle-like reticulate macules on the dorsal hands are accompanied by palmar pits and breaks in the palmar rete ridge pattern. In dermatopathia pigmentosa reticularis (DPR), there is widespread reticulate pigmentation that begins in early childhood and persists throughout life. Adermatoglyphia and a punctate palmoplantar keratoderma are seen. Lacrimal keratosis are also seen. Naegeli–Franceschetti–Jadassohn syndrome is allelic to DPR. This manifests with acral bullae in the in the first few days after birth. Reticulate pigmentation begins in the second or third decade and is seen mainly on the neck, in the axillae, and periorificially. There may be sparse hair, hypohidrosis, enamel pitting, adermatoglyphia and a

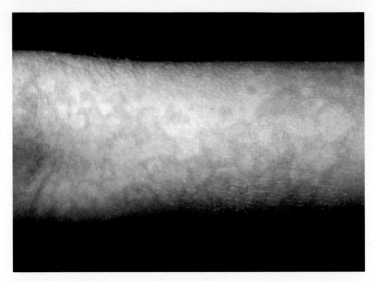

FIGURE 11.39 · Erythema infectiosum displaying a pink reticulate eruption on the arm.

punctate keratoderma. In dyskeratosis congenita, there is reticulated hyperpigmentation on the face, neck, and trunk with associated palmar hyperkeratosis, oral leukoplakia, and nail dystrophy. Epidermolysis bullosa simplex (EBS) with mottled pigmentation is a rare type of EBS with superficial blistering that may be localized or generalized. The reticulate pigmentation may also be localized to the upper body, or it may be generalized. In dyschromatosis universalis hereditaria, there is a diffuse pattern of reticulate pigmentation with associated hypopigmentation. In X-linked reticulate pigmentary disorder (X-linked cutaneous amyloidosis), there are similar findings along with hypohidrosis; corneal opacification; and respiratory, urologic, and gastrointestinal manifestations.

HERPETIFORM

This adjective is used to describe grouped lesions on an erythematous base, including papules, vesicles, pustules, erosions, or crusts. These are the stages of development of lesions of the herpes simplex virus, or of the varicella zoster virus. *Herpetiform* may refer to a configuration or a grouping (Figure 11.40). Herpes simplex and herpes zoster are classic examples of the herpetiform configuration or grouping. Impetigo herpetiformis, or pustular psoriasis in pregnancy, manifests herpetiform pustules; pemphigus herpetiformis, a rare subtype of pemphigus, manifests grouped herpetiform vesicles, erosions and crusts; and dermatitis herpetiformis manifests grouped urticarial papules, vesicles, erosions, and crusts. In pemphigus herpetiformis, the intraepidermal split is superficial, and so it may be difficult to find a primary vesicle on examination. Tables 11.14 and 11.15 list the herpetiform differential diagnosis by primary lesion and by reaction pattern, respectively. As discussed in Chapter 3, the physical findings of round erosions and crusts can provide clues to the presence of a primary vesicobullous disorder.

> **Clinical Tip** The presence of round erosions and crusts implies the presence of a preceding vesicle or bulla. These secondary lesions may be a clue to the presence of a vesicobullous disorder.

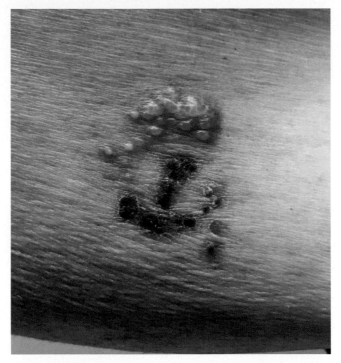

FIGURE 11.40 • A close-up of herpes simplex showing grouped vesicles and pustules, and nearby grouped crusts at the site of a previous, healing episode.

TABLE 11.14. Herpetiform Grouping by Primary Lesion

VESICLES
- Herpes simplex
- Herpes zoster
- Pemphigus herpetiformis
- Dermatitis herpetiformis

PUSTULES
- Impetigo herpetiformis

TABLE 11.15. Herpetiform Grouping by Reaction Pattern

VESICOBULLOUS REACTION PATTERN
- Herpes simplex
- Herpes zoster
- Pemphigus herpetiformis
- Dermatitis herpetiformis

VASCULAR REACTION PATTERN
- Urticarial plaques of dermatitis herpetiformis

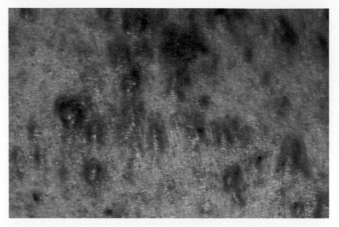

FIGURE 11.41 • A close-up of leiomyomas, showing a cluster of elongated pink and brown papules.

AGMINATE (OR AGMINATED)

The term *agminate* refers to the fact that lesions are clustered together at a specific site. Spitz nevi, pyogenic granulomas, melanoma metastases (Figure 9.52), and leiomyomas (Figure 11.41) can manifest in this way. Lupus miliaris disseminatus faciei is also known as *acne agminata*. Here, small red-orange papules are clustered periorbitally or on the lower face. Lupus miliaris disseminatus faciei was previously thought to be a tuberculide; however, current understanding is that it is a form of granulomatous rosacea or periorbital dermatitis. In the case of pigmented lesions or leiomyomas, agminated lesions may also represent a developmental phenomenon in that it may be a variant of a segmental distribution. Table 11.16 lists the differential diagnosis of agminate by primary lesion.

TABLE 11.16. Differential Diagnosis of Agminated/Clustered Papules and Nodules
PAPULES
• Lupus miliaris disseminatus faciei
• Pyogenic granulomas
• Leiomyomas
• Spitz nevi
• Melanoma metastases: satellitosis
NODULES
• Melanoma metastases: satellitosis

SUMMARY

- Eruptions may manifest lesions with characteristic shapes or characteristic configurations or arrangements of lesions.
- The differential diagnosis of each type of shape, configuration and arrangement is discussed here.
- The approach for each may be etiologic or morphologic (by primary lesion, color, or reaction pattern).

More on Distribution

12

Distribution in the present context refers to the body location of any eruption. This chapter focuses on differential diagnoses for each distribution. Classic and variant distribution patterns for eruptions will be discussed. Sites of predilection for neoplasms will also be mentioned. These differential diagnoses will be divided by reaction pattern and other morphologic attributes, such as pustules or macules of different colors, when useful. Some of the classic distribution patterns that eruptions tend to follow were mentioned in Chapter 1. In this chapter, these and additional locations will be considered, as are listed in the textbox below.

Distribution of Primary Lesions

- Photoexposed
- Flexures
- Intertriginous
- Seborrheic
- Extensors
- Truncal
- Acral
- Palms and soles
- Dorsal hands
- Digits
- Webspaces
- Periorbital
- Ear
- Nose
- Face
- Generalized

PHOTOEXPOSED ERUPTIONS

In *photoexposed* eruptions, light plays a role in the pathogenesis of the eruption. As mentioned previously, the sites that are most commonly involved in photoexposed eruptions include one or more sites on the face, neck, the "V" of the chest, the upper back, and the dorsal arms and hands. Other sites, such as dorsal feet and lower legs, may also be involved.

Photoexposed Sites

- Face
- Neck
- "V" of the chest
- Upper back
- Dorsal arms and hands
- Dorsal feet and lower legs

Also note spared areas such as the eyelid creases, the area of the upper neck that is in shadow from the chin, and Wilkonson's triangle (a triangular area behind the earlobe).

Photoprotected Sites

- Eyelid creases
- Upper neck that is in shadow from the chin
- Triangle behind the earlobe

An etiologic classification of the photoexposed differential diagnosis appears in Table 1.6. Many dermatoses that occur in photoexposed areas are rarely encountered.

Some are rare genetically inherited syndromes. Phototoxic and photoallergic eruptions are more common, and medications as a cause, or underlying lupus or some of the porphyrias should always be borne in mind. A comprehensive morphologic differential diagnosis of eruptions with a predilection for photoexposed sites is listed in Table 1.7 by primary lesion. Table 12.1 outlines the photoexposed differential diagnosis

---

TABLE 12.1. Photoexposed Distribution, by Reaction Pattern

PAPULOSQUAMOUS
- Discoid lupus erythematosus
- Subacute cutaneous lupus erythematosus: psoriasiform variant
- Photoexacerbated psoriasis
- Pellagra
- Photolichenoid eruption
- Lichen planus actinicus

VESICOBULLOUS
- Porphyria cutanea tarda
- Variegate porphyria
- Erythropoietic protoporhyria
- Gunther disease
- Phytophotodermatitis—in severe cases, vesicle and bulla formation occurs
- Juvenile spring eruption
- Polymorphous light eruption, vesicular type
- Hydroa vacciniforme

ECZEMATOUS
- Photoallergic dermatitis
- Chronic actinic dermatitis
- Actinic reticuloid
- Actinic prurigo
- Polymorphous light eruption, eczematous type

DERMAL
- Tumid Lupus
- Subacute cutaneous lupus erythematosus: annular polycyclic variant

VASCULAR
- Erythema
  - Sunburn
  - Phototoxic reactions due to drugs
  - Phototoxicity that accompanies connective tissue disease, including subacute or systemic lupus, and dermatomyositis
  - Poikiloderma
    - Poikiloderma of Civatte
    - Poikiloderma associated with dermatomyositis or systemic lupus erythematosus
  - Reticulate erythema in Bloom syndrome
- Urticaria/urticarial
  - Solar urticaria
  - Erythropoietic protoporphyria
  - Polymorphous light eruption

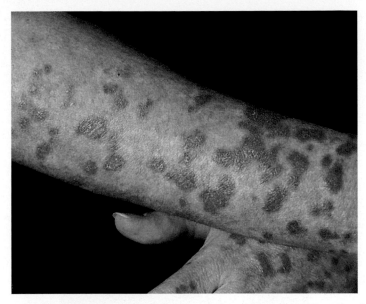

FIGURE 12.1 • Subacute cutaneous lupus on the arm, displaying psoriasiform plaques on the forearm and hand. (Reproduced with permission from Kang S, Amagai M, Bruckner AL, et al: *Fitzpatrick's Dermatology,* 9th ed. New York, NY: McGraw Hill; 2019.)

by reaction pattern. Psoriasis may be photoacentuated. Some lichenoid drug eruptions (classically from tetracyclines, hydrochlorothiazide, and furosemide) as well as lichen planus actinicus have a photodistribution. Lichen planus actinicus is lichen planus that is localized to sun-exposed areas. There are four subtypes, including a classic plaque type, an annular variant, a dyschromic variant and a pigmented variant. Discoid lupus erythematosus (DLE) and the psoriasiform variant of subacute lupus erythematous (SCLE; see Figure 12.1 and 1.5D) both present with papulosquamous morphology. The annular, polycyclic type of SCLE lacks scale and falls into the dermal reaction pattern category. Tumid lupus is also a dermal reaction pattern disease. Systemic lupus erythematous (SLE) may present with a malar rash or a more widespread photosensitive eruption (both vascular reaction pattern). In severe SLE, there may be epidermal necrosis, and so an eroded presentation is also possible (Figure 12.2). Pellagra is seen in vitamin B_3 deficiency. A scaly photoexposed eruption with shellac-like scales in seen. Secondary erosions may occur (Figure 12.3). "Casal's necklace" is the term given to pellagra at the V of the neck; a V-shaped plaque has a rim of darker scales (see Figure 6.27). Regarding the porphyrias, porphyria cutanea tarda (PCT) presents with bullae on photoexposed areas. Bullae heal with scarring and milia formation (see Figure 7.31). Hypertrichosis and sclerodermoid plaques are two further features that do not necessarily involve photoexposed skin. The findings in porphyria variegata (variegate porphyria) are subtle. There is usually minimal vesicle and bulla formation, and scarring is seen. In erythropoietic protoporphyria (EPP), vesicles and bullae are rarely seen. More typically, there is edema and erythema, and occasionally purpura that follows sun exposure. This is accompanied by extreme skin pain. Wheals may be seen (a vascular reaction pattern morphology). EPP typically has onset in early childhood. In Gunther disease (congenital erythropoietic protoporhyria), there is early onset of

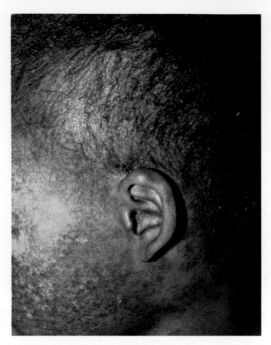

FIGURE 12.2 • Severe systemic lupus erythematosus showing full-thickness necrosis in some areas, and erosions and superficial peeling in others. Note the associated *lupus hair*: thinning and shortened hairs at the anterior scalp margin.

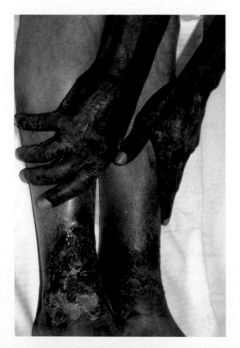

FIGURE 12.3 • Pellagra, presenting with erythematous and hyperpigmented plaques in photoexposed areas with shiny, large scales and secondary erosions.

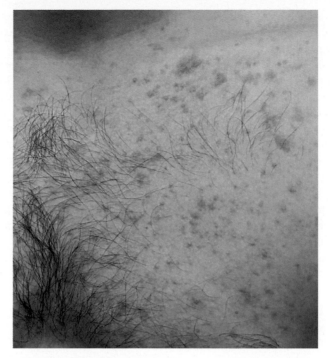

FIGURE 12.4 • Polymorphous light eruption presenting with erythematous papules on the chest.

skin fragility, vesicle and bulla formation with subsequent scarring, and loss of acral structures, including nasal tip and fingers. This phenomenon is termed photomutilation. Further features include erythrodontia (red teeth), liver abnormalities, and red urine. Polymorphous light eruption (PMLE) may present with erythematous papules (vascular reaction pattern; see Figure 12.4), an eczematous morphology, or a vesicular morphology. Onset is in the third or fourth decade typically, and women are affected more frequently than men. PMLE erupts after the first sun exposure of the season and occurs less frequently as the summer continues (the phenomenon of "hardening"). The face is spared (similarly assumed to be secondary to "hardening"), but all other photoexposed sites may be affected. Juvenile spring eruption is believed to be a variant of PMLE that predominantly affects boys. When exposed to sunlight, in the presence of cold, such as in the spring, papulovesicles and frank vesicles appear on the ears. The eruption heals without scarring. Hydroa vacciniforme is a more severe photoexposed dermatosis of childhood. It also is seen more frequently in boys. Papulovesicles and frank vesicles occur on sunexposed sites. They then crust over and heal with depressed scars. A severe form that occurs on sun-covered areas as well has been rarely reported. Vesicle and bulla formation occurs in severe cases of phytophotodermatitis.

In the eczematous category, photoallergic dermatitis is usually of a subacute or chronic morphology. Topical applications, such as sunscreen constituents (benzophenones) and fragrances, or oral drugs, such as nonsteroidal anti-inflammatory drugs, may be responsible. Chronic actinic dermatitis is a similar eruption that usually has a chronic eczematous morphology. It occurs in the absence of a known drug or other antigen. Actinic reticuloid is chronic actinic dermatitis with a histopathologic pattern that resembles mycosis fungoides. Actinic prurigo occurs in childhood and is thought to be familial. Intensely pruritic photodistributed papules are quickly excoriated and may become pruriginous.

Photosensitive erythema is seen in sunburn and phototoxic eruptions due to drugs or accompanying connective tissue disease, including SCLE, SLE, or dermatomyositis. The erythema in dermatomyositis may have a violaceous color. Poikiloderma is the constellation of atrophy, telangiectasias, hypo- and hyperpigmentation. Poikiloderma of Civatte is seen in the sun-exposed areas of the lateral neck and upper chest. Erythema is prominent given a significant telangiectatic component. Poikiloderma is also seen in association with dermatomyositis and SLE, amongst other causes. In Bloom syndrome, photodistributed reticulated erythema may be seen. Urticarial eruptions that respect photoexposed areas include solar urticaria, PMLE, and EPP (as mentioned previously). In solar urticaria, itchy hives erupt a few minutes after sun exposure. It may be a primary condition, or it may be secondary to lupus or porphyria. PMLE may present with urticarial papules.

Conditions with photoinduced or exacerbated pigmentary alteration are summarized in Table 12.2. Generalized hyperpigmentation is seen in a variety of disease states.

TABLE 12.2. Photoexposed Distribution: Dermatoses with Predominant Color Changes

DIFFUSE
- Generalized hyperpigmentation with photoaccentuation
  - Chronic renal insufficiency
  - Primary biliary cirrhosis
- Photoaccentuated drug pigmentation
  - Slate-gray: amiodarone, tricyclic antidepressants
  - Blue-gray: phenothiazines, minocycline
  - Brown-gray: antimalarials
  - Magenta: gold
- Phototoxic drug eruption
  - Antiarrhythmics (amiodarone, quinidine), antifungals (voriconazole), diuretics (furosemide, thiazides), NSAIDs (nabumetone, naproxen, piroxicam), phenothiazines (chlorpromazine, prochlorperazine), psoralens (5-methoxypsoralen, 8-methoxypsoralen), quinolones (ciprofloxacin, lomefloxacin, nalidixic acid, sparfloxacin), tetracyclines (doxycycline, demeclocycline), St. John's wort, topical tar
- Hyper- and hypopigmented macules
  - Xeroderma pigmentosum

LOCALIZED
- Brown
  - Phytophotodermatitis
  - Melasma
- Gray-brown
  - Lichen planus actinicus: pigmented type
- White
  - Idiopathic guttate hypomelanosis
  - SCLE
- Brown and white
  - DLE

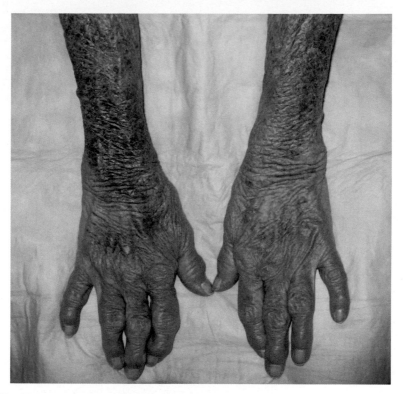

FIGURE 12.5 • Extensive deep brown-gray pigmentation on the dorsal forearms secondary to chronic minocycline use.

In chronic renal insufficiency as well as primary biliary cirrhosis, there is generalized hyperpigmentation that is accentuated in the photoexposed areas. In photoaccentuated drug pigmentation, pigmentary changes may be various shades of brown, blue, or gray, or even a magenta color in the case of pigmentation secondary to gold salts. Figure 12.5 shows extensive deep brown-gray pigmentation on the dorsal forearms secondary to chronic minocycline use. Phototoxic drug eruptions and phytophotodermatitis heal with postinflammatory hyperpigmentation that is seen in photoexposed areas. In phytophotodermatitis, linear and geometric shapes are seen. In xeroderma pigmentosum, a rare autosomal recessive dermatosis, there is early onset of photodistributed lentigines and hypopigmented macules, giving rise to a mottled appearance of the skin. The pigmentary changes precede the similarly early onset of skin cancers. Localized photoaccentuated pigmentation is also seen in melasma; tan, well-demarcated macules are seen over the cheeks, forehead, and upper lip. Lichen planus actinicus, as mentioned, is lichen planus that is localized to sun-exposed areas. The pigmented subtype presents with grayish-brown macules on the face and neck. In idiopathic guttate hypomelanosis, hypopigmented macules measuring between 3 and 5 mm are seen on the chronically sun-exposed aspects of the arms and legs. SCLE may also heal with hypo- or depigmented, photodistributed macules. DLE leaves behind prominent pigmentary changes in its wake (Figure 12.6). Depigmented macules and scarred-down plaques, often with hyperpigmented rims, are a fairly common presentation of DLE on scalp, face, and forearms.

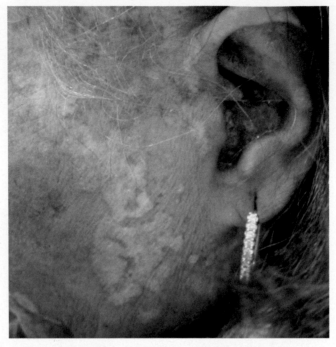

FIGURE 12.6 · Discoid lupus erythematosus (DLE) with pink scaly facial plaques, resolving with depigmented macules. Note also scaling in the conchal bowl—a site of predilection for DLE.

FLEXURES

The *flexures* are the skin areas that are found where the limbs bend and include the antecubital and the popliteal fossae.

> **Clinical Tip** Flexures = antecubital and popliteal fossae

A circumscribed group of dermatoses favor these areas. These are listed in Table 12.3 by reaction pattern, pustules, and macules. Erythrasma is a superficial infection with *Corynebacterium minutissimum*. It presents as thin, scaly, and well- demarcated plaques that are usually located in the intertriginous folds, including axillae, inguinal folds, and inframammary skin. The flexures are also a site of predilection but are less frequently involved that the intertriginous zones. The toe webs may be involved. Hailey–Hailey disease favors the intertriginous areas. In widespread or severe cases, the antecubital fossa may be involved (Figure 12.7). Macerated plaques with small linear erosions that are classic for the disease are seen. Acanthosis nigricans is usually seen in the neck and in the intertriginous areas. The flexures may be uncommonly involved. The flexures are a site of predilection of atopic dermatitis in childhood (Figure 12.8). Initially, during infancy, the scaly plaques of atopic dermatitis occur on the extensors of the extremities. Beyond infancy, predilection changes to the flexural surfaces. In adulthood, atopic dermatitis may be found anywhere on the skin surface, including the flexures. Formaldehyde is ubiquitous in the environment. It is also used to treat fabrics, such as permanent press and antiwrinkle clothing. Sites of predilection for contact dermatitis from formaldehyde

TABLE 12.3. Differential Diagnosis of Eruptions That Favor the Flexures, by Reaction Pattern, Pustules, and Macules

PAPULOSQUAMOUS
- Erythrasma
- Hailey–Hailey disease
- Acanthosis nigricans

ECZEMATOUS
- Atopic dermatitis
- Allergic contact dermatitis from formaldehyde and clothing dyes
- Systematized contact dermatitis (baboon syndrome)

PUSTULES
- Subcorneal pustular dermatosis

DERMAL
- Pseudoxanthoma elasticum
- Fibroelastolytic papulosis
- Flexural variant of granuloma annulare
- Xanthoma disseminatum
- Intertriginous xanthomas
- Erdheim–Chester disease

VASCULAR
- SDRIFE

MACULES
- Dowling-Degos disease

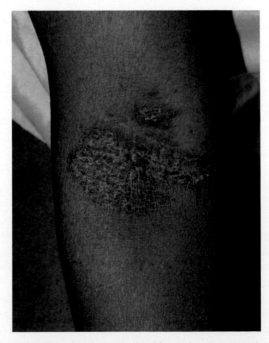

FIGURE 12.7 • Hailey–Hailey disease in the antecubital fossa, showing crusted and scaly plaques.

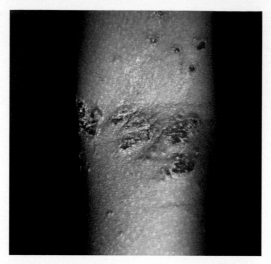

FIGURE 12.8 • Atopic eczema in the antecubital fossa, displaying a subacute eczematous morphology.

are areas that may be in contact with tight-fitting clothing, including flexures, around the axillae, the upper back, and the waistband. Textile dermatitis from clothing dyes also occurs in this distribution. "Baboon syndrome" refers to an eruption that involves the buttocks and the symmetric involvement of at least one flexural or intertriginous area. It may occur as a result of a systematized contact dermatitis or systemic drug-related intertriginous and flexural exanthema (SDRIFE). Systematized contact dermatitis usually occurs after ingestion of an antigen that the affected individual has previously been sensitized to. Systematized contact dermatitis usually has a subacute eczematous morphology. SDRIFE presents with well-demarcated erythema of the buttocks, thighs, intertriginous areas, and the flexures following exposure to systemic drugs, such as β-lactams and mercury. It subsumes a vascular reaction pattern morphology. In subcorneal pustular dermatosis, flaccid pustules arise in the axillae, around inguinal folds, and in the flexures and may spread to the trunk.

Pseudoxanthoma elasticum (PXE) is an autosomal recessively inherited. There is abnormal calcification of elastic tissue in the skin, the eye, and blood vessels. Yellowish, 2–3-mm papules with a "plucked chicken" appearance appear most prominently on the neck, axillae, inguinal folds, and the antecubital and popliteal fossae. Mucous membranes may be affected. Fibroelastolytic papulosis (FEP) is a similarly appearing acquired disorder, where white or yellowish 2–3-mm papules appear on the trunk, on the posterior neck, and in the axillae in later life. The flexures and extremities may also be involved. There is no systemic involvement in FEP. While granuloma annulare is typically located on the extensors, a flexural variant can occur (Figure 12.9). In xanthoma disseminatum, red-brown papules and plaques involve the flexures, trunk, and proximal arms and legs. They become yellower with time. There may be associated infiltration of the oral mucosa and respiratory tract, meninges, and bones. Diabetes insipidus is a common concomitant. Intertriginous xanthomas are seen in finger webs, palmar creases, axillae, buttocks, and the antecubital and popliteal fossae. They occur in the setting of type IIA hyperlipidemia. In Erdheim–Chester disease, xanthoma

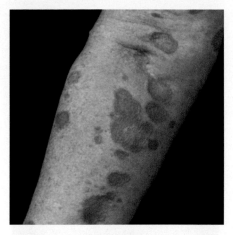

FIGURE 12.9 • Granuloma annulare on the volar forearm, showing slightly atrophic, annular plaques. (Reproduced with permission from Wolff K, Johnson RA, Saavedra AP, et al: *Fitzpatrick's Color Atlas and Synopsis of Clinical Dermatology*, 8th ed. New York, NY: McGraw Hill; 2017.)

disseminatum–like plaques and nodules are seen in the minority of cases. Systemically, there may be sclerosis of long bones, and infiltration of viscera, the retroperitoneum and the orbit.

Dowling-Degos disease (also known as *reticular pigmented anomaly of the flexures*) is an autosomal dominantly inherited dermatosis. Axillae and flexures manifest brown discrete and reticulated macules, and comedonal papules have also been reported in these areas. The face may have similar findings.

Interestingly, in ichthyosis vulgaris, the flexures are classically spared (Figure 12.10).

> **Clinical Tip** The flexures are spared in ichthyosis vulgaris.

INTERTRIGINOUS

Intertriginous areas are those areas in which two skin surfaces are closely opposed to each other. They include the axillary and the inguinal folds, the inframammary regions, and the intergluteal cleft. The lower abdominal fold is an additional intertriginous site in a very overweight individual. Additionally, the flexures can become intertriginous in this population, in that they may be partially or completely occluded. The toe webspaces may at times be very closely opposed, so this area can be classified as an intertriginous area. The dermatoses of the toe webs are considered separately later in the section titled "Webspaces."

Intertriginous Areas Include:	
• Axillary and inguinal folds	• Lower abdominal fold, flexural skin in
• Inframammary regions	obesity
• Intergluteal cleft	• Toe webs

Many dermatoses that favor the intertriginous areas also occur in the flexures as seen above. Additionally, numerous other dermatoses tend to occur here. Table 12.4

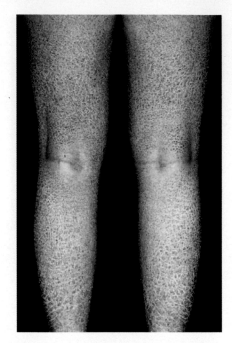

FIGURE 12.10 • Ichthyosis vulgaris, showing sparing of the popliteal fossae. (Reproduced with permission from Wolff K, Johnson RA, Saavedra AP, et al: *Fitzpatrick's Color Atlas and Synopsis of Clinical Dermatology*, 8th ed. New York, NY: McGraw Hill; 2017.)

TABLE 12.4. Dermatoses Favoring Intertriginous Areas, by Reaction Pattern, Pustules, and Macules

PAPULOSQUAMOUS
- Inverse psoriasis
- Tinea cruris
- Erythrasma
- Pityriasis circinata et marginata of Vidal
- Acanthosis nigricans
- Hailey–Hailey disease
- Darier disease
- Pemphigus vegetans
- Extramammary Paget disease
- Granular parakeratosis
- Acrodermatitis enteropathica
- Langerhans cell histiocytosis
- Lichen sclerosus
- Condyloma lata

VESICOBULLOUS
- Herpes simplex
- Herpes zoster
- Pemphigus vegetans
- Darier disease
- Acrodermatitis enteropathica
- Hailey–Hailey disease

(Continued)

TABLE 12.4.   Dermatoses Favoring Intertriginous Areas, by Reaction Pattern, Pustules, and Macules (continued)

ECZEMATOUS
- Intertrigo
- Seborrheic dermatitis
- Irritant dermatitis
- Allergic contact dermatitis
- Systematized contact dermatitis
- Baboon syndrome

PUSTULES
- Folliculitis
- Candidal intertrigo
- Subcorneal pustular dermatosis
- Amicrobial pustulosis of the folds
- Eosinophilic folliculitis of Ofuji

DERMAL
- Furuncle
- Epidermal cyst
- Hidradenitis suppurativa
- Fox-Fordyce disease
- Pseudoxanthoma elasticum
- Fibroelastolytic papulosis
- Intertriginous xanthomas

VASCULAR
- Intertrigo
- Erythema migrans
- Systemic drug-related intertriginous and flexural exanthema (SDRIFE)
- Toxic erythema of chemotherapy

MACULES
- Neurofibromatosis
- Dowling-Degos disease

provides a comprehensive list of these dermatoses, classified by reaction pattern, pustules, and macules. Intertrigo is the prototypic eruption in the folds (Figure 12.11; see also Figure 1.7A). Scaly or shiny pink or red are seen under the breasts, in the inguinal folds, in the intergluteal fold, in the axillae or under the pannus. Intertrigo may be a manifestation of seborrheic dermatitis (Figure 12.12). Sometimes erythema without scale is seen—this intertrigo can also be classified as a vascular reaction pattern. The differential diagnosis of scaly intertriginous eruptions is quite broad. In this location scale may be minimal or macerated, given that there is close proximity of skin surfaces and lack of evaporation of moisture. In the papulosquamous category, inverse psoriasis presents as well-demarcated salon-pink plaques with scale or overlying maceration when it is in this location (Figure 12.13). In tinea cruris, an active scaly edge is seen on the inner upper thighs or extending onto the suprapubic skin. It may be unilateral or bilateral. Erythrasma commonly occurs on intertriginous skin. It fluoresces under Wood's lamp with a coral red color. Figure 12.14A shows a light brown and pink

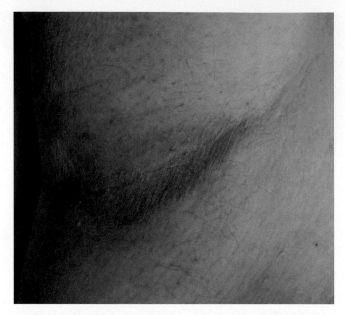

FIGURE 12.11 · Intertrigo, showing a scaly and macerated light pink plaque in the axilla.

plaque of erythrasma extending onto the inner upper thigh from the inguinal fold. Figure 12.14B shows the same area fluorescing a coral red color under Wood's lamp illumination. Pityriasis circinata et marginata of Vidal is a variant of pityriasis rosea in which large ovoid plaques preferentially cluster in and around the inguinal and axillary folds. Acanthosis nigricans may be seen in the setting of obesity, glucose intolerance, or malignancy. It presents as velvety plaques on the neck and in the axillae (Figure 12.15; see also Figure 1.7E). Inguinal folds and inner thighs may be involved, and in malignancy-associated cases, the dorsal hands, cheeks, and lips may also be involved. Both Hailey–Hailey disease and Darier disease may involve the folds, the former more frequently than the latter. Hailey–Hailey disease may be scaly (Figure 12.16) or macerated with tiny linear erosions (Figures 1.7C and 7.3). Darier disease presents with scaly and greasy papules. The classic distribution of Darier disease is seborrheic,

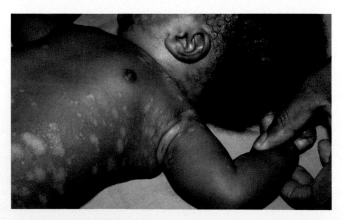

FIGURE 12.12 · Seborrheic dermatitis in an infant, showing a well-demarcated pink plaque in the axilla.

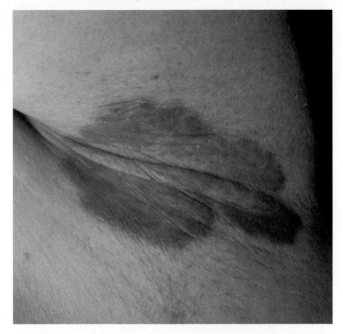

FIGURE 12.13 • Inverse psoriasis, showing a well-demarcated pink plaque with overlying maceration in the axilla.

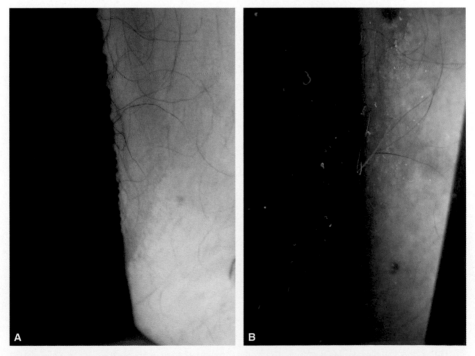

FIGURE 12.14 • (A) A light brown and pink plaque of erythrasma extending from the inguinal fold onto the inner upper thigh; (B) a plaque of erythrasma on the inner upper thigh displaying coral red fluorescence under Wood's lamp illumination.

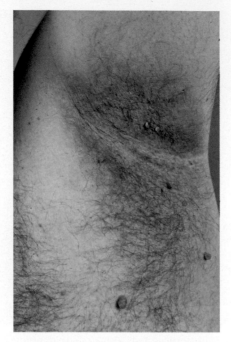

FIGURE 12.15 • Acanthosis nigricans showing a large, velvety, hyperpigmented plaque in the axilla.

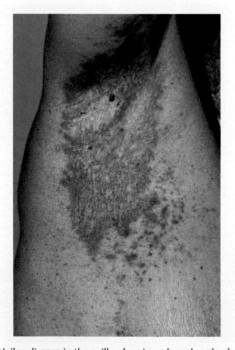

FIGURE 12.16 • Hailey–Hailey disease in the axilla, showing a broad, scaly plaque.

including the central chest, upper back, scalp, and postauricular skin. The lateral neck is a further site of predilection, as are the folds. It may be more widespread, and it may involve palms and soles with pits, the oral mucosa with a cobblestone appearance, and nails with longitudinal red and white lines (alternating red and white lines are called a "candy cane" appearance or the "sandwich sign"). Further findings include acrokeratosis verruciformis–like papules on the distal extremities (flat verrucous papules) and leukodermic macules (a rare finding, most commonly seen in darker-skinned individuals). A rare bullous variant of Darier disease can be seen in the intertriginous location. Pemphigus vegetans is a vegetating form of pemphigus vulgaris that occurs in the folds (see Figure 1.7D) and occasionally on the scalp. Vegetating plaques are seen in these anatomic locations. These plaques may have a macerated surface, and bullae or "footprints" of bullae may be difficult to discern, leading one to consider a papulosquamous disorder. Erosions may be seen outside the folds, which may provide a clue to the presence of a blistering disease. Extramammary Paget disease is a rare cutaneous adenocarcinoma, an extension of an underlying adenocarcinoma, or one that has arisen in a pelvic organ. It presents as one or more well-demarcated scaly plaques in or around the inguinal folds. Occasionally these may be eroded and therefore they may resemble eczema or Hailey–Hailey disease. An important management approach is to trial 2–3 weeks of topical steroids on any scaly groin eruption that resembles eczema or Hailey–Hailey disease. If there is no response to this treatment, a biopsy is indicated.

> **Clinical Tip** Extramammary Paget disease can look like eczema or Hailey-Hailey disease.

Granular parakeratosis is a rare skin-limited dermatosis. It was initially recognized in the axillae and assigned the name *axillary granular parakeratosis*. Subsequently, it has been described in other intertriginous sites as well. Look for well-demarcated scaly plaques that may have small mounds of adherent scale on their surface. Histopathologically, the hallmark is retention of keratohyalin granules with parakeratosis in the stratum corneum. Acrodermatitis enteropathica typically presents with scaly plaques with or without bullae, in the diaper area, including the inguinal folds. The face, especially the perioral location, and the acral areas also affected. Acrodermatitis enteropathica is usually seen in infants who have recently been weaned from breast milk, but it may also be seen in adults who have been on total parenteral nutrition. Another childhood disease of the folds is Langerhans cell histiocytosis. Scaly and crusted papules and plaques preferentially affect the seborrheic areas, including the intertriginous areas. Also consider lichen sclerosus in the papulosquamous category. White, atrophic, scaly, and macerated plaques can involve inguinal and intergluteal folds, along with the vulval, penile, or perianal mucosa. A rare but "do not miss" diagnosis is condyloma lata. They are a manifestation of secondary syphilis. They present as moist, eroded, and sometimes vegetating papules and plaques on genital skin or the intergluteal fold. Condyloma lata may rarely occur in other folds, such as the inframammary area (Figure 12.17) and the toe webs.

In the vesicobullous category, consider Darier disease, pemphigus vegetans, and acrodermatitis enteropathica, as outlined above. Herpes simplex and herpes zoster are two "do not miss" diseases in this location. HSV in the perianal location occurs with sacral nerve involvement. L1 zoster involves the inguinal fold, T1 zoster involves the axillary fold, and zoster in the perianal area is due to lower sacral dermatome involvement. Finally, in Hailey–Hailey disease, vesicles are rarely encountered. The classic

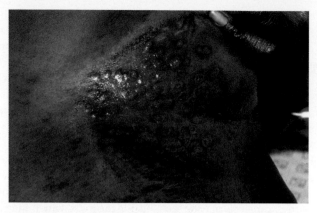

FIGURE 12.17 · Condyloma lata, showing moist, eroded papules in the inframammary area.

small linear erosions that accompany macerated plaques in this location provide a clue to the presence of underlying acantholysis.

In the eczematous category, seborrheic dermatitis is a common cause. Irritant dermatitis may be seen in the axillae secondary to deodorant use, and allergic contact dermatitis may also be encountered in this location, including allergies to deodorant or fragrance. Formaldehyde and textile contact dermatitis typically occur on the anterior and posterior axillary folds and spare the axillary vault. Systematized contact dermatitis and baboon syndrome involve the intertriginous folds, as outlined above.

Regarding pustules, there are a handful of dermatoses that present with intertriginous pustules. The most commonly seen are folliculitis (Figure 12.18) and candidiasis.

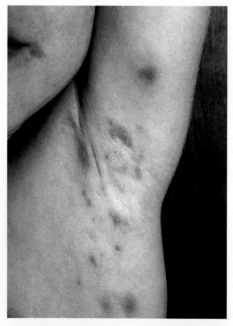

FIGURE 12.18 · Folliculitis and furunculosis in the axilla. (Image appears with permission from VisualDx. Copyright VisualDx.)

Classically, in candidiasis, there are brightly erythematous ("beefy-red") plaques with outlying satellite papules and pustules but candidiasis may present with lighter pink erythema (see Figure 1.7B), or papules and pustules only. Severe candidiasis may also be eroded. In subcorneal pustular dermatosis, flaccid pustules occur in axillae, around inguinal folds, in the flexures and may spread to the trunk. A pus-fluid level is a classical clinical sign here. Impetigo herpetformis is pustular psoriasis in pregnancy. This eruption typically arises in the intertriginous areas in the third trimester and can generalize (see Figure 11.6). Amicrobial pustulosis of the folds is a very rare eruption in patients with underlying SLE. Superficial pustules, erosions, and crusts are seen. Besides the folds, the scalp may also be involved. Another rare eruption is eosinophilic folliculitis of Ofuji. It is usually seen in Japan. It starts in and around the intertriginous areas. Pustules form annular patterns in these areas.

In the dermal reaction pattern, the axillae are a common site for furuncles (see Figure 12.18) and epidermal cysts. Hidradenitis suppurativa is also commonly seen (Figure 12.19). Tender erythematous nodules are the initial lesions. These may drain and lead to secondary changes, including sinus tract formation and cribriform scarring. Fox–Fordyce disease is the presence of perifollicular flesh-colored papules in the axillae and around the areolae (see Figure 1.7F). These are apocrine-rich sites. PXE, FEP, and intertriginous xanthomas, as mentioned previously, favor the axillae and inguinal areas.

In the vascular reaction pattern, intertrigo is the prototype. SDRIFE involves inter-triginous areas (Figure 12.20), as does toxic erythema of chemotherapy. In the latter eruption, erythematous and edematous plaques develop on intertriginous skin and hands and feet a few weeks after chemotherapy. Erythema migrans frequently, but by no means always, occurs around a fold.

In the macule category, an important "do not miss" item is axillary freckling (Figure 12.21); it is one of the diagnostic signs of neurofibromatosis (Crowe's sign).

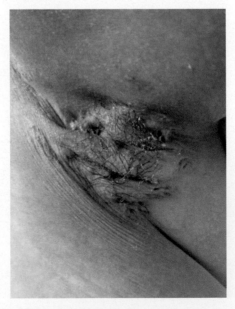

FIGURE 12.19 · Hidradenitis suppurativa, displaying papules, sinus tracts, and scarring.

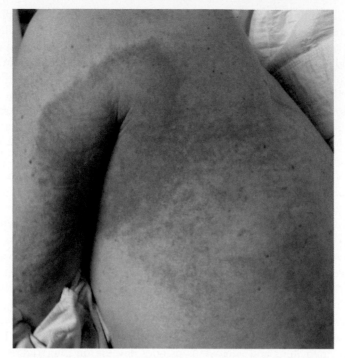

FIGURE 12.20 • Symmetric drug-related intertriginous and flexural exanthema (SDRIFE) from a systemic medication, showing a well-demarcated erythematous plaque surrounding the axilla and similar outlying papules.

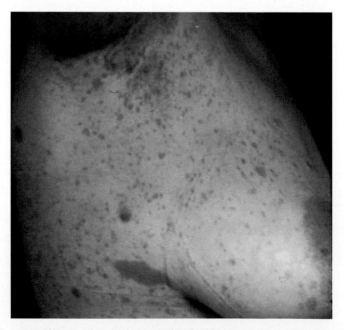

FIGURE 12.21 • Neurofibromatosis, displaying axillary freckling. Note the nearby café-au-lait macules.

TABLE 12.5. Seborrheic Distribution, by Reaction Pattern

PAPULOSQUAMOUS
- Seborrheic dermatitis
- Darier disease
- Pemphigus foliaceus
- Vitamin B_6 deficiency
- Langerhans cell histiocytosis

VESICOBULLOUS
- Pemphigus foliaceus

VASCULAR
- Purpuric macules can be seen in Langerhans cell histiocytosis

SEBORRHEIC

The differential diagnosis of eruptions that occur in the *seborrheic* distribution is presented in Table 12.5. The seborrheic areas include the scalp, the postauricular skin, the concave surfaces of the external ear, eyebrows, glabella, nasolabial folds, beard area, central chest, upper back, and the intertriginous areas.

Seborrheic Areas		
• Scalp	• Nasolabial folds	• Upper back
• In and behind the ear	• Beard area	• Intertriginous areas
• Eyebrows and glabella	• Central chest	

Seborrheic dermatitis is the prototype. Erythema with overlying greasy scales in these locations is typical. On the central chest, petaloid plaques (annular plaques with a flower-like configuration) are a unique finding. In vitamin B_6 deficiency, patients develop a seborrheic dermatitis-like eruption. In Darier disease, the morphology is different, but the distribution is the same. Scaly, brownish papules are seen. Langerhans cell histiocytosis is typically a disease of infancy. The seborrheic areas are preferentially affected with scaly and crusted papules (Figure 12.22). Langerhans cell histiocytosis may have many morphologies, including purpuric macules (see Figure 10.2). This is a "do not miss" diagnosis and should be considered in cases with a typical morphology or cases of seborrheic dermatitis in this age group that are recalcitrant to therapy. Pemphigus foliaceus typically starts in the seborrheic areas (see Figure 7.18). As it is a superficial blistering disease, flaccid bullae are quickly replaced by superficial exfoliative scaling. It may be easy to miss any "footprints" of bullae and so, including pemphigus foliaceus in the papulosquamous category of the seborrheic distribution will allow for diagnosis of this "do not miss" item.

EXTENSORS

Numerous dermatoses favor the extensor aspects of the extremities, as is seen in Table 12.6. These areas include the elbows and adjacent arm and forearm extensors, knees and adjacent thighs and shins, and the dorsal feet and hands.

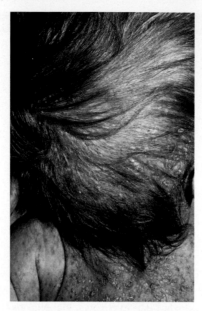

FIGURE 12.22 • Langerhans cell histiocytosis showing scaly papules and plaques on the posterior scalp.

Extensors

- Elbows and adjacent arms and forearms
- Knees and adjacent thighs and shins
- Dorsal feet, hands, and dorsal digits

Psoriasis is the prototypic extensor disease (Figure 12.23). Well-demarcated silvery plaques are typically seen. The classic childhood form of pityriasis rubra pilaris (PRP; type IV) displays well-demarcated plaques with follicular prominence over the elbows and knees. Frictional lichenoid dermatitis is a form of eczema that presents with slightly violaceous plaques over the elbows in a child. It presents with a papulosquamous morphology. The palmoplantar keratodermas that display the transgrediens phenomenon also fall into this category; hyperkeratotic plaques occur over the elbows and knees in Papillion–Lefevre syndrome, Haim–Munk syndrome, and Vohwinkel disease, among others. In Vohwinkel syndrome, these plaques are characteristically starfish-shaped. Metacarpophalangeal and metatarsophalangeal joints may also be involved. A further extremely rarely encountered entity is lipoid proteinosis. In this autosomal recessively inherited abnormality in ECM1, also known as *Urbach–Wiethe disease*, there is abnormal deposition of amorphous hyaline material in the skin, mucosa, larynx, and viscera. It presents with a hoarse cry in infancy due to laryngeal infiltration. Skin infiltration leads to beaded papules along the eyelid margin known as blepharosis moniliformis. Verrucous plaques occur at sites of friction, such as over the knees and elbows (see Figure 9.26). Acral verrucous keratoses, skin fragility, and erosion are further cutaneous features, and there is associated macroglossia. Acrokeratosis paraneoplastica occurs in the setting of an upper aerodigestive tract malignancy. There are psoriasiform or lichenoid papules and plaques that present on acral areas, including the fingers, toes, nose, penis, and ears. The palms,

TABLE 12.6. Dermatoses That Favor the Extensors, by Reaction Pattern, Pustules, and Macules

PAPULOSQUAMOUS
- Psoriasis: well-demarcated plaques with silvery scale
- Pityriasis rubra pilaris
- Frictional lichenoid dermatitis
- Palmoplantar keratodermas with transgrediens
- Lipoid proteinosis
- Acrokeratosis paraneoplastica

VESICOBULLOUS
- Epidermolysis bullosa acquisita
- Dermatitis herpetiformis

PUSTULES
- Bowel-associated dermatitis arthrosis syndrome (BADAS)
- Papulonecrotic tuberculide

ECZEMATOUS
- Atopic dermatitis in infancy
- Frictional lichenoid dermatitis

DERMAL
- Papular urticaria
- Granuloma annulare
- Erythema elevatum diutinum
- Palisaded and neutrophilic granulomatous dermatitis
- Tuberous xanthomas
- Eruptive xanthomas
- Gouty tophi
- Rheumatoid nodules
- Papulonecrotic tuberculide

VASCULAR
- Dermatomyositis
- Erythema

MACULES
- Vitiligo

soles, and elbows may be involved (see Figure 6.33C). Nails may be brittle or dystrophic and may be lost.

Vesicobullous diseases with a preferential extensor distribution include dermatitis herpetiformis (DH) and epidermolysis bullosa acquisita (EBA). In DH, the elbows and knees, along with the scalp and buttocks, are sites of predilection. Itchy urticarial plaques subsequently develop overlying small, discrete, and confluent vesicles, which are rarely intact at presentation, given the degree of associated pruritus. DH is seen in the setting of gluten-sensitive enteropathy. The mechanical subtype of EBA presents with bullae and ulcers and subsequent scarring over extensor aspects of the extremities, especially over joints (areas that are prone to trauma). Bullous erythema multiforme is a subtype of erythema multiforme that is usually associated with HSV.

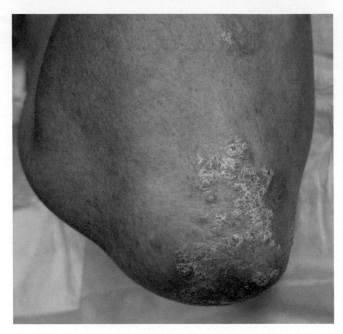

FIGURE 12.23 • Psoriasis, displaying typical well-demarcated papules with overlying silvery scales on the elbow.

Erythema multiforme may subsume a palmoplantar presentation, an extensor presentation (elbows and dorsal hands) or a combination.

Regarding pustules on the extensors, bowel-associated dermatitis arthrosis syndrome (BADAS) is a symmetric eruption of large pustules over extensor aspects of extremities. It is seen in patients with underlying inflammatory bowel disease or short-bowel syndrome. Papulonecrotic tuberculide is one of a group of reactions that occurs in response to the presence of tuberculosis antigens. It typically presents as a symmetric eruption of firm papules that cover the extensor aspects of the extremities, face, ears, palms, and soles. Pustules may also be seen. Papules ulcerate, crust, and leave varioliform scars.

In the eczematous category, atopic dermatitis in infancy favors the extensors. The flexures become preferentially involved as the child becomes a toddler.

Papular urticaria is a hypersensitivity reaction to the presence of insect bites. Many smooth erythematous papules are seen over the extensor aspects of the extremities (see Figure 10.14). A classic dermal disease that favors extensor surfaces is granuloma annulare. Smooth papules and annular plaques that may be pink, flesh-colored, or red-brown are seen. Erythema elevatum diutinum is a chronic leukocytoclastic vasculitis that may occur in association with HIV disease, streptococcal infection or an underlying IgA gammopathy. Red-brown papules, plaques, and nodules are seen over extensors. In the late fibrotic stage, nodules can become large and may resemble keloids. Palisaded and neutrophilic granulomatous dermatitis is a rare entity that is usually seen in the setting of connective tissue disease. It presents with substantive smooth papules and plaques over the extensor surfaces. Tuberous xanthomas are yellowish firm papules and nodules that are seen over the knees and elbows, usually in inherited

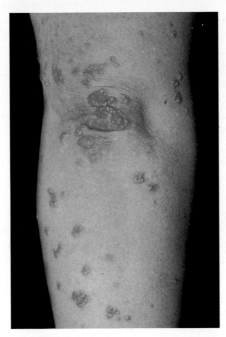

FIGURE 12.24 • Tuberous and eruptive xanthomas over the elbow and extensor forearm, displaying nodules with a yellowish hue and similar smaller papules, respectively. (Reproduced with permission from Kang S, Amagai M, Bruckner AL, et al: *Fitzpatrick's Dermatology*, 9th ed. New York, NY: McGraw Hill; 2019.)

forms of hyperlipidemia. Eruptive xanthomas occur in the setting of inherited or acquired hypertriglyceridemia and also favor the extensors, along with the buttocks and trunk. Occasionally, the two coexist when both triglyceride and cholesterol levels are high, as in familial hypercholesterolemia, type IIb (Figure 12.24). Gouty tophi are typically are seen on the ears but may also cluster around elbows and around the small joints of the hands. Tophi may appear as white, yellow, or orangey papules or nodules. They feel firm or hard. Rheumatoid nodules appear as flesh-colored or reddish deep nodules, and sometimes papules, around the elbows and on the dorsal aspects of the interphalangeal joints.

In the vascular reaction pattern, one of the cutaneous manifestations of dermato-myositis favors the extensors; linear pink to violaceous macules may be seen extending from the elbows down the forearms, from the knees toward the thighs, or from the ulnar styloid up the forearm. Erythema over the knuckles is another diagnostic sign. Superficial abrasion and scaling of these areas may occur, giving rise to a papulosqua-mous or eczematous morphology. Erythema multiforme has a typically vascular reaction pattern morphology. Finally, with respect to extensors, vitiligo commonly occurs over joints and so can be classified here.

TRUNCAL LESIONS

Some dermatoses preferentially occur on the trunk. Many viral exanthems and drug eruptions begin on the trunk. After a prodromal period, SJS/TEN presents with tender macules on the chest that signify early necrosis. These then spread centrifugally out-ward. Pityriasis rubra pilaris classically begins as discrete scaly follicular papules on the upper back. These then become confluent and spread downward and outward. The upper chest is a site of predilection for photoexposed eruptions; the central chest, for seborrheic eruptions; and reticular erythematous mucinosis and the lower back, for psoriasis. Pityriasis rosea typically occurs on the trunk and proximal extremities. Dermatitis herpetiformis favors the buttocks along with the elbows, knees, and scalp. Grover disease (transient acantholytic dermatosis) is the presence of scaly papules and sometimes vesicles in older individuals with lighter skin phototypes. It is often pruritic but may be asymptomatic. The upper back and upper abdomen are sites of predilection, but other aspects of the trunk may also be involved. Unilateral laterothoracic exanthem is also known as *asymmetric periflexural exanthem of childhood*. It presents with asymmetrically distributed truncal erythematous papules and plaques. These begin near intertriginous folds on one side, and the eruption may become more generalized over subsequent weeks. In seabather's eruption, there is a self-limited erythematous papular eruption in areas that have been exposed to the nematocysts of the sea anemone or jellyfish. While melanoma can occur anywhere on the skin surface, the back is the most common site for melanoma in men, whereas the calf is the predilection site in women.

ACRAL LESIONS

The palms and soles, along with the fingers, toes, ears, nose, and tip of penis, can be classified as acral sites.

> **Clinical Tip** Acral areas include fingers and toes, ears and nose, and the tip of the penis.

In this section, we will discuss eruptions that involve more acral sites than just fingers and toes. These are usually vasculopathic in nature. Dermatoses that affect fingers and/or toes in isolation or as part of a wider, nonacral process, will be discussed separately below. Cocaine levamisole toxicity is a mixed vasculopathy and vasculitis that is seen in users of levamisole-adulterated cocaine. There is an acute onset of tender purpuric macules and papules that involve helices of the ears and other acral areas. Retiform purpura may occur more widely also. Leukopenia and antineutrophil cytoplasmic antibody (ANCA) positivity are frequent concomitants. In septic vasculopathy, asymmetric small purpuric macules or papules occur on acral sites, including fingertips, toes, helices, and earlobes. In disseminated intravascular coagulopathy, there may be ischemia and necrosis of digits (see Figure 10.34), ears, nose, and sometimes the distal penis. In type 1 cryoglobulinemia, precipitation of cryoglobulins occurs in colder regions of body, including all the acral areas mentioned above (see also Figure 10.33). Mottled angulated plaques may progress to necrosis. Type 1 cryoglobulinemia is associated with an underlying monoclonal gammopathy or myeloma. Cryofibrinogenemia presents in a similar fashion. Acrokeratosis paraneoplastica, as described under "Extensors" (above), is a papulosquamous eruption that preferentially involves the acral areas. Figure 12.25 shows a case of acrokeratosis paraneoplastica with well-demarcated hyperkeratotic plaques on the fingers and palms. Acrodynia is another nonvasculopathic acral disease. It is part of a constellation of findings that are seen in mercury toxicity. Painful erythema on the tips of digits and nose may be seen. Palms and soles may be globally involved, and edema may be a concomitant finding. Systemically, there may be irritability, loss of appetite, and drowsiness. Hyperhidrosis

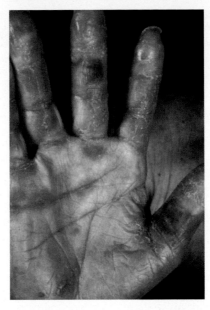

FIGURE 12.25 • Acrokeratosis paraneoplastica, showing small hyperkeratotic plaques on fingers and palm.

and alopecia may occur. Children who play with mercury from broken mercury thermometers and sphygmomanometers are usually affected, but mercury toxicity is extremely rare nowadays, given that these mercury-containing devices are very infrequently used these days.

Dermatoses Affecting Acral Areas	
• Cocaine levamisole toxicity	• Type I cryoglobulinemia
• Septic vasculopathy	• Cryofibronogenemia
• Disseminated intravascular coagulopathy	• Acrokeratosis paraneoplastica
	• Acrodynia

PALMS AND SOLES

Palms and soles manifest a variety of heterogeneous dermatoses, either as part of an acral eruption, as part of a more diffuse eruption, or as a limited phenomenon. There are a multitude of dermatoses that occur in this location. Table 12.7 lists a comprehensive differential diagnosis of eruptions and neoplasms that favor palms and soles in terms of reaction pattern and pustules.

In the papulosquamous category, tinea manuum and tinea pedis are a "do not miss" diagnosis. *Trichophyton rubrum* tinea presents with powdery scales (see Figure 12.26; see also Figures 1.8B and 6.13). An asymmetric plantar scaly eruption or a "one-hand, two-foot" dermatosis is a diagnostic clue to the presence of tinea.

> **Clinical Tip** Asymmetric plantar involvement or a "one-hand, two-foot" dermatosis is suggestive of the diagnosis of dermatophytosis.

TABLE 12.7. Differential Diagnosis of Palmoplantar Eruptions, by Reaction Pattern and Pustules

PAPULOSQUAMOUS
- Tinea manuum, tinea pedis
- Psoriasis
- Mycosis fungoides
- Lichen planus
- Discoid lupus
- LE/LP overlap
- Scabetic burrow
- Crusted scabies
- Inherited and acquired palmoplantar keratodermas
- Pityriasis rubra pilaris
- Acral erythema
- Hand–foot syndrome
- Reactive arthritis
- Secondary syphilis
- Acral verrucous keratoses
- Porokeratosis palmaris et plantaris
- Palmar pits of basal cell nevus syndrome, Cowden syndrome
- Pitted keratolysis
- Keratolysis exfoliativa
- Peeling skin syndrome
- Keratolytic winter erythema
- Acrokeratosis paraneoplastica
- Tripe palms
- Aquagenic wrinkling of the palms

VESICOBULLOUS
- Severe irritant or allergic contact dermatitis
- Dyshidrotic eczema
- Dyshidrosiform variant of bullous pemphigoid
- Hand, foot, and mouth disease
- Milker's nodule
- Epidermolysis bullosa simplex
- Dystrophic epidermolysis bullosa
- Epidermolysis bullosa acquisita
- Unilateral: think zoster
- Unilateral or bilateral: bullous tinea pedis

PUSTULES
- Palmoplantar pustular psoriasis
- SAPHO syndrome
- Dyshidrotic eczema
- Gonococcemia
- Fire ant bites
- Infantile acropustulosis
- Transient neonatal pustular melanosis

ECZEMATOUS
- Severe irritant or allergic contact dermatitis
- Dyshidrotic eczema
- Keratolysis exfoliativa

(Continued)

TABLE 12.7. Differential Diagnosis of Palmoplantar Eruptions, by Reaction Pattern and Pustules (continued)

DERMAL
- Compound or intradermal nevi
- Calcinosis cutis
- Eccrine poroma
- Kaposi sarcoma
- Palmar crease xanthomas (xanthoma striatum palmare)
- Palmar xanthomas
- Amelanotic melanoma

VASCULAR
- Erythema
  - Palmar erythema
    - Inherited
      - Erythema palmare hereditarium
    - Acquired
      - Physiologic in the setting of pregnancy
      - Smoking
      - Liver cirrhosis
      - SLE and rheumatoid arthritis
      - Thyrotoxicosis
      - Diabetes mellitus
  - Kawasaki disease
  - Raynaud disease
  - Raynaud phenomenon
  - Erythromelalgia
  - Complex regional pain syndrome
  - Acrodynia
  - Viral exanthems
  - Acute graft-versus-host disease
- Urticaria/urticarial
  - Urticaria
  - Serum sickness and serum sickness–like reaction
- Target lesions
  - Erythema multiforme
- Round macules
  - Fixed drug eruption
- Telangiectasias
  - Osler–Rendu–Weber disease
- Plaques
  - Secondary syphilis
- Purpura
  - Leukocytoclastic vasculitis
  - Septic vasculitis
    - Asymmetric purpura on distal digits
    - Janeway lesions
  - Rocky Mountain spotted fever

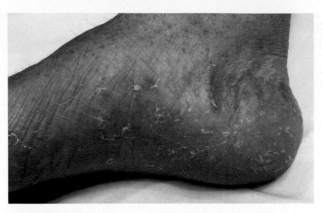

FIGURE 12.26 • Tinea pedis, showing collarettes and superficial scaling on the sole, bordered by an annular rim at the medial heel.

Psoriasis may have its usual classic features on the palms and soles with well-demarcated plaques and micaceous scale (Figure 12.27), but it may lose these features and be difficult to differentiate from hyperkeratotic eczemas, such as is seen in cases of chronic allergic contact dermatitis or chronic dyshidrotic eczema (see Figure 1.8C) in this location. Look for the presence of sago grain-type vesicles to diagnose eczema, but sometimes these are not present.

> **Clinical Tip** It may be difficult to differentiate psoriasis and eczema on palms and soles.

Mycosis fungoides may lead to scaly or hyperkeratotic plaques on palms (see Figure 1.8D) or soles. Lichen planus may rarely occur on palms or soles; it presents as a hyperkeratotic plaque with a violaceous appearance. Discoid lupus is a rare finding in this location, but in LE/LP overlap—a form of lupus with lichenoid histology—palmoplantar involvement is a common presentation (Figure 12.28). Atrophic or hyperkeratotic plaques may be seen. Inherited or acquired keratodermas may be

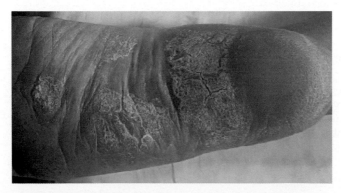

FIGURE 12.27 • Psoriasis on the sole, showing thin plaques topped by micaceous, somewhat silvery, scales.

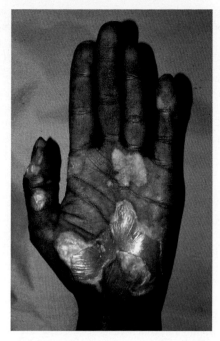

FIGURE 12.28 • LE/LP overlap showing shiny pink plaques with overlying thick scales on the palm.

global, focal, or punctate. Crusted scabies is another "do not miss" diagnosis in this group. This may manifest with crusts and erosions in the finger and toe webs and more globally over palms and soles, or it may manifest with thick, powdery scales. Patients are either extremely itchy, or not at all. Crusted scabies is highly contagious, and a high level of suspicion is needed to entertain this diagnosis. In pityriasis rubra pilaris, a keratoderma with an orange color is typical. Acral erythema from traditional chemotherapeutic agents, such as doxorubicin or 5-fluorouracil presents as tender lichenoid papules and plaques on palms and soles that extend to the lateral aspects of fingers and toes, and sometimes to the dorsal hands and feet. The hand–foot syndrome from multikinase inhibitors (sunitinib and sorafenib) manifests with painful hyperkeratotic plaques and nodules with an erythematous rim on weight-bearing areas or in areas of friction. Keratoderma blennorhagicum is the keratoderma seen in reactive arthritis; tender hyperkeratotic plaques with thick, towering, limpet-like scales or ostracious scales (see Figure 6.17) are seen on soles predominantly. Secondary syphilis has a predilection for palms and soles; tender erythematous or violaceous scaly plaques are seen (see Figure 1.8A). Ollendorff sign is the presence of tenderness on palpation of a lesion of secondary syphilis. Acral verrucous keratoses of Cowden syndrome, Rothmund–Thompson syndrome, and lipoid proteinosis (see Figure 6.8B) present as scaly small plaques on the palmoplantar surfaces and the lateral aspects of palms and fingers.

Punctate keratodermas may manifest pits or keratotic papules, or both, as is summarized in Table 12.8. There are two types of inherited keratodermas that present with pits. Both are inherited in an autosomal dominant fashion. The diffuse type presents with pits, as well as keratotic papules that may coalesce to form hyperkeratotic or

TABLE 12.8. Punctate Keratodermas, by Pits or Keratotic Papules

CONDITIONS WITH PITS	CONDITIONS WITH KERATOTIC PAPULES
• Diffuse punctate keratoderma	• Verrucae
• Punctate keratoderma of palmar creases	• Diffuse punctate keratoderma
• Darier disease	• "Music box" keratoderma
• Hailey–Hailey disease	• Cowden syndrome
• Basal cell nevus syndrome	• Arsenical keratoses
• Pitted keratolysis	• Porokeratosis of palms and soles

verrucuous plaques in wear-and-tear areas. The second type is punctate keratoderma of the palmar creases where 1–2-mm pits, translucent papules, and keratotic papules are confined to palmar creases. Both Darier disease (see Figure 6.36) and Hailey–Hailey disease may display keratin-filled pits on palms and soles. In basal cell nevus syndrome, palmoplantar pits occur in association with multiple basal cell cancers. Pitted keratolysis is a corynebacterial infection of the soles. Superficial pits appear in the stratum corneum. These measure 2–3 mm and can be confluent. A musty odor and background hyperhidrosis may accompany these findings.

Regarding keratotic papules in this location, verrucae are common (Figure 12.29). A rare inherited spiny keratoderma, also known as "music box" keratoderma, presents with thin keratotic spines that arise from palmoplantar keratotic papules. Sporadic cases also occur. In Cowden syndrome, palmoplantar keratotic papules and acral verrucous keratoses are seen in concert with trichilemmomas. Individuals with Cowden syndrome are at increased risk for various internal malignancies. Naegeli–Franceschetti–Jadassohn syndrome is the constellation of punctate palmoplantar keratotic papules, reticulate hyperpigmentation, hypohidrosis, and nail dystrophy. Arsenical keratoses are one of the cutaneous findings of arsenic exposure. Porokeratosis of palms and soles is a subset of porokeratosis that is limited to palms and soles; 1–3-mm translucent and keratotic papules bounded by thready porokeratotic rims are seen. The latter finding clinches the diagnosis, but it may be difficult to discern clinically.

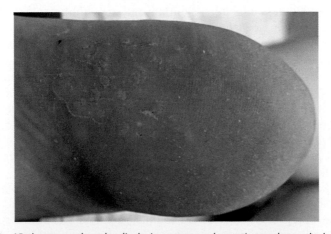

FIGURE 12.29 · Viral warts on the soles displaying verrucous keratotic papules on the heel.

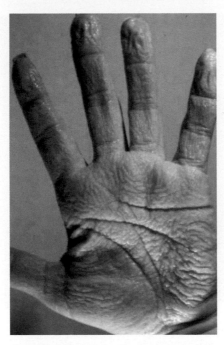

FIGURE 12.30 • Aquagenic wrinkling of the palms, showing a macerated, wrinkled appearance of the palm that has had a short exposure to tap water.

Fine peeling may be seen in a few conditions: Keratolysis exfoliativa is a mild form of dyshidrotic eczema that presents predominantly with superficial scaling, including collarettes of scale (see Figure 6.32). Peeling skin syndrome is a group of inherited keratinizing disorders marked by superficial peeling. Some forms are generalized, and others are localized to palms and soles. Keratolytic winter erythema is a very rare inherited peeling dermatosis that occurs in the Afrikaner population in an area in the Cape Province in South Africa. Centrifugal peeling of palms and soles is more marked in the winter months. It is exacerbated by alcohol or fever. Scaly eruptions on palms and soles may be a paraneoplastic phenomenon; acrokeratosis paraneoplastica (Bazex syndrome) usually involves fingers and toes, but palms and soles may be affected (see Figure 12.25). In tripe palms, the palms are thickened and velvety with accentuation of skin markings. Tripe palms are a manifestation of acanthosis nigricans on the palms. In aquagenic wrinkling of the palms, there is rapid wrinkling of the palms on exposure to water (Figure 12.30). Some cases have been seen in association with cystic fibrosis, and an increased salt content of the stratum corneum has been postulated as a mechanism for this curious finding.

Vesicles and bullae on palms or soles may signify a severe irritant or allergic contact dermatitis. In dyshidrotic eczema, the lateral aspects of fingers and toes only may be involved, or palmar and plantar involvement in more severe cases may be seen. Vesicles are typically "sago grain" size, but may be larger especially on palms and soles, and bullae may also be seen (Figure 12.31). If bullae or vesicles are unilateral, think zoster (Figure 12.32), especially if they are clustered on an erythematous base, and examine the forearm or leg for further similar findings. Another cause of unilateral vesicles or bullae is bullous tinea pedis. This is usually itchy, and it flares in hot weather. *Trichophyton mentagrophytes* is the typical culprit. Numerous autoimmune bullous

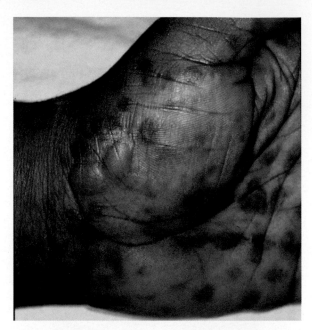

FIGURE 12.31 • Severe dyshidrotic eczema, showing vesicles and larger bullae on the palm. (Reproduced with permission from Kelly AP, Taylor SC, Lom HW, et al: *Taylor and Kelly's Dermatology for Skin of Color*, 2nd ed. New York, NY: McGraw Hill; 2016.)

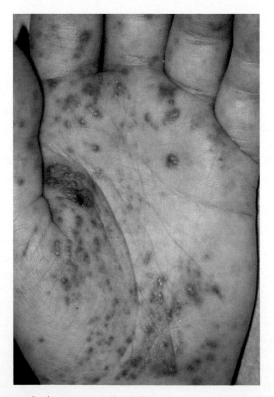

FIGURE 12.32 • C7 zoster displaying grouped vesicles and purpuric macules on the palm.

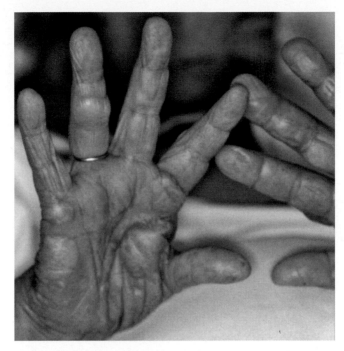

FIGURE 12.33 · Bullous pemphigoid resembling severe dyshidrotic eczema, with scattered bullae on the palm. (Used with permission from Dr. Deepak Modi, University of the Witwatersrand, Johannesburg, South Africa.)

disorders may be seen in this anatomic location. The dyshidrosiform variant of bullous pemphigoid resembles dyshidrotic eczema (Figure 12.33; see also Figure 7.24). Hand–foot–mouth disease is an acute viral illness of early childhood predominantly, but non-immune adults may also develop the disease. There is a high fever that is accompanied by small oral erosions and vesicles on lateral aspects of fingers and toes and palms and soles. The vesicles are typically oval and may have a grayish appearance. Sometimes papules only are seen. Coxsackie viruses and other enteroviruses are responsible. Enterovirus A71 has been associated with more severe disease, including an exanthem that spreads more proximally on the limbs and the possible presence of internal organ inflammation, such as encephalitis and pneumonitis. Milker's nodule is a parapox infection that usually occurs after milking an infected cow. A papule or nodule may vesiculate and crust before healing over weeks. The dorsal hand, fingers, palm, or other areas of the distal forearm may be affected. Epidermolysis bullosa simplex presents in childhood with vesicles and bullae occurring after minor trauma predominantly on the palms and soles. The generalized, or Dowling–Meara, variant presents as widespread blistering that may display herpetiform grouping of vesicles and bullae and an associated palmoplantar keratoderma. In the recessive form of dystrophic EB (DEB), severe skin fragility, and widespread bulla formation and erosions appear shortly after birth. Scarring is common, and severe and milia are a feature. Scarring of the hands leads to "mitten" deformities. The mechanobullous variant of acquired epidermolysis bullosa presents with bullae that occur in response to trauma. Both dorsal hands and feet and palmoplantar surfaces may be affected.

Superficial pustules on palms and soles may be seen in palmoplantar pustular psoriasis. They are accompanied by brown incipient crusts (see Figure 2.37). SAPHO

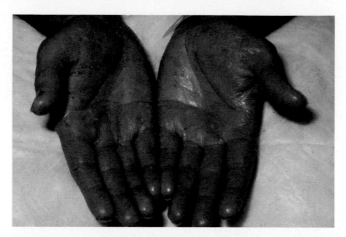

FIGURE 12.34 • Severe irritant dermatitis, displaying diffuse shiny erythema, scaling, and erosions on the palms.

(synovitis, acne, pustulosis, hyperostosis, osteitis) syndrome may also present with palmoplantar pustulosis. In dyshidrotic eczema, longstanding vesicles may become cloudy and resemble pustules. In gonococcemia, acral, asymmetric large tender pustules on purpuric bases may be seen. Fire ant bites are extremely itchy. Pustules may be seen. Exposed areas, such as palms, soles, and other parts of the distal extremities may be affected. The onset of infantile acropustulosis is around 3–6 months of age. Crops of pustules and vesicles occur on the palms and soles until the age of 3 years. Transient neonatal pustular melanosis is seen at birth. Scattered superficial pustules, collarettes of scale, and postinflammatory hyperpigmentation are seen on the face and trunk and less commonly on the palms and soles.

Palmoplantar eczematous dermatoses include irritant and allergic contact dermatitides, dyshidrotic eczema, and keratolysis exfoliativa. Irritant eczema may be dry and scaly, or if there has been exposure to a strong acid or alkali, it may display shiny, erythematous plaques that may be eroded (Figure 12.34). Longstanding dyshidrotic eczema may become hyperkeratotic (see Figure 1.8C).

In the dermal reaction pattern, compound or intradermal nevi may be seen in this location. Palms and soles are the most common sites of presentation of eccrine poromas. They present as friable reddish nodules with a collarette of scale around the edge. In Kaposi sarcoma, (KS), violaceous plaques or nodules are seen. Palms and soles are sites of predilection for KS. Palmar crease xanthomas (xanthoma striatum palmare) are typically seen in seen in mixed hypertriglyceridemia and hypercholesterolemia (such as in familial dysbetalipoproteinemia), and more diffuse palmar xanthomas may be seen in primary biliary cirrhosis and multiple myeloma. Melanoma is a "do not miss" diagnosis on palms and soles. These acral melanomas may either be pigmented or amelanotic, in which case they may appear flesh-colored, pink or reddish in color.

In terms of the vascular reaction pattern, a variety of morphologies may be seen in this anatomic location. Diffuse erythema of the palms (palmar erythema) may be inherited, but is usually acquired and is secondary to an underlying systemic disorder. The palmar erythema of SLE may have a reticulate appearance (Figure 12.35). One of the diagnostic criteria for Kawasaki disease is erythema and edema of palms and soles. Fever, lymphadenopathy, a polymorphic rash, and conjunctival and oropharyngeal

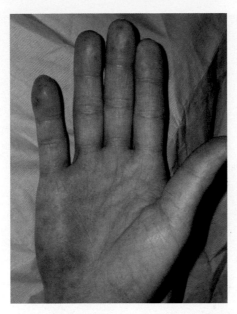

FIGURE 12.35 • Palmar erythema in SLE displaying a reticulated appearance.

involvement are further criteria. In Raynaud disease, symmetric episodic vasospasm occurs secondary to cold exposure. Fingers and sometimes palms turn white, then blue, then red. In Raynaud phenomenon, similar changes to Raynaud disease occur in the setting of connective tissue disease, usually in scleroderma. Vasospasm is typically asymmetric, nail fold capillary changes may be seen, and digital necrosis may occur. Erythromelalgia is the episodic occurrence of erythema and burning of bilateral feet more frequently than hands. Symptoms are worse at night. In complex regional pain syndrome, pain in an affected limb may be accompanied by red or purplish discoloration, textural changes in skin, and abnormal sweating. Many viral exanthems have palmar involvement. In acute graft-versus-host disease (GVHD), palms and soles are a site of predilection (Figure 12.36; see also Figure 10.32).

Urticaria can involve the palms and soles (Figure 12.37). In serum sickness and serum sickness–like reactions, bilateral palmar or plantar involvement of urticarial plaques may be a feature.

> **Clinical Tip** Urticarial plaques of bilateral palms or soles may signify the presence of serum sickness or a serum sickness–like reaction.

Target lesions are seen symmetrically on palms and soles in erythema multiforme. In fixed drug eruption, a single round plaque may involve numerous fingers. Secondary syphilis may present early in the disease course with tender thin plaques without scale. Later, the typical papulosquamous appearance evolves.

Purpura may also be seen on palms and soles. In leukocytoclastic vasculitis, palmoplantar involvement is rare. In septic vasculitis, asymmetric and stellate purpura is seen on the distal digits. Janeway lesions are hemorrhagic, painless macules, usually found on thenar and hypothenar eminences. They are a sign of acute bacterial endocarditis. Rocky Mountain spotted fever (RMSF) is caused by *Rickettsia rickettsiae*. A few days to over a

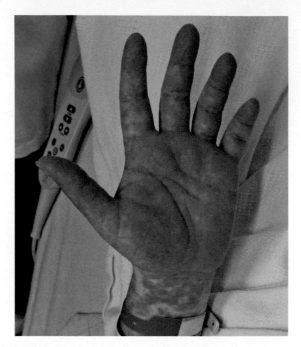

FIGURE 12.36 · Acute graft-versus-host disease, displaying significant palmar involvement.

week after inoculation of the organisms by a tick bite, there is fever, nausea, vomiting, and abdominal pain. Blanching macules and papules occur on the distal extremities, including palms and soles. Later in the disease course, these become petechial or purpuric. If untreated, RMSF can cause a sepsis-like syndrome with acute organ failure.

Table 12.9 displays the differential diagnosis of pigmented macules in this anatomic location. If multiple pigmented macules are seen, think normal variant in a darker skin phototype, postinflammatory hyperpigmentation from a preceding

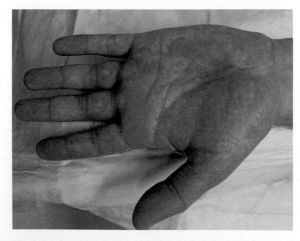

FIGURE 12.37 · Urticaria on the palm, displaying edematous and erythematous plaques with an accentuated arcuate border.

TABLE 12.9. Pigmented Macules on Palms or Soles

MULTIPLE
- Normal variant
- Postinflammatory hyperpigmentation
- Vitamin B$_{12}$ deficiency
- Junctional nevi

SINGLE
- Junctional nevus
- Talon noir
- Tinea nigra
- Acral melanoma

eruption such as secondary syphilis, or vitamin B$_{12}$ deficiency. Junctional nevi are usually medium or dark brown in this location. One of more may be seen. Talon noir is a superficial subcorneal hemorrhage caused by frictional trauma. It may appear black and can mimic a pigmented lesion (see Figure 4.17E). On close-up inspection, a deep maroon color may be appreciable. Talon noir can be pared down with a blade and removed completely in this way. Tinea nigra is a rarely encountered superficial fungal infection that is seen predominantly in the tropics. It presents as a dark brown to black macule on the sole or palm and may mimic melanoma. Finally, acral melanoma is a "do not miss" diagnosis. It may present with a macule that is any shade of brown or a combination of shades of brown. It may also be amelanotic and present with a pink or reddish color.

DORSAL HANDS

The differential diagnosis of eruptions and neoplasms on the dorsal hands differs substantially from that on the palms. In general, dermatoses that occur on the dorsal hands are those that occur on extensors (including psoriasis and dermatomyositis over knuckles); on acute and habitually sun-exposed sites (including porphyria cutanea tarda, actinic keratoses, and squamous cell carcinoma), from inoculation of microorganisms (such as erysipeloid or sporotrichosis), as a result of contactants (such as airborne contact dermatitis) or bites, or those that are induced by friction (such as epidermolysis bullosa acquisita or vitiligo).

Some of the Dermatoses on the Dorsal Hands Are Those That Occur:

- As a result of inoculation of microorganisms
- On acutely and habitually sun-exposed sites
- On extensors
- As a result of contactants or bites
- As a result of friction

Table 12.10 lists a comprehensive differential diagnosis for this location by etiology, and in Table 12.11, a differential diagnosis by reaction pattern, pustules, and macules is outlined. The differential diagnosis of conditions that preferentially affect the

TABLE 12.10. Differential Diagnosis of Dermatoses with a Predilection for the Dorsal Hands, by Etiology

INHERITED
- Xeroderma pigmentosum
- Reticulate acropigmentation of Dohi
- Amyloidosis cutis dyschromica
- Dyschromatosis universalis hereditaria
- Acrokeratosis verruciformis of Hopf
- Darier disease with acrokeratosis verruciformis–like papules
- Bazex–Dupre–Christol syndrome
- Porphyria cutanea tarda
- Variegate porphyria

ACQUIRED
- Infectious
  - Bacterial
    - Cellulitis
    - Erysipelas
    - Erysipeloid
    - *Vibrio vulnificans* infection
    - Cat scratch disease
  - Viral
    - Flat warts
    - Common warts
    - Milker's nodule
    - Orf
  - Mycobacterial
    - *Mycobacterium marinum* infection
    - Primary inoculation tuberculosis
    - Tuberculosis verrucosa cutis
  - Fungal
    - Sporotrichosis
- Inflammatory/autoimmune
  - Granuloma annulare
  - Rheumatoid nodules
  - Erythema multiforme
  - Epidermolysis bullosa acquisita
  - Porphyria cutanea tarda
  - Variegate porphyria
  - Pseudoporphyria
  - Erythropoeietic protoporphyia
  - SLE
  - SCLE
  - Generalized DLE
  - Dermatomyositis
  - Scleroderma
  - Psoriasis
  - Irritant dermatitis
  - Pityriasis rubra pilaris
  - Vitiligo
  - Allergic contact dermatitis
  - Photoallergic dermatitis

(Continued)

TABLE 12.10. Differential Diagnosis of Dermatoses with a Predilection for the Dorsal Hands, by Etiology (continued)

ACQUIRED (CONT.)
- Chronic actinic dermatitis
- Airborne contact dermatitis
- Insect bites
- Metabolic
  - Porphyria cutanea tarda
- Depositional
  - Tuberous xanthomas- over MCPs
  - Acral persistent papular mucinosis
  - Lipoid proteinosis
- Neoplastic
  - Seborrheic keratosis
  - Actinic keratosis
  - Squamous cell cancer in situ
  - Squamous cell cancer
  - Melanoma in situ
  - Melanoma
  - Multinucleate cell angiohistiocytoma
- Paraneoplastic
  - Acanthosis nigricans
  - Multicentric reticulohistiocytoma
  - Neutrophilic dermatosis of the dorsal hands
- Drug/chemical-related
  - Chemical leukoderma
  - Pseudoporphyria
  - Fixed drug eruption
  - Phytophotodermatitis
  - Phototoxic drug eruption

TABLE 12.11. Differential Diagnosis of Dorsal Hand Dermatoses, by Reaction Pattern, Pustules, and Macules

PAPULOSQUAMOUS
- Psoriasis
- Pityriasis rubra pilaris
- Generalized DLE
- SCLE
- Seborrheic keratosis
- Flat wart
- Common wart
- Actinic keratosis
- Squamous cell cancer in situ
- Squamous cell cancer
- Acrokeratosis verruciformis of Hopf
- Darier disease with acrokeratosis verruciformis–like papules
- Acanthosis nigricans
- Tuberculosis verrucosa cutis

(Continued)

TABLE 12.11. Differential Diagnosis of Dorsal Hand Dermatoses, by Reaction Pattern, Pustules, and Macules (continued)

VESICOBULLOUS
- Allergic contact dermatitis
- Photoallergic dermatitis
- Phytophotodermatitis
- Phototoxic drug eruption
- Bullous insect bite
- Erythema multiforme
- Erysipelas
- Bullous Sweet syndrome
- *Vibro vulnificans* infection
- Porphyria cutanea tarda
- Variegate porphyria
- Pseudoporphyria
- Epidermolysis bullosa acquisita—mechanobullous type

PUSTULES
- Neutrophilic dermatosis of the dorsal hands
- Fire ant bites

ECZEMATOUS
- Irritant dermatitis
- Allergic contact dermatitis
- Photoallergic dermatitis
- Chronic actinic dermatitis
- Airborne contact dermatitis

DERMAL
- Granuloma annulare
- *Mycobacterium marinum* infection
- Primary inoculation tuberculosis
- Cat scratch disease
- Multinucleate cell angiohistiocytoma
- Melanoma
- Tuberous xanthomas
- Multicentric reticulohistiocytoma
- Rheumatoid nodules
- Acral persistent papular mucinosis
- Lipoid proteinosis
- Scleroderma

VASCULAR
- Erythropoeietic protoporphyia
- Insect bites

WHITE MACULES
- Vitiligo: over MCPs, dorsal hands
- Contact or drug-induced leukoderma
- Idiopathic guttate hypomelanosis

(Continued)

TABLE 12.11. Differential Diagnosis of Dorsal Hand Dermatoses, by Reaction Pattern, Pustules, and Macules (continued)

BROWN MACULES
- Reticulate acropigmentation of Kitamura
- Degos–Dowling disease
- Ephelides
- Lentigines
- Nevi
- Melanoma in situ
- Melanoma
- Phytophotodermatitis
- Fixed drug eruption

WHITE AND BROWN MACULES: "MOTTLED PIGMENTATION"
- Xeroderma pigmentosum
- Reticulate acropigmentation of Dohi: starts on dorsal hands and spreads proximally
- Amyloidosis cutis dyschromica: hyper- and hypopigmented macules, not limited to dorsal hands; biopsy shows amyloid deposition
- Dyschromatosis universalis hereditarian: hyper- and hypopigmented macules, widespread distribution, autosomal dominant, onset in first year of life

PITS
- Bazex–Dupre–Christol syndrome

knuckles is found in Table 12.14 and discussed below. In Bazex–Dupre–Christol syndrome, an X-linked dominant condition, affected individuals develop follicular atrophoderma that is most marked on the dorsal hands. It manifests as tiny follicle-based pits (Figure 12.38). It also can affect the elbows. There is associated hypohidrosis, milia formation, and an increased propensity to form basal cell cancers.

The dorsal hands and fingers are common sites of inoculation of cutaneous infections. Erysipeloid is caused by the *Erysipelothrix rhusiopathiae*, a Gram-positive

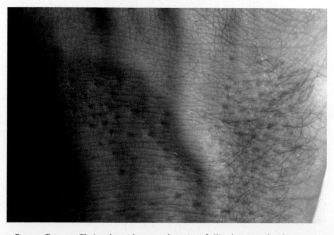

FIGURE 12.38 • Bazex–Dupre–Christol syndrome, showing follicular atrophoderma on the dorsal hand.

bacillus that infects fish and other animals. A well-demarcated erythematous plaque develops at the site of inoculation. Bullae may occur, and the infection can become more widespread or cause endocarditis. *Vibrio vulnificans* is a Gram-negative bacillus that can cause severe cellulitis and necrotizing fasciitis. It spreads rapidly and can be fatal, especially in immunocompromised hosts. It is acquired through contact with raw shellfish. In cat scratch disease, *Bartonella henselae*, a Gram-negative bacillus, is inoculated through a cat scratch or bite. Locally, there is a dermal papule or nodule or pus formation. There may be associated local lymphadenopathy. Milker's nodule (as mentioned previously) and orf commonly occur on the fingers. They are viral diseases caused by parapox viruses. They occur through inoculation of infected animal products. Orf occurs after contact with infected goats or sheep. Fingers and thumbs are most frequently affected but the hand—typically the dorsal hand—may be involved. *Mycobacterium marinum* is an atypical mycobacterium that affects people with fish tanks or who have been in contact with other sources of freshwater, such as in swimming pools, or occasionally, saltwater. Sporotrichosis is a deep fungal infection that is usually inoculated from an infected thorn, soil, or other plant matter. These infections also cause a dermal papule or nodule at the site of inoculation, and lymphocutaneous spread may be seen. Primary inoculation tuberculosis presents as an ulcer ("chancre"). It occurs in an individual who has no underlying immunity to tuberculosis. Tuberculosis verrucosa cutis (TB verrucosa cutis) is a form of inoculation TB in a sensitized individual. It presents as a verrucous or vegetating plaque.

In the inflammatory category, pityriasis rubra pilaris on the dorsal hands is described as having a "nutmeg grater appearance." Tiny papules with peripheral accentuation of scale are seen. Granuloma annulare has a propensity for this location. It may be seen over the metacarpophalangeal joints, or it may occur more broadly (Figure 12.39).

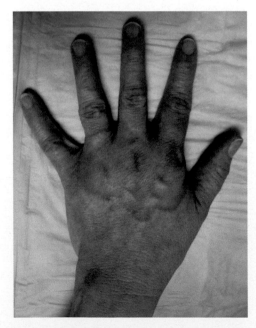

FIGURE 12.39 · Granuloma annulare on the dorsal hand, showing an arcuate plaque that encompasses the metacarpophalangeal joints.

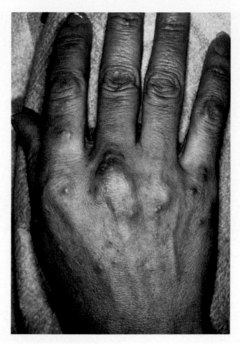

FIGURE 12.40 · Bullous erythema multiforme on the dorsal hand, showing scattered raised atypical target lesions (erythematous small plaques with central vesicles). (Used with permission from Dr. Miguel Sanchez, New York University, New York, NY.)

The dorsal hands are a site of predilection for erythema multiforme, as mentioned previously (Figure 12.40).

In the neoplastic group, acrokeratosis verruciformis of Hopf presents with flat verrucous-appearing papules on the distal extremities. Similar papules have been seen in Darier disease (see Figure 6.8A), and both conditions have now been recognized to be allelic. Multinucleate cell angiohistiocytoma is an extremely rare benign vascular and histiocytic proliferation that is seen on the dorsal hands and wrists of predominantly women. Actinic keratoses (see Figure 6.22) and all forms of skin cancer may be seen in this location, given that it is a chronically sun-exposed site (Figure 12.41). It appears as a reddish or maroon papule or plaque. Lesions are typically solitary but may be multiple. In the paraneoplastic group, malignant acanthosis nigricans in particular (but also severe acanthosis nigricans from other causes) may present with velvety plaques over the knuckles. Multicentric reticulohistiocytoma is associated with an underlying, usually solid-organ malignancy in around a quarter of cases. Reddish-brown smooth papules and, occasionally, nodules are seen scattered over the dorsal fingers and over the metacarpophalangeal joints (Figure 9.33). "Coral beading" is the clustering of tiny papules in a line around the nail fold—a phenomenon that is typical for this disease. There is an associated arthritis in most individuals. Neutrophilic dermatosis of the dorsal hands is a bullous variant of Sweet syndrome that occurs in this location. Sweet syndrome–like plaques, purulent eroded plaques with a bluish appearance, and boggy plaques have been described. The associations of Sweet syndrome should be sought. An underlying hematologic malignancy has been more frequently found in neutrophilic dermatosis of the dorsal hands than with other forms of Sweet syndrome.

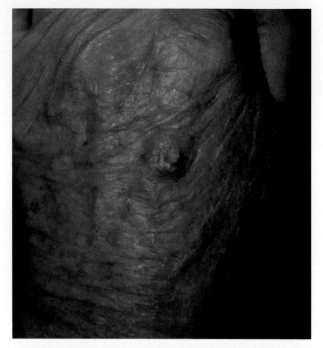

FIGURE 12.41 · A squamous cell cancer on the dorsal hand, showing an infiltrated erythematous plaque with an overlying cutaneous horn.

DIGITS

The differential diagnosis of dermatoses on digits recapitulates that of palms and soles, as well as the dorsal hands, and is listed in Table 12.12. The periungual location is considered separately in Table 12.13. In Kawasaki disease, fingers may be involved with erythema and edema (vascular reaction pattern). Later in the disease course, desquamation of fingertips occurs. The finger is a common site for herpetic whitlow. Rarely, a toe may be affected. In herpetic whitlow, there is primary inoculation of HSV into the skin. Infants are commonly affected, but any age may be afflicted with the primary disease. There may be coexistent HSV elsewhere. Initially, herpetic whitlow is seen as erythema and edema of part of a digit. Grouped vesicles eventuate and crust over (see Figure 7.5). Pain and tenderness are frequent concomitants. Recurrences are rare. Blistering distal dactylitis is a bacterial infection caused by group A streptococcus. This manifests as a cloudy bulla on the distal digit. More proximal involvement may infrequently occur.

In the dermal reaction pattern category, periungual fibromas are firm, small flesh-colored or pinkish papules that arise at the lateral or proximal nail fold, usually on a toe. They may be an isolated finding, or they may be a cutaneous finding of tuberous sclerosis (Figure 12.42). Erythema elevatum diuntinum may also be seen on dorsal aspects of digits (see Figure 9.8).

In the vascular category, Osler–Rendu–Weber disease (hereditary hemorrhagic telangiectasia), with telangiectasias manifest as bright red macules and papules over the fingers (Figure 12.43), toes, palms, soles, face, and oral cavity (including the lips and tongue) and in the nose may occur. Epistaxis is a common occurrence. Internal organs may have telangiectasias and larger vascular neoplasms, such as arteriovenous malformations.

TABLE 12.12. Differential Diagnosis of Conditions that Occur on Digits, by Reaction Pattern and Pustules

PAPULOSQUAMOUS
- Warts
- Tinea manuum, tinea pedis
- Psoriasis
- Mycosis fungoides
- Lichen planus
- Discoid lupus
- LE/LP overlap
- Scabetic burrow
- Crusted scabies
- Inherited and acquired palmoplantar keratodermas
- Pityriasis rubra pilaris
- Acral erythema
- Hand–foot syndrome
- Reactive arthritis
- Secondary syphilis
- Acral verrucous keratoses
- Porokeratosis palmaris et plantaris
- Palmar pits of basal cell nevus syndrome, Cowden syndrome
- Pitted keratolysis
- Keratolysis exfoliativa
- Peeling skin syndrome
- Keratolytic winter erythema
- Acrokeratosis paraneoplastica
- Tripe palms
- Aquagenic wrinkling of the palms

VESICOBULLOUS
- Herpetic whitlow
- Blistering distal dactylitis
- Severe irritant or allergic contact dermatitis
- Dyshidrotic eczema
- Dyshidrosiform variant of bullous pemphigoid
- Hand, foot, and mouth disease
- Epidermolysis bullosa simplex
- Dystrophic epidermolysis bullosa
- Epidermolysis bullosa acquisita
- Unilateral–think zoster
- Unilateral or bilateral: bullous tinea pedis
- Milker's nodule
- Orf
- Erysipeloid
- *Vibrio vulnificans* infection

PUSTULES
- Herpetic whitlow
- Blistering distal dactylitis
- Orf
- Milker's nodule

(Continued)

TABLE 12.12. Differential Diagnosis of Conditions that Occur on Digits, by Reaction Pattern and Pustules (continued)

PUSTULES (CONT.)
- Cat scratch disease
- Tularemia
- Palmoplantar pustular psoriasis
- Acrodermatitis continua of Hallopeau
- SAPHO syndrome
- Dyshidrotic eczema
- Gonococcemia
- Fire ant bites
- Infantile acropustulosis
- Transient neonatal pustular melanosis

ECZEMATOUS
- Dyshidrotic eczema
- Irritant dermatitis
- Allergic contact dermatitis
- Keratolysis exfoliativa
- Lichen simplex chronicus

DERMAL
- Infantile digital fibromatosis
- Juvenile hyaline fibromatosis
- Myxoid pseudocyst
- Glomus tumor
- Periungual fibroma
- Eponychial fibrokeratoma
- Enchondroma
- Maffucci's syndrome
- Granuloma annulare
- Erythema elevatum diutinum
- Giant cell tumor of the tendon sheath
- Dermatofibroma
- Orf
- Milker's nodule
- Tularemia
- *Mycobacterium marinum*
- Sporotrichosis
- Insect bites
- Gouty tophi
- Multicentric reticulohistiocytosis
- Scleroderma
- Calcinosis cutis

VASCULAR
- Palmar erythema—erythema frequently involves palmar aspect of digits
- Acrodynia
- Kawasaki disease
- Complex regional pain syndromes
- Erythromelalgia
- Raynaud disease

(Continued)

TABLE 12.12.   Differential Diagnosis of Conditions that Occur on Digits, by Reaction Pattern and Pustules (continued)

VASCULAR (CONT.)
- Raynaud phenomenon
- Chilblains
- Chilblain lupus
- Pseudo-chilblains of Covid-19 infection
- Acute gout
- Osler–Rendu–Weber disease
- Septic vasculitis
- Gonococcemia
- Rocky Mountain spotted fever
- Janeway lesions
- Osler's nodes
- Cryoglobulinemia
- Cryofibroinogenemia
- Cholesterol emboli
- Thrombotic vasculopathies
  - Antiphospholipid syndrome
- Erysipeloid
- *Vibrio vulnificans* infection

WHITE MACULES
- Vitiligo: over MCPs, dorsal hands
- Contact or drug-induced leukoderma
- Idiopathic guttate hypomelanosis

BROWN MACULES
- Reticulate acropigmentation of Kitamura
- Degos–Dowling disease
- Ephelides
- Lentigines
- Nevi
- Melanoma in situ
- Melanoma
- Phytophotodermatitis
- Fixed drug eruption
- Postinflammatory hyperpigmentation
- Vitamin B_{12} deficiency
- Talon noir
- Tinea nigra

WHITE AND BROWN MACULES: "MOTTLED PIGMENTATION"
- Xeroderma pigmentosum
- Reticulate acropigmentation of Dohi
- Amyloidosis cutis dyschromica
- Dyschromatosis universalis hereditaria

PITS
- Bazex–Dupre–Christol syndrome

TABLE 12.13. Differential Diagnosis of Conditions that Frequently Occur in the Periungual Location, by Reaction Pattern and Pustules

PAPULOSQUAMOUS
- Keratolysis exfoliativa
- Warts
- Acrokeratosis paraneoplastica

VESICOBULLOUS
- Herpetic whitlow
- Blistering distal dactylitis
- Dyshidrotic eczema
- Severe irritant or allergic contact dermatitis

PUSTULES
- Acute paronychia
- Acrodermatitis continua of Hallopeau
- Gonococcemia
- Septic vasculitis

ECZEMATOUS
- Dyshidrotic eczema
- Irritant dermatitis
- Allergic contact dermatitis
- Lichen simplex chronicus
- Keratolysis exfoliativa

DERMAL
- Infantile digital fibromatosis
- Juvenile hyaline fibromatosis
- Myxoid pseudocyst
- Glomus tumor
- Periungual fibroma
- Eponychial fibrokeratoma
- Multicentric reticulohistiocytois
- Granuloma annulare
- Giant cell tumor of the tendon sheath
- Dermatofibroma

VASCULAR
- Chronic paronychia
- Periungual erythema is a sign of connective tissue disease: SLE and dermatomyositis
- Nail fold capillary changes of connective tissue disease may be seen with the naked eye and these findings are accentuated on dermoscopy–in dermatomyositis, giant capillary loops, tortuous vessels, and capillary dropout are seen; while in scleroderma, dilated vessels, large capillaries ("megacapillaries"), and microhemorrhages may be seen
- Nail fold infarcts—typically seen in scleroderma; may also be seen in severe forms of dermatomyositis; findings include nail fold hemorrhages and small ulcerations
- In hereditary hemorrhagic telangiectasia, there may be giant nail fold capillary loops, subungual telangiectasias, and splinter hemorrhages
- Splinter hemorrhages: small linear red to dark purple subungual macules
- Pseudo-chilblains of COVID-19 infection

MACULES
- Hutchinson sign
- Pseudo-Hutchinson sign

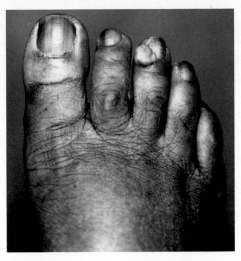

FIGURE 12.42 • A periungual fibroma, showing a large pink and brown periungual papule arising from the proximal nailfold. (Reproduced with permission from Kelly AP, Taylor SC, Lom HW, et al: *Taylor and Kelly's Dermatology for Skin of Color*, 2nd ed. New York, NY: McGraw-Hill Education; 2016.)

An important "do not miss" diagnosis in the vascular reaction pattern category of the digits is that of pseudo-chilblains of Covid-19 infection. These erythematous or violaceous papules and plaques may be painful, itchy or asymptomatic. They typically occur in younger individuals who have experienced a mild form of the disease within the preceding few weeks.

In the macule category, Hutchinson sign is the presence of brown, black or variegated pigment on periungual skin. It signifies extension of a nail matrix or subungual melanoma. Pseudo-Hutchinson sign is the presence of periungual brown pigment that arises from a benign lesion of the nail apparatus, such as a nevus.

A subset of dermatoses favor the knuckles (metacarpophalangeal and interphalangeal joints), and these are listed for conciseness in Table 12.14. Figures 12.44–12.46

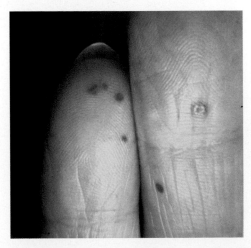

FIGURE 12.43 • Osler–Rendu–Weber disease showing bright red telangiectasias on the distal digits.

TABLE 12.14. Differential Diagnosis of Dermatoses that Favor the Knuckles, by Reaction Pattern

PAPULOSQUAMOUS

- Psoriasis
- Knuckle pads
- Inherited keratodermas
  - Epidermolytic keratoderma of Vorner
  - Vohwinkel keratoderma: starfish-shaped
  - Mal de Meleda
  - Acrokeratoelastoidosis: papules, along with papules on insteps or thenar eminences
- Dermatomyositis
- Acanthosis nigricans

VESICOBULLOUS

- Epidermolysis bullosa acquisita: mechanobullous type

ECZEMATOUS

- Irritant dermatitis

DERMAL

- Granuloma annulare
- Tuberous xanthomas
- Multicentric reticulohistiocytoma
- Rheumatoid nodules

VASCULAR

- Dermatomyositis
- SLE often, but not always, spares interphalangeal joints

WHITE MACULES

- Vitiligo: over MCPs, dorsal hands

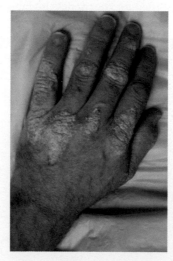

FIGURE 12.44 · Psoriasis over the metacarpophalangeal joints, showing well-demarcated plaques with ostraceous scale.

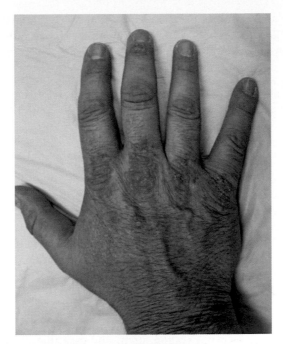

FIGURE 12.45 • Subacute eczema affecting the metacarpophalangeal joints, showing scaly plaques with tiny round erosions and crusts.

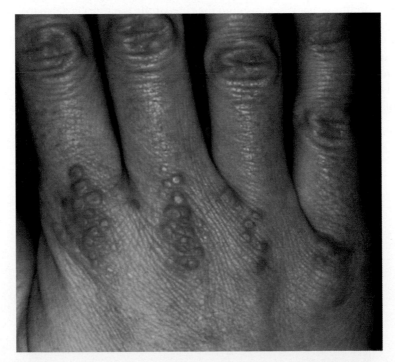

FIGURE 12.46 • Dermatomyositis, showing pink and violaceous papules over the metacarpophalangeal joints. (Reproduced with permission from Soutor C, Hordinsky MK: *Clinical Dermatology*. New York, NY: McGraw Hill; 2013.)

show the similar appearance of psoriasis, eczema, and dermatomyositis in this anatomic location. Note that in SLE knuckles are typically spared, rather than involved. This rule is not absolute, however.

> **Clinical Tip**
> - Dermatomyositis is a "do not miss" diagnosis for a dermatosis favoring the knuckles.
> - SLE on the dorsal fingers tends to spare the knuckles.

WEBSPACES

Webspaces may be affected by a circumscribed group of diseases. Irritant dermatitis involves webspaces and other parts of the hand with dryness and scaling. Erosio interdigitalis blastomycetica is a candida infection of the webspaces (Figure 12.47). It occurs most frequently in the finger webs and only rarely is seen in toe webs. It presents as a reddish thin plaque that is frequently macerated. One or more webspaces may be involved. The most common cause of a macerated toe web is tinea pedis. The third and fourth toe webs are involved most frequently, either unilaterally or bilaterally. Erythrasma may also occur in between the toes. There may be associated surrounding yellowish scale, but erythrasma may be difficult to distinguish clinically from the more common tinea pedis. Consider this diagnosis in any severe case of toe web maceration, or in any case that does not respond to topical antifungal therapy. A potassium hydroxide preparation is not always positive in cases with macerated scale (maceration lowers the sensitivity of the test). Another condition that is seen around the rims of the toe webs is dermatitis neglectica, otherwise known as *terra firma dermatosis*. It is a retention hyperkeratosis that occurs when individuals do not vigorously wash this area with a facecloth or the like. Sometimes macerated scale in webspaces reflects this phenomenon, rather than tinea pedis. If so, the scale will come away easily and the webspace will appear normal underneath it. Wood's lamp illumination will yield coral red fluorescence in cases of erythrasma. Corns in toe webspaces are typically macerated and are known

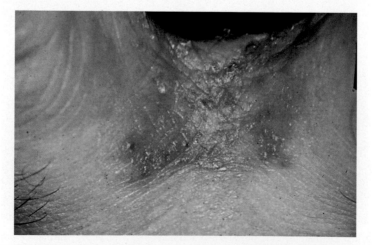

FIGURE 12.47 · Erosio interdigitalis blastomycetica, showing a red plaque at the finger web with tiny erosions and scale.

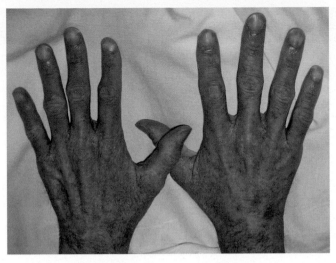

FIGURE 12.48 · Crusted scabies, showing crusting at the webspaces and over the dorsal hands.

as "soft corns." They usually arise in between two closely opposed interphalangeal joints. Condyloma lata may be seen in the toe webs as this is an intertriginous site. Condyloma lata may mimic soft corns in that they are well-demarcated, macerated papules. One or more may be seen in a webspace and they are typically malodorous in addition. Scabetic burrows frequently cluster in webspaces. They are linear scaly papules that measure 1 or 2 mm. Crusted scabies presents in this location with larger crusts or powdery scales (Figure 12.48). Intertriginous xanthomas are pathognomonic for familial type 2A hypercholesterolemia. Webspaces may also be involved with yellowish plaques in this condition.

Nevi and acral melanoma can occur in a webspace, so always carefully examine the webspaces as part of a total body skin examination. Acral melanomas may be amelanotic. Look for a flesh-colored, pink or reddish papule, plaque, or nodule in this location.

Conditions Found in Webspaces Include the Following:	
• Irritant dermatitis: fingers > toes	• Soft corn: toes
• Tinea pedis: toes	• Condyloma lata: toes
• Erosion interdigitalis blastomycetica: fingers > toes	• Intertriginous xanthomas: fingers or toes
• Erythrasma: toes	Do not miss:
• Dermatitis neglectica: toes	• Nevi and atypical nevi
• Scabies: fingers or toes	• Melanoma

PERIORBITAL

Certain dermatoses have a predilection for eyelid skin. These are listed in Table 12.15 by reaction pattern and color. Table 12.16 houses the subcategory of papules that occur on the eyelid margin. In the papulosquamous category, small seborrheic keratoses may be seen in this location in older individuals. Squamous cell cancers are a rare finding here. Both herpes simplex and herpes zoster are "do not miss" diagnoses in this location.

TABLE 12.15. Differential Diagnosis of Periorbital Dermatoses and Neoplasms by Reaction Pattern and Color

PERIORBITAL
- Papulosquamous
  - Seborrheic keratosis
  - Squamous cell carcinoma
  - Acanthosis nigricans
- Vesicobullous
  - Herpes simplex
  - Herpes zoster
- Eczematous
  - Allergic contact dermatitis
  - Irritant contact dermatitis
  - Atopic dermatitis
  - Lichen simplex chronicus
- Dermal
  - Hordeolum
  - Chalazion
  - Xanthelasma
  - Plane xanthoma
  - Necrobiosis xanthogranuloma
  - Orbital xanthogranuloma
  - Periorbital dermatitis
  - Rosacea
  - Sarcoidosis
  - Nevi
  - Milia
  - Apocrine hidrocystoma
  - Eccrine hidrocystoma
  - Syringomas
  - Trichilemmoma
  - Trichoepithelioma
  - Sebaceous carcinoma
  - Basal cell carcinoma
  - Lipoid proteinosis
  - Primary amyloidosis
- Vascular
  - Dermatomyositis: heliotrope
  - "Raccoon eyes"
- White
  - Vitiligo

The eyelid is not a common site for herpes simplex, but V1 zoster typically involves the upper eyelid and the ipsilateral forehead with grouped vesicles and edema. In the eczematous category, allergic contact dermatitis frequently manifests here. Allergens that contact the eyelid skin directly, such as those in cosmetics or eye medicaments, as well as allergens that are carried by the fingertips, such as nail varnish, for example, may be responsible. Atopic individuals may also develop eczema in this location, and sometimes, irritant dermatitis is responsible. The heliotrope rash of dermatomyositis may be erythematous or violaceous. It is typically smooth (vascular reaction pattern), but it

TABLE 12.16. Differential Diagnosis of Papules on the Eyelid Margin

SOLITARY
- Hordeolum
- Chalazion
- Apocrine hidrocystoma
- Nevus
- Sebaceous carcinoma

MULTIPLE
- Eccrine hidrocystomas
- "Beading" along eyelid margin
  - Primary amyloidosis: occur along with "pinch" purpura
  - Lipoid proteinosis: *blepharosis moniliformis*

may be superficially abraded or scaly (Figure 12.49), and so, it may mimic eczema. It is typically bilateral but may be unilateral. It may be accompanied by edema. Acanthosis nigricans can rarely occur in this location (Figure 12.50).

In the dermal reaction pattern category, a hordeolum or stye is an acute infection, usually with *Staphylococcus aureus*, of follicles on the eyelid margin. It presents as a painful red papule at the eyelid margin. A chalazion is chronic inflammation of the eyelid margin caused by a blocked Meibomian gland duct. It also presents as a reddish papule that lasts for weeks. Yellow eyelid papules and plaques are most commonly xanthelasma. Less commonly, they may represent plane xanthomas, necrobiotic xanthogranuloma, or orbital xanthogranuloma. In xanthelasma, a normal lipid profile is seen in up to half of patients. In those with hypercholesterolemia, any inherited hyperlipoproteinemia or acquired forms, such as cholestasis, may be present. In planar

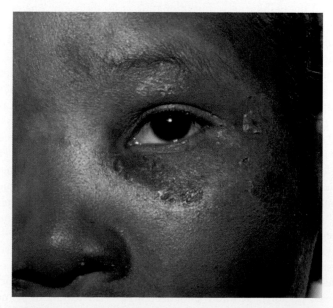

FIGURE 12.49 • A heliotrope rash of dermatomyositis, showing violaceous erythema and overlying scale on the eyelids.

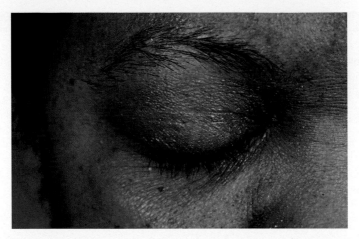

FIGURE 12.50 · Acanthosis nigricans on the eyelid, showing a light brown velvety plaque.

xanthomas, diffuse yellow plaques are seen. An underlying type III hyperlipoproteine-mia, or an IgA monoclonal gammopathy, or myeloma may be present. In necrobiotic xanthogranuloma, yellow, orange, or yellow-red plaques, papules, and nodules occur initially on periorbital skin. Subsequently, the face, trunk, and limbs may be involved. Lesions may ulcerate. It is usually associated with an IgGκ gammopathy, but IgGλ or IgA gammopathy are more rarely seen. Orbital xanthogranuloma resembles the peri-orbital plaques of necrobiotic xanthogranuloma, but there is slow extension over the years, and there is no systemic involvement. In periorificial dermatitis, perioral and periorbital skin may manifest tiny pink or reddish papules. These are typically smooth but may be scaly. Fluorinated topical steroids and fluorinated toothpastes are thought to contribute to the pathogenesis, but idiopathic cases do occur. The eyelid skin is a rare locale for the inflammatory papules of rosacea and of lupus miliaris disseminata faceii (granulomatous rosacea). Further in the granulomatous category, papular and micropapular sarcoid may be seen on the lids.

Nevi and milia may be seen on and around the eyelid margins. Apocrine and eccrine hidrocystomas present as one or more translucent and sometimes somewhat bluish papules on and around the eyelid margin. Apocrine hidrocystomas are usually soli-tary and are typically located on the eyelid margin. Eccrine hidrocystomas are usually multiple and occur on or around the eyelid skin. Eyelid margins may also be involved. Syringomas present as flesh-colored small papules on the lower lids. These slowly enlarge over decades and may reach a size of ≥5–6 mm in later years. One of the sites or predilection of sebaceous carcinoma is the upper eyelid margin. It typically occurs in older women. Basal cell cancers are a rare finding on eyelid skin. The phenomenon of "beading"—the formation of a line of contiguous tiny papules—along the eyelid margin is seen in two infiltrative diseases: lipoid proteinosis (as mentioned above) and primary amyloidosis. In primary amyloidosis, diffuse infiltration of the skin with AL amyloid occurs in the setting of an underlying monoclonal gammopathy or myeloma. Beaded papules along eyelid margin and associated macroglossia also occur. "Pinch purpura"— easy hemorrhage into traumatized areas—is a feature of primary amyloi-dosis and may occur on eyelid skin as well (see Figure 9.18).

"Raccoon eyes" are the phenomenon of periorbital ecchymoses occurring in the setting of a fracture of the base of the skull. Finally, eyelid skin is frequently involved in vitiligo.

The differential diagnosis of periorbital edema is broad, as seen in Table 12.17. Periorbital edema may accompany infections or inflammatory conditions of eyelid skin, or it may be secondary to underlying systemic disease. It may be bilateral or unilateral as is outlined in the table. The heliotrope rash of dermatomyositis may, on occasion, be accompanied by edema. Solid facial edema is a rare consequence of acne. There is centrofacial lymphedema that may involve the eyelids. In chronic cases, dermal fibrosis ensues. Solid facial edema of rosacea has also been termed

---

TABLE 12.17. Differential Diagnosis of Periorbital Edema

BILATERAL
- Angioedema
- Allergic contact dermatitis
- Heliotrope of dermatomyositis
- Lymphedema
- Solid facial edema of acne
- Morbihan syndrome
- Systemic causes
  - Cardiac: heart failure
  - Renal: nephrotic syndrome, chronic renal insufficiency
  - Hepatic: hepatic failure (decreased albumin production)
  - Superior vena cava syndrome
- Infections
  - Trichinosis
  - Onchocerciasis
- Blepharochalasis
- Ascher syndrome
- Cavernous sinus thrombosis: more commonly, unilateral

UNILATERAL
- Trauma
  - Internal or external stye
  - Allergic contact dermatitis
  - Angioedema: more commonly, bilateral
  - Heliotrope of dermatomyositis: more commonly, bilateral
  - Infection
    - Erysipelas
    - Orbital cellulitis
    - Herpes simplex
    - Herpes zoster (V1)
    - Anthrax
    - Onchocerciasis
    - Trypanosomiasis (Romana's sign)
    - Cat scratch disease
- Cavernous sinus thrombosis
- Orbital tumors
- Insect bite

Morbihan syndrome. Here, usually the upper face, including the eyelids is affected. In blepharochalasis, there are idiopathic intermittent episodes of eyelid edema and erythema. This inflammation affects elastic tissue and leads to an atrophic and wrinkled appearance of the lids. Ascher syndrome is the association of blepharochalasis with duplication of the upper lip and thyroid goiter.

In trichinosis, a roundworm infestation, *Trichinella* larvae, penetrate the gut and invade other organs. This phase is accompanied by peripheral eosinophilia, bilateral eyelid edema, and occasionally by an exanthematous eruption. Onchocerciasis, also known as *river blindness,* is a parasitic infection with a nematode, *Onchocerca volvulus.* Diffuse pruritus leads to widespread lichenification and pigmentary changes on the skin. Periorbitally, there may be subcutaneous nodules (in which the female adult produces microfilariae) and associated edema. These may be unilateral or bilateral. Ultimately microfilariae invade the orbit and lead to a host of ophthalmologic findings, including blindness in untreated cases. Unilateral periorbital edema is seen in a host of rare infections. Cutaneous anthrax leads to significant periorbital edema if inoculated near the eye. Inoculation of microorganisms into the eye leads to periorbital edema in the case of *Trypanosoma cruzi* (South American trypanosomiasis, also called *Chagas disease*). Parinaud's oculoglandular syndrome is the presence of conjunctivitis and preauricular lymphadenopathy. It occurs from inoculation of *Bartonella henselae* (cat scratch disease) into the eye.

THE EAR

Table 12.18 contains a comprehensive list of eruptions and neoplasms that favor the ear, divided up by reaction pattern. The ear is an acral site, so vasculopathies from

TABLE 12.18. Differential Diagnosis of Dermatoses on the Ear, by Reaction Pattern and Macules

PAPULOSQUAMOUS
- Psoriasis: well-made plaques with silvery scale behind ears
- Seborrheic dermatitis
- Acanthoma fissuratum (postauricular)
- Seborrheic keratosis (postauricular)
- Chondrodermatitis nodularis helicis
- Actinic keratoses
- Squamous cell cancer in situ
- Invasive squamous cell cancer
- Myeloma-associated follicular spicules of nose and ears

VESICOBULLOUS
- Hydroa vacciniforme
- Juvenile spring eruption
- Phytophotodermatitis
- Phototoxic reactions

ECZEMATOUS
- Allergic contact dermatitis: earrings, hair products
- Photoallergic contact dermatitis
- Chronic actinic dermatitis

(Continued)

TABLE 12.18. Differential Diagnosis of Dermatoses on the Ear, by Reaction Pattern and Macules (continued)

ECZEMATOUS (CONT.)
- Airborne contact dermatitis (eg, aerosolized lichen)
- Seborrheic dermatitis
- Juvenile spring eruption can resemble subacute eczema

DERMAL
- Primary cutaneous amyloidosis of the external ear
- Lichen scrofulosorum
- Tuberous xanthomas
- Chiclero ear
- Relapsing polychondritis
- Angiolymphoid hyperplasia with eosinophils
- Cartilaginous pseudocyst
- Weathering nodules
- Familial trichodiscoma syndrome
- Keloid (earlobe from ear piercing)
- Epidermal inclusion cyst (postauricular)
- Accessory tragus (preauricular)
- Nevus sebaceous (postauricular)
- Melanoma

VASCULAR
- Cocaine levamisole toxicity
- Septic vasculopathy
- Type 1 cryoglobulinemia
- Cryofibrinogenemia
- Reactive angioendotheliomatosis
- Venous lake

BROWN MACULES
- Lentigines
- Lentigo maligna

cryoprecipitants, such as type I cryoglobulinemia and cryofibrinogenemia, will manifest here. Similarly, septic vasculopathy that usually presents with acral asymmetric small purpuric macules and papules will also be seen in this body location. Cocaine levamisole toxicity characteristically involves the helices. Reactive angioendotheliomatosis is an extremely rare condition in which a reactive increase in endothelial cells is seen. It occurs in the setting of a range of different primary diseases, such as chronic infections (infective endocarditis, tuberculosis), monoclonal gammopathies, and cryoglobulinemia. Earlobes are involved with erythematous or violaceous plaques, which may become purpuric or necrotic. The abdomen and lower extremities are also preferentially involved.

The ear is also classified as a seborrheic location; the postauricular skin, conchal bowl, and other concave surfaces of the external ear (Figure 12.51) are sites of predilection of seborrheic dermatitis and seborrheic eruptions, such as Darier disease and vitamin B_6 deficiency. Psoriasis presents as well-formed plaques with silvery scale behind the ears. A site of predilection for DLE is the conchal bowl (Figure 12.52).

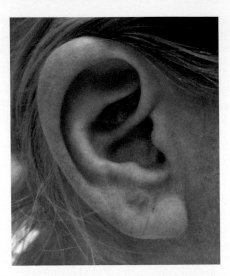

FIGURE 12.51 · Seborrheic dermatitis, displaying scaling at the triangular fossa.

Additionally, the ear is frequently a site of acute and chronic sun exposure, so photoinduced and photoexacerbated dermatoses are seen in this location. Hydroa vacciniforme and juvenile spring eruption commonly involve the ear. Photoallergic contact dermatitis, chronic actinic dermatitis, and phototoxic eruptions, including phytophotodermatitis, can also affect the ear. The benign (weathering nodules, lentigines), premalignant (actinic keratoses), and malignant [basal cell cancer (BCC; Figure 12.53)], squamous cell carcinoma in situ (SCCIS), squamous cell carcinoma (SCC; Figure 12.54), lentigo maligna, melanoma] sequelae of chronic photodamage

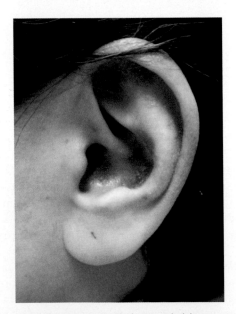

FIGURE 12.52 · Discoid lupus erythematosus (DLE), showing dark brown scaly plaques with follicular prominence in the conchal bowl and near the helix.

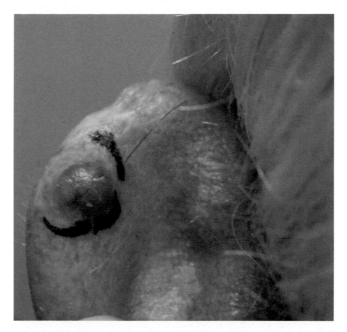

FIGURE 12.53 · Basal cell carcinoma, presenting as pearly papules on the posterior helix.

also present on the ears. Weathering nodules are actually papules: one or more 2–3-mm cartilaginous papules occur on the ear helix. They are usually seen in older men. Sun damage is thought to play a role in their development. The ear is a site that is exposed to bites and airborne allergens. Chiclero ulcer is the presence of an ulcerative plaque on the ear caused by *Leishmania mexicana* complex. There may be associated surrounding edema and erythema (Figure 12.55). It predominantly affects forest workers who collect gum from rubber trees in Central America. Airborne contact dermatitis can involve this location (Figure 12.56).

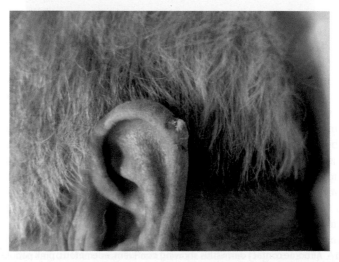

FIGURE 12.54 · Squamous cell carcinoma on the helix presenting as a hyperkeratotic, infiltrated papule.

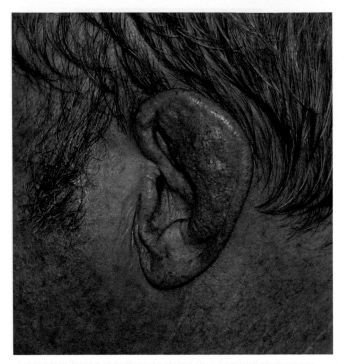

FIGURE 12.58 • A cartilaginous pseudocyst showing a broad plaque with an uneven surface, involving the scaphoid and triangular fossae.

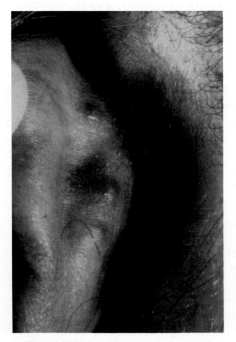

FIGURE 12.59 • Angiolymphoid hyperplasia with eosinophils presenting with reddish papules in the postauricular location.

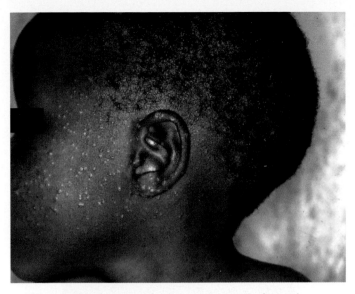

FIGURE 12.60 · Lichen scrofulosorum showing fine papules over the face and ear.

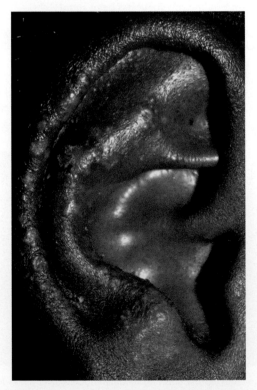

FIGURE 12.61 · Papulonecrotic tuberculide, showing smooth papules on the helix and antihelix.

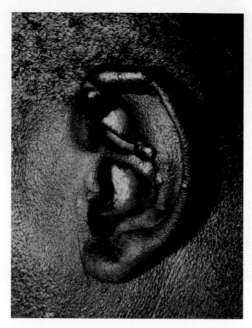

FIGURE 12.62 • Tuberous xanthomas, presenting as yellowish papules and plaques on the ear.

the familial trichodiscoma syndrome. It is a rare inherited dermatosis, and other sites are also involved, but no internal involvement has been reported.

Dermatoses on the Ear Are Those That Occur:

- On acral surfaces
- In the seborrheic distribution
- On acutely and habitually sun-exposed sites
- On exposed sites
- In cartilage
- As a result of repetitive pressure
- As developmental phenomena

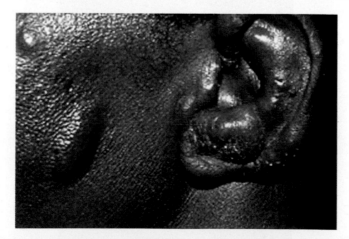

FIGURE 12.63 • Lepromatous leprosy, showing infiltrated nodules over the lower ear and cheek.

THE NOSE

The differential diagnosis for conditions on the nose is broad. The conditions are listed by etiology in Table 12.19 and by reaction pattern, pustules, and macules in Table 12.20. Any number of infections may occur in this location. Bacterial folliculitis, *Demodex*

TABLE 12.19. Differential Diagnosis of Dermatoses on the Nose, by Etiology

INFECTIOUS
- Bacterial
  - Folliculitis
  - Impetigo
  - Rhinoscleroma
  - Septic vasculopathy
- Mycobacterial
  - Lupus vulgaris
  - Lepromatous leprosy
- Viral
  - HSV
  - V1 zoster
  - warts
  - mollusca
  - Trichodysplasia spinulosa
- Fungal
  - Tinea faciei
  - *Pityrosporum* folliculitis
  - Blastomycosis
  - Coccidiodomycosis
  - Paracoccidiodomycosis
- Parasitic
  - *Demodex* folliculitis
  - Mucocutaneous leishmaniasis
  - Rhinosporidiosis

INFLAMMATORY/AUTOIMMUNE
- Acne
- Rosacea
- Perioral dermatitis
- Eosinophilic folliculitis
- Sarcoidosis
  - Lupus pernio: around nares and columella
  - Angiolupoid variant
  - Micropapules, papules, plaques, nodules
- Granuloma faciale
- DLE
- SLE
- Scleroderma: "pinched" nose
- Hydroa vacciniforme
- Phytophotodermatitis

(Continued)

TABLE 12.19. Differential Diagnosis of Dermatoses on the Nose, by Etiology (continued)

INFLAMMATORY/AUTOIMMUNE (CONT.)
- Phototoxic reactions
- Allergic contact dermatitis
- Photocontact dermatitis
- Chronic actinic dermatitis
- Airborne contact dermatitis e.g. aerosolized lichen
- Seborrheic dermatitis: glabella, nasolabial folds
- Relapsing polychondritis

DEPOSITIONAL
- Scleremyxedema: early sign is infiltration at glabella

RETENTION KERATOSIS
- Trichostasis spinulosa

CRYOPROTEINS
- Type 1 cryoglobulinemia
- Cryofibrinogenemia

NEOPLASTIC
- Benign
  - Lentigines
  - Nevi
  - Fibrous papule
  - Seborrheic keratosis
  - Angiofibromas of tuberous sclerosis
  - Trichilemmomas of Cowden syndrome: nose, upper lip, central face
  - Multiple trichoepitheliomas cluster on and around nose
  - Mixed tumor (chondroid syringoma)- one of the sites of predilection
  - Milia, epidermal cyst
  - Sinonasal papilloma
- Premalignant
  - Actinic keratosis
- Malignant
  - Squamous cell cancer in situ
  - Invasive squamous cell cancer
  - Basal cell cancer
  - Merkel cell cancer
  - Atypical fibroxanthoma
  - Microcystic adnexal carcinoma
  - Melanoma in situ
  - Melanoma
  - Kaposi sarcoma
  - Angiosarcoma

PARANEOPLASTIC
- Myeloma-associated follicular spicules of nose and ears

DRUG/TOXIN
- Cocaine levamisole toxicity

TABLE 12.20. Differential Diagnosis of Dermatoses on the Nose, by Reaction Pattern, Pustules, and Macules

PAPULOSQUAMOUS
- Actinic keratosis
- Squamous cell cancer in situ
- Invasive squamous cell cancer
- Warts
- Seborrheic keratosis
- Tinea faciei
- DLE
- Lupus vulgaris: may be scaly or smooth; around nares and columella
- Spines
  - Trichostasis spinulosa
  - Trichodysplasia spinulosa
  - Myeloma-associated follicular spicules of nose and ears
- Polypoid mass from nares
  - Sinonasal papilloma
  - Rhinosporidiosis
- Vegetating plaques
  - Blastomycosis
  - Coccidiodomycosis
  - Paracoccidiodomycosis
  - Mucocutaneous leishmaniasis

VESICOBULLOUS
- HSV
- V1 zoster
- Hydroa vacciniforme
- Phytophotodermatitis
- Phototoxic reactions

PUSTULES
- Bacterial folliculitis
- Impetigo
- Acne
- Rosacea
- Perioral dermatitis: nasolabial folds
- *Demodex* folliculitis
- Eosinophilic folliculitis
- *Pityrosporum* folliculitis
- HSV
- VI zoster

ECZEMATOUS
- Allergic contact dermatitis
- Photocontact dermatitis
- Chronic actinic dermatitis
- Airborne contact dermatitis (eg, aerosolized lichen)
- Seborrheic dermatitis: glabella, nasolabial folds

(Continued)

TABLE 12.20. Differential Diagnosis of Dermatoses on the Nose, by Reaction Pattern, Pustules, and Macules (continued)

DERMAL

- Nevi
- Fibrous papule
- Angiofibromas of tuberous sclerosis
- Trichilemmomas of Cowden syndrome: nose, upper lip, central face
- Multiple trichoepitheliomas cluster on and around nose
- Mixed tumor (chondroid syringoma)—one of the sites of predilection
- Milia, epidermal cyst
- Granulomatous rosacea
- Granuloma faciale
- Sarcoidosis
  - Lupus pernio: around nares and columella
  - Angiolupoid variant
  - Micropapules, papules, plaques, nodules
- Lupus vulgaris: may be scaly or smooth; around nares and columella
- Rhinoscleroma
- Scleromyxedema: early sign is infiltration at glabella
- Scleroderma: "pinched" nose
- Relapsing polychondritis
- Basal cell cancer
- Merkel cell cancer
- Atypical fibroxanthoma
- Microcystic adnexal carcinoma
- Melanoma
- Kaposi sarcoma
- Angiosarcoma

VASCULAR

- Rosacea
- SLE—malar rash can involve the nose
- Cocaine levamisole toxicity
- Septic vasculopathy
- Type 1 cryoglobulinemia
- Cryofibrinogenemia

BROWN MACULES

- Ephelides
- Lentigines
- Lentigo maligna

folliculitis, and *Pityrosporum* folliculitis favor the face, and pustules can be seen on the nose. Impetigo favors the upper cutaneous lip just beneath the nasal sills. Rhinoscleroma is caused by the Gram-negative bacillus *Klebsiella pneumoniae* var. *rhinoscleromatis*. Rhinorrhea is superseded by papules and nodules in the nose, and on and around the nares. Untreated disease leads to sclerosis and deformity. It is extremely rare.

Lupus vulgaris is a form of cutaneous tuberculosis. It presents with dermal papules around the nasal alar rims. Plaques may enlarge, become scaly, and atrophy. Lupus vulgaris may also occur on the face, or off the face less frequently.

Lepromatous leprosy presents as diffuse infiltration of the face. It is one cause of a leonine facies.

Viral infections, such as HSV and V1 zoster, may be seen on the nose. If the tip of the nose is involved, this indicates nasociliary branch involvement and also the presence of ophthalmic involvement. Warts and molluscum contagiosum are frequently encountered on all facial areas. Trichodysplasia spinulosa is seen in immunosuppressed individuals. Recently, it has been discovered that trichodysplasia spinulosa is caused by the trichodysplasia spinulosa–associated polyoma virus. Spiny flesh-colored or erythematous follicle-based papules arise on the central face, including the nose. In the fungal category, tinea faceii presents as an annular plaque on any facial surface. Various deep fungal infections favor the nose. These typically present as vegetating plaques. Blastomycosis is a deep fungal infection caused by *Blastomyces dermatitidis*. It spreads hematogenously from underlying pulmonary disease. One or more dermal or scaly papules, plaques, or nodules are seen. They may be ulcerated or crusted, and they heal with scarring. Coccidiodomycosis is caused by *Coccidioides immitis*. It presents with an ulcerated dermal or hyperkeratotic plaque or nodule. The nasolabial fold is the site of predilection, and other facial and more widespread sites may be involved.

Paracoccidiodomycosis is also a deep fungal infection. The mucocutaneous form affects oral mucosa, palate, and less often the nose. There are destructive, hyperkeratotic or eroded plaques. Mucocutaneous leishmaniasis ("New World" leishmaniasis) is seen in Central and South America. Initial inoculation of organisms by the sand flea may occur on the body. Up to years later, destructive granulomatous disease occurs in the nose and around the nares. Ulceration of cartilage and the hard palate may be seen. Rhinosporidiosis is most commonly seen in India. It is caused by *Rhinosporidium seeberi*, a parasite. It presents as a polypoid mass from anterior nose.

Inflammatory conditions include rosacea and perioral dermatitis. Rosacea occurs over the nose and on the other convex areas of the face. Perioral dermatitis favors the nasolabial folds as well as other perioral sites. Discoid lupus may involve the nose, as may the malar rash of SLE. Other photosensitive eruptions and allergic, irritant, airborne, and photocontact eruptions occur here. Seborrheic dermatitis favors the glabella and nasolabial folds. In the granulomatous category, lupus pernio is a subtype of cutaneous sarcoidosis. It also has a predilection for the nasal alar rims (Figures 12.64

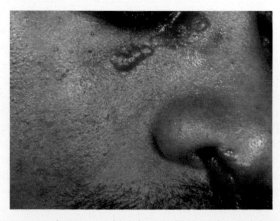

FIGURE 12.64 • Lupus pernio, showing a reddish-brown plaque at the nasal alar rim.

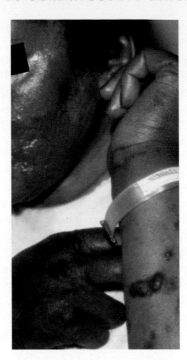

FIGURE 12.65 • Lupus pernio, showing reddish violaceous plaques at the nasal alar rim and on the cheek.

and 12.65). Plaques and nodules may be seen anywhere on the face and scattered over the trunk and extremities also. Lupus pernio is associated with severe underlying systemic sarcoidosis in many cases. The angiolupoid variant typically presents as pink, smooth plaques on the sides of the nasal bridge. Other forms of sarcoidosis may also be seen in this location. Also included in the granulomatous category is granuloma faciale. The nose may be involved.

Regarding depositional disease, an early sign of scleromyxedema is infiltration at the glabella. Both the limited and systemic forms of scleroderma lead to a bound-down appearance of facial skin, including the nose ("pinched nose").

Trichostasis spinulosa is a common condition where multiple vellus hairs become trapped in a keratinaceous plug within hair follicles, rather than being shed. The nose is a site of predilection for this phenomenon, as are the forehead and lower back. These tiny hairs appear as black spines growing out of hair follicles. The two other spiny conditions are exceedingly rare.

The nose is an acral area and, as such, is a site that is involved in acral vasculopathic conditions, as outlined above. Various benign and malignant conditions occur here. Fibrous papules of the nose are firm pink papules that occur on and around the nose (Figure 12.66). The nose is a site of predilection for the angiofibromas of tuberous sclerosis. Trichilemmomas may be associated with Cowden syndrome; they favor the nose, upper lip, and other central areas of the face. Multiple trichoepitheliomas tend to cluster on and around the nose. The nose is a site of predilection of mixed tumors (chondroid syringomas). Sinonasal papillomas develop from the pseudostratified ciliated epithelium that lines the nose and sinuses. The exophytic type of sinonasal papilloma may present as a polypoid verrucous mass at the anterior nare.

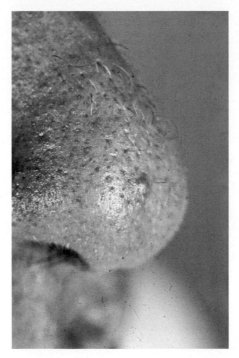

FIGURE 12.66 · Fibrous papule of the nose, presenting as a tiny pink papule at the nasal tip.

This is extremely rare. Actinic keratoses and all forms of skin cancer may occur here (Figures 12.67 and 12.68), as may Kaposi sarcoma (Figure 12.69) and angiosarcoma. Myeloma-associated follicular spicules of the nose and ears are a paraneoplastic phenomenon. Follicular spines occur on the nose and ears. They may appear fine or coarse. They consist of precipitated monoclonal proteins.

The differential diagnosis of destructive nasal septal lesions is listed in Table 12.21. They may occur without cutaneous findings, or in concert with cutaneous findings that are seen at the nares. Infectious causes include rhinoscleroma and late congenital syphilis (which leads to a "saddle nose" deformity). In the tertiary stage of yaws (caused

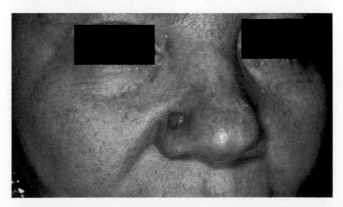

FIGURE 12.67 · A basal cell cancer, presenting as a pearly nodule at the nasal alar groove.

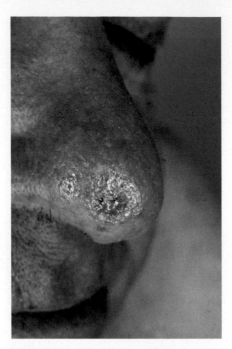

FIGURE 12.68 · A squamous cell cancer, presenting as an eroded papule on the nasal tip.

by *Treponema pallidum* ssp. *pertenue*), there is mutilation of the central face, which begins at the base of the septal nasal fossa. This is known as *gangosa*. Bejel is caused by *T. pallidum* ssp. *pallidum*. Its tertiary stage also has nasal destruction as one of its concomitants. It is less destructive than gangosa. Mucocutaneous leishmaniasis has cutaneous findings outlined above. It can also lead to destruction of the nasal septum. In terms of inflammatory causes, in granulomatosis with polyangiitis, the upper respiratory tract is an area of predilection. Early on, there is persistent crusting and hemorrhagic granuloma of the nostril, nasal septum, pharynx, or larynx. This may eventuate in nasal septal

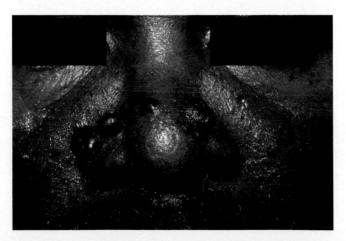

FIGURE 12.69 · Kaposi sarcoma, presenting as deep purple nodules on and around the nose.

TABLE 12.21. Differential Diagnosis of Destructive Nasal Septal Lesions
INFECTIOUS
• Rhinoscleroma
• Late congenital syphilis
• Tertiary yaws
• Bejel
• Mucocutaneous leishmaniasis
INFLAMMATORY
• Granulomatosis with polyangiitis
• Sarcoidosis
• Noma

destruction. Nasal septum infiltration and destruction is a rare manifestation of sarcoidosis. In noma, there is extensive centrofacial destruction of tissue. It is usually seen in malnourished children. Oral fusobacteria and spirochetes are thought to play a role in the pathogenesis. Finally, in the neoplastic category, the nasal type extranodal natural killer (NK)/T-cell lymphoma (formerly known as *lethal midline granuloma*) presents as an ulcerative, necrotic, and destructive process within the nose. The palate may be destroyed as well.

THE FACE

The differential diagnosis of dermatoses on the face is exceedingly broad. A contracted differential diagnosis recapitulates that of the nose, as listed above. A further important differential diagnosis here is that of *leonine facies*. This term refers to diffuse infiltration of the face by an inflammatory, and sometimes, a neoplastic process. Leonine facies may be scaly (papulosquamous reaction pattern), or smooth (dermal reaction pattern). Table 12.22 lists this differential by reaction pattern. It is also useful to consider the differential of flesh-colored papules of the face. These lesions are listed in Table 12.23.

TABLE 12.22. Differential Diagnosis of Leonine Facies
PAPULOSQUAMOUS
• Chronic actinic dermatitis
• Actinic reticuloid
• Mycosis fungoides
• Trichodysplasia spinulosa
DERMAL
• Lepromatous leprosy
• Pachydermoperiostosis
• Multicentric reticulohistiocytosis
• Scleromyxedema
• Post-kala-azar dermal leishmaniasis
• Primary amyloidosis
• Lipoid proteinosis

TABLE 12.23. Causes of Flesh-Colored Facial Papules

SOLITARY
- Intradermal nevus
- Epidermal inclusion cyst—has a central punctum
- Fibrous papule
- Trichoepithelioma
- Trichilemmoma
- Trichofolliculoma—has a central hair
- Mixed tumor: firm or hard
- Pilomatricoma: hard
- Palisaded and encapsulated neuroma
- Amelanotic melamoma
- Merkel cell tumor
- Atypical fibroxanthoma

MULTIPLE
- Depositional
  - Amyloidosis
  - Lipoid proteinosis
  - Osteoma cutis: multiple hard flesh-colored or whitish papules
- Neoplastic
  - Syringomas (infraorbital)
  - Trichilemmomas (centrofacial)
  - Trichoepitheliomas (lateral aspects nose, nasolabial folds, infraorbital)
  - Angiofibromas (can be pink; centrofacial)
  - Trichodiscomas, fibrofolliculomas (can be white)

GENERALIZED

Some eruptions occur on all or most body parts. These may start in one location and progress to involve all locations. Examples include viral exanthems, such as measles or rubella that start on the face and spread caudally. Pityriasis rubra pilaris typically starts on the upper back and generalizes. Stevens–Johnson syndrome/toxic epidermal necrolysis (SJS/TEN) begins on the upper chest and may generalize. Erythroderma is the global or near-global involvement of the entire cutaneous surface. Erythroderma may be scaly, in which case the term "exfoliative dermatitis" can be used. Scaly erythroderma can be classified as having a papulosquamous or eczematous reaction pattern. Alternatively, erythroderma may be smooth, in which case it can be classified as having a vascular reaction pattern. Eruptions that have the propensity to cause erythroderma are listed in Table 12.24 by reaction pattern. Psoriasis and eczema (atopic dermatitis, allergic contact dermatitis, and seborrheic dermatitis) are most frequently seen. Mycosis fungoides may become erythrodermic. *Sezary syndrome* refers to erythrodermic mycosis fungoides with associated circulating atypical T cells. Noncutaneous lymphomas and leukemias and HIV can also lead to an exfoliative dermatitis. While erythrodermic drug eruptions are typically nonscaly (eg, diffuse exanthematous drug reaction, DRESS, or "red man" syndrome), any longstanding drug eruption may become scaly. Rarer causes of exfoliative erythroderma include pityriasis rubra pilaris, lichen planus, dermatomyositis, and nonbullous congenital ichthyosiform

TABLE 12.24. Causes of Erythroderma, by Reaction Pattern

PAPULOSQUAMOUS
- Psoriasis
- Eczema
  - Atopic dermatitis
  - Allergic contact dermatitis
  - Seborrheic dermatitis
- Mycosis fungoides
- Sezary syndrome
- Lymphoma/leukemia
- Drug-induced
- PRP
- Lichen planus
- Dermatomyositis
- Tinea corporis
- Crusted scabies
- HIV-related
- Leiner disease
- Omenn disease
- Netherton syndrome
- Bullous congenital ichthyosiform erythroderma
- Nonbullous congenital ichthyosiform erythroderma

VESICOBULLOUS
- Pemphigus foliaceus
- Bullous pemphigoid
- TEN

VASCULAR
- Exanthematous drug eruption
- DRESS
- "Red man" syndrome

erythroderma. Very rarely, tinea corporis may become generalized, and longstanding crusted scabies certainly can. In infancy, rare syndromes such as Netherton syndrome, Leiner disease (generalized seborrheic dermatitis, diarrhea, and failure to thrive), and Omenn disease (severe combined immunodeficiency, high IgE, lymphadenopathy). Nonbullous congenital ichthyosiform erythroderma can lead to persistent waxing and waning erythroderma throughout life. Vesicobullous disease may also rarely be generalized. Examples include pemphigus foliaceus, bullous pemphigoid, and toxic epidermal necrolysis.

SUMMARY

- Eruptions and neoplasms may manifest predilections for specific body locations.
- The differential diagnoses of many distribution patterns are discussed here.
- The approach for each may be etiologic or morphologic (by primary lesion, color, and reaction pattern).

Examining Scalp, Hair, Nails, Mucous Membranes, and Lymph Nodes

13

Examination of the scalp, hair, nail, mucous membranes, and lymph nodes can provide additional diagnostic clues for any given eruption. Furthermore, the scalp, hair, nails, and mucous membranes may be the sole site of disease involvement. A former resident of mine, now a respected colleague, coined the mnemonic "GIFTs" for this diagnostic box of the wheel of diagnosis, where GIFT stands for "*gleaning information from the*" scalp, hair, nails, and mucous membranes, as well as from examining the lymph nodes. Examining these areas can be like gifts to the diagnostician, in that they may be replete with diagnostic information. Each of these anatomic sites and structures will be considered in turn in this chapter.

THE SCALP

Some dermatoses characteristically involve the scalp and may cause alopecia. Diagnostic clues can be found in the expression of the disease itself. Examples here include papulosquamous presentations, such as the perifollicular scale and erythema of lichen planopilaris, or dermal reaction pattern presentations, such as the brownish or sometimes reddish plaques of scalp sarcoidosis.

Additionally, scalp disease may lead to scarring or nonscarring alopecia, and each disease state has a characteristic outcome, such as the scarring alopecia that accompanies discoid lupus erythematosus (DLE) or the nonscarring alopecia that may eventuate in tinea capitis. Some dermatoses can cause nonscarring loss early in the disease course, and ultimately scarring alopecia if the disease is severe or untreated, such as in kerion. Of note, the distinction between scarring and nonscarring alopecia is not always easy to discern. When examining the scalp, look for preservation of hair follicle openings at regular intervals in the affected area and compare this to a nonaffected area. In the earliest forms of scarring alopecia, there may be "follicular dropout"—an interruption to the regularity of follicles and the presence of small, scarred areas where no follicles can be seen. A dermatoscope can assist greatly in this determination.

> **Clinical Tip** Follicular dropout is an early sign of scarring alopecia. This sign may be difficult to discern. A dermatoscope can help.

Table 13.1 provides a differential diagnosis of scalp dermatoses by reaction pattern. Each reaction pattern is further subdivided according to whether scarring or nonscarring

TABLE 13.1. Differential Diagnosis of Scalp Dermatoses and Their Typical Patterns of Alopecia

DISEASE	NONSCARRING ALOPECIA	SCARRING ALOPECIA	NO ALOPECIA
Papulosquamous			
Tinea capitis	✓		Early
Kerion	Early or mild	✓	
Favus		✓	
Scabies			✓
Secondary syphilis	✓		
Psoriasis	If severe		✓
Pityriasis rubra pilaris	If severe		✓
Lichen planopilaris		✓	Early
Frontal fibrosing alopecia		✓	Early
DLE		✓	
Follicular mucinosis	✓		
Dermatomyositis	✓		✓
Reactive arthritis			✓
Acrokeratosis paraneoplastica			✓
Seborrheic keratosis	✓		✓
Common or flat wart	✓		✓
Actinic keratosis			✓
Squamous cell cancer in situ	✓	✓	Early
Squamous cell cancer		✓	
Atypical fibroxanthoma		✓	
Vesicobullous			
Herpes zoster V1			✓
Junctional epidermolysis bullosa		✓	
Dystrophic epidermolysis bullosa		✓	
Pemphigus vulgaris	If severe		✓
Pemphigus foliaceus	If severe		✓
Bullous pemphigoid		✓	
Dermatitis herpetiformis			✓
Mucous membrane pemphigoid		✓	
Epidermolysis bullosa acquisita		✓	
Eczematous			
Seborrheic dermatitis	Severe		✓
Allergic contact dermatitis	Severe		✓
Atopic dermatitis	Severe		✓
Pustules			
Folliculitis			✓
Acne			✓
Rosacea			✓

(Continued)

TABLE 13.1. Differential Diagnosis of Scalp Dermatoses and Their Typical Patterns of Alopecia (continued)

DISEASE	NONSCARRING ALOPECIA	SCARRING ALOPECIA	NO ALOPECIA
Pustules (cont.)			
Herpes zoster			✓
Kerion	Early or mild	✓	
Folliculitis decalvans		✓	
Acne keloidalis nuchae	✓	✓	
Dissecting cellulitis		✓	
Erosive pustular dermatosis of the scalp		✓	
Pyoderma gangrenosum: rare in this location		✓	
Amicrobial pustulosis of the folds	✓		✓
Neonatal cephalic pustulosis			✓
Erythema toxicum			✓
Transient neonatal pustular melanosis			✓
Eosinophilic pustular folliculitis of infancy			✓
Dermal			
Sarcoidosis	✓	✓	
Follicular mucinosis	✓		
Lipedematous scalp			✓
Milia			✓
Nevi			✓
Epidermal cyst	If large		✓
Pilar cyst	If large		✓
Cherry angioma			✓
Cylindroma	✓		
Mixed tumor	If large		✓
Proliferating trichilemmal tumor	✓		
Basal cell cancer	✓	✓	✓
Squamous cell cancer		✓	
Melanoma	✓	✓	✓
Merkel cell tumor		✓	
Atypical fibroxanthoma		✓	
Lymphoma/leukemia	✓		
Angiosarcoma		✓	
Scalp metastasis		✓	
Vascular			
Systemic lupus erythematosus	✓		✓
Dermatomyositis	✓		✓

alopecia is characteristically present. The scalp dermatosis itself or the accompanying alopecia may be the primary presenting manifestation of scalp disease, or both may be equally prominent. In some cases, as in folliculitis, or the presence of small benign neoplasms, no alopecia is seen. This third category is also outlined in Table 13.1.

Presenting Features of Scalp Disease

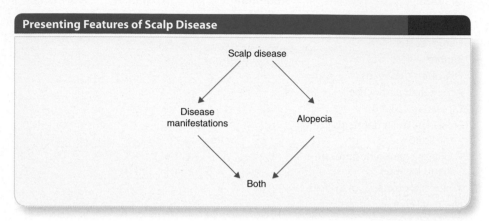

In the papulosquamous category, tinea capitis presents with small scaly plaques with or without nonscarring alopecia. Sometimes hairs may be broken off as in endothrix infection caused by *Trichophyton tonsurans* and other *Trichophyton* species. Tinea capitis is more common in children. Inflammatory forms may present with pustules in addition. Kerion is a type of tinea capitis that presents with marked inflammation. This is usually caused by zoophilic or geophilic dermatophytes. There may be boggy plaques, pustules, and crusting and loss of the papulosquamous appearance. Because of the pustules, a bacterial infection may be intuited, and so a high index of suspicion is needed to make the diagnosis.

> **Clinical Tip** Consider the diagnosis of dermatophyte infection for pustules occurring on the scalp, especially in children.

Untreated kerion may lead to scarring alopecia. Favus is another tinea capitis variant. It is caused by *Trichophyton schoenleinii*. Cup-shaped crusts (*scutula*) develop around affected hair shafts, and ultimately hairs are lost and scarring alopecia results. Scabies rarely occurs on the scalp. It is usually seen in this location in immunosuppressed individuals. It presents with scaling, crusting, and excoriations and may be accompanied by crusted scabies elsewhere. The classic appearance of secondary syphilis on the scalp is that of a "moth-eaten" alopecia. Small areas of nonscarring hair loss occur focally or globally on the scalp.

In the inflammatory papulosquamous category, scalp psoriasis presents as it does off the scalp with well-demarcated papules and plaques with silvery scales. Scales can also be micaceous. Scalp psoriasis is rarely accompanied by alopecia; however, nonscarring alopecia may be seen in severe cases. In the classical type of pityriasis rubra pilaris (type 1), scaly follicular papules begin on the scalp, become confluent to form plaques, and generalize in a caudal fashion. The scalp may also be involved in the atypical type (type 2), and nonscarring alopecia is rare. As discussed previously, lichen planopilaris (LPP) appears as perifollicular erythema and scale. Usually, the vertex is involved, and the condition may spread more broadly. Scarring alopecia is a typical

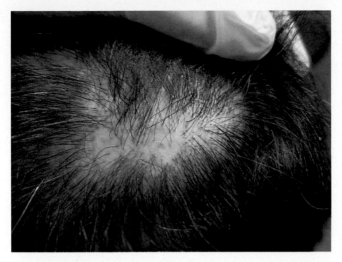

FIGURE 13.1 • Lichen planopilaris showing scarring alopecia with perifollicular erythema and scale on the scalp.

sequela (Figure 13.1). Frontal fibrosing alopecia (FFA), a variant of LPP, involves the anterior and lateral hairline with similar findings. Some cases are smoldering, but in others, progressive scarring hair loss is seen. FFA can be accompanied by flesh-colored perifollicular papules on the forehead and temples (Figure 13.2), and the eyebrows and eyelashes may be involved. The scalp, face, and conchal bowls are predilection sites of DLE, as described earlier in this chapter. Active DLE presents as a well-demarcated

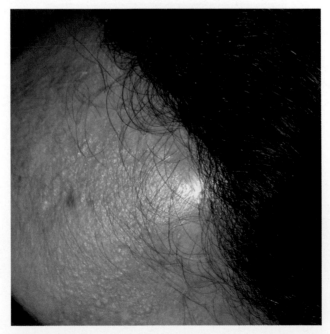

FIGURE 13.2 • Frontal fibrosing alopecia showing a shiny atrophic plaque of scarring alopecia at the anterior hairline, along with numerous tiny flesh-colored papules on the forehead.

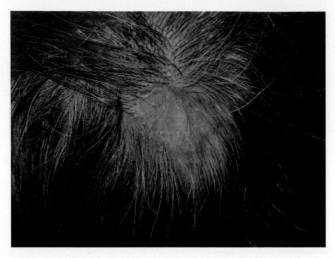

FIGURE 13.3 · A pink plaque of discoid lupus erythematosus (DLE) on the scalp showing scarring alopecia.

scaly erythematous plaque. Initially scarring alopecia may not be appreciable, but this appears with chronicity, as is seen in Figure 13.3. Ultimately, atrophic, scarred, depigmented plaques eventuate (Figure 13.4). Follicular mucinosis may be a primary process or secondary to mycosis fungoides. It presents with follicular papules and infiltrated plaques that may be scaly or smooth (dermal reaction pattern). The scalp, face,

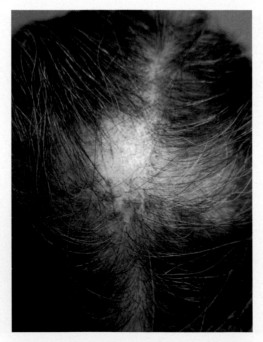

FIGURE 13.4 · Burned-out DLE appearing as depigmented atrophic plaques with scarring alopecia on the vertex scalp.

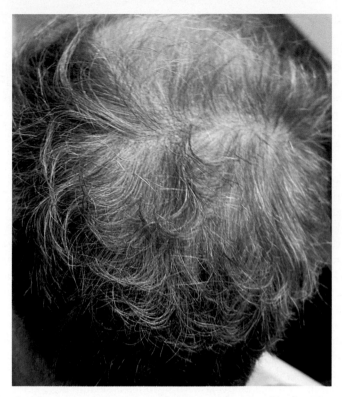

FIGURE 13.5 • Dermatomyositis of the scalp appearing as a thin pink and faintly violaceous plaque on the vertex.

and neck are frequently affected, although generalized forms may occur. Nonscarring alopecia may be present. Dermatomyositis on the scalp presents as very itchy, scaly (or sometimes nonscaly), pink, violaceous, or poikilodermatous plaques. This may or may not be accompanied by nonscarring alopecia (Figure 13.5).

> **Clinical Tip** Consider dermatomyositis of the scalp for any pruritic pink, violaceous, or poikilodermatous scalp eruption.

Scalp involvement is not uncommon in reactive arthritis. Psoriasiform plaques may manifest ostraceous or limpet-like scales. In acrokeratosis paraneoplastica, scalp involvement occurs late in the disease course. Lichenoid or psoriasiform plaques may be seen.

Seborrheic keratoses are frequently seen on the scalp, and warts may occur here as well. Actinic keratoses, squamous cell cancer in situ, and invasive squamous cell cancers are seen in this location, especially in the presence of androgenetic or other longstanding alopecia.

In the vesicobullous category, most conditions are autoimmune, but V1 zoster may also give rise to vesicles in the scalp. The pemphigus family may present with flaccid vesicles and bullae, or just erosions and crusting in the scalp. Hair loss is rarely seen, but when it is present, alopecia is typically nonscarring. Its presence has been associated in the literature with more severe disease. For the subepidermal autoimmune blistering diseases that involve the scalp, most may be accompanied by scarring alopecia. The term *Brunsting–Perry variant of mucous membrane pemphigoid* refers to a skin-dominant presentation (mild or with no mucous membrane involvement), and this typically involves the scalp with scarring alopecia. In dermatitis herpetiformis, scalp involvement with itchy urticarial plaques and resulting vesicles and erosions is typical but hair loss rare. Of note, toxic epidermal necrolysis classically spares the scalp, for unclear reasons.

> **Clinical Tip** Toxic epidermal necrolysis usually spares the scalp.

The scalp is a predilection site in seborrheic dermatitis. Mild forms present with dandruff only. This may progress to scaling and erythema of the scalp, and the classical finding of greasy yellow scales may also be seen. The scalp is frequently involved in atopic dermatitis. Itchy, scaly plaques with or without lichenification are seen. In allergic contact dermatitis occurring secondary to a product that is being used on the scalp, there is typically initial involvement of the skin around the scalp, such as on the face, ears, or neck. It is only in severe or persistent cases that the scalp becomes involved. Hair loss is unusual in scalp eczemas, but if the condition is severe or longstanding, nonscarring alopecia can occur.

Regarding pustules in the scalp, folliculitis is common. Acne can occur on the scalp and rosacea, less commonly so. Consider V1 zoster for pustules in a dermatome on the scalp. As mentioned above, the possibility of an inflammatory tinea capitis or kerion should be considered when pustules are seen on the scalp, especially in children. Scarring alopecia with pustules is seen in acne keloidalis nuchae (where keloidal papules and plaques accompany pustules at the posterior hairline, and ultimately keloidal plaques and nodules only are seen, as in Figure 13.6), folliculitis decalvans (where pustules eventuate in areas of scarring alopecia), and dissecting cellulitis (where boggy, sometimes cerebriform, plaques are associated with draining sinuses and rare pustules, as seen in Figure 13.7). A rarer cause of scarring alopecia is erosive pustular dermatosis. This condition usually occurs on

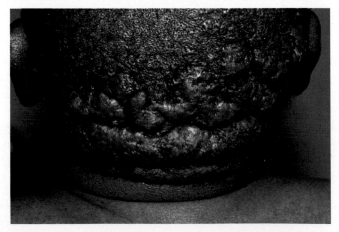

FIGURE 13.6 · Advanced acne keloidalis nuchae manifesting confluent keloidal nodules and plaques on the occiput.

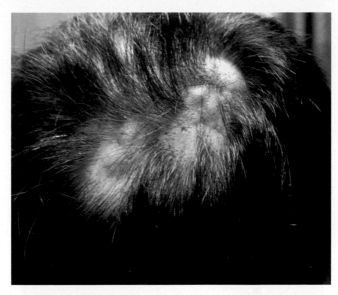

FIGURE 13.7 · Dissecting cellulitis showing a scarring alopecia with a cerebriform topography and a single nondraining sinus on the central scalp.

the sun-damaged scalp of a patient who has undergone cryotherapy or other treatment for actinic keratoses or keratinocyte carcinomas. Pustules are superseded by crusts, which give rise to atrophic plaques when they resolve. Pyoderma gangrenosum begins as perifollicular pustules, and although this does cause scarring, it is very rarely seen on the scalp. Another rare condition that causes pustules on the scalp is amicrobial pustulosis of the folds. It is seen in the setting of underlying connective-tissue disease, usually systemic lupus erythematosus (SLE). The intertriginous areas and the scalp are affected by pustules and erosive plaques. If alopecia is present, this is usually nonscarring. In the neonatal period, consider neonatal acne (or *neonatal cephalic pustulosis*) as a cause of pustules on the scalp, or erythema toxicum neonatorum, which may occur on almost any part of the skin and in which pustules may be associated with wheals. Transient neonatal pustular melanosis may also involve the scalp. Throughout infancy, eosinophilic pustular folliculitis is a cause of scalp pustules. Affected babies are itchy, and although any body part may be affected, scalp involvement is usual.

In the dermal category, consider scalp sarcoidosis or follicular mucinosis (as mentioned above). Scalp sarcoidosis is uncommon and is usually seen in cases with more severe, systemic involvement. Typical orange-brown plaques, or violaceous or hypopigmented plaques, occur that may lead to nonscarring or scarring alopecia. Lipedematous scalp is an extremely rare condition in which a thickened subcutaneous layer gives rise to a boggy feeling on palpation of the scalp. This may be accompanied by itching. Milia, nevi, pilar cysts, epidermal inclusion cysts, and cherry angiomas are commonly seen on the scalp. The scalp is a predilection site for cylindromas, mixed tumors, and proliferating trichilemmal tumors. Consider the diagnosis of keratinocyte carcinomas, melanoma, Merkel cell carcinoma, and atypical fibroxanthoma, especially on a chronically sun-damaged scalp. Angiosarcoma typically arises on the head, including the scalp or neck of older individuals. It presents as a rapidly growing pink, red, or

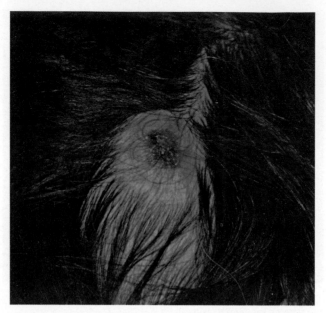

FIGURE 13.8 • A scalp metastasis from breast cancer showing a scarred down pink plaque with central crusting.

maroon plaque or tumor that may ulcerate. Pink or purple dermal nodules may represent lymphoma or leukemia in the skin. Furthermore, the scalp is a common site for cutaneous metastases that present as new-onset papules or nodules in an adult with known or occult malignancy (Figure 13.8). Alopecia neoplastica is a rare form of cutaneous metastasis to the scalp that presents with scarring alopecia. One or (rarely) more patches or thin flesh-colored or pinkish plaques may evolve in a patient with known or occult malignancy. These may clinically resemble alopecia areata.

> **Clinical Tip** Consider the diagnosis of alopecia neoplastica for any new-onset focal alopecia that resembles alopecia areata, especially in someone with a known history of malignancy.

In the vascular reaction pattern, SLE and dermatomyositis may present with erythema in the scalp. As mentioned above, a hallmark of dermatomyositis is its intense itch.

Finally, with respect to scalp disease, alopecia may occur with no obvious scalp disease, and this category will be discussed below in the section on hair.

HAIR

Diagnostic clues can be found in scalp hair, as outlined above, but also in hair elsewhere on the body, such as the eyebrows, eyelashes, and body hair.

Alopecia

Regarding hair loss on the scalp, this may accompany a scalp dermatosis as listed in Table 13.1, or it may be secondary to alterations in hair growth, such as androgenetic alopecia and telogen effluvium. If scalp alopecia is the sole presenting sign, determination of whether a scarring or nonscarring process is present is the next step. Examining the pattern of the alopecia and looking for hair shaft abnormalities are further features that can assist in diagnosis.

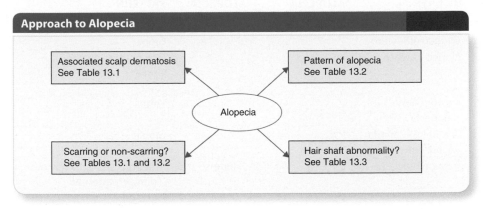

Approach to Alopecia

Associated scalp dermatosis
See Table 13.1

Pattern of alopecia
See Table 13.2

Alopecia

Scarring or non-scarring?
See Tables 13.1 and 13.2

Hair shaft abnormality?
See Table 13.3

Table 13.2 lists alopecic conditions on the scalp that present with minimal skin findings, along with the type (scarring or nonscarring) and pattern of alopecia that is typically seen. Some of these conditions may be scarring or nonscarring, and if this is the case, the same condition might be listed in the table under each category. Sometimes, hair shafts are primarily affected, such as in inherited or acquired hair shaft disorders, or when there are concretions around hair shafts. Hair shaft disorders may also lead to alopecia.

In anagen effluvium, there is usually a rapid loss of hair as the anagen phase of the hair cycle is abruptly truncated, usually from a chemotherapeutic drug. Hair is lost within weeks of the initial insult. In telogen effluvium, an illness, surgery, or other traumatic event precipitates the initiation of catagen of all scalp hair. This phase lasts for 3 months and is followed by telogen, which is experienced as hair fall. This resolved within months. The hair pull test will be positive in both conditions; firmly grasp a 1-cm^2 area of hair in each of four quadrants and pull. The proximal ends of anagen hairs are pigmented and not rounded, as opposed to telogen hairs, which display a whitish rounded proximal end.

Clinical Tip A hair pull test can help to differentiate anagen from telogen hairs; the former has a pigmented, tapered proximal end and the latter, a whitish, rounded end.

Another example of a nonscarring alopecia that presents without other overt clinical features is alopecia areata. Here one or more hairless patches are seen on the scalp. The scalp looks normal and feels normal or slightly softer than the surrounding scalp. Hair follicles are preserved. An "exclamation point" hair is a hair that is wider toward its free edge and thinner at its root. Exclamation point hairs are a sign of alopecia areata and are usually found on the periphery of the patches. Alopecia areata may be found off the scalp, too, for example, involving the eyebrows or eyelashes, the beard area, or anywhere else on the body. Alopecia areata may be static and readily responsive to therapy, or progressive (Figure 13.9) and even global, involving the entire scalp (alopecia totalis; see Figure 13.10) or the entire body (alopecia universalis). The term *ophiasis* refers to a severe variant of alopecia areata where the scalp margin is involved with a band of nonscarring loss. This subtype responds less readily to therapeutic intervention. When hair regrows in alopecia areata, it may be white initially, but this is rarely a permanent phenomenon (Figure 13.11).

TABLE 13.2. Alopecia with Limited or Absent Scalp Findings

DISEASE	NONSCARRING ALOPECIA	SCARRING ALOPECIA	PATTERN
Anagen effluvium	✓		Global
Telogen effluvium	✓		Global
Alopecia areata	✓		One or more patches Ophiasis Total
Androgenetic alopecia	✓		Vertex
Cronkhite–Canada syndrome	✓		Global
Traction alopecia	✓	✓ (late)	Anterior scalp line; may be diffuse/patterned
Trichotillomania	✓		Patchy
Syphilis	✓		"Moth-eaten"
Follicular mucinosis	✓		
Alopecia neoplastica	✓		Anywhere
Pressure alopecia	✓	✓ (severe)	Sites of chronic pressure
Halo scalp ring	✓	✓ (severe)	Circumferential or a part thereof—occiput, temporal scalp above ears, frontal scalp
Neonatal occipital alopecia	✓		Occiput
Cutis aplasia		✓	Vertex
Temporal triangular alopecia	✓		Temporal area
Hair shaft abnormalities	✓		Patchy or diffuse thinning
Loose anagen syndrome	✓		Diffuse thinning
Incontinentia pigmenti		✓	Following Blaschko lines
Pseudopelade of Brocq		✓	Vertex and central scalp
Central centrifugal cicatricial alopecia		✓	Broad patch on vertex; may be numerous scattered patches

In androgenetic alopecia, patterned loss on the vertex and anterior scalp is seen. Male pattern alopecia often shows bitemporal loss and thinning at the vertex. Female pattern loss most commonly presents with diffuse thinning on the anterior scalp, but bitemporal loss may also be a feature. Cronkhite–Canada syndrome is an acquired disorder of unknown etiology that comprises polyposis of the gastrointestinal tract, diarrhea, and cutaneous manifestations, such as rapid global hair loss, patchy hyperpigmentation, and nail changes (thinned nails, onychomadesis, and koilonychia). This hair loss was previously considered telogen effluvium; however, newer research suggests that it is a form of alopecia areata.

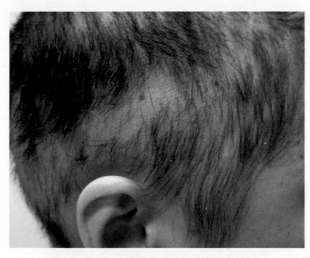

FIGURE 13.9 · Progressive alopecia areata showing smooth areas of nonscarring hair loss and intervening more patchy loss—the beginning of an ophiasis pattern.

In traction alopecia, nonscarring hair loss is seen in areas of the scalp that were previously subjected to chronic low-grade trauma as a result of repeated pulling back or styling of the hair. Examples here include anterolateral hairline involvement in girls or women who keep their hair pulled back in tight ponytails (Figure 13.12) or buns, or a patterned loss throughout the scalp in those who keep their hair in braids for prolonged periods of time. If chronic and longstanding, traction alopecia may ultimately lead to scarring. Trichotillomania is the compulsive pulling out of scalp or other hair (some people favor pulling eyebrow, eyelash, or pubic hair). Focal or larger areas of scalp hair pulling may occur, resulting in one or more patches of thinned hair. The classic diagnostic sign is the presence of hairs of different lengths in the affected area. While the underlying skin is usually normal, there may be associated excoriations, crusts, or eczematization.

> **Clinical Tip** In trichotillomania, look for hairs of differing lengths in the affected area. The underlying skin may be normal or may have excoriations, crusts, or eczematization.

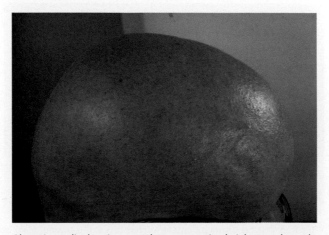

FIGURE 13.10 · Alopecia totalis showing complete nonscarring hair loss on the scalp.

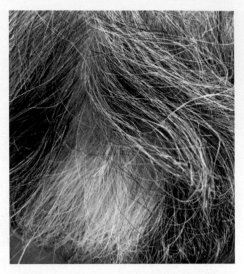

FIGURE 13.11 · Alopecia areata with white hairs at sites of hair regrowth.

Secondary syphilis may cause nonscarring patchy hair loss that is termed "moth-eaten" alopecia (Figure 13.13). This resolves with treatment.

> **Clinical Tip** The presence of patchy, "moth-eaten" alopecia should prompt a search for secondary syphilis.

Pressure alopecia may be seen in adults and children when the scalp is immobilized for long periods of time, such as after surgery or stay in an intensive care unit. Milder cases are nonscarring and result from localized anagen effluvium. In more severe cases, scalp ischemia can lead to ulceration, in which case scarring will eventually develop.

Alopecia may manifest in the neonatal period or in early childhood. Halo scalp ring is a form of alopecia that manifests shortly after birth. It results from prolonged labor caused by caput succedaneum. It manifests as a ring that entirely or partially encircles the

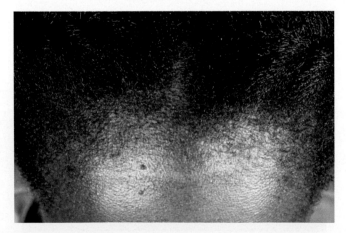

FIGURE 13.12 · Traction alopecia showing nonscarring hair loss at the anterior scalp, secondary to hair being repeatedly pulled back from the face.

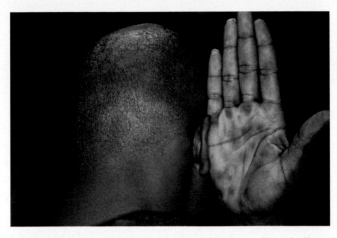

FIGURE 13.13 • Secondary syphilis showing "moth-eaten" alopecia on the scalp. (Reproduced with permission from Kang S, Amagai M, Bruckner AL, et al: *Fitzpatrick's Dermatology*, 9th ed. New York, NY: McGraw Hill; 2019.)

scalp. Most cases are nonscarring; scarring is seen only in severe cases. Neonatal occipital alopecia was previously also assumed to be a pressure-induced phenomenon, where occipital hairs are lost during the first few months of life. This is currently assumed to be due to the occipital scalp hair undergoing telogen effluvium at birth (the other areas of the scalp will have undergone this in utero). Aplasia cutis is the congenital absence of skin that usually is seen on the scalp, but other anatomic areas may also be affected. At birth, a moist ulceration or a scar may have already eventuated. The "hair collar" sign is the presence of coarse dark terminal hairs around the edge of the affected area. The presence of this sign has been associated with an underlying neural tube defect.

> **Clinical Tip** "Hair collar" sign: terminal hairs encircling aplasia cutis, which may signal an underlying neural tube defect.

Aplasia cutis may be isolated or may occur in syndromes such as trisomy 13 or Goltz syndrome. Non–scalp hair may also be affected. Temporal triangular alopecia is a rare condition that appears in childhood on the temporal scalp. It is usually unilateral, although bilateral cases have been reported. It is a form of nonscarring alopecia with miniaturization of hairs confined to this anatomic area of the scalp. Some of the inherited hair shaft abnormalities, (as is seen in Table 13.3), may present in childhood with patchy or global thinned scalp hair. Loose anagen syndrome is usually inherited, although it may be acquired. The primary defect is thought to be an abnormality in how the hair cuticle attaches to the inner root sheath. It is usually seen in infants or children with blond or white hair. Diffuse nonscarring alopecia is seen. The hair pull test will result in copious numbers of anagen hairs. Examination of the hair bulb under trichoscopy or light microscopy will reveal a ruffled cuticle. In incontinentia pigmenti, scarring alopecia may occur in the fourth stage, and it may be the only presenting sign in adolescence or adulthood. It has been described as "whorled" alopecia, and it follows Blaschko lines.

An example of scarring hair loss with no other features is pseudopelade of Brocq. This entity is thought to represent the end stage of any scarring process where confluent, atrophic hairless patches, usually round or oval in shape, are seen on the central scalp in particular. The term "footprints in the snow" has been applied to the appearance of these thin, scarred plaques; it refers to their round or oval shape that bears resemblance to footprints.

> **Clinical Tip** The term "footprints in the snow" refers to the round or oval appearance of the thin, scarred plaques in pseudopelade

Central centrifugal cicatricial alopecia also most commonly presents with minimal overt scalp findings (occasionally pustules and scaling are seen). Scarring alopecia eventuates on the vertex, but patterned cases may occur. An autosomal dominant mutation in the inner root sheath has recently been identified in affected patients of African descent. Trauma from hair grooming, such as hair relaxers, hot combs, glues, and braiding, precipitate the condition in those who are genetically predisposed.

Hair Shaft Disorders

Hair shaft disorders may be inherited or acquired. Inherited disorders have a structural defect, whereas acquired conditions may have either structural changes (such as trichorrhexis nodosa, which results from trauma from hair care practices), or peripilar concretions (such as from an infection or keratinaceous material attached to the shaft).

> **Clinical Tip** Hair shaft disorders include those with structural abnormalities or those involving peripilar concretions.

Table 13.3 outlines the inherited hair shaft disorders and their associations. Clinical suspicion of an inherited hair shaft disorder can be confirmed by trichoscopy or light microscopy, and in some cases scanning electron microscopy may be needed. Some of these disorders cause fragile hair that leads to hair breakage and is accompanied by alopecia that is seen early in life. These conditions are indicated by asterisks in Table 13.3.

Table 13.4 outlines the acquired disorders that affect the hair shaft. In the category of acquired structural defects, trichorrhexis nodosa, "bubble hair," and trichoptilosis occur secondary to hair-grooming practices, including excessive heat from hairdryers and curling irons, or from application of chemicals. Trichorrhexis nodosa may also be seen in the setting of thyroid disease and malnutrition. "Bubble hair" is the presence of air pockets or bubbles within the hair cortex. These conditions lead to hair breakage. Trichoptilosis is the presence of "split ends," where the free end of the hair shaft frays. Pili torti is usually inherited, as mentioned above. It may be an acquired finding in the setting of malnutrition, and it has been associated with oral retinoid therapy. Tufted folliculitis (also known as "tufted hair" or pili multigemini) refers to multiple hair shafts egressing from a single follicle. This phenomenon may be seen in scarring alopecia, such as folliculitis decalvans and dissecting cellulitis.

In ectothrix tinea capitis, fungal spores and hyphae are seen around the hair shaft under light microscopy. The usual causative organisms of ectothrix are *Microsporum* species and *Trichophyton verrucosum*. In endothrix, these fungal structures invade the hair shaft and classically cause broken-off hairs. This is known as "black-dot" tinea capitis. It is usually caused by *Trichophyton* species, such as *Trichophyton tonsurans*.

The differential diagnosis of concretions (material or organisms) attached to hair shafts encompasses a succinct list of conditions. Infectious causes include bacterial and fungal diseases. *Trichomycosis axillaris* is the presence of yellowish material that ensheathes the axillary hair. Less frequently, pubic hair is involved. *Corynebacterium* species are

TABLE 13.3. Inherited Hair Shaft Disorders and Their Associated Conditions

HAIR SHAFT ABNORMALITY	DESCRIPTION	SYNDROMES IN WHICH THIS CAN BE SEEN
Pili torti*	Hair shafts are flattened and twisted; shiny, "spangled" appearance	Isolated finding Bjornstad syndrome (bilateral hearing loss) Crandall syndrome (hearing loss, hypogonadism) Bazex–Dupré–Christol syndrome (X-linked dominant, follicular atrophoderma, hypotrichosis with hair shaft abnormalities, basal cell cancers) Menkes kinky hair syndrome (X-linked, defect in copper transport Also reported in Netherton syndrome; see under trichorrhexis invaginata
Monilethrix*	Hair shafts have elliptical nodes that give rise to a beaded appearance	Autosomal dominant
Trichorrhexis invaginata* ("bamboo hair")	Nodes along hair shaft sit in widened cup-shaped portions: "ball-and-socket" appearance	Netherton syndrome (ichthyosiform erythroderma at birth, ichthyosis linearis circumflexa, atopic diathesis, high IgE; usually the frontal scalp hair and the eyebrows are affected)
Trichorrhexis nodosa*	Fraying of hair shaft through weakest areas	Netherton syndrome Acquired secondary to excessive hair grooming
Trichothiodystrophy*	Brittle hair Tiger tail banding under polarized light	There may be associated photosensitivity, ichthyosis, intellectual impairment, short stature, and decreased fertility.
Pili bifurcati	Hair shafts may be bifurcated	Bazex–Dupré–Christol syndrome
Pili trianguli et canaliculi ("uncombable hair" syndrome)	Silvery "spangled" hair A groove runs along one side (light microscopy) Hair appears triangular (scanning electron microscopy)	Isolated finding, usually autosomal dominant
Woolly hair nevus	A localized portion of scalp hair is tightly curled, thinner than the surrounding hair and sometimes a lighter color	Isolated Skin fragility: woolly hair nevus syndrome (palmoplantar keratoderma, dystrophic nails, bullae)
Pili annulati	Alternating light and dark bands along hair shaft, caused by intermittent air spaces within shafts	Isolated finding, autosomal dominant

*Connotes those disorders that lead to hair fragility.

TABLE 13.4. Acquired Disorders That Affect the Hair Shaft

ACQUIRED STRUCTURAL DEFECTS
- Trichorrhexis nodosa
- Bubble hair
- Trichoptilosis
- Pili torti
- Tufted folliculitis

TINEA CAPITIS
- Ectothrix
- Endothrix
- Favus; see under concretions

CONCRETIONS AROUND HAIR SHAFTS
- Infection
  - Corynebacterial
    - Trichomycosis axillaris
  - Fungal
    - White piedra
    - Black piedra
    - Favus
- Infestation
  - Nits
- Inflammatory
  - Pityriasis amianatacea
- Other
  - Hair casts

responsible. Lack of frequent washing may be a predisposing factor. White piedra is caused by *Trichosporon* species. Loosely adherent white, light brown, or yellowish powdery grains are found on pubic, facial, and axillary hair most frequently. Widespread cases may be seen in HIV disease, in which case a *Trichosporon* fungemia may ensue. In black piedra, firmly adherent small black grains are most commonly found on scalp hair. *Piedraia hortae* is the responsible organism. The term *scutula* refers to the presence of thick yellow crusts surrounding the base of the hair shafts in favus, a type of tinea capitis caused by *Trichophyton schoenleinii*. In pediculosis capitis, nits are seen around a centimeter from the scalp. These are the eggs or egg casings of the lice and are firmly adherent to the hair. Pityriasis amiantacea presents as thick whitish-yellow scales that form concretions around groups of hair shafts on the scalp (Figure 13.14). This condition is believed to represent a form of seborrheic dermatitis or psoriasis. It has rarely been seen in association with atopic dermatitis or tinea capitis. Hair casts are loosely adherent clumps of keratin.

Hair Color

Hair color or a change in hair color on the scalp may also be diagnostically relevant. This may be global or focal as is outlined in Table 13.5. Completely white hair may be seen in normal or premature ageing and is also seen in type 1 oculocutaneous albinism (OCA), where patients lack tyrosinase and so no pigment is produced in skin or hair. A number of medications have been reported to cause onset of graying including tyrosine kinase inhibitors, ipilimumab and the antimalarials. Imatinib mesylate, a

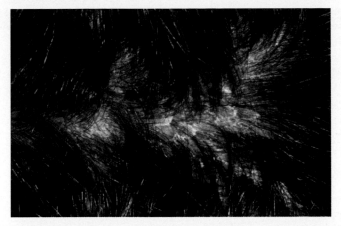

FIGURE 13.14 • Pityriasis amiantacea showing yellowish concretions around hair shafts.

tyrosine kinase inhibitor may cause graying, but has been reported to reverse graying more frequently. The phenomenon of one or more focal patch of gray or white hair is known as poliosis circumscripta. This may be inherited or acquired. If inherited, it may be an isolated or syndromic. A white forelock may be an isolated finding or

TABLE 13.5. Differential Diagnosis of Hair Color

WHITE, GRAY
- Global
  - Normal or premature ageing
  - Albinism, OCA type 1
  - Drug-induced
    - Tyrosine kinase inhibitors
      - imatinib
      - dasatinib
      - sunitinib
      - pazopanib
    - Anti-CTLA4 antibody
      - ipilimumab
    - Antimalarials
      - chloroquine
      - hydroxychloroquine
- Focal
  - Inherited
    - Isolated white forelock
    - Isolated occipital white lock
    - Piebaldism
    - Waardenburg syndrome
    - Tuberous sclerosis
  - Acquired
    - After regrowth of alopecia areata
    - Post-inflammatory phenomenon
    - Vitiligo

(Continued)

TABLE 13.5.   Differential Diagnosis of Hair Color (continued)

WHITE, GRAY (CONT.)
- Halo nevus
- Alezzandrini syndrome
- Vogt-Koyanagi-Harada syndrome

SILVERY-GRAY
- Chediak-Higashi syndrome
- Griscelli syndrome
- Elejade syndrome

REPIGMENTATION OF HAIR
- Global
  - Drug-induced
    - imatinib
    - latanoprost
    - adalimumab
    - thalidomide
    - etretinate
    - erlotinib
    - Anti-PD-1 therapy
      - nivolumab
      - pembrolizumab
      - atezolizumab
    - brentuximab
- Focal
  - Lentigo maligna
  - Melanoma

RED, GINGER
- Rufous albinism, OCA type 3

YELLOW
- Albinism, OCA type 2
- Tar products change the color of gray hair to yellow

GREEN
- Copper

it may be seen in three autosomal dominantly inherited conditions: Waardenburg syndrome, piebaldism or tuberous sclerosis. There are 4 subtypes of Waardenburg syndrome. Each may be accompanied by a white forelock and a depigmented patch on the forehead. Synophrys and a broad nasal root (secondary to dystopia canthorum) are further findings. In piebaldism, a white forelock is accompanied by depigmented patches on around the elbows and knees, on the forehead and on the central trunk. In tuberous sclerosus, hypopigmented patches (such as ash leaf or confetti macules) are seen on the skin, along with other cutaneous features of the syndrome (such as a shagreen patch, fibrous forehead plaque, periungual fibromas and adenoma sebaceum). A white forelock is present in a minority of individuals with tuberous sclerosis. It is reported to develop as early as the neonatal period and so may be an early diagnostic sign. Acquired poliosis circumscripta is seen when vitiligo affects the scalp; the hair in the affected areas will also be depigmented. When a halo nevus occurs in the scalp, the hairs in the depigmented area around the nevus may be similarly depigmented. As alopecia areata resolves, some of the new hairs may grow in white at first, and then develop color later on. In Vogt-Koyanagi-Harada syndrome there is autoimmune destruction of melanocytes in the leptomeninges, uvea, inner ear and skin. Aseptic meningitis, uveitis and possible subsequent visual loss, as well as hearing loss precede development of vitiliginous patches and poliosis. In Alezzandrini syndrome, skin and hair depigmentation, usually of the face and scalp, accompany ipsilateral visual and auditory loss.

Shiny gray, or silver-gray hair is an early finding in the triad of gray hair syndromes, including Chediak-Higashi, Griscelli and Elejade syndrome. In these rare inherited syndromes, there are a variety of defects in intracellular protein transport, including melanosomes, that give rise to melanin clumping in the hair and pigmentary dilution in the skin. Neurological, immunological and hematological effects are seen, depending on the syndrome.

Repigmentation of gray hair is an infrequent side effect of numerous medications, the newest class being the anti- PD1 inhibitors. Focal hair repigmentation has been reported as a diagnostic sign of melanoma in-situ, as well as melanoma of the scalp; this is a "do not miss" diagnostic sign.

> **Clinical Tip:** Consider the diagnosis of melanoma in-situ or melanoma underlying the spontaneous development of focal repigmentation of gray scalp hair.

In type 3 OCA, the rufous type, hair may appear orange or red, whereas in type 2 OCA, hair appears yellow. The use of tar shampoo and other tar-containing products may stain gray or white hair yellow. Finally, copper in swimming pool water, not chlorine as once suspected, is responsible for the greenish color of blond hair in swimmers.

Eyebrows and Eyelashes

The term *madarosis* encompasses eyebrow and eyelash loss. *Milphosis* is the term applied to eyelash loss alone. The differential diagnosis of madarosis is very broad because almost any condition that affects these anatomic areas can lead to hair loss that is either nonscarring or scarring, depending on the disease process. Table 13.6 lists some of the most common and classic causes of madarosis, subclassified according to whether the condition is scarring or nonscarring. Additional causes of milphosis include inflammatory disorders of the eyelid margins, such as blepharitis or rosacea, and neoplasms of the eyelid margins, such as sebaceous carcinoma.

Trichomegaly can be congenital. It can be caused by chronic disease states, and has been reported in tuberculosis, human immunodeficiency virus (HIV) disease, systemic lupus erythematosus (SLE), and dermatomyositis. It is the epidermal growth factor receptor inhibitors (EGFR) inhibitors (cetuximab, gefitinib, panitumumab, and erlotinib), cyclosporin, interferon α-2b, topiramate, and latanoprost have all been reported to cause trichomegaly. Latanoprost is a prostaglandin F2α analog, which is used to treat glaucoma. Trichomegaly is a common side effect. There is an increased length of anagen and increased conversion of telogen to anagen hairs. It can also stain the iris brown. Other prostaglandin F2α analogs, bimatoprost and travoprost, have been noted to do the same.

TABLE 13.6. Differential Diagnosis of Madarosis

NONSCARRING
- Inherited
  - Hair shaft disorders: patchy or diffuse
- Acquired
  - Hair growth disorders
    - Telogen effluvium
    - Anagen effluvium
  - Infectious
    - Lepromatous leprosy: diffuse
    - Secondary syphilis: "moth-eaten"
    - Tinea faciei
  - Inflammatory
    - Atopic dermatitis: patchy or diffuse
    - Seborrheic dermatitis: patchy or diffuse
    - Alopecia areata: patchy or diffuse
    - Ulerythema ophryogenes: lateral third of eyebrow thinned
    - Follicular mucinosis
    - Cronkhite–Canada syndrome
  - Metabolic
    - Hypothyroidism: lateral third of eyebrow is thinned
    - Hyperthyroidism
  - Traumatic
    - Trichotillomania: patchy or diffuse
  - Neoplastic
    - Benign neoplasms occurring in the eyebrow, such as nevi
    - Mycosis fungoides

SCARRING
- Inherited
  - Junctional and dystrophic epidermolysis bullosa
  - Lamellar ichthyosis
- Infectious
  - Lupus vulgaris
  - Paracoccidioidomycosis
- Inflammatory
  - DLE
  - Frontal fibrosing alopecia
  - En coup de sabre
  - Sarcoidosis
- Neoplastic
  - Malignant tumors that affect the eyebrow or eyelid margin

Hair Loss on the Body

A nonscaring decreased density of hair on the body, including axillae and pubic hair, may be seen with senescence. Alopecia areata may affect any hair-bearing area in a patchy or global fashion (alopecia universalis). Anterolateral alopecia of the shins is a fairly common finding in men; this, too, is nonscarring. It is thought to occur secondary to minor trauma to skin areas that become irritated by rubbing against clothing. Trichotillomania can affect eyebrows, eyelashes, and pubic hair. Follicular mucinosis may occur anywhere on the body. Lichen planopilaris may affect non–scalp hair and cause a scarring alopecia.

Excess Hair Growth

Excess hair growth may be seen in hirsutism and hypertrichosis. *Hirsutism* is the growth of terminal hairs in androgen-dependent areas, such as the beard area, the periareolar skin, and the central chest and abdomen. This pattern of hair growth is seen in the presence of inherited or acquired conditions of excess androgen secretion, such as in congenital adrenal hyperplasia, polycystic ovarian syndrome, or an androgen-secreting tumor of the adrenal or ovary. Milder cases may be familial and may have no underlying abnormality. Hirsutism may also be induced by exogenous testosterone, such as that used as a part of transgender care. *Hypertrichosis* may be inherited or acquired and may be either localized or generalized. In inherited hypertrichosis, there may be terminal, vellus, or lanugo hairs. The hypertrichosis may be an isolated finding, and there are a handful of rare genetic syndromes with hypertrichosis as a finding. An example is Cantu syndrome, where chondrodysplasia, cardiomegaly, and facial abnormalities are accompanied by hypertrichosis. Localized hypertrichosis may be seen over a Becker nevus, for example, or it may be syndromic, such as in Cornelia de Lange syndrome, where terminal hair growth is seen on the upper back and around the anterior and lateral hairline. A faun tail nevus describes the presence of terminal hairs over the lumbosacral area or posterior neck. This finding may signal an underlying spinal cord defect such as dysraphism. Localized hypertrichosis accompanies some of the forms of porphyria, such as porphyria cutanea tarda and variegate porphyria. Acquired generalized hypertrichosis may be seen in acromegaly, POEMS (polyneuropathy–organomegaly–endocrinopathy–monoclonal gammopathy–skin changes) syndrome, or in the setting of drug therapy such as corticosteroids or cyclosporin. Acquired hypertrichosis lanuginosa may be seen in anorexia nervosa or as a paraneoplastic phenomenon. Localized hypertrichosis may arise in anatomic areas that are subject to chronic trauma or friction, or rarely after strong topical steroid use. Facial hypertrichosis is a known side effect of topical minoxidil therapy.

Bedside Diagnostic Maneuvers and Tests for Scalp and Hair Disease

For a scaly scalp, especially in a child, and in adult cases where tinea capitis is suspected, perform a potassium hydroxide (KOH) preparation of the proximal portions of a few hairs. A Wood's lamp will reveal a greenish or bluish-green color in *Microsporum* tinea capitis and a blue color in favus. Perform Gram stain and culture of pustules and consider performing a KOH preparation of pus for any suspected case of kerion. Perform a polymerase chain reaction (PCR) test on a vesicle or pustule, looking for zoster. For any patient presenting with alopecia, examine the path width on the vertex and anterior scalp, and compare it to the path width on the occiput. In androgenetic alopecia, it will be wider on the vertex and anterior scalp than the occiput. Perform a hair pull test by tugging on approximately 1 cm^2 of hair in four quadrants. The presence of more than five telogen hairs signifies telogen effluvium. In anagen effluvium, numerous anagen hairs will come out.

Trichoscopy is the application of dermoscopy for hair disorders. Characteristic scalp findings have been described for any condition that causes alopecia. The dermatoscope or light microscope in the clinic can also help identify hair shaft disorders. Some centers are equipped with an electron microscope; this can also assist in the diagnosis of hair shaft disorders. Ordering bloodwork for TSH, iron studies, and a hormone panel can assist in the diagnosis of alopecia and scalp lupus. Biopsy for H and E (hematoxylin and eosin), as well as perilesional biopsy of normal skin, can assist with the diagnosis of an autoimmune blistering disease.

Bedside Diagnostic Maneuvers and Tests for Scalp and Hair Disease

- Wood's lamp, KOH for scales
- Gram, KOH, and Wright stains for pustules
- PCR for vesicles and pustules
- Path width, hair pull test for alopecia
- Examine scalp under dermatoscope
- Examine hairs under light microscope or dermatoscope; hair shaft abnormalities

- Hormone panel for hirsutism
- Thyroid-stimulating hormone (TSH) and connective- tissue labs for alopecia areata
- Biopsy for H and E and direct immunofluorescence (DIF) in case of blistering disease
- Electron microscopy of hair

NAILS

Nail findings can provide clues to the presence of an associated dermatosis or underlying systemic disease. They may also herald a nail bed or nail matrix tumor, or may be benign, isolated findings. Additionally, characteristic nail findings from medications have been described. Some of the classic nail and periungual signs that are indicative of specific diseases are listed in the textbox below.

Nail Signs and Periungual Signs

Nail Signs
- Oil-drop sign: distal brown spot that is a sign of incipient onycholysis
- Sandwich sign: alternating red and white lines of the nails in Darier disease (Figure 13.15)

Periungual Signs
- Samitz sign: ragged cuticles seen in dermatomyositis
- Hutchinson sign: brown or black pigmentation on a nail fold from a subungual melanoma
- Pseudo-Hutchinson sign: brown or black pigmentation on a nail fold from conditions other than melanoma, such as lentigines or nevi of the nail matrix

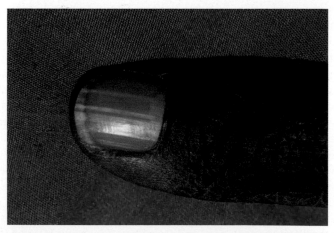

FIGURE 13.15 • The sandwich sign of Darier disease showing alternating red and white lines of the fingernail.

TABLE 13.7. Nail Abnormality Definitions

NAIL FINDING	DEFINITION
Anonychia	Absent nail
Beau line	A transverse ridge in the nail
Dorsal pterygium	The proximal nail fold attaches to the nail matrix; as the nail grows, a triangular wedge of nail fold forms down the center of the nail, dividing the nail into two
Erythronychia	Red color of the nail
Leukonychia	White color of the nail
Lindsay nail ("half-and-half" nail)	Proximal portion is white and distal portion has a brownish color; seen in chronic kidney disease
Mees' lines	Transverse white lines just distal to the matrix; seen in arsenic toxicity, thallium toxicity, chronic kidney disease, and heart failure and in patients receiving chemotherapy
Melanonychia	Brown or black color of the nail
Muerhcke lines	A double white transverse line; seen in hypoproteinemic states, such as liver failure, nephrotic syndrome, malnutrition
Onychodermal band	The distal 2–3-mm portion of the nail, seen just before the nail separates from the nail bed
Onychogryphosis	Markedly thickened, curved, and elongated nails
Onycholysis	Distal lifting of the nail plate off the nail bed
Onychomadesis	Proximal detachment of nail plate from nail matrix
Onychorrhexis	Longitudinal ridging
Nail pitting	Pock marks in the nail plate
Photoonycholysis	Onycholysis induced by sunlight
Splinter hemorrhage	Small linear red to dark purple subungual macules
Subungual hyperkeratosis	Increased keratin beneath the nail plate
Subungual red comets	Elongated tortuous capillaries under nail plate, as seen in tuberous sclerosis
Terry nail	Nail is globally white, except for the distalmost 0.5–3 mm (onychodermal band that can be pink or brown); seen in hypoproteinemic state, such as cirrhosis, and in heart failure and diabetes
Trachyonychia	Nails have a roughened surface
Twenty-nail dystrophy	All nails display trachyonychia
Ventral pterygium	The distal part of the nail bed is attached to the undersurface of the nail plate

Table 13.7 encapsulates the definitions for the nail findings that are included in this section. Table 13.8 defines the disease entities of the nail that are mentioned later in this section. Table 13.9 (see also Figures 13.16–13.22) delineates the nail findings in selected dermatoses by reaction pattern, pustules, and macules, and, where important, the periungual findings are listed as well. Important clues to the presence of connective-tissue disease may be found in the appearance of nails and periungual tissues. These findings are presented in Table 13.9 and summarized in Table 13.10.

TABLE 13.8. Definitions of Disease Entities of the Nail

DISEASE ENTITY	EXPLANATION
Dermatophytoma	Fungal abscess under the nail plate composed of fungal spores, filaments, or both; rare form of onychomycosis presenting as a white-yellow or orange-brown longitudinal streak in the nail plate
Onychopapilloma	A benign subungual neoplasm caused by an abnormality in the nail matrix
Twenty-nail dystrophy	All nails display trachyonychia; may be an isolated finding or may be seen in lichen planus, psoriasis, or alopecia areata

TABLE 13.9. Typical Nail Changes Seen in Various Common and Rare Dermatoses, by Reaction Pattern and Macules

PAPULOSQUAMOUS
- Psoriasis
  - Nail bed disease (Figure 13.16)
    - Onycholysis
    - Subungual hyperkeratosis
    - Splinter hemorrhages
    - Oil-drop sign
    - Twenty-nail dystrophy
    - Acrodermatitis continua of Hallopeau: painless pustules around and under the nail persist and recur and lead to anonychia
    - Psoriatic onychopachydermoperiostitis: terminal phalanges display a periostitis; the overlying nail manifests onycholysis and subungual hyperkeratosis, and the surrounding soft tissue is edematous and thickened
  - Nail matrix disease
    - Pits: coarse, irregular (Figures 13.16 and 13.17)
- Lichen planus (Figure 13.18)
  - Onychorrhexis
  - Dorsal pterygium
  - "Sandpapered" nail dystrophy: fine onychorrhexis
  - Twenty-nail dystrophy
  - Anonychia
- DLE
  - Periungual erythema is a sign of SLE
- Onychomycosis
  - Distal lateral subungual onychomycosis
  - Superficial white onychomycosis (Figure 13.19)
  - Total dystrophic onychomycosis
- Pityriasis rubra pilaris
  - Subungual hyperkeratosis
  - Onychorrhexis
- Reactive arthritis: nail changes may resemble those seen in psoriasis
  - Pits
  - Subungual hyperkeratosis
  - Changes seen in acrodermatitis continua of Hallopeau

(Continued)

TABLE 13.9. Typical Nail Changes Seen in Various Common and Rare Dermatoses, by Reaction Pattern and Macules (continued)

PAPULOSQUAMOUS (CONT.)

- Darier disease
  - Distal V-shaped nick is characteristic
  - Longitudinal red lines
  - Longitudinal white lines
  - Alternating longitudinal red and white lines: known as the "sandwich sign" or "candy cane"
- Hailey–Hailey disease
  - Longitudinal white lines
- Inflammatory linear verrucous epidermal nevus (ILVEN)
  - Trachyonychia
- Chronic graft versus host disease (Figure 13.20)
  - Transverse ridging
  - Trachyonychia
  - Onychorrhexis
  - Longitudinal erythronychia
  - Dorsal pterygium
  - Thin nail plates
- Subungual keratoacanthoma/SCC
  - Longitudinal erythronychia
  - Longitudinal melanonychia
  - Painful subungual mass
  - Longitudinal split in nail
  - Loss of nail plate
  - Verrucous papule/ plaque/nodule on or around nail bed
  - Ulcerated/friable papule/plaque/ nodule on nail bed
  - Scaly papule/plaque on or around nail bed

VESICOBULLOUS

- Porphyria cutanea tarda, pseudoporphyria
  - Photoonycholysis
- Epidermolysis bullosa acquisita
  - Painful onycholysis from subungual bulla formation
- Subungual blistering disease that scar (eg, junctional and dystrophic forms of epidermolysis bullosa)
  - Anonychia
- Herpetic whitlow
  - Grouped vesicles or pustules around and sometimes under the nail

ECZEMATOUS

- If the proximal nail fold is involved with eczema that is severe enough to interfere with keratinization in the nail matrix
  - Transverse ridging and/or coarse pits

PUSTULES

- Acrodermatitis continua of Hallopeau
  - Periungual lakes of pus and eventual anonychia
- Felon
  - Subungual pus and pain
- Herpetic whitlow
  - Grouped vesicles or pustules around and sometimes under the nail

(Continued)

TABLE 13.9. Typical Nail Changes Seen in Various Common and Rare Dermatoses, by Reaction Pattern and Macules (continued)

DERMAL
- Sarcoidosis
  - Onycholysis and subungual hyperkeratosis
  - Dorsal pterygium
  - Painful clubbing
- Primary amyloidosis
  - Dense onychorrhexis
  - Longitudinal erythronychia
  - Anonychia
- Leprosy
  - Longitudinal ridging (paucibacillary)
  - Anonychia, brittle nails, thinned nails (multibacillary)
- Multicentric reticulohistiocytoma
  - Ridging and grooves if papules affect proximal nail fold
- Scleroderma
  - Thickened, beaked nails
  - Hyperkeratosis of hyponychium
  - Inverse pterygium
  - Splinter hemorrhages
  - Nail fold capillary loop abnormalities
- Tuberous sclerosis
  - Periungual fibroma
    - Longitudinal groove
  - Subungual fibroma
    - Longitudinal groove
    - Oval white or red patch
  - Splinter hemorrhages
  - Subungual red comets

MELANOMA
- Pigmented
  - Longitudinal melanonychia
  - Longiudinal erythronychia
  - Subungual pigmented papule or nodule
  - Hutchinson sign
  - Ulcerated or bleeding papule or nodule
  - Destruction of nail plate
  - Loss of nail plate
- Amelanotic
  - Longitudinal erythronychia
  - Subungual colorless, pink, red, bluish or purplish mass
  - Ulcerated or bleeding papule or nodule
  - Destruction of nail plate
  - Loss of nail plate

(Continued)

TABLE 13.9. Typical Nail Changes Seen in Various Common and Rare Dermatoses, by Reaction Pattern and Macules (continued)

VASCULAR
- SLE
  - Nail changes
    - Onycholysis
    - Transverse or longitudinal ridging
    - Red lunulae
    - Transverse leukonychia
    - Ventral pterygium
  - Periungual changes
    - Periungual erythema
    - Nail fold capillary loop abnormalities
    - Nail fold infarcts
- Dermatomyositis
  - Periungual changes (Figure 13.21)
    - Nail fold capillary loop abnormalities
    - Ragged cuticles
    - Nail fold infarcts
- Toxic epidermal necrolysis
  - Onychomadesis
  - Anonychia as a sequela
- Septic vasculitis
  - Splinter hemorrhages
- Osler–Rendu–Weber disease
  - Subungual red streaks; macules and papules 1–4 mm
  - Nail fold telangiectasias
- Kawasaki disease
  - Periungual desquamation
  - Orange-brown or white discoloration of nails
  - Beau lines
  - Onychomadesis

MACULES
- Cronkhite–Canada syndrome (Figure 13.22)
  - Thinned nails
  - Onycholysis
  - Onychomadesis
  - Koilonychia

In Table 13.11 (see also Figures 13.23–13.27), nail findings and their skin and systemic associations are categorized by color and pattern. Splinter hemorrhages are small linear red to dark purple subungual macules that occur secondary to bleeding in the nail bed. Table 13.12 (see also Figure 13.28) outlines the causes of splinter hemorrhages by etiology. Table 13.13 describes some structural nail defects along with their disease

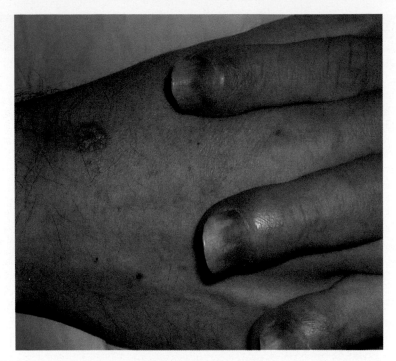

FIGURE 13.16 • Psoriasis affecting the nail bed and nail matrix showing onycholysis and subungual hyperkeratosis, as well as nail pitting of the fingernails. (Used with permission from Dr Miguel Sanchez, Bellevue Hospital, New York University School of Medicine, New York, NY.)

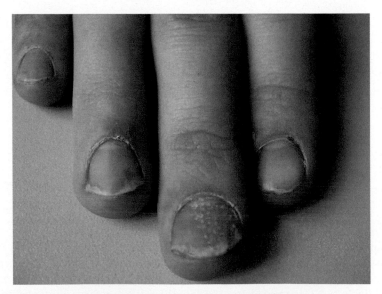

FIGURE 13.17 • Psoriasis affecting the nail matrix showing coarse pits on the nail. (Reproduced with permission from Kang S, Amagai M, Bruckner AL, et al: *Fitzpatrick's Dermatology*, 9th ed. New York, NY: McGraw Hill; 2019.)

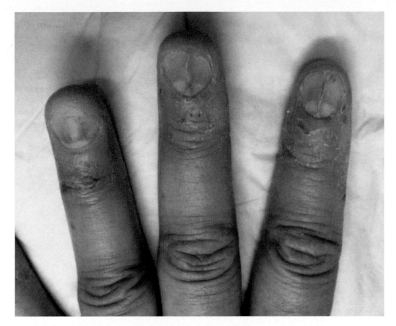

FIGURE 13.18 • Lichen planus of the fingernails showing onychorrhexis and early dorsal pterygium formation.

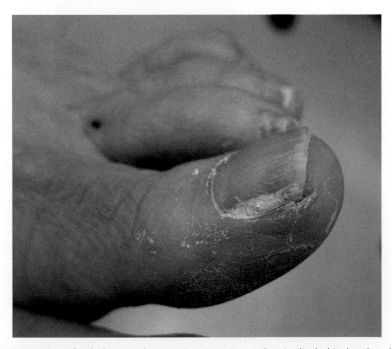

FIGURE 13.19 • Superficial white onychomycosis presenting as a longitudinal white band on the great toenail. Note also the surrounding scaling of tinea pedis.

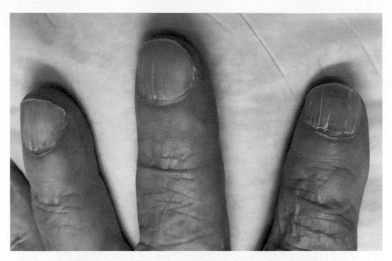

FIGURE 13.20 • Chronic graft versus host disease manifesting with onychorrhexis and onychomadesis.

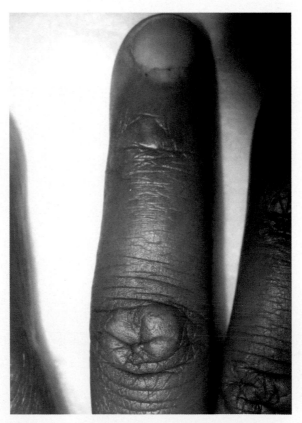

FIGURE 13.21 • Dermatomyositis showing a thickened ragged cuticle and nail fold infarcts. Note also the atrophic dermal papules of dermatomyositis over the interphalangeal joints.

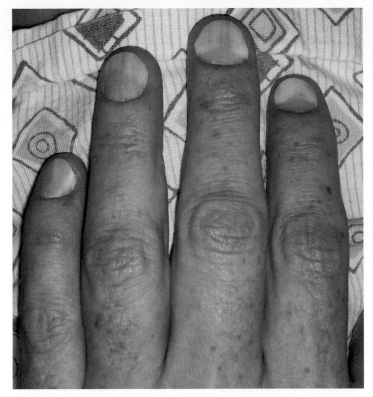

FIGURE 13.22 • Cronkhite–Canada syndrome showing onycholysis and early koilonychias of the fingernails as well as pigmentary macules on the dorsal fingers.

TABLE 13.10. Nail and Periungual Findings in Connective-Tissue Disease

NAIL OR PERIUNGUAL FINDING	SLE	DERMATOMYOSITIS	SCLERODERMA
Red lunula	+++	+	No
Ventral pterygium	+	+	+++
Hyperkeratosis of the hyponychium	+	No	+++
Splinter hemorrhages	++, especially in the setting of antiphospholipid syndrome	+	+
Thickened, ragged cuticles	++	+++	+
Periungual erythema	+++	++	+
Nail fold infarcts	+++	++	+
Proximal nail fold telangiectasia	++	+++	+

TABLE 13.11. Differential Diagnosis of Causes of Nail Conditions That Affect Nail Color

PINK, RED
- Red lunula
  - SLE
  - Rheumatoid arthritis
  - Chronic obstructive pulmonary disease (COPD) and other pulmonary diseases
  - Cardiac failure
  - Cirrhosis
  - Carbon monoxide poisoning
  - Alopecia areata
- Longitudinal erythronychia
  - Single
    - Onychopapilloma
    - Glomus tumor
    - Wart
    - SCCIS, SCC
    - Amelanotic melanoma
  - Multiple
    - Darier disease
    - Lichen planus
    - Graft versus host disease
    - Primary amyloidosis
- Red streaks, macules, papules
  - Osler–Rendu–Weber disease
  - Subungual red comets of tuberous sclerosis

ORANGE OR LIGHT BROWN
- Oil-drop sign in psoriasis

BROWN, BLACK
- Subungual pigment
- Melanoma
- Longitudinal melanonychia
  - Single
    - Lentigo
    - Nevus
    - Dermatophytoma
    - Atypical lentiginous melanocytic proliferation
    - Melanoma
    - SCC
  - Multiple
    - Normal variant
    - Drug-related, including AZT (Figure 13.23), hydroxyurea, chemotherapy
    - Endocrine disorder (eg, Addison disease)
    - Lentiginosis (eg, Laugier–Hunziker syndrome, Peutz–Jegher syndrome)
    - Lichen planus
    - SLE
- Transverse melanonychia
  - From chemotherapy such as hydroxyurea, etoposide
  - Radiation-induced

(Continued)

TABLE 13.11. Differential Diagnosis of Causes of Nail Conditions That Affect Nail Color (continued)

BROWN, BLACK (CONT.)
- Subungual heme
  - Splinter hemorrhages (see Table 13.12)
  - Subungual hematoma (Figure 13.24)
- Other subungual pigments
  - Onychomycosis: brown, black
  - Pseudomonal nail infection: brown, green, sometimes black
  - Drug-related: hydroxychloroquine leads to diffuse brown discoloration

WHITE
- Longitudinal white lines
  - Superficial white onychomycosis
  - Darier disease
  - Hailey–Hailey disease
  - Dermatophytoma
- Transverse white lines
  - Trauma
  - Mees' lines
  - Muerhcke lines
  - Lindsay nails
  - Terry nails
  - SLE
- Global leukonychia
  - Inherited
  - Hypoproteinemic states
- Other patterned leukonychia
  - Trauma, including excessive manicuring
  - Onychomycosis
    - Superficial white onychomycosis
    - Proximal white subungual onychomycosis
    - White can also be seen in other forms of onychomycosis
    - Dermatophytoma

YELLOW
- Longitudinal yellow line(s)
  - Onychomycosis
  - Onychopapilloma
  - Onychomycosis, including dermatophytoma
- Other yellow conditions
  - Onychogryphosis
  - Yellow nail syndrome
  - Discoloration from prolonged nail varnish application, darker colors
  - Transverse yellow lines may occur secondary to tetracyclines
  - Yellow nails may be seen in SLE

BLUE, PURPLE
- Usually single
  - Subungual hematoma, can be more than one (Figure 13.25)
  - Glomus tumor, can be more than one
  - Amelanotic melanoma

(Continued)

TABLE 13.11. Differential Diagnosis of Causes of Nail Conditions That Affect Nail Color (continued)

BLUE, PURPLE (CONT.)
- Usually multiple
  - Raynaud phenomenon, primary or secondary
  - Splinter hemorrhages
  - Exogenous pigmentation such as from blue dye in footwear (Figure 13.26)
  - Drug-induced
    - Diffuse blue-gray pigmentation: minocycline
    - Blue-black discoloration: chloroquine, sparfloxacin (blue lunulae)
  - Argyria: diffuse blue pigmentation of nail bed

GREEN
- Pseudomonal nail infection (Figure 13.27)

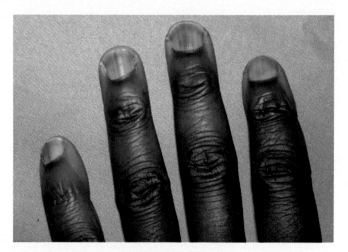

FIGURE 13.23 • Longitudinal melanonychia of nails from AZT.

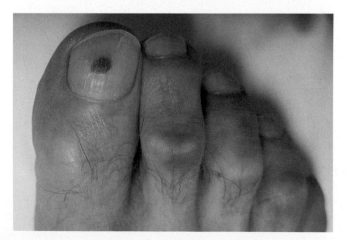

FIGURE 13.24 • A subungual hematoma presenting as a brownish discoloration of the great toenail.

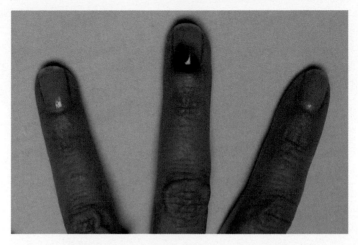

FIGURE 13.25 • A subungual hematoma presenting as a bluish mass underneath the third fingernail.

and drug associations. Nail pitting may occur as a result of psoriasis, eczema, or alopecia areata. Coarse pits are seen in the former two entities and fine, "grid-like" pits, in the latter.

Differential Diagnosis of Nail Pitting

- Alopecia areata: fine, grid-like pits
- Psoriasis: coarse pits
- Eczema: may cause coarse pitting if it involves the proximal nail fold

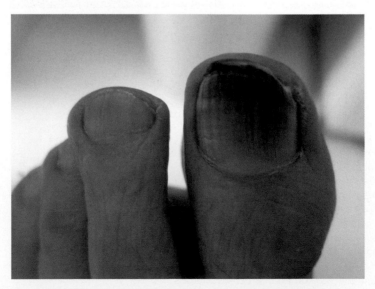

FIGURE 13.26 • Bright blue nail pigmentation from an exogenous blue dye, from socks.

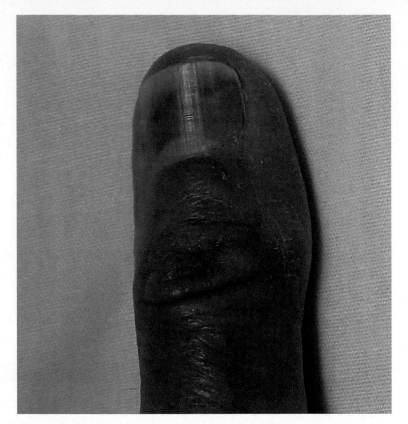

FIGURE 13.27 • Greenish discoloration of nails from pseudomonal infection.

TABLE 13.12. Causes of Splinter Hemorrhage

- Distal hemorrhage due to trauma
- Bleeding disorders (eg, thrombocytopenia)
- Embolic
  - Acute and subacute bacterial endocarditis
  - Bacterial sepsis (Figure 13.28)
  - Rheumatic fever
  - Nonbacterial endocarditis of SLE
  - Antiphospholipid syndrome
  - Atrial myxoma
  - From thrombi forming within an arterial aneurysm
- Vasculitic
  - Leukocytoclastic vasculitis
  - Types II and II cryoglobulinemia
  - Connective tissue diseases
  - Trichinosis
- Dilated superficial dermal capillaries in the nail bed
  - Psoriasis
  - Osler–Rendu–Weber disease
  - Subungual red comets in tuberous sclerosis

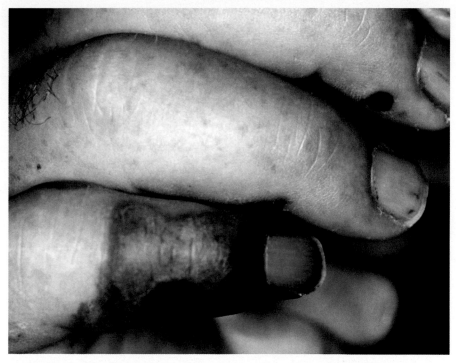

FIGURE 13.28 · Splinter hemorrhages of nails, as seen in a case of bacterial sepsis with disseminated intravascular coagulopathy.

Pain under the nail is an uncommon symptom. It may be associated with subungual pus collection, vesicle or bulla formation, or painful neoplasms of skin or bone in a subungual location. The differential diagnoses of the most frequent causes of subungual pain are listed in the textbox below.

Differential Diagnosis of Subungual Pain

- Felon
- Ingrown toenail
- Retronychia
- Subungual hematoma
- Vesicle, bulla
  - Photoonycholysis
  - Porphyria cutanea tarda
  - Pseudoporphyria
  - Epidermolysis bullosa acquisita
  - Junctional and dystrophic forms of epidermolysis bullosa
- Neoplasm
  - Benign
    - Glomus tumor
    - Warty dyskeratoma
    - Exostosis
    - Osteochondroma
  - Malignant
    - Keratoacanthoma/squamous cell carcinoma (SCC)

Periungual changes may be associated with nail changes. A comprehensive list of these changes is seen in Table 13.14 (see also Figures 13.29–13.34).

TABLE 13.13. Structural Nail Defects and Their Associated Conditions

NAIL FINDING	ISOLATED FINDING?	SKIN/NAIL/ PERIUNGUAL DISEASE	SYSTEMIC CONDITION	MEDICATION
Onycholysis	Yes; from trauma	Psoriasis Lichen planus Irritant or allergic contact dermatitis Onychomycosis	Hyper- or hypothyroidism Porphyria cutanea tarda Pseudoporphyria	Photoonycholysis from doxycycline, PUVA, oral contraceptives Oral retinoids, chemotherapy
Koilonychia	Yes	Psoriasis Lichen planus	Iron deficiency Plummer–Vinson syndrome (iron deficiency, dysphagia from esophageal web, predisposition to esophageal SCC) Nail–patella syndrome Cronkhite–Canada syndrome	
Onychorrhexis	Yes; "wear and tear" nails from excessive hand washing, use of nail cosmetics	Lichen planus Psoriasis PRP Darier disease	SLE Hypothyroidism Malnutrition Dyskeratosis congenita	Oral retinoids
Dorsal pterygium	Yes; from local trauma	Lichen planus, graft vs host disease Mucous membrane pemphigoid After TEN	Raynaud phenomenon Nail–patella syndrome Dyskeratosis congenita	
Ventral pterygium	Yes; may be familial or due to trauma	Scleroderma	Scleroderma SLE Raynaud phenomenon	
Onychomadesis	Yes; sometimes no cause found	Acute paronychia Pemphigus vulgaris Alopecia areata Erythroderma After SJS/TEN	After hand–foot–mouth disease After severe infections After Kawasaki disease Cronkhite–Canada syndrome	Chemotherapy Retinoid therapy Anticonvulsants
Anonychia: any condition that causes scarring or infiltration of the nail matrix	Yes; congenital cases reported, secondary to trauma	Lichen planus Acrodermatitis continua of Hallopeau Junctional/dystrophic EB	Nail–patella syndrome Dyskeratosis congenita Hidrotic ectodermal dysplasia Primary amyloidosis	

Bedside Diagnostic Maneuvers and Tests for Nails

Nail scrapings can assist with diagnosis of fungus. In cases of distal lateral subungual onychomycosis, obtain the specimen from the subungual hyperkeratosis. In superficial white onychomycosis, scrape the dorsal nail in the affected area. In proximal subungual onychomycosis, scrape the dorsal nail over the affected area, discard the initial specimen, and scrape again. For any evolving longitudinal melanonychia or erythronychia, or for any presumed neoplasm, nail matrix biopsy is warranted. This may also be needed for diagnosis of subungual painful processes, along with imaging. In the clinic, order bloodwork to rule out systemic disease, in the case of leukonychia, onycholysis, or where findings suggest connective tissue disease, among other presentations.

Bedside Diagnostic Maneuvers and Tests for Nail Disease	
• Nail scrapings and clippings for H and E • Nail matrix biopsy for diagnosis of nail disease and nail matrix lesion (longitudinal melanonychia or erythronychia)	• Bloodwork to rule out systemic disease • Imaging for suspected subungual neoplasm

MUCOUS MEMBRANES, LIPS, AND ORAL CAVITY

Mucous membranes are epithelia that secrete mucus. They line the gastrointestinal, respiratory, and urogenital tracts, including the mouth, nose, trachea, larynx, esophagus, urethra, and vulva. The conjunctiva is also a mucous membrane that lines the inner eyelids and the sclera.

Mucous Membranes Line the:	
• Gastrointestinal tract from mouth to anus • Respiratory tract from nasal passages to alveola	• Urogenital tract to urethra in men and including vulva in women • Eyelids and sclera (conjunctiva)

This section of the chapter focuses on the diagnostic clues of oral mucous membrane findings and also touches on disease manifestations of nasal, laryngeal, esophageal, conjunctival, and genital mucosa.

The vermillion of the lip has a keratinized, non-mucus-secreting epidermis. Examination of the vermillion may provide rich diagnostic information in both dermatologic and oral disease, so diagnostic findings of the vermillion have been included in this section.

Table 13.14 describes the classic oral and vermillion manifestations of a wide range of dermatologic conditions by reaction pattern, pustules, and macules. Some intraoral findings, such as candidiasis and warts, may not be accompanied by cutaneous disease, and thus they are not listed in the table and are discussed here instead. The intraoral manifestations of candidiasis are manifold. The typical presentation is that of creamy white plaques on any intraoral surface that can be rubbed off with a cotton-tipped

TABLE 13.14. Oral and Lip Findings by Reaction Pattern

DISEASE	ORAL FINDING
Papulosquamous	
Lichen planus	Reticulate white plaques on the buccal mucosa
	White plaques and erosions on the lips
	Erosive oral disease; seen especially on the tongue
	Violaceous plaques are also seen on the tongue
DLE	Plaques resemble those on the skin, typically found on the palate (Figure 13.29)
	Oral ulcers may also be seen in cases of SLE; smaller, aphthous-like
Secondary syphilis	Mucous patches (Figure 13.30)
	"Snail-track" ulcers
	"Split papules" at oral commissures: papules with a linear fissure running laterally through them
Reactive arthritis	Geographic tongue
Acanthosis nigricans	Velvety or corrugated plaques on the lips, usually in the setting of the malignant variant
Darier disease	White corrugated cobblestoned plaques on the palate or buccal mucosa
	Cobblestone appearance to the lips
Vitamin B_2, B_3, or B_6 deficiency	Glossitis
Tertiary syphilis	Destruction of palate
Histoplasmosis	Destruction of palate
Vesicobullous	
Junctional epidermolysis bullosa	Widespread oral ulceration; scarring leads to ankyloglossia and microstomia
	Periorificial granulation tissue
Dystrophic epidermolysis bullosa	Widespread oral ulceration; scarring leads to ankyloglossia and microstomia
Acquired autoimmune bullous diseases	See Table 7.8
HSV, VZV	See Table 13.16
Acrodermatitis enteropathica	Stomatitis, glossitis, angular cheilitis
Necrolytic migratory erythema	Stomatitis, glossitis
Eczematous	
Atopic dermatitis	Angular cheilitis
Lip licker's dermatitis	An irritant dermatitis, scaling with or without erythemaon and around the vermillion
Allergic contact dermatitis	Scaling, crusting, erythematous papules and plaques on or around the vermillion
Exfoliative cheilitis	Scaling, crusting, erosion of the vermillion
Pustules	
Pustular psoriasis	Geographic tongue
Behcet disease	Oral aphthae

(Continued)

TABLE 13.14. Oral and Lip Findings by Reaction Pattern (continued)

DISEASE	ORAL FINDING
Dermal	
Myxedema	Macroglossia
Primary amyloidosis	Macroglossia (Figure 13.31)
Lipoid proteinosis	Macroglossia, yellowish or whitish papules and plaques of all oral mucosal surfaces (Figure 13.32)
	Cobblestone appearance of lips
Xanthoma disseminatum	Yellow papules and plaques
Kaposi sarcoma	Purple patches, plaques, or nodules on any oral surface (Figure 13.33)
Leukemia	Gingival hyperplasia
Multicentric reticulohistiocytoma	Papules on tongue, gums, buccal mucosa, and lips
Multiple endocrine neoplasia type 2b	Mucosal neuromas present as papules or nodules on the tongue and lips
Vascular	
SLE	Erosions, ulcerations, erythema; less commonly, features resembling lichen planus are seen, such as whitish plaques or lacy network
	DLE can involve the vermillion: well-demarcated erythematous or white scaly papules or plaques
Dermatomyositis	Rarely reported: oval palatal patch is an erythematous patch on the posterior hard palate
Osler–Rendu–Weber disease	Bright red macules and papules on the tongue and lips (Figure 13.34)
Scurvy	Gingival friability and bleeding
Scarlet fever	Strawberry tongue
Kawasaki disease	Strawberry tongue early and later, raspberry tongue; dry, red, and fissured lips
Acute graft versus host disease	Intraoral and lip ulceration, erythema in the mouth, crusted lips
Other viral exanthems	See Table 13.16
Macules	
Laugier–Hunziker syndrome	Brown or gray macules on the vermillion, buccal mucosa, soft palate, and other mucosal sites
Peutz–Jeghers syndrome	Periorificial small brown macules, including the vermillion
	Intraorally, the gums, buccal mucosa, and hard palate are predilection sites

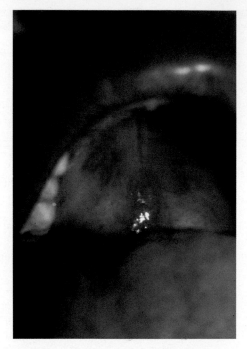

FIGURE 13.29 • Discoid lupus erythematosus in the mouth showing a palatal plaque that resembles cutaneous DLE.

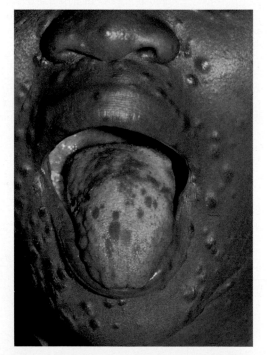

FIGURE 13.30 • Secondary syphilis with mucous patches showing eroded flat papules on the dorsal tongue, as well as copper-colored papules on the face.

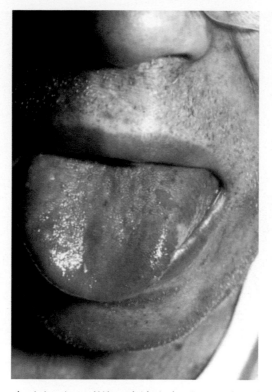

FIGURE 13.31 • Macroglossia in primary (AL) amyloidosis showing an enlarged tongue.

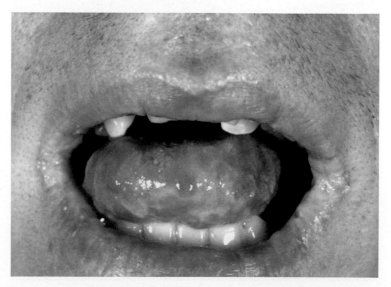

FIGURE 13.32 • Macroglossia in lipoid proteinosis showing an enlarged tongue with grooves laterally from pressure from the teeth. Note also the perioral shiny papules.

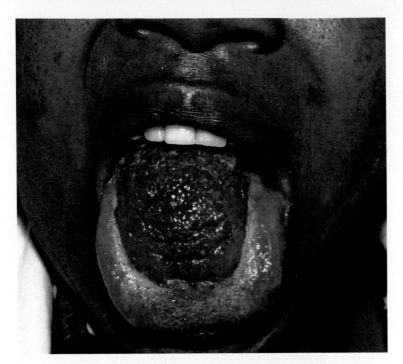

FIGURE 13.33 · Oral Kaposi sarcoma presenting as a purple tumor on the dorsal tongue.

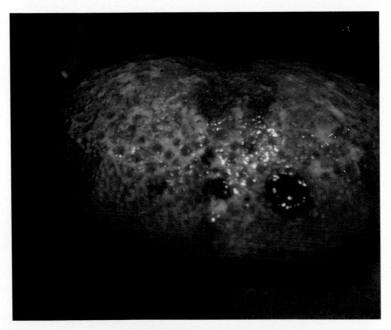

FIGURE 13.34 · Osler–Rendu–Weber syndrome showing bright red papules on the distal tongue.

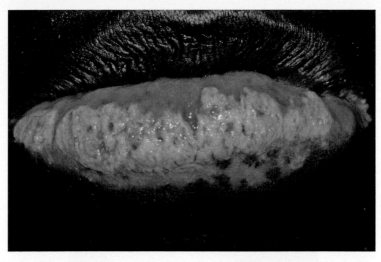

FIGURE 13.35 • Pseudomembranous candidiasis presenting as white plaques on the labial mucosa.

swab (also known as the *pseudomembranous* type; see Figure 13.35). A chronic form of this, known as *hyperplastic candidiasis*, presents as a localized thickened white plaque that resembles leukoplakia. Angular cheilitis resulting from candidiasis is known as *perleche* (Figure 13.36). It is typically seen in the setting of ill-fitting dentures that may harbor *Candida* spp. and may be accompanied by intraoral manifestations of candidiasis. Erythematous candidiasis may present acutely with painful depapillated tongue and erythema of other intraoral surfaces. It may be associated with recent antibiotic use and is known colloquially as "antibiotic sore mouth." *Median rhomboid glossitis*

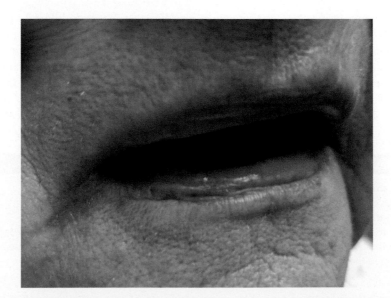

FIGURE 13.36 • Perleche showing a triangular thin erythematous plaque with overlying white streaks at the oral commissure.

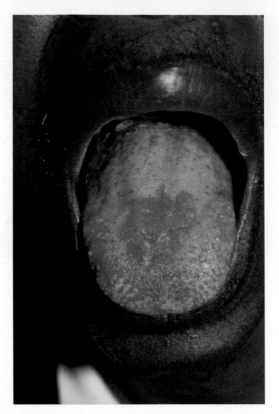

FIGURE 13.37 • Median rhomboid glossitis showing a depapillated patch on the central tongue. Note also the pseudomembranous candidiasis (white papules) on the distal tongue.

is the presence of localized erythematous candidiasis on the central dorsal tongue. It forms a rhomboidal shape (Figure 13.37). The acronym "CITNIP" (candida infection of the tongue associated with nonspecific inflammation of the palate) is found in the oral medicine literature. It refers to the presence of median rhomboid glossitis with palatal erythema. The acronym "CITCIP" refers to the presence of candida infection of the tongue and candida infection of the palate. It is usually seen in HIV-positive patients. Finally, a hyperplastic form of erythematous candidiasis may be localized to any oral surface.

Manifestations of Oral Candidiasis	
• Creamy white plaques: pseudomembranous candidiasis	• CITNIP
	• CITCIP
• Perleche	• Hyperplastic candidiasis
• Acute erythematous candidiasis: "antibiotic sore mouth"	• White plaque resembling leukoplakia
	• Localized erythematous plaque
• Median rhomboid glossitis	

Intraoral warts may resemble common warts (Figure 13.38) or condyloma acuminata and resemble a cauliflower. Heck's disease (also known as *focal epithelial*

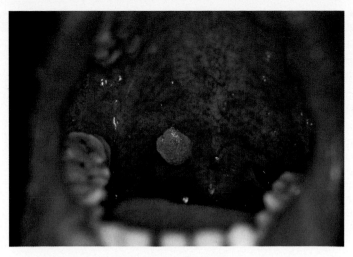

FIGURE 13.38 • An intraoral wart presenting as a white papule near the uvula.

hyperplasia) is caused by human papillomavirus (HPV) types 13 and 32. Multiple small erythematous or whitish papules are seen on any oral surface, especially in children. Oral florid papillomatosis is a form of verrucous carcinoma that presents in the mouth. It presents as a confluence verrucous papules and plaques on any intraoral surface.

Manifestations of Intraoral Warts

- Common wart
- Condyloma acuminata
- Heck's disease

Differential Diagnosis
- Oral florid papillomatosis

The differential diagnosis of mucous membrane erosions and ulcers, as well as white and red papules and plaques in the mouth, is considered next.

Important Differential Diagnoses to Consider in the Mouth

- Erosions and ulcers
- White papules and plaques
- Red papules and plaques
- Oral pigmented macules

Mucous Membrane Erosions and Ulcers

The differential diagnosis of oral erosions and ulcers is broad. An etiologic approach is seen in Table 13.15. In the inherited category, severe forms of junctional and dystrophic epidermolysis bullosa (EB) manifest widespread oral ulceration. The resultant scarring leads to ankyloglossia and microstomia. Perioral granulation tissue is another finding in severe junctional EB.

In the bacterial category, gonococcal pharyngitis may present with ulceration. Any form of syphilis may manifest oral ulceration. In primary syphilis, an oral chancre may occur on the lip, on the tongue, or in the pharynx. It is painless,

TABLE 13.15. Differential Diagnoses of Oral Erosions and Ulcers

INHERITED
- Junctional epidermolysis bullosa
- Dystrophic epidermolysis bullosa

INFECTIOUS
- Gram-negative cocci
  - Gonococcal pharyngitis
- Treponemal
  - Primary syphilis: chancre
  - Secondary syphilis: mucous patches, "snail-track" ulcers
  - Malignant secondary syphilis: atypical mucous patches
  - Tertiary syphilis: gummas, perforated palate
- Mixed bacterial, treponemal
  - ANUG
- Viral
  - HSV
    - Primary herpetic gingivostomatitis
    - Secondary HSV in an immunocompromised individual
  - Varicella
  - Zoster
    - V2: uvula and tonsillar area
    - V3: floor of mouth and buccal mucous membrane
    - Ramsay–Hunt: ipsilateral vesicles/erosions on soft palate
  - CMV: oral ulcers
  - Coxsackie
    - Herpangina
    - Hand–foot–mouth disease
    - Foot–mouth disease
  - HIV: acute seroconversion disease
  - Chikungunya
- Deep fungal
  - Histoplasmosis
  - Mucormycosis
  - Paracoccidioidomycosis
- Parasitic
  - Leishmaniasis

INFLAMMATORY
- Aphthous ulcers
  - Minor
  - Major
  - Herpetiform
  - Complex aphthosis
- Behcet disease
- MAGIC syndrome
- Erosive lichen planus
- Chrnoic graft versus host disease
- Systemic lupus erythematosus

(Continued)

TABLE 13.15. Differential Diagnoses of Oral Erosions and Ulcers (continued)

INFLAMMATORY (CONT.)
- Erythema multiforme
- MIRM
- Acute graft versus host disease
- Granulomatosis with polyangiitis
- Autoimmune blistering disease
  - Pemphigus vulgaris
  - Paraneoplastic pemphigus
  - Mucous membrane pemphigoid
  - Bullous pemphigoid

NEOPLASTIC
- Squamous cell cancer
- Kaposi sarcoma

DRUG-RELATED
- Methotrexate and other chemotherapeutic agents cause oral ulcers in the setting of leukopenia
- SJS/TEN

PHYSICAL FACTORS
- Trauma: bite line
- Caustic agents such as strong acids cause a whitish slough
- Radiation: mucositis and ulceration

with a raised border, and it may be accompanied by cervical lymphadenopathy. In secondary syphilis, mucous patches are eroded papules or plaques on the tongue that may or may not be covered by a whitish slough, also known as a *pseudomembrane*. Snail-track ulcers occur when many mucous patches become confluent, thereby forming a serpiginous configuration. (A third, rare, intraoral manifestation of secondary syphilis is the presence of verrucous plaques that are white and resemble leukoplakia.) Malignant syphilis (lues maligna) is an uncommon form of secondary disease, often seen in the HIV-positive population. Purulent or necrotic papules and nodules are accompanied by large, atypical and sometimes crateriform mucous patches in up to a third of patients. In tertiary syphilis, intraoral gummas may be seen on the tongue or palate most frequently. One or more mucosal nodules ulcerate and in the case of a palatal ulcer, may erode bone and give rise to perforation. Acute necrotizing ulcerative gingivostomatitis (ANUG) is the rapid onset of fulminant ulceration of the gums. It is seen in young people who do not brush their teeth frequently. Oral anaerobic bacteria and spirochetes (such as *Fusobacterium nucleatum* and *Borrelia vincentii*, respectively) are assumed to be responsible.

In the viral category, primary herpes simplex virus (HSV) infection typically occurs as painful, scattered, small intraoral erosions or ulcers. In recurrent HSV in an immunocompromised individual, a similar picture, or grouped vesicles or erosions intraorally may be seen (recurrent HSV is rarely seen inside the mouth in an immunocompetent individual). In varicella, an enanthem is common. Vesicles and erosions may be seen on any oral surface. In zoster of the maxillary branch of the trigeminal nerve (V2), grouped vesicles or erosions are seen unilaterally on the uvular–tonsillar area; in zoster of the mandibular branch of the trigeminal nerve (V3), the floor of mouth and buccal mucous membrane are affected; and in Ramsay–Hunt syndrome (zoster of the seventh cranial nerve, also affecting the eighth nerve at the geniculate ganglion, and characterized facial nerve palsy, vesicles of the ear, along with tinnitus and possible hearing loss), ipsilateral vesicles or erosions may be seen on the soft palate. In cytomegaloviral infection, which typically occurs in immunosuppressed individuals such as those with AIDS, intraoral or perianal ulcers may be seen.

Enanthems may accompany numerous viral exanthems. These findings are encapsulated in Table 13.16. Viruses that cause oral erosions and ulcers are discussed here. Coxsackie virus causes a wide range of viral syndromes. For instance, in herpangina, which may be caused by Coxsackie types A5, 6, 8, 10, and 16, approximately 15–20 vesicles or ulcers may be seen on the soft palate and more posteriorly. These heal in 4–7 days. In hand–foot–mouth disease, typically caused by Coxsackie virus A16 (although other types of enteroviruses can be responsible, in which case disease is more severe), the palate and areas more anterior to that (tongue, gums, buccal mucous membranes) may be involved, along with distal extremity papulovesicles. Foot–mouth disease, a disease of livestock, has rarely affected humans. Intraoral vesicles give rise to ragged ulcers. Acute seroconversion disease occurs in 50–80% of patients with primary HIV infection. In approximately 70% of cases, oropharyngeal erythema and ulceration are seen.

TABLE 13.16. Examples of Viral Enanthems	
DISEASE	**ORAL FINDING**
Measles	Koplik spots: whitish 1–2-mm papules on a background of erythema on the buccal and sometimes lower labial mucosa
Rubella	Forchheimer spots: tiny erythematous macules on the soft palate or uvula
Roseola	Nagayama spots: erythematous papules on the soft palate and uvula
Hand–foot–mouth disease	Vesicles are transient and rupture to form painful erosions and may be large (1–2 cm); any intraoral surface may be affected
Herpangina	Painful shallow erosions with yellowish slough and surrounding bright red erythema on the soft palate, uvula, and around the tonsils
Other enteroviruses	Vesicular or papular enanthems may be seen
Papular purpuric gloves and socks syndrome	Petechiae may be seen on the tongue, hard palate, and pharynx; intraoral vesicles and erosions may occur
Acute HIV disease	Erosions on the posterior palate and pharynx
Varicella	Vesicles and erosions may be seen
Chikungunya	Aphthous ulcers, erosions, cheilitis in a few patients
Smallpox	The enanthem parallels the exanthem; erythematous macules and papules progress rapidly to umbilicated pustules and erode

Genital ulceration is seen in approximately a third of patients. Other concomitants include high fever and a sore throat. Oral thrush, lymphadenopathy, and meningoencephalitis may be seen. Chikungunya may cause oral aphthae or erosions in a minority of cases.

Deep fungal infections involve the oral cavity in a variety of presentations. In histoplasmosis, an oral ulcer, usually of the palate, may be a presenting feature. Mucormycosis is a rare and fulminant fungal infection of immunocompromised individuals, caused by that may present with a rapidly enlarging necrotic ulcer of the palate that spreads to involve sinuses and possibly the brain. In paracoccidioidomycosis, there may be painful ulcerated plaques in and around the mouth and nose, including the palate. Fungating and hyperkeratotic plaques are also seen on the central area of the face. Similar findings are seen in mucocutaneous leishmaniasis.

In the inflammatory category, the most common cause of intraoral ulcers is aphthosis. Minor aphthous ulcers measure 2–4 mm and occur on the buccal mucosa, floor of the mouth, and the ventral tongue. One or a few lesions may be present at any given time. They heal over 7–10 days. Major aphthae measure up to 1 cm. They may be seen on any area of the mouth, including the palate and the dorsal tongue. There may be one or a few present at any given time, and they typically take longer to heal, approximately 10–40 days. A herpetiform variant of aphthae has also been described. This variant affects females most frequently; it presents as multiple 2-mm ulcers that coalesce and recur frequently. Complex aphthosis is the presence of almost constant, multiple oral or oral and genital aphthae in the absence of systemic manifestations. In Behcet disease, oral aphthae present at least 3 times over the course of 12 months. This is accompanied by at least two of the following: genital aphthae, synovitis, posterior uveitis, cutaneous pustular vasculitis, and meningoencephalitis. MAGIC syndrome (mouth and genital ulcers and inflamed cartilage) is an overlap syndrome with features of both Behcet disease and relapsing polychondritis.

Many other inflammatory skin diseases have intraoral erosions and ulcers as part of their presentation. Oral lichen planus is commonly erosive. White plaques inside the mouth are accompanied by one or more erosions or ulcers on any intraoral surface. Chronic graft versus host disease presents most commonly with lichenoid or sclerodermatous features. Lichenoid intraoral changes may be seen. Oral erosions or ulcers of systemic lupus erythematosus (SLE) can occur on any oral surface. They are symmetric or asymmetric. They may be accompanied by erythematous patches, and lichenoid features may be present. In erythema multiforme and mycoplasma pneumonia–induced rash and mucositis (MIRM), the lips may be characteristically affected with diffuse hemorrhagic crusting. In Stevens–Johnson syndrome/toxic epidermal necrolysis (SJS/TEN), similar lip involvement may be seen. This finding is typical of these three diagnoses as well as paraneoplastic pemphigus (PNP) (also known as PAMS—paraneoplastic autoimmune multiorgan syndrome). Focal lip erosions and crusts are also possible. Painful intraoral erosions and ulcers are also seen in the aforementioned diseases. Acute graft versus host disease may manifest with intraoral and lip erosions or ulcers. There may also be intraoral erythema and crusting of lips.

Differential Diagnosis of Hemorrhagic Crusting of Both Lips	
• Erythema multiforme	• SJS/TEN
• MIRM	• PNP/PAMS

Granulomatosis with polyangiitis may manifest oral ulceration, perforation of the palate, and "strawberry gums." The latter term describes the presence of gingival hyperplasia studded with papules and superimposed petechiae. The characteristic intraoral findings of the autoimmune blistering diseases are listed in Table 7.8.

Intraoral squamous cell carcinoma presents as an intraoral plaque or nodule that is frequently ulcerated.

In the drug-induced category, methotrexate and other chemotherapeutic agents cause oral ulcers in the setting of leukopenia. Radiation also leads to ulceration and mucositis. Other physical factors such as trauma or caustic agents may lead to erosions.

Oral ulceration may rarely extend to involve the larynx. This can be seen in pemphigus vulgaris, PNP/PAMS, SJS/TEN, and mucous membrane pemphigoid.

Conditions in Which Laryngeal Erosive or Ulcerative Disease Can Occur	
• Pemphigus vulgaris	• SJS/TEN
• PNP/PAMS	• Mucous membrane pemphigoid

Additionally, the presence of a subtype of erosion or ulceration known as *marginal gingivitis* (or *desquamative gingivitis*) is seen in a short list of diseases, as is contained in the textbox below.

Marginal Gingivitis	
• Erosive oral lichen planus	• Mucous membrane pemphigoid
• Pemphigus vulgaris	

A further differential diagnosis to consider, when looking at intraoral erosions or ulcerations, is that of oral and genital ulceration. The presence of oral erosions or ulcers should prompt questioning about genital involvement. Table 13.17 provides a list of diseases, listed by the etiologic classification, to consider when both oral and genital forms of ulceration are present.

Oral White and Red Papules and Plaques

The differential diagnoses of white and red papules and plaques in the mouth are listed in Tables 13.18 and 13.19, respectively. Leukoplakia and erythroplakia are premalignant conditions that will always require a biopsy. They present as white and red plaques, respectively. Any intraoral surface may be affected. Additionally, leukoplakia may involve the vermillion. Leukoplakia may just represent hyperkeratosis, but up to 40% of cases will go on to become squamous cell cancer in situ or invasive squamous cell cancer. *Erythroleukoplakia* refers to the presence of white and red areas within one plaque. Often, a speckled appearance is seen. These lesions have a higher risk of malignant transformation. In erythroplakia, malignant transformation approaches 100% (Figure 13.39).

TABLE 13.17. Differential Diagnosis of Orogenital Erosions or Ulcerations

INFECTIOUS
- HIV seroconversion disease

INFLAMMATORY
- Erosive lichen planus
- SLE
- Aphthous ulcers
- Behcet disease
- MAGIC syndrome
- Autoimmune blistering diseases
  - Pemphigus vulgaris
  - PNP/PAMS
  - Mucous membrane pemphigoid
- Chronic graft versus host disease may present with an erosive lichen planus–type picture on mucous membranes
- Nutritional
  - Pellagra
- Drug
  - SJS/TEN

TABLE 13.18. Differential Diagnosis of White Papules or Plaques in the Mouth

INFECTIOUS
- Viral wart
- Candidiasis
- Oral hairy leukoplakia

INFLAMMATORY
- Contact stomatitis (eg, caused by reaction to cinnamon)
- Lichen planus
- Chronic graft versus host disease
- SLE

TRAUMATIC
- Frictional keratoses, such as morsicatio buccarum or linguarum
- Leukedema: white discoloration of mucosa that disappears when mucosa stretched; secondary to mild irritation, such as from mouthwash
- Chemical burn, such as from acids (eg, vinegar) or alkalis

NEOPLASTIC
- Benign
  - Oral white sponge nevus (eg, in pachyonychia congenita)
- Premalignant
  - Leukoplakia, isolated or in dyskeratosis congenita; malignant transformation in ≤40% of cases
  - Erythroleukoplakia: speckled red and white areas; carries a higher risk of malignant transformation
  - Proliferative verrucous leukoplakia; malignant transformation in 70–100% of cases
- Malignant
  - Oral florid papillomatosis (verrucous carcinoma)
  - SCCIS, SCC

DRUG-RELATED
- Lichenoid drug eruption
- Aspirin-induced burn of oral mucosa

TABLE 13.19.   Differential Diagnosis of Red Papules or Plaques in the Mouth

INFECTIOUS
- Viral wart
- Erythematous candidiasis

INFLAMMATORY
- Contact stomatitis (eg, caused by reaction to cinnamon)
- Lichen planus
- Chronic graft versus host disease
- SLE

TRAUMATIC
- Chemical burn, such as from acids (eg, vinegar) or alkalis

NEOPLASTIC
- Benign
  - Hemangioma
  - Osler–Rendu–Weber disease
- Premalignant
  - Erythroplakia, erythroleukoplakia: malignant transformation in ≤100% of cases
- Malignant
  - Oral florid papillomatosis (verrucous carcinoma)
  - SCCIS, SCC
  - Kaposi sarcoma

DRUG
- Lichenoid drug eruption
- Aspirin-induced burn of oral mucosa

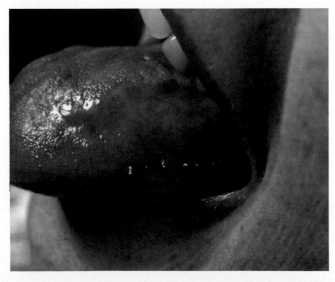

FIGURE 13.39 • Erythroplakia presenting as an erythematous plaque on the lateral tongue, biopsied to reveal squamous cell carcinoma.

TABLE 13.20. Causes of Intraoral and Vermillion Pigmented Macules

INTRAORAL
- Single
  - Mercury amalgam tattoo
  - Oral melanoacanthoma
  - Oral melanotic macule
  - Nevus
  - Melanoma
- Multiple
  - Normal variant in darker skin phototype
  - Drug-induced pigmentation (eg, minocycline, hydroxychloroquine, amiodarone)
  - LEOPARD syndrome
  - Laugier–Hunziker syndrome
  - Peutz–Jeghers syndrome
  - Addison disease
  - HIV disease

VERMILLION
- Single
  - Labial melanotic macule
- Multiple
  - Drug-induced (eg, minocycline)
  - LEOPARD syndrome
  - Laugier–Hunziker syndrome
  - Peutz–Jeghers syndrome
  - Addison disease
  - Carney complex

Table 13.20 lists the causes of pigmented macules on the vermillion and intraorally. Oral pigmented macules may be single or multiple. They may be brown, gray-brown, dark gray, or blue-black. A mercury amalgam tattoo is usually gray or blue-gray. It is seen near a tooth filled with a mercury filling. An oral melanoacanthoma is dark brown or black. It is a benign growth akin to a pigmented seborrheic keratosis. It usually occurs on the buccal mucosa. Nevi can occur intraorally as well. They are usually found on the hard palate. Intraoral melanoma is exceedingly rare. However, these lesions are typically far advanced at the time of diagnosis, and prognosis is poor. Color variegation, asymmetry, and irregular borders may be seen as in cutaneous melanoma. Labial melanotic macules are lentigines seen on the vermillion. Intraoral lentigines are termed *oral melanotic macules*. These, too, are usually solitary. One or more may be present.

Multiple intraoral, pigmented macules are a normal finding in individuals with darker skin phototypes. Drug causes include minocycline (where blue-black or dark gray macules are seen on the lower lip and in the mouth), hydroxychloroquine (with diffuse brown pigmentation of the hard palate), and amiodarone (indicated by bluish pigmentation). Rarer causes include LEOPARD syndrome (lentiginosis, EKG abnormalities, ocular hypertelorism, pulmonary stenosis, abnormal genitalia, growth retardation of growth, deafness), Laugier—Hunziker syndrome (lips, intraoral surfaces, nails, and acral areas have pigmented macules), Peutz–Jegher syndrome (periorificial and vermillion lentiginosis that fade with time, persistent intraoral pigmented macules, and the presence of hamartomatous polyps in the gastrointestinal tract), Addison disease (diffuse cutaneous pigmentation accompanied by intraoral pigmented macules), and HIV disease (where intraoral pigmented macules are seen without cutaneous pigmentation). In Carney complex, diffuse lentiginosis may also affect the lips. There are accompanying blue nevi, atrial and cutaneous myxomas, and endocrine abnormalities.

Differential Diagnosis by Anatomic Region

In the remainder of this section, the causes of a spectrum of findings by anatomic site are enumerated, including lips, gums, the tongue, and the conjunctiva, and the causes of a nasal septal lesion are also discussed. Table 13.21 lists the differential diagnosis of

---

TABLE 13.21. Differential Diagnosis of Vermillion and Oral Commissure Findings

SCALING OF LIPS
- Lip-licking dermatitis
- Allergic contact dermatitis
- Exfoliative cheilitis
- Morsicatio labiorum
- Kawasaki disease

CRUSTING OF LIPS
- Lip-licking dermatitis
- Allergic contact dermatitis
- Exfoliative cheilitis
- Morsicatio labiorum
- Impetigo
- HSV
- Kawasaki disease

DIFFUSE HEMORRHAGIC CRUSTING OF LIPS
- Erythema multiforme
- MIRM
- SJS/TEN
- PAMS

LIP ULCERATION AND CRUSTING
- HSV
- V3 zoster
- Erythema multiforme
- MIRM
- SJS/TEN
- PAMS
- Acute graft versus host disease
- Morsicatio labiorum

(Continued)

TABLE 13.21. Differential Diagnosis of Vermillion and Oral Commissure Findings (continued)

ANGULAR CHEILITIS
- Perleche
- Eczema: commonly atopic, also lip-licking dermatitis
- Vitamin B2 deficiency
- Acrodermatitis enteropathica
- Cystic fibrosis

PAPULES AT ORAL COMMISSURES
- Milia
- Fordyce spots
- Warts
- Split papules of secondary syphilis

LIP SWELLING
- Angioedema
- Acute allergic contact dermatitis
- Melkersson–Rosenthal syndrome
- Cheilitis glandularis
- Ascher syndrome

WHITE PAPULES/PLAQUES ON THE VERMILLION
- Lichen planus
- DLE
- Actinic cheilitis
- Leukoplakia

vermillion and oral commissure findings. The term *cheilitis* connotes inflammation of the lips. Scaling and crusting may be seen. The differential diagnosis of each of these findings is outlined separately in the table. As mentioned above, there is a short list of diseases that present with diffuse hemorrhagic erosion and crusting of the lips. However, more diseases may present with focal lip ulceration and crusting, such as HSV, V3 zoster, acute graft versus host disease, and morsicatio labiorum. The latter condition refers to the erosion, crusting, hemorrhagic crusting, scaling, and plaque formation that may be induced by lip picking, pulling, or biting. A different set of conditions may affect the oral commissures. Atopic dermatitis is a common cause of angular cheilitis in childhood, and perleche, which is a candidal infection, is a common cause on older adults, as outlined above. Nutritional deficiencies, including some of the vitamin B_2 deficiency and acrodermatitis enteropathica, should be considered in the differential diagnosis. Patients with cystic fibrosis also develop angular cheilitis. Papules at the oral commissures might be milia, Fordyce spots, warts, or "split papules" of secondary syphilis.

The most frequent causes of lip swelling include allergic contact dermatitis and angioedema. In the former, scaling and crusting may be present. Rarer causes include Melkersson–Rosenthal syndrome (Figure 13.40A,B), cheilitis glandularis, and Ascher syndrome. In Melkersson–Rosenthal syndrome (also known as *granulomatous cheilitis* or *cheilitis granulomatosa*), the upper lip is involved more frequently. Initially edema waxes and wanes, and then becomes permanent. Facial nerve palsy and a scrotal

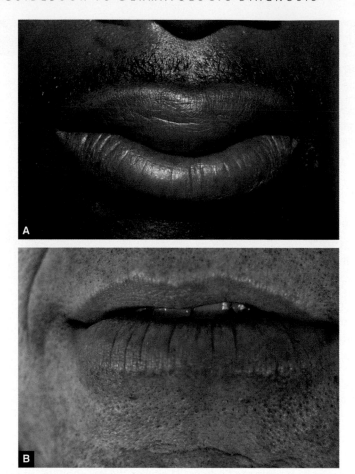

FIGURE 13.40 • Melkersson–Rosenthal syndrome presenting as swelling of (A) both lips and (B) the lower lip only.

tongue are seen in approximately a third of patients. In cheilitis glandularis, the lower lip is involved more frequently. There is edema, and there may also be lower lip eversion. Fluid egressing from the minor salivary glands on the lower buccal mucosa may be seen. In Ascher syndrome, the upper lip is involved more frequently. It may appear as a double lip when the oral mucosa is intensely edematous and may be seen below the vermillion. Acute episodes of edema affect the periorbital areas and lead to eyelid atrophy (known as *blepharochalasis*).

Table 13.22 lists the differential diagnoses of gum findings. The presence of gingival hyperplasia suggests a differential diagnosis that includes both inherited and acquired entities. In the inherited category, it is a frequent finding in tuberous sclerosis and juvenile hyaline fibromatosis, where onset occurs in early life and is accompanied by skin infiltration, joint contractures, and lytic lesions of the bones. In this condition, there is an autosomal recessively inherited abnormality of collagen synthesis that leads to the deposition of hyaline material in skin, mucosa, and joints. Intraoral trichilemmomas lead to bulky gingiva in Cowden syndrome, and mucosal neuromas do the same in multiple endocrine

TABLE 13.22. Differential Diagnosis of Gum Findings

GINGIVAL HYPERPLASIA
- Inherited
  - Tuberous sclerosis
  - Juvenile hyaline fibromatosis
  - Intraoral trichilemmomas in Cowden syndrome
  - Mucosal neuromas in MEN 2b
- Acquired
  - Poor oral hygiene
  - Scurvy
  - Granulomatosis with polyangiitis
  - Sarcoidosis
  - Granulomatous cheilitis
  - Kaposi sarcoma
  - Leukemic infiltrates; seen especially in AML M4 and M5
  - Medications
    - Cyclosporine
    - Nifedipine, verapamil
    - Phenytoin
- Marginal gingivitis
  - Pemphigus vulgaris
  - Erosive lichen planus
  - Mucous membrane pemphigoid

neoplasia (MEN) type 2b. Acquired conditions may also be causative. The commonest cause of gingival hyperplasia is poor oral hygiene, where it may be seen along with gingival retraction. In scurvy, the gums are friable and bleed. They may be hypertrophic and hemorrhagic. In granulomatosis with polyangitis, gingival hypertrophy is known as "strawberry gums" because of their resemblance to the fruit. Granulomatous cheilitis may be accompanied by gingival hypertrophy. Kaposi sarcoma frequently involves the mouth, which usually signals underlying gastrointestinal disease. Purple papules, plaques, and nodules may affect the gums. Also, in the neoplastic category, leukemic infiltrates of the gums are seen in the setting of acute myeloid leukemia (AML) types M4 and M5. A range of medications can cause hyperplastic gingiva, including cyclosporine, calcium channel blockers, and phenytoin. The causes of marginal gingivitis are outlined above.

The differential diagnosis of a variety of tongue findings is seen in Table 13.23. Macroglossia may be inherited or acquired. "Geographic tongue" is also known as benign migratory glossitis (Figure 13.41A,B). It is usually an isolated finding, but it may accompany psoriasis, especially pustular psoriasis, and reactive arthritis. A fissured tongue is also known as a *scrotal tongue*. It has been reported in association with Melkersson–Rosenthal syndrome (Figure 13.42), Down syndrome, and acromegaly. *Atrophic glossitis* refers to the loss of filiform and fungiform papillae on the dorsal tongue. It may occur as a result of a nutritional deficiency or in erythematous candidiasis. It is a secondary finding in individuals affected by dry mouth of any cause (such as radiation, medications, Sjogren syndrome, HIV disease, and diabetes). It may also be seen in celiac disease. The term "strawberry tongue" connotes the presence of edema of the fungiform papillae.

TABLE 13.23. Differential Diagnosis of Tongue Findings

MACROGLOSSIA
- Inherited
  - Lipoid proteinosis
  - Beckwith–Wiedemann syndrome
  - Congenital infiltrating lipomatosis of the face (CILF)
  - Down syndrome
  - Mucopolysaccharidoses
    - Hurler
    - Hunter
    - Sanfillipo
    - Maroteaux–Lamy
- Acquired
  - Acromegaly
  - Myxedema
  - Primary amyloidosis
  - Melkersson–Rosenthal syndrome
  - Granulomatous cheilitis

GEOGRAPHIC TONGUE
- Isolated
- Psoriasis, especially pustular psoriasis
- Reactive arthritis

SCROTAL (FISSURED) TONGUE
- Isolated
- Melkersson–Rosenthal syndrome
- Down syndrome
- Acromegaly

ATROPHIC GLOSSITIS
- Nutritional
  - Iron
  - Vitamin B_2, B_3, B_6, B_{12} deficiency
  - Acrodermatitis enteropathica
  - Necrolytic migratory erythema
- Xerostomia
- Infectious
  - Candidiasis
- Celiac disease

STRAWBERRY TONGUE
- Scarlet fever
- Kawasaki disease
- Toxic shock syndrome

A white strawberry tongue implies a superadded white coating, and the edematous papillae appear at regular intervals through the coating, thus resembling a strawberry. A red strawberry tongue has no coating and is also called a "raspberry tongue."

Some dermatologic conditions that affect the conjunctiva are listed in Table 13.24 by etiology. In the infectious category, HSV and V1 zoster may lead to conjunctivitis and keratitis that is usually unilateral. Mycoplasma-induced rash and mucositis

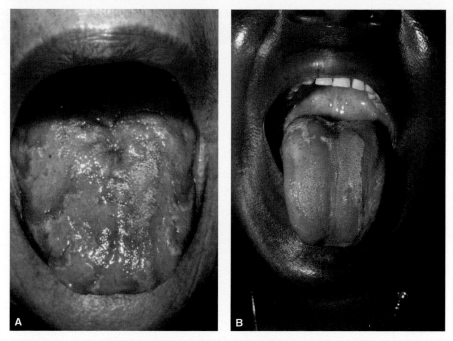

FIGURE 13.41 • Geographic tongue presenting as (A) multiple red, arcuate depapillated plaques with whitish borders on the dorsal tongue and (B) a single large depapillated plaque with a geographic outline on the dorsal tongue.

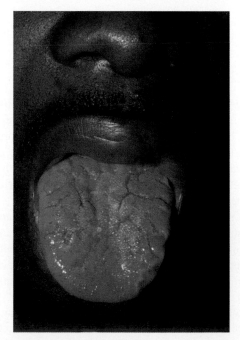

FIGURE 13.42 • Melkersson–Rosenthal syndrome showing a fissured tongue (Used with permission from Dr Deepak Modi, University of the Witwatersrand, Johannesburg, South Africa.).

TABLE 13.24. Differential Diagnosis of Conjunctivitis Seen in Association with Dermatologic Disease

INFECTIOUS
- HSV
- Ophthalmic zoster
- MIRM
- Chlamydia
- Parinaud oculoglandular syndrome
  - Cat scratch disease
  - Tularemia
  - Sporotrichosis
  - Primary chancre of tuberculosis
  - American trypanosomiasis

INFLAMMATORY
- Ocular rosacea
- Reactive arthritis
- Kawasaki disease
- Mucous membrane pemphigoid
- Pemphigus vulgaris
- Behcet disease
- Sarcoidosis
  - Anterior uveitis most common, but any part of the eye may be affected
  - Reported to cause Parinaud oculoglandular syndrome
- Sweet syndrome

PARANEOPLASTIC
- PNP/PAMS

DRUG
- SJS/TEN

may affect the eye as well. It has been reported to cause conjunctivitis, conjuntival ulceration, and conjunctival pseudomembranes. Chlamydia infrequently affects the eye, causing bilateral conjunctivitis, and in reactive arthritis, conjunctivitis is a more freuqent occurrence. Parinaud oculoglandular syndrome is the association of a conjunctival granuloma in one eye and ipsilateral preauricular lymphadenopathy. Various infectious causes have been associated with the syndrome, as outlined in the table, and sarcoidosis has also been reported as cause.

Of the inflammatory causes of conjunctivitis, rosacea is perhaps the most common cutaneous disease culprit. Besides conjunctivitis, rosacea can cause blepharitis. Conjunctivitis and conjunctival erosions or ulcers may be seen in autoimmune blistering diseases, such as pemphigus vulgaris, mucous membrane pemphigoid, and paraneoplastic pemphigus. In the latter two conditions, scarring is a sequela, which may lead to symblepharon and entropion. Behcet disease and sarcoidosis typically cause uveitis, but both may lead to conjuncitivis as well. Sweet syndrome may be accompanied by conjunctivitis and episcleritis, and SJS/TEN may cause conjunctivitis, iritis, corneal erosion, scarring, and ultimately, vision loss.

TABLE 13.25. Differential Diagnosis of a Nasal Septal Lesion

INFECTIOUS
- Rhinoscleroma
- Late congenital syphilis
- Yaws
  - Gangosa
  - Goundou
- Bejel
- Mucocutaneous leishmaniasis
- Paracoccidioidomycosis
- Rhinosporidiosis
- Noma

INFLAMMATORY
- Granulomatosis with polyangiitis
- Sarcoidosis

NEOPLASTIC
- Lethal midline granuloma

Finally, with respect to the mucous membranes, nasal septal lesions are typical of a wide range of rare infectious, inflammatory, and neoplastic diseases, as outlined in Table 13.25. Rhinoscleroma is caused by *Klebsiella pneumonia* spp. *rhinoscleromatis*. An initial rhinorrheal stage is superseded by an infiltrative stage that presents with nodules in and around the nose. Late-stage rhinoscleroma is marked by sclerosis and deformity of the nose. Saddle-nose deformity is a classic finding of late congenital syphilis. It is caused by underdevelopment of nasal cartilage. Yaws is caused by *Treponema pallidum* spp. *pertenue*. Gangosa is a manifestation of the tertiary stage of yaws. Mutilation of central face begins at the base of the nasal fossa of the septum. *Goundou* is the term applied to yaws that has been superinfected secondarily, resulting in exposed nasal bones. Bejel is caused by *T. pallidum* spp. *pallidum*. Nasal destruction is also concomitant with the tertiary stage; this causes less destruction than is typically seen in gangosa. As mentioned above, mucocutaneous leishmaniasis may involve the entire centrofacial area and may cause nasal septal destruction. Rhinosporidiosis is a mycosis caused by *Rhinosporidium seeberi*. Exuberant nondestructive nasal masses occur and may extend beyond the nares. The nasopharynx or soft palate is involved in most cases. Noma is a rare disease that is usually seen in malnourished children. It is characterized by extensive centrofacial destruction of tissue. Oral fusobacteria and spirochetes are believed to play a role in the pathogenesis.

In the inflammatory category, the upper respiratory tract is a predilection site in granulomatosis with polyangiitis. Early on there is crusting and hemorrhagic granulomas of the nostril, nasal septum, pharynx, or larynx. Epistaxis may occur. There is eventual destruction of the nasal septum. Infiltration of the nasal septum is a rare manifestation of sarcoidosis. Lethal midline granuloma (nasal-type extranodal natural killer T-cell lymphoma) presents with a destructive necrotic ulcers of the nasal septum and hard palate. Cutaneous papules and plaques may be seen.

Bedside Diagnostic Maneuvers and Tests for Mucous Membrane Disease

Rub the tip of a cotton-tipped applicator over an intraoral white plaque. In cases of candidiasis, a whitish material will come off the mucosa, thus differentiating it from other white conditions. Perform PCR to look for HSV or zoster. Perform Gram stain and culture for pustules or crusting on the vermillion. Biopsy with or without DIF may be necessary for diagnosis of many intraoral conditions.

Bedside Diagnostic Maneuvers and Tests for Mucous Membranes

- Firmly swab a white lesion; if it is candidiasis, plaques will come off
- Perform PCR for HSV and VZV
- Perform Gram stain and culture for pustules and crusting
- Biopsy for H and E, and DIF where necessary

TABLE 13.26. Rash and Generalized Lymphadenopathy

DISEASE	LOCALIZED/GENERALIZED
Papulosquamous	
Tinea capitis	Localized
Any erythroderma	Generalized
Mycosis fungoides	Generalized or localized*
Sezary syndrome	Generalized*
Secondary syphilis	Generalized
Squamous cell cancer	Localized†
Vesicobullous	
Paraneoplastic pemphigus	Generalized or localized (in accompanying non-Hodgkin lymphoma)†
Eczematous	
Erythrodermic eczema	Generalized
Dermal	
Merkel cell carcinoma	Localized†
Melanoma	Localized†
Lymphoma	Generalized or localized†
Leukemia	Generalized or localized†
Any cutaneous metastasis	Generalized or localized†
Vascular	
Infectious mononucleosis	Generalized
Acute CMV	Generalized
Primary HIV seroconversion disease	Generalized
Other viral exanthems	Generalized
Rubella	Primarily occipital and postauricular
DRESS	Generalized
AESOP	Localized
Kikuchi disease	Localized

*Indicates either malignant or reactive involvement.
†Indicates malignant involvement.

LYMPH NODES

Lymph nodes reside in the subcutaneous tissue, and so can be readily palpated during a skin examination, including in the submental, supraclavicular, anterior, and posterior cervical chains and the postauricular, epitrochlear, axillary, inguinal, and popliteal basins. Additionally, lymph nodes that are extremely enlarged may be visually appreciable. Enlarged lymph nodes may be seen in a variety of reactive and malignant conditions. Enlarged, tender nodes may be seen in lymphadenitis, such as that accompanying cat scratch disease or the other ulceroglandular syndromes, as seen in Table 3.3. Table 13.26 lists some of the dermatologic conditions that may be accompanied by lymphadenopathy versus the reaction pattern.

SUMMARY

- Examining the scalp, hair, nails, mucous membranes, and lymph nodes can be like gifts to the clinician in that these areas are replete with diagnostic information.
- Scalp disease may be accompanied by scarring or nonscarring alopecia, and alopecia may be the sole presenting sign.
- Body hair changes may indicate underlying dermatologic or systemic disease.
- Nail changes may signify nail infection, a dermatologic disease, systemic disease, or a benign or malignant subungual or periungual neoplasm, or they may be isolated.
- Each mucous membrane may hold diagnostic findings, and each finding may have numerous possible causes.
- Lymphadenopathy that accompanies dermatologic disease may be either localized or generalized and either reactive or malignant.
- Bedside diagnostics can be employed to help pinpoint a diagnosis. Serologic tests can also add diagnostic information.

Numerous bedside diagnostic tests and maneuvers can be employed to help narrow down differential diagnoses, and their use may even obviate the need for biopsy. The clinical signs outlined below are not 100% sensitive, but if present, they can help to clinch specific diagnoses.

FINGERTIPS: PALPATION MANEUVERS THAT CAN HELP CLINCH DIAGNOSES

Palpating lesions, as has been mentioned and outlined previously, will render a wealth of clinical information. Palpating lesions can help to assess their depth and consistency, and can elicit tenderness, all of which can guide diagnosis. There are some further specific palpation maneuvers that can yield diagnostic information:

In patients with suspected SJS/TEN or the pemphigus group of diseases, place sideways pressure, using a thumb, on areas that seem to be necrotic (display tender, red macules), or on the edge of a bulla or erosion. If there is lateral extension of the bulla, or if there is detachment of epidermis from dermis, this is a deemed to be positive and is known as the *Nikolsky sign*. The *Asboe–Hansen sign* refers to lateral extension of a bulla after downward pressure on its surface. It is similarly positive in SJS/TEN and the pemphigus group. In any case of suspected tinea versicolor, the typical fine white branny scales may not be immediately evident, and macules may appear smooth. Skin can be stretched laterally over or at the edges of an affected macule by using two thumbs, or a thumb and an index finger. This will allow for the scales to cleave and to become more apparent. Finally, placing firm inward pressure on the sides of a dermatofibroma will cause dimpling. This is called the *dimple sign* (see Figure 9.55). It will not be positive in older, more atrophic dermatofibromas, or in dermatofibromas that are raised papules or nodules.

> **Palpation Maneuvers**
>
> - Press laterally on the edge of a bulla or on suspected necrotic epidermis in SJS/TEN or pemphigus vulgaris.
> - Place downward pressure on a bulla in the same conditions.
> - Place sideways pressure over a suspected macule of tinea versicolor.
> - Push the edges of a suspected dermatofibroma together.

EMPLOYING A COTTON-TIPPED APPLICATOR

The back of a cotton-tipped applicator can assist in a handful of diagnostic maneuvers; the first is to gently scrape incipient scales over a suspected plaque of psoriasis. This raises the scales, and a diagnostic bright white or silvery color becomes apparent. I call this the *modified Auspitz sign*. An *Auspitz sign* describes the bleeding points that eventuate when plaques of psoriasis are firmly scraped with the back of a cotton-tipped applicator. The bleeding points represent tips of the papillary dermis that are unroofed when the thinned rete ridges that are classic of psoriasis are removed. Lighter scraping will not cause bleeding and will make for a more comfortable patient. The second maneuver is to create wheals in a suspected case of dermographism or urticaria. Run the back of the cotton-tipped applicator over normal skin; a positive test will take a few minutes to appear. Red dermographism is the presence of a linear red macule after this maneuver—it may be seen in a mild or partially treated case. White dermographism refers to the presence of a white wheal surrounded by a red "flare," and dermographism is the presence of a raised, red wheal (see Figure 10.26). This exact maneuver can be applied in cases of suspected cutaneous mastocytosis. Scrape the back of the cotton-tipped applicator across lesional skin in a suspected case. A positive test—inducement of an urticarial plaque—is known as the *Darier sign*. A bulla may result in an exuberant case. Another form of cutaneous mastocytosis, urticaria pigmentosa, displays a positive Darier sign less frequently (see Figure 9.54) and telangiectasia macularis eruptiva perstans, not much at all. Finally, using the back of the cotton-tipped applicator to lift the sheet of hyperkeratotic scales from a plaque of discoid lupus erythematosus (DLE) will reveal widened follicular openings on the plaque and follicular plugs (so-called *carpet-tack sign*) on the undersurface of the scaly sheet.

Use the Back of a Cotton-Tipped Applicator:

- Raise bright white/silvery scales over a suspected plaque of psoriasis.
- Elicit dermographism in a suspected case of dermographism or urticaria.
- Elicit a wheal in mastocytosis.
- Remove surface scale in suspected DLE.

EMPLOYING A MICROSCOPE SLIDE: DIASCOPY

Diascopy refers to firmly pressing a piece of flat, transparent glass (usually a microscope slide) against the skin. This maneuver temporarily compresses blood vessels and will blanch out erythematous lesions that are nonpurpuric. In purpura, blood has egressed in to the dermis from the vessels, and so, purpuric lesions will not blanch (Figure 14.1). An exception to this rule is that thicker vascular plaques, such as a port wine stain or a hemangioma, will not blanch, owing to the depth of the lesion and the fact that not all blood vessels can be occluded by the superficial pressure of diascopy. Diascopy can also be used in cases in which cutaneous sarcoidosis or tuberculosis (lupus vulgaris) is suspected. The pressure from the microscope slide blanches out any erythema in the lesion under examination, and a granulomatous infiltrate will become the color of apple jelly.

Press Down on a Lesion with a Microscope Slide:

- To see if it blanches in cases of suspected purpura
- To look for an "apple jelly" color in cases of suspected sarcoidosis or lupus vulgaris

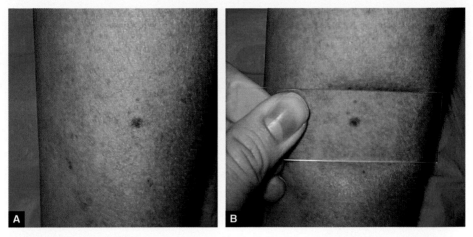

FIGURE 14.1 · Diascopy of a purpuric macule showing lack of blanching on application of pressure.

PERFORMING SKIN, HAIR, AND NAIL SCRAPINGS FOR FUNGAL EVALUATION

Skin, hair, and nail scrapings may be collected for microbiologic examination. In cases of suspected dermatophyte or tinea versicolor infection, a potassium hydroxide (KOH) or similar preparation containing a stain (such as a Swartz–Lamkins preparation) can be performed. Remember the adage "If it scales, scrape it," and have a high index of suspicion to perform a KOH on any scaly eruption to rule out fungus. For skin scrapings, scrape the active scaly edge of a suspected plaque of tinea for highest yield. On the feet, macerated scale may yield a false negative, so try to scrape the sole instead, if there is active disease there. For suspected nail fungus, scrape under the nail and procure subungual debris in the case of distal lateral subungual and total dystrophic onychomycosis. For superficial white onychomycosis, scrape the top of the nail, and in cases of suspected proximal subungual onychomycosis, scrape the nail over the affected area, discard that specimen, and use the second scraping specimen for evaluation. For suspected tinea capitis, remove hairs for microscopic examination. A Wood's lamp may also be diagnostic (see discussion below).

Place the specimen on a microscope slide and cover with a coverslip. Place a drop of KOH or KOH with stain underneath the coverslip. Flame with a match but not to the point of boiling (at which time, bubbling will occur). Hyphal structures are branched and have cross-striations. Tinea versicolor is a yeast and has yeast forms and pseudohyphae (when the yeasts start to bud), the so-called "spaghetti and meatball" appearance (Figure 14.2). Tinea versicolor will invariably be teeming with organisms. In cases of tinea incognito, a similar picture, full of hyphae, will be seen (Figure 14.3). But for a typical case of dermatophytosis, one will need to scan the entire field to find hyphae (Figure 14.4). The specimen is not always immediately positive, and coming back to it an hour or so later, may then yield a positive result. In a negative result, where suspicion is high, send skin scrapings to the microbiology laboratory. In suspected nail fungus, the sensitivity of KOH preparation is lower. In any suspected case of nail fungus that is not immediately confirmed under the microscope, send a nail clipping to the laboratory. Histopathologic examination of nail clippings with a periodic acid schiff (PAS) stain can yield a higher positive rate than microbiologic examination; however,

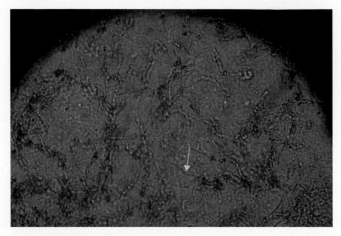

FIGURE 14.2 • "Spaghetti and meatball" appearance of tinea versicolor under light microscopy. The red arrow points to the "meatballs" (yeast forms of *Pityrosporum ovale*), and the blue arrow points to the "spaghetti" (pseudohyphal forms of *P. ovale*).

in cases where it is difficult to obtain a clipping, and only scraping is possible (such as proximal subungual onychomycosis), the specimen will need to be sent for microbiologic examination (as scrapings would be lost in histopathologic processing). For hairs, there may be ectothrix or endothrix infections. In ectothrix, the fungal hyphae and spores cover the outside of the lower part of the hair near the root. Ectothrix is seen in *Microsporum* infections as well as *Trichophyton verrucosum*. In endothrix the fungal hyphae and spores will be seem coursing through the inside of the hair shaft. Examples include *Trichophyton tonsurans* and *Trichophyton violaceum*. Ectothrix infections will also fluoresce under Wood's lamp, whereas endothrix infections do not.

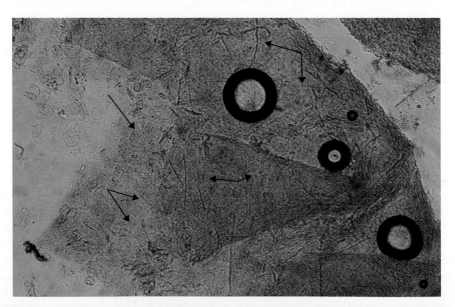

FIGURE 14.3 • A low-power view of scrapings from a case of tinea incognito, showing a high density of hyphae crisscrossing the field, as highlighted by the black arrows.

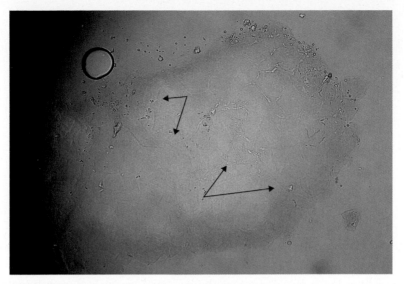

FIGURE 14.4 • A low-power view of a case of non-tinea incognito tinea corporis, showing scattered hyphae, as highlighted by the black arrows.

USE OF MINERAL OIL IN THE DERMATOLOGY CLINIC

In cases of suspected scabies, perform a mineral oil preparation. Look for a burrow to scrape. This is a tiny scaly linear papule. These papules can be found in webspaces, around wrists, and around the axillae. In crusted scabies, scraping any mound of scales will yield positive results. Apply mineral oil to the microscope slide, to the blade, and directly to the skin to be scraped, and scrape firmly over the burrow. Cover with a coverslip and examine under the microscope. There are only a few mites in any given case of scabies (Figure 14.5), so often, this test will be negative and it will be necessary to treat the patient

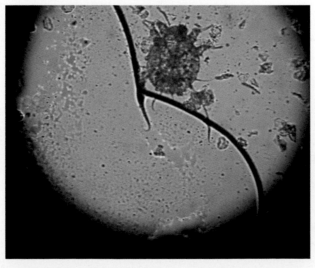

FIGURE 14.5 • A microscopic view of a scabies mite in a case of scabies.

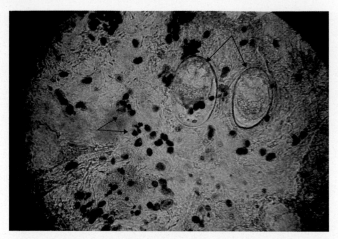

FIGURE 14.6 · A microscopic view of scrapings from a patient with crusted scabies, showing two mites within eggs (black arrows) and a high density of scybala (red arrows).

on clinical suspicion. Sometimes eggs may be seen (oval structures) or scybala (mite feces, which appear as small dark structures). On the other hand, in cases of crusted scabies, many mites will be seen. Additionally, eggs and scybala will be copious (Figure 14.6).

Mineral oil can also be applied onto a plaque of lichen planus. This maneuver will attenuate the appearance of any surface scales and will enhance the appearance of Wickham's striae. These are white lines that course along the surface of lesions of lichen planus. They represent the areas of hypergranulosis that are characteristic of the disease histopathologically.

PERFORMING A TZANCK PREPARATION

With the advent of the polymerase chain reaction (PCR) test for herpes simplex and zoster infections that can yield a result within hours, Tzanck tests are no longer being performed in some centers. The Tzanck preparation still has the advantage of immediate results. In any suspected case of HSV or zoster, scrape the base of an unroofed vesicle or bulla and place the scraping on a microscope slide. When dry, apply a Giemsa stain and cover with a coverslip. Examine the slide, looking for multinucleate giant cells, which are diagnostic.

PERFORMING A TAPE-STRIPPING TEST

An alternative for the diagnosis of scabies is the adhesive tape-stripping test. Firmly place the transparent tape over suspected burrows, ensure its adherence, and pull it off. Apply this tape directly to a microscope slide, adhesive side down, and examine under the microscope.

PERFORMING A WRIGHT'S STAIN

Wright's stain comprises eosin and methylene blue. It is used to stain peripheral blood smears, and it can assist in identification of the different types of white cells. In any suspected case of erythema toxicum neonatorum, smear the contents of a pustule onto a microscope slide and allow it to dry. Add a drop of Wright's stain and a coverslip. This test will reveal many eosinophils that supports this diagnosis.

EMPLOYING AN ALCOHOL SWAB TO REMOVE SCALES

While scales render a wealth of diagnostic information, removing them can reveal the morphology of their underlying papules and plaques more fully. An alcohol wipe can be used to accomplish this. An example is revealing the violaceous color of lichen planus once scales have been removed.

IMMERSION IN WATER

In a suspected case of aquagenic wrinkling of the palms, immerse the patient's hands in a receptacle of tap water or run them under the tap for 2–3 minutes. Rapid wrinkling along with a whitish macerated appearance of the palms will result (see Figure 12.30). Accentuated eccrine duct openings are also a feature.

EMPLOYING WOOD'S LAMP

Wood's lamp (also known as a *long-wave ultraviolet lamp* or a "black light") is a medium-pressure mercury lamp with a nickel–chromium oxide silica glass filter that filters out all visible light and transmits light in the 320–420-nm range, maximally at 365 nm. It is a useful adjunct in the diagnosis of a variety of dermatologic conditions.

Wood's lamp may be used to diagnose a broad array of infections. Table 14.1 summarizes these infections and their characteristic fluorescence colors.

TABLE 14.1. Uses of a Wood's Lamp

INFECTIONS
- Fungal infections
  - Tinea capitis
    - *Microsporum* spp.—affected hairs fluoresce a greenish color
    - *Trichophyton schoenleinii* (favus)—affected hairs fluoresce a blue color
  - *Pityrosporum ovale*
    - Tinea versicolor—scaly macules fluoresce a yellowish color
    - Pityrosporum folliculitis—affected follicles fluoresce yellow
- Bacterial infections
  - *Pseudomonas*—fluoresces green
  - *Corynebacterium* species
  - Erythrasma—affected scales fluoresce coral-red
  - Trichomycosis axillaris—affected hair shafts fluoresce pink
  - *Propionibacterium acnes*—pink flurorescence is seen in affected follicles

PORPHYRIAS
- Porphyria cutanea tarda—urine, feces, and blister fluid fluoresce
- Congenital erythropoetic porphyria—erythrocytes and teeth fluoresce
- Erythropoetic protoporphyria—erythrocytes fluoresce

PIGMENTARY DISORDERS
- Depigmented versus hypopigmented
  - Depigmented conditions appear milk-white
  - Hyopigmented conditions are a dull white color
- Hyperpigmented conditions—variations in epidermal pigment become more apparent under Wood's lamp (eg, melasma) whereas dermal pigment (eg, postinflammatory change) does not

In tinea capitis, infected hairs produce a chemical known as *pteridine*, which is responsible for their fluorescence. *Microsporum* species fluoresce a greenish or bluish-green color. *Trichophyton schoenleinii* causes favus. It fluoresces blue. Of note, a false-positive blue color is imparted by topical preparations that contain salicylic acid. Wood's lamp may also be used to measure response to therapy; serial evaluations will reveal increasing negative fluorescence on proximal hair shafts if therapy has been effective. *Pityrosporum ovale* infections, such as tinea versicolor and *Pityrosporum* folliculitis, fluoresce yellow or yellow-green under Wood's lamp. *Pseudomonas* produces pyoverdins, which give rise to green fluorescence of infected areas. *Corynebacterium* species produce coproporphyrin III, which imparts a coral-red fluorescence, such as may be seen in erythrasma (Figure 12.14) and pitted keratolysis. Coproporphyrin II accumulates on the epidermal surface, and so a false-negative Wood's lamp fluorescence may be obtained if the patient has recently bathed or showered. *Propionibacterium acnes* produces coproporphyrin, which fluoresces pink. Pink hair follicles may be seen in acne and in progressive macular hypomelanosis.

Excess porphyrin accumulation in various body fluids, cells, or teeth occurs in various forms of porphyria and may be highlighted by Wood's lamp fluorescence. Typically a pink or red color is seen. Table 14.1 outlines the body fluids or structures that fluoresce in the porphyrias (Figure 14.7).

Wood's lamp can help accentuate differences in pigmentation that cannot be easily appreciated with the naked eye. This is true for both hypopigmentation and hyperpigmentation. An example of the application of this is the use of Wood's lamp to pick up the ash-leaf and other macules in a case of suspected tuberous sclerosis. These may otherwise be subtle and difficult to appreciate, but Wood's lamp accentuates their whiteness. Depigmented conditions such as vitiligo, chemical leukoderma, melanoma-associated leukoderma, piebaldism, and tyrosinase-negative albinism appear bright white (or milk-white) under Wood's lamp (Figure 14.8), whereas hypopigmented conditions, such as postinflammatory hypopigmentation, ash-leaf macules and other macules of tuberous sclerosis, and nevus depigmentosus are a dull white color. The color of nevus anemicus does not accentuate at all as it is not primarily a pigmentary disorder. Wood's

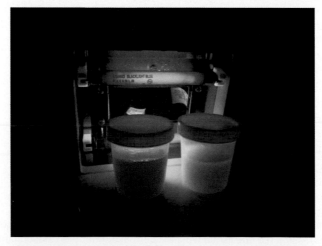

FIGURE 14.7 · Pinkish red fluorescence under Wood's lamp of urine from a patient with porphyria cutanea tarda in the vial on the left; normal control urine in the vial on the right.

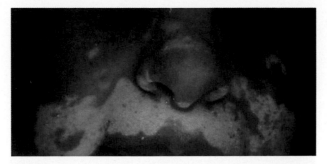

FIGURE 14.8 • Wood's lamp examination of vitiligo on the face showing a bright white appearance.

lamp can also be used to differentiate melasma from other brown macules, such as postinflammatory hyperpigmentation, as variations in epidermal pigment become more apparent under Wood's lamp, whereas those in dermal pigment do not.

PERFORMING DERMOSCOPY

A *dermatoscope* is a vital tool in the assessment cutaneous neoplasms, including pigmented lesions, seborrheic keratoses, and skin cancers. Dermoscopy requires dedicated training and use for proficiency. There is a plethora of recent literature about the dermoscopic findings in other diseases, including hair disorders. An in-depth discussion about dermoscopic findings in different lesions and hair disorders is beyond the scope of this book, but we will address the findings in general terms. Pigmented lesions may have a pigment network, dots and globules. If these features are regularly and symmetrically distributed in the lesion, a benign nevus is the likely diagnosis (Figure 14.9). If they are irregularly distributed in the lesion, an atypical nevus is likely. Early melanoma can be difficult to discern from an atypical nevus. A well-developed

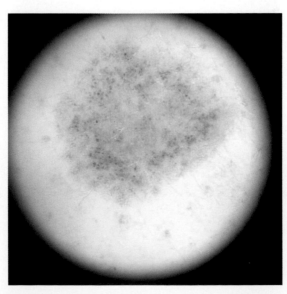

FIGURE 14.9 • A dermoscopic view of a congenital nevus, showing symmetric distribution of dots and peripheral regular pigment network.

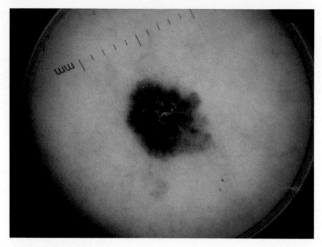

FIGURE 14.10 · A dermoscopic view of a melanoma, showing a central blue-white veil, milky red areas, and asymmetric, irregular pigment network.

melanoma has asymmetry, with white and red areas signifying regression, blue areas signifying dermal pigment, and marked network irregularity (Figure 14.10). Other network features, such as radial streaming, may be seen. Amelanotic melanoma is a diagnostic challenge, even dermoscopically. Polymorphic vessels and milky-red areas may be present. Seborrheic keratoses lack network. They have milia and comedo-like openings and may display a cerebriform pattern. They may have irregular crypts, fissures, and ridges (Figure 14.11). Basal cell cancers have arborizing telangiectasias. Squamous cell cancers display polymorphic vessels and white perifollicular circles.

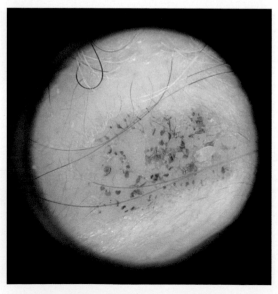

FIGURE 14.11 · A dermoscopic view of a seborrheic keratosis, showing comedo-like openings, ridges, and an early cerebriform pattern. Note the lack of pigment network.

Dermoscopy of hair-bearing skin in the evaluation of hair disorders has been termed *trichoscopy*. Yellow dots may be seen in affected areas in alopecia areata and androgenetic alopecia. White perifollicular dots may be seen in lichen planopilaris or decalvans folliculitis. Black dots are seen in alopecia areata and black dot tinea capitis. Various vascular patterns have been described, and in their absence, atrophy or scarring should be suspected.

SKIN BIOPSY

Histopathologic examination renders definitive diagnosis almost all the time. Shave and punch biopsy techniques need to be learned and practiced for proficiency. In cases of suspected autoimmune blistering disease, a biopsy of normal skin, adjacent to a bulla, should be sent in Michel's medium for direct immunofluorescence. For suspected Henoch–Schonlein purpura, biopsy lesional skin for immunofluorescence and to look for the presence of IgA in vessels. In cases of suspected deep fungal or atypical mycobacterial examination, perform an extra biopsy and send it in saline to the microbiology laboratory for culture.

SUMMARY

- Bedside diagnostics can enhance diagnostic accuracy and narrow down differential diagnoses.
- In most cases, they are straightforward to perform.
- Practice and study are needed for proficiency in microscopic assessment of scrapings, dermoscopy, and skin biopsy technique.

Index

Note: Page numbers followed by "f" and "t" refer to figures and tables respectively.